Pulmonary Aspergillosis

Chen Qiu • Pu-Xuan Lu • Shi-Ping Wu
Editors

Pulmonary Aspergillosis

Diagnosis and Cases

PMPH PEOPLE'S MEDICAL PUBLISHING HOUSE

Springer

Editors
Chen Qiu
Shenzhen People's Hospital
Shenzhen
China

Pu-Xuan Lu
Shenzhen Center for Chronic Disease Control
Shenzhen
China

Shi-Ping Wu
Shenzhen People's Hospital
Shenzhen
China

ISBN 978-981-13-3434-4 ISBN 978-981-13-3435-1 (eBook)
https://doi.org/10.1007/978-981-13-3435-1

Library of Congress Control Number: 2019934206

This Springer imprint is published by the registered company Springer Nature Singapore Pte Ltd.
The registered company address is: 152 Beach Road, #21-01/04 Gateway East, Singapore 189721, Singapore

Preface

Pulmonary aspergillosis is a lung disease caused by *Aspergillus fumigati*. Based on the large-scale multicentered study in China directed by Professor Youning Liu, the cases of pulmonary aspergillosis account for 37.9%, ranking the first, in all cases of pneumomycosis in patients with non-hematologic malignancies. In recent years, along with wide application of broad-spectrum antibiotics, cytotoxic drugs, immunosuppressants, and adrenocortical hormone as well as increasing cases of organ transplantation and HIV/AIDS, the incidence of pulmonary aspergillosis has been increasing. Aspergillus infection has been the important causative factor of other diseases and the cause of death in immunocompromised populations such as patients with persistent granulocytic deficiency, HIV infection, and hereditary immunodeficiency as well as receivers of allogeneic hematopoietic stem cell transplantation and lung transplantation.

In order to help clinicians and specialists diagnosing pulmonary aspergillosis and formulating rational therapeutic protocol, our team, consisted of 60 middle-aged and young clinicians and specialists working in respiratory department, infectious diseases department, intensive care unit, diagnostic radiology department, pathology department, and microbiology department, compiled this book. We collected cases of pulmonary aspergillosis definitively diagnosed by microbiology and pathology and especially selected those typical cases that tend to be misdiagnosed and difficult in therapeutic decision-making. We present these cases in this book with figures and texts to narrate the case history, laboratory tests, imaging features, clinical diagnosis, key points for differential diagnosis, and therapeutic principles of pulmonary aspergillosis. The experienced specialists wrote introductions and summaries about cases of pulmonary aspergillosis resembling to pulmonary tuberculosis and about cases of pulmonary aspergillosis presenting with chest distress and chest pain, with fever, and with hemoptysis to guide your reading. Meanwhile, comments on each case presented in this book were given for more extensive and intensive discussion about each case, which are intended to improve clinical reasoning and clinical practice of the readers.

This book has rich, detailed, and practical content about diagnosis and treatment of pulmonary aspergillosis with important points foregrounded. It provides reference for clinicians, specialists, and medical students working or studying in respiratory department, infectious diseases department, oncology department, intensive care unit, diagnostic radiology department, pathology department, and microbiology department.

All of the editors and contributors committed to compiling this book by referring to large quantity of domestic and international references and guidelines. We present our heartfelt thanks to the editors and contributors. We also thank the People's Medical Publishing House for their planning, guiding, and promoting the editing of this book. We thank each professional who contributed to the publication of this book.

During the compiling of this book, we tried to trace the latest development of the specialty and elucidate each case in detail. However, the techniques of diagnosing and treating pulmonary aspergillosis are developing rapidly, and the corresponding clinical guidelines are continually updated. In addition to the limited knowledge of the editors and the time limits, errors are hardly avoided. We appreciate your pointing out the mistakes so that they can be corrected.

Shenzhen, China
July 20, 2018

Chen Qiu
Pu-Xuan Lu
Shi-Ping Wu

Contents

About the Editors

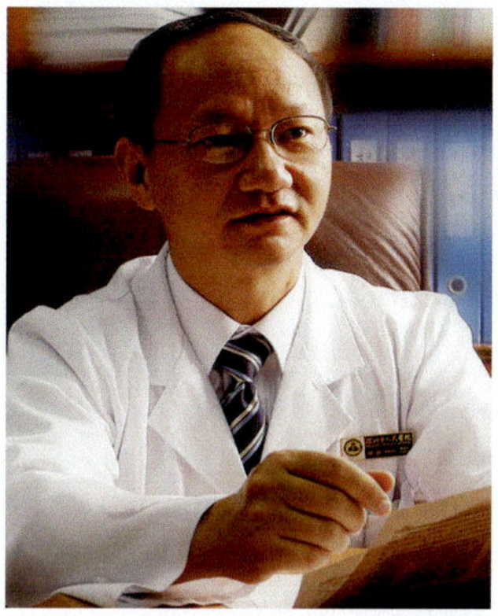

Chen Qiu is the discipline leader of respiratory medicine, discipline leader of respiratory and critical medicine, and dean at the Second Clinical Medicine School of Jinan University (Shenzhen People's Hospital). Professor Qiu is also the director at the Institute of Shenzhen Respiratory Disease and the director of the National Drug Clinical Trial institute.

His academic titles include committee member, Asthma group at the respiratory branch of Chinese Medical Society; review expert, Medicine branch of National Natural Science Funding Commission, China; review expert, Education Development Center for Degree and Postgraduate at Ministry of Education, China; review expert, Provincial Science and Technology Planning Project, Guangdong, China; associate director, Provincial Hospital Association of Guangdong, China; deputy chair, Respiratory branch of Provincial Medical Society of Guangdong, China; deputy chair, Respiratory Physician Branch of Provincial Physician Association of Guangdong, China; deputy chair, Expert Committee for Respiratory Medication of Provincial Pharmacy Society of Guangdong, China; deputy chair, Respiratory Disease Control and Prevention Branch of Provincial Preventive Medicine Society of Guangdong, China; deputy chair, Respiratory Rehabilitation Branch of Provincial Thoracic Disease Society of Guangdong, China; and chair, Respiratory Branch of Shenzhen Medical Society.

Professor Qiu is the editorial committee member of *Chinese Journal of Tuberculosis and Respiration*, Chinese edition of *Chest*, Chinese edition of the *Lancet* (*Respiratory Medicine*), and *Journal of Guangdong Medicine*; standing editorial committee member of Medicine Review and Modern Hospital; and associate editor of *Electronic Journal of Emerging Infectious Disease*. He has edited and translated three academic treaties, finished five academic treaties as associate editor, and contributed to four academic treaties.

He also directed six projects funded by the National Natural Science Foundation of China and the Provincial Natural Science Foundation of Guangdong, China. He owns seven patents for invention and six patents for utility models.

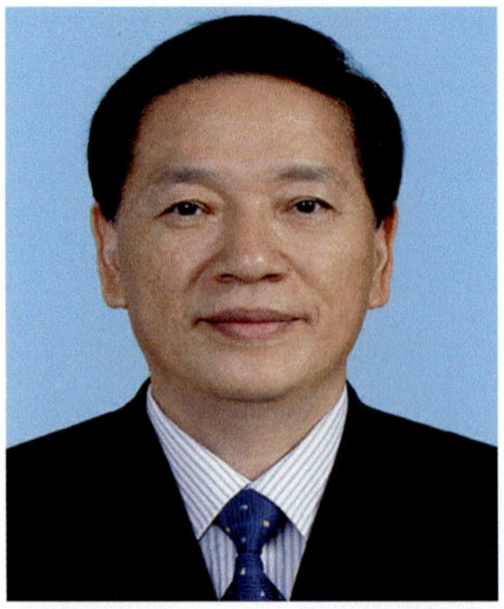

Pu-Xuan Lu is a professor and graduate supervisor of Guangdong Medical University and the radiology department director of Shenzhen Center for Chronic Disease Control.

His academic titles include chief editor of *Electronic Journal of Emerging Infectious Disease*; deputy chair, Radiology of Infectious Disease group at radiology branch of Chinese Medical Society; deputy chair, Radiology of Infectious Disease group at Chinese Radiology Society; deputy chair, Radiology branch of Chinese Sexually Transmitted Disease and HIV/AIDS Society; deputy chair, Beijing Diagnostic Imaging Technology Innovation Alliance; deputy chair, Radiology branch of Provincial Health Management Society of Guangdong, China; and editorial committee member of the *Journal of Radiology of Infectious Disease*.

His research fields include diagnostic imaging and differential diagnosis of emerging infectious diseases, such as SARS, MERS, AIDS, human infected avian influenza, tuberculosis, hepatitis, and other infectious diseases as well as clinical and basic sciences of emerging infectious diseases.

Professor Lu has edited or co-edited more than ten academic treaties. *Diagnostic Imaging of Emerging Infectious Diseases* has been published by Springer in November 2015, which obtained national key award for book output in May 2017 by the General Administration of News and Publishing, China. In the last 5 years, he has directed and finished five national and provincial as well as international collaborative research projects. Pu-Xuan Lu has published more than 150 papers. 33 of these papers were published in SCI-indexed journals. He received 12 awards from Chinese Medical Society, Chinese Preventive Medicine Society, Guangdong provincial government, and Shenzhen city government.

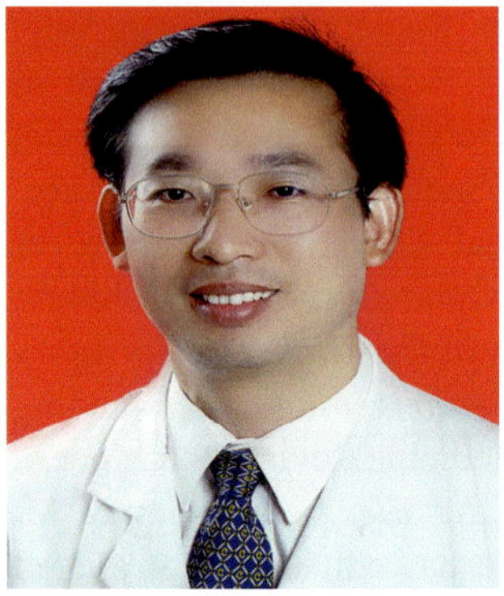

Shi-Ping Wu is the director of the Department of Infectious Disease at the Second Clinical Medical college of Jinan University (Shenzhen People's Hospital).

Academic titles include standing committee member, Infection branch of Guangdong Medical Society, China; standing committee member, Practitioner in Infection Medicine Branch of Guangdong Practitioner Society; deputy chair, Practitioner in Infection Medicine Branch of Shenzhen Practitioner Society; deputy chair, Infection Branch of Shenzhen Medical Society; deputy chair, Hepatopathy Branch of Shenzhen Medical Society; deputy chair, Integrated Chinese Medicine with Western Medicine for Hepatopathy Branch of Shenzhen Medical Society; Professor at Shenzhen Health and Family Planning and Medical Continuing Education Center; and associate editor of *Electronic Journal of Emerging Infectious Disease*.

Professor Wu has worked as physician, teacher, and researcher for more than 30 years. He has published more than 90 research papers internationally and nationally. He has also edited, co-edited, and contributed to seven academic treaties, including Infectious Atypical Pneumonia, Human Infected Avian Influenza, Diagnostic Imaging of Emerging Infectious Disease, and Viral Hepatitis.

Contributors

Associate Editors

Dong-Na Su Second Clinical Medical College of Jinan University, Shenzhen, Guangdong, China

Ling-Wei Wang Second Clinical Medical College of Jinan University, Shenzhen, Guangdong, China

Ying-Yun Fu Second Clinical Medical College of Jinan University, Shenzhen, Guangdong, China

Guan-Xun Cheng Shenzhen Hospital of Beijing University, Shenzhen, Guangdong, China

Wei-Dong Song Shenzhen Hospital of Beijing University, Shenzhen, Guangdong, China

Editorial Board Members

Yazhou Cai Shenzhen Hospital of Beijing University, Shenzhen, Guangdong, China

Budong Chen Affiliated Beijing Chest Hospital, Capital Medical University, Beijing, China

Dandan Chen Second Clinical Medical College of Jinan University, Shenzhen, Guangdong, China

Hongtao Chen Second clinical medical college of Jinan University, Shenzhen, Guangdong, China

Huaisheng Chen Second clinical medical college of Jinan University, Shenzhen, Guangdong, China

Peifen Chen Third People's Hospital of Shenzhen, Shenzhen, Guangdong, China

Yanwei Chen Sixth People's Hospital of Shenzhen, Shenzhen, Guangdong, China

Guan-Xun Cheng Shenzhen Hospital of Beijing University, Shenzhen, Guangdong, China

Zhiqiang Cheng Second clinical medical college of Jinan University, Shenzhen, Guangdong, China

Guofang Deng Third People's Hospital of Shenzhen, Shenzhen, Guangdong, China

Qiwen Deng Sixth People's Hospital of Shenzhen, Shenzhen, Guangdong, China

Qunyi Deng Third People's Hospital of Shenzhen, Shenzhen, Guangdong, China

Jiezhu Ding Shenzhen Hospital of Beijing University, Shenzhen, Guangdong, China

Mengjie Feng Second clinical medical college of Jinan University, Shenzhen, Guangdong, China

Ying-Yun Fu Second clinical medical college of Jinan University, Shenzhen, Guangdong, China

Wei Gao Second clinical medical college of Jinan University, Shenzhen, Guangdong, China

Jingshan Gong Second clinical medical college of Jinan University, Shenzhen, Guangdong, China

Xiaojing Guo Second clinical medical college of Jinan University, Shenzhen, Guangdong, China

Hui Han Shenzhen Hospital of Beijing University, Shenzhen, Guangdong, China

Xuemei Han Second clinical medical college of Jinan University, Shenzhen, Guangdong, China

Yulin He Affiliated First Hospital of Nanchang University, Nanchang, Jiangxi, China

Zhengqiang He Second clinical medical college of Jinan University, Shenzhen, Guangdong, China

Chengying Hong Second clinical medical college of Jinan University, Shenzhen, Guangdong, China

Guoxin Huang Second clinical medical college of Jinan University, Shenzhen, Guangdong, China

Rong Huang Shenzhen Hospital of Beijing University, Shenzhen, Guangdong, China

Wendi Huang Shenzhen Hospital of Beijing University, Shenzhen, Guangdong, China

Xia Huang Second clinical medical college of Jinan University, Shenzhen, Guangdong, China

Xiaoyan Huang Affiliated First Hospital of Guangzhou Medical University, Shenzhen, Guangdong, China

Chang'e Jin Second clinical medical college of Jinan University, Shenzhen, Guangdong, China

Hongtao Jin Second clinical medical college of Jinan University, Shenzhen, Guangdong, China

Jingjing Li Affiliated People's Hospital of Shiyan, Hubei Medical and Pharmaceutical College, Shiyan, Hubei, China

Na Li Central Hospital of Longgang District, Shenzhen, Guangdong, China

Xiaofen Li Provincial People's Hospital, Nanchang, Jiangxi, China

Xiaohe Li Third People's Hospital of Shenzhen, Shenzhen, Guangdong, China

Qin Liu Affiliated First Hospital of Guangzhou Medical University, Guangzhou, Guangdong, China

Xueyan Liu Second clinical medical college of Jinan University, Shenzhen, Guangdong, China

Pu-Xuan Lu Centre for Chronic Diseases Control of Shenzhen, Shenzhen, Guangdong, China

Yuemei Lu Second clinical medical college of Jinan University, Shenzhen, Guangdong, China

Wei Ma Longgang Third People's Hospital, Shenzhen, Guangdong, China

Shusong Peng Second clinical medical college of Jinan University, Shenzhen, Guangdong, China

Wanling Qi Affiliated First Hospital of Nanchang University, Nanchang, Jiangxi, China

Chen Qiu Second clinical medical college of Jinan University, Shenzhen, Guangdong, China

Fei Shi Second clinical medical college of Jinan University, Shenzhen, Guangdong, China

Shi-Ling Song Second clinical medical college of Jinan University, Shenzhen, Guangdong, China

Wei-Dong Song Shenzhen Hospital of Beijing University, Shenzhen, Guangdong, China

Dong-Na Su Second clinical medical college of Jinan University, Shenzhen, Guangdong, China

Xiongfei Sun Second clinical medical college of Jinan University, Shenzhen, Guangdong, China

Wenhui Tang Shekou People's Hospital, Shenzhen, Guangdong, China

Li Tu Shenzhen Hospital of Beijing University, Shenzhen, Guangdong, China

Guangsuo Wang Second clinical medical college of Jinan University, Shenzhen, Guangdong, China

Hui Wang Third People's Hospital of Shenzhen, Shenzhen, Guangdong, China

Ling-Wei Wang Second clinical medical college of Jinan University, Shenzhen, Guangdong, China

Junmin Wen Second clinical medical college of Jinan University, Shenzhen, Guangdong, China

Di Wu Second clinical medical college of Jinan University, Shenzhen, Guangdong, China

Fucheng Wu Second clinical medical college of Jinan University, Shenzhen, Guangdong, China

Senquan Wu People's Hospital of Dongguan, Dongguan, Guangdong, China

Shi-Ping Wu Second clinical medical college of Jinan University, Shenzhen, Guangdong, China

Ruming Xie Affiliated Beijing Ditan Hospital of Capital Medical University, Beijing, China

Jin Xu School of Foreign Languages, Southern Medical University, Guangzhou, Guangdong, China

Ping Xu Shenzhen Hospital of Beijing University, Shenzhen, Guangdong, China

Jian Yang Second clinical medical college of Jinan University, Shenzhen, Guangdong, China

Minjie Yang Second clinical medical college of Jinan University, Shenzhen, Guangdong, China

Hui Yin Shenzhen Hospital of Beijing University, Shenzhen, Guangdong, China

Qing Yu Affiliated Zhujiang Hospital of Southern Medical University, Guangzhou, Guangdong, China

Zhijian Yu Sixth People's Hospital of Shenzhen, Shenzhen, Guangdong, China

Jing Yuan Third People's Hospital of Shenzhen, Shenzhen, Guangdong, China

Hui Zeng Third People's Hospital of Shenzhen, Shenzhen, Guangdong, China

Jianfeng Zeng Third People's Hospital of Shenzhen, Shenzhen, Guangdong, China

Qingsi Zeng Affiliated First Hospital of Guangzhou Medical University, Guangzhou, Guangdong, China

Lukun Zhang Third People's Hospital of Shenzhen, Shenzhen, Guangdong, China

Ping Zhang People's Hospital of Dongguan, Dongguan, Guangdong, China

Qianqian Zhang People's Hospital of Zhoukou, Zhoukou, Henan, China

Jian Zheng Third People's Hospital of Shenzhen, Shenzhen, Guangdong, China

Jiaxuan Zhou Affiliated First Hospital of Guangzhou Medical University, Guangzhou, Guangdong, China

Fuqiang Zhu Second clinical medical college of Jinan University, Shenzhen, Guangdong, China

Songming Zhuo Central Hospital of Longgang, Shenzhen, Guangdong, China

Part I

Basics and Clinical Management of Pulmonary Aspergillosis

Introduction to Pulmonary Aspergillosis

1

Dong-Na Su, Chen Qiu, Pu-Xuan Lu, and Shi-Ping Wu

Aspergillus is categorized into fungus that is extensively existing in the natural world. Aspergillosis is an infectious, allergic, and toxic disease caused by aspergillus. Pulmonary aspergillosis is caused by inhalation of airborne spores of aspergillus. Based on the immune state and potential pulmonary basic disease, the spores of aspergillus can cause different types of lung lesions, therefore different clinical manifestations and imaging demonstrations. Due to the extensive existence of the risk factors contributing to the occurrence of pulmonary aspergillosis, such as the prevalence of HIV/AIDS and tuberculosis, wide use of glucocorticoid, and wide application of organ transplantation as well as increasingly improved diagnostic techniques, the incidence and detection rate of pulmonary aspergillosis has been increasing recently. The disease has been fatal infectious disease in immunocompromised patients [1]. Due to the improved diagnostic technique, pulmonary aspergillosis is clinically diversifying, which presents challenges to the clinicians and specialists. Therefore, it is vitally important for clinicians and specialists to know about the key points for its diagnosis and the therapeutic principles.

Pulmonary aspergillosis is a bronchial and/or lung disease caused by aspergillus, mainly *Aspergillus fumigatus*. A joint effort was made by the European Society of Clinical Microbiology and Infectious Diseases (ESCMID) and European Respiratory Society (ERS) in the year 2015 to summarize previous research findings about chronic aspergillosis. The *Chronic Pulmonary Aspergillosis: Rationale and Clinical guidelines for Diagnosis and Management* (2015) [2] was hence published to replace the *2014 ECCMID Aspergillus Guideline* [3]. Another effort was made by the Infectious Diseases Society of America (IDSA) to summarize the relevant evidence of different types of aspergillosis based on the hot issues of its clinical diagnosis and management. And hence the new edition of the *Guideline for Diagnosis and Management of Aspergillosis* was published in 2016 [4] to replace the previous edition published in 2008 [5]. Starting with the basic theory, this chapter provides readers with a comprehensive understanding of the etiology, epidemiology, pathology and pathogenesis, clinical manifestations, diagnosis, and treatment of pulmonary aspergillosis in a short period of time. At the same time, it also lays a solid theoretical foundation for readers to correctly analyze and understand the wonderful case after the chapter.

References

1. Cunha C, Aversa F, Lacerda JF, et al. Genetic PTX3 deficiency and aspergillosis in stem-cell transplantation. N Engl J Med. 2014;370:421–32.
2. Denning DW, Cadranel J, Beigelman-Aubry C, et al. Chronic pulmonary aspergillosis: rationale and clinical guidelines for diagnosis and management. Eur Respir J. 2016;47:45–68.
3. Godet CL, Philippe B, Laurent F, Cadranel J. Chronic pulmonary aspergillosis: an update on diagnosis and treatment. Respiration. 2014;88(2):162–74.
4. Patterson TF, Thompson GR III, Denning DW, et al. Practice guidelines for the diagnosis and management of aspergillosis: 2016 update by the Infectious Diseases Society of America. Clin Infect Dis. 2016;63(4):e1–60.
5. Walsh TJ, Anaissie EJ, Denning DW, et al. Treatment of aspergillosis: clinical practice guidelines of the Infectious Diseases Society of America. Clin Infect Dis. 2008;46:327–60.

D.-N. Su · C. Qiu (✉) · S.-P. Wu
Second Clinical Medical College of Jinan University, Shenzhen, Guangdong, China

P.-X. Lu
Centre for Chronic Diseases Control of Shenzhen, Shenzhen, Guangdong, China

C. Qiu et al. (eds.), *Pulmonary Aspergillosis*, https://doi.org/10.1007/978-981-13-3435-1_1

Etiology of Pulmonary Aspergillosis

2

Dong-Na Su, Chen Qiu, Pu-Xuan Lu, and Shi-Ping Wu

Aspergillus widely exists in the natural world, accounting for about 12% of all the fungi in the air. It is provided by dead plants, animal feces, and dead bodies of animals and is a saprophytic fungus parasitizing in the soil. Aspergillus is a general term for filamentous fungi with resembling properties which is categorized into the genus *Aspergillus*. Its nutrient hypha has septum, and part of the hypha grows into long and coarse conidiophore with apical flask-shaped or sphere-shaped vesicle and surface sterigmata. The sterigmata are commonly two-layer structure, with strands of spherical conidia of coarse surfaces attached. The conidiophore, apical vesicle, sterigmata, and conidium constitute spore head (Fig. 2.1). There are at least 170 kinds of *Aspergillus* within human knowledge. The conidium may be yellow, green, black, brown, or orange, and the color is the basis for identification of its strain. The conidiophore grows on the Sertoli cell and connects to the nutrient hypha via the Sertoli cell. The morphology of aspergillus spore panicle includes the length of conidiophores, shape of the apical vesicle, and single or double small peduncle. The shape, size, surface structure, and color of the conidium are the basis for identification of its strain. The most optimal temperature for the growth of

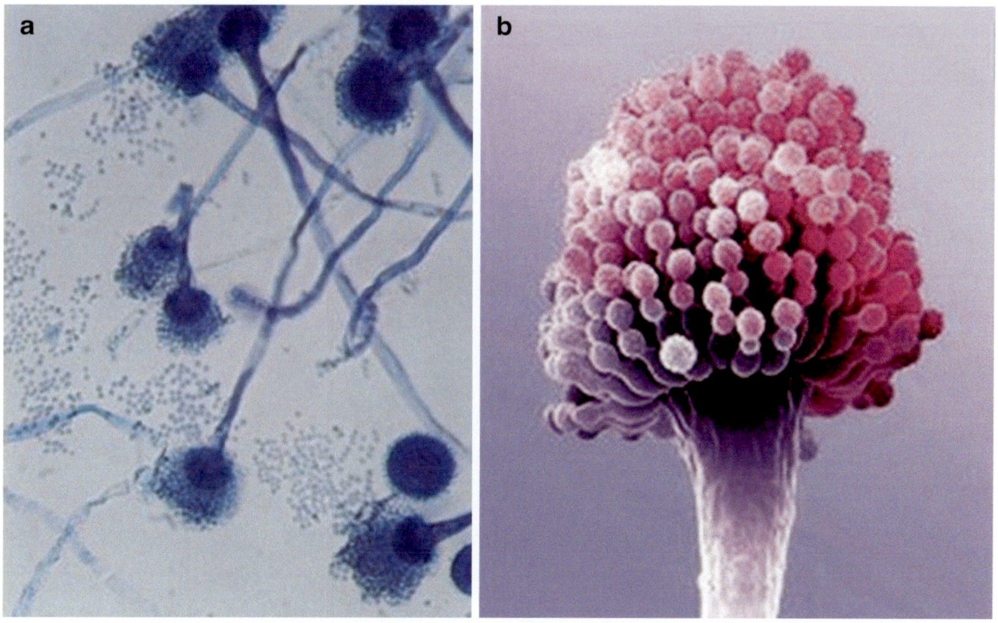

Fig. 2.1 (**a**, **b**) Morphology of aspergillus

D.-N. Su · C. Qiu · S.-P. Wu
Second Clinical Medical College of Jinan University, Shenzhen, Guangdong, China

P.-X. Lu (✉)
Centre for Chronic Diseases Control of Shenzhen, Shenzhen, Guangdong, China

C. Qiu et al. (eds.), *Pulmonary Aspergillosis*, https://doi.org/10.1007/978-981-13-3435-1_2

aspergillus is 25–30 °C. The most common pathogenic aspergillus is *Aspergillus fumigatus*, followed by *Aspergillus flavus* and *Aspergillus niger*. Other rarely found aspergilla include *Aspergillus candidus*, *Aspergillus glaucus*, *Aspergillus parasiticus*, *Aspergillus terreus*, *Aspergillus versicolor*, and *Aspergillus oryzae*.

The conidium scattering in the air can reproduce via elongation of the hypha at favorable conditions. The formation of hypha septum indicates production of two separate cells. In addition, the anisospore called ascospore is also capable of reproducing. Under a microscope, infiltration of a large quantity of neutrophil granulocytes at the lesion can be observed. And Y-shaped hypha at 45° angle with septal wall can also be observed (Fig. 2.2).

Large quantities of hyphae and spores with the hyphae twining into the mass and septum of the hypha in 45° angle (PAS staining).

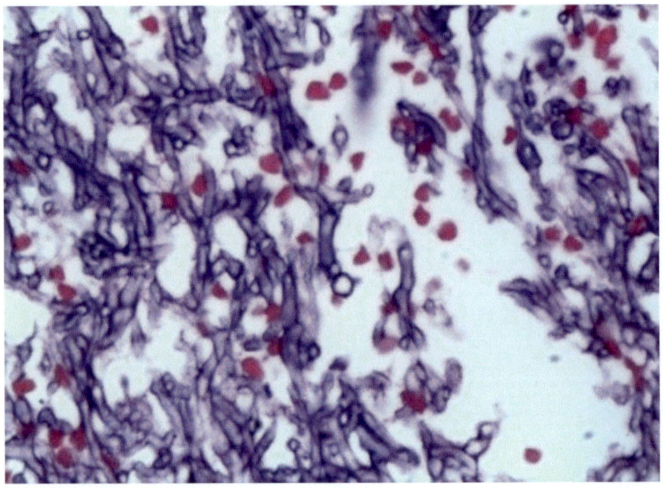

Fig. 2.2 Aspergillus smear

Epidemiology of Pulmonary Aspergillosis

3

Dong-Na Su, Chen Qiu, Pu-Xuan Lu, and Shi-Ping Wu

Aspergillus exists extensively in the natural world that may be found in the soil, air, plants, wild or domestic fowl, and feathers of flying birds. It can also be commonly found at farms, stables, stalls, and barns. Aspergillus can parasite at human skin and upper respiratory tract but is not pathogenic due to human resistance to it. Aspergillosis is mostly secondary. When the immunity is compromised, the pathogenic aspergillus invades human lungs via the respiratory tract. It may also invade the skin and mucosa. In severe cases, septicemia occurs to involve other tissues and systems. Recent studies have shown that some strains of aspergillus may be carcinogenic. IgE-mediated allergic reaction may be triggered in anaphylactic person after inhalation of aspergillus spores to induce bronchial spasm.

Inhalation of aspergillus by individuals with normal immunity does not cause the disease. However, pulmonary aspergillosis occurs in immunocompromised individuals. It commonly occurs on the basis of diabetes, blood diseases, malignancies, large area burn, serious malnutrition, and other chronic wasting diseases. In other cases, pulmonary aspergillosis is induced due to long-term use of antibiotics, glucocorticoid, and/or immunosuppressant. In addition, it is commonly secondary to bronchiectasis, cavernous pulmonary tuberculosis, pulmonary cyst, pulmonary abscess, lung carcinoma, and other structural lung diseases.

In all the fungal infections following lung transplantation surgery, pulmonary aspergillosis accounts for about 44%, and the incidence of pulmonary aspergillosis after parenchymal organ transplantation surgery is 21%. It has been reported that the incidence of pulmonary aspergillosis after hematopoietic stem cell transplantation is 14–25% in China and 31% in the USA. The large-scale multicentered study in China directed by Prof. Liu [1] in the year 2011 has demonstrated that the lung fungal infections in patients with non-hematologic malignancies include pulmonary aspergillosis (180 cases, 37.9%), pulmonary candidiasis (162 cases, 34.2%), pulmonary cryptococcosis (74 cases, 15.6%), pneumocystis (23 cases, 4.8%), pulmonary mucormycosis (10 cases, 2.1%), pulmonary penicilliosis marneffei (4 cases), and histoplasmosis (2 cases). However, there is no latest report about the incidence of pulmonary aspergillosis.

It is well known that *Mycobacterium tuberculosis* infection is the most common risk factor of chronic pulmonary aspergillosis across the world. A previous study in the UK have found that in patients with sputum *Mycobacterium tuberculosis* negative for 1 year after antituberculosis treatment, 14% was detected with sputum aspergillus and the aspergillus detection rate rose to 22% in patients with sputum *Mycobacterium tuberculosis* negative for 4 years after antituberculosis treatment. Another study found that the aspergillus antibody positive rate was 25% in patients with sputum *Mycobacterium tuberculosis* negative for 1 year. The data is possibly underestimated. Research indicated that the total case of chronic pulmonary aspergillosis secondary to tuberculosis may be up to 1.2 million. In some poorly equipped hospitals, chronic pulmonary aspergillosis may be misdiagnosed as complication of previous tuberculosis or relapse of tuberculosis because its presenting symptoms resemble to those of tuberculosis.

Reference

1. Liu Y, She D, Sun T, et al. Multicentered retrospective analysis of clinically defined cases of pneumomycosis during 1998 to 2007 in China. Chin J Tuberc Respir. 2011;34(2):86–90.

D.-N. Su · C. Qiu · S.-P. Wu (✉)
Second Clinical Medical College of Jinan University, Shenzhen, Guangdong, China

P.-X. Lu
Centre for Chronic Diseases Control of Shenzhen, Shenzhen, Guangdong, China

C. Qiu et al. (eds.), *Pulmonary Aspergillosis*, https://doi.org/10.1007/978-981-13-3435-1_3

4 Pathology and Pathogenesis of Pulmonary Aspergillosis

Dong-Na Su, Chen Qiu, Pu-Xuan Lu, and Shi-Ping Wu

In its early stage, the lesion of pulmonary aspergillosis is diffuse infiltrative and exudative change, and in its advanced stage, the lesion is necrosis, suppuration, or granuloma. In the lesion, a large quantity of hyphae can be found. Penetration of the hyphae into vascular vessel may cause vasculitis, perivasculitis, and thrombus (fungal embolus) formation. Thrombus (fungal embolus) formation further induces tissue ischemia and necrosis. Pathologically, based on invasion of aspergillus hyphae into lung tissue (invasion of basilar membrane of bronchial epithelium in the airway), pulmonary aspergillosis is classified into invasive and noninvasive types. Invasive pulmonary aspergillosis is commonly acute and can be further grouped into vascular invasive and airway-invasive subtypes. Noninvasive pulmonary aspergillosis is commonly chronic, with the hyphae confined within original lung cavities that do not invade other lung tissues. There is intermedius type in invasive and noninvasive pulmonary aspergillosis, which is known as subacute invasive pulmonary aspergillosis or chronic necrotizing pulmonary aspergillosis.

Acute invasive pulmonary aspergillosis presents with extensive infiltrative pneumonia or localized granuloma. In some cases, the lesions are necrosis, suppuration, and multiple small abscesses (Fig. 4.1).

In early stage of typical aspergillus infection, diagnostic imaging demonstrates subpleural high-density nodular consolidation opacity. Several days later, the lesion may be demonstrated with halo sign. The consolidated nodule by CT scan is demonstrated with lower surrounding density but still higher than lung tissue density to show ground-glass-like ring-shaped opacity. The underlying pathophysiological mechanism is that aspergillus destroys minor blood vessels in the lungs to cause hemorrhagic infarction of the lung parenchyma and early central necrotic nodule is then surrounded by hemorrhagic area. The halo sign is commonly demonstrated in the early stage of pulmonary aspergillosis, which is characteristic of the disease (Figs. 4.2 and 4.3).

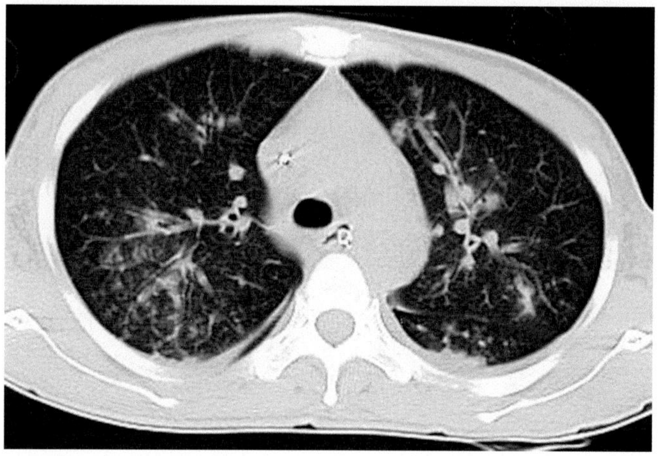

Fig. 4.1 Acute invasive pulmonary aspergillosis

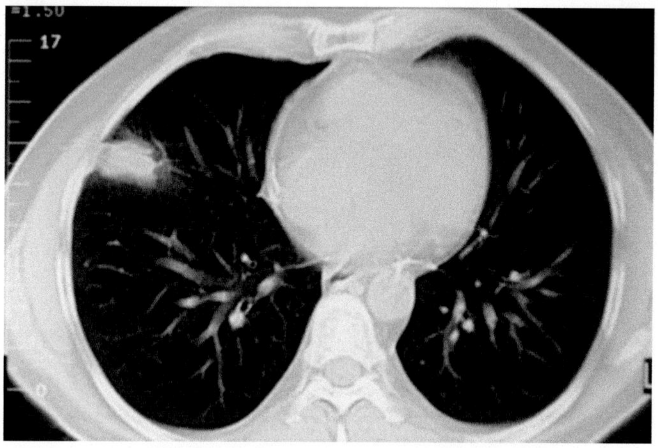

Fig. 4.2 Aspergillosis. Aspergillus nodule accompanied by halo sign

D.-N. Su (✉) · C. Qiu · S.-P. Wu
Second Clinical Medical College of Jinan University, Shenzhen, Guangdong, China

P.-X. Lu
Centre for Chronic Diseases Control of Shenzhen, Shenzhen, Guangdong, China

C. Qiu et al. (eds.), *Pulmonary Aspergillosis*, https://doi.org/10.1007/978-981-13-3435-1_4

About 10–15 days after aspergillus infection, the lung consolidation area is subject to liquefaction and necrosis to show typical air crescent sign. Air crescent sign was believed to be a specific sign of aspergilloma which is located in the cavity and mobile along with changes of body postures but remains proximal to the ground. The underlying mechanism of air crescent sign has been believed to be shrinkage of infarct lung tissue in the lung consolidation area (Fig. 4.4) or formation of spherical lesion in previously existing cavity.

The noninvasive or extremely slight localized invasive aspergillus infection in the previously existing cavitary lung lesion may induce formation of aspergilloma or other types of chronic aspergillosis. Aspergilloma commonly occurs and grows larger in the lung cavity caused by bronchiectasis, lung neoplasm, tuberculosis, or other chronic lung infections (Fig. 4.5). In rare cases, aspergilloma gradually progresses into chronic necrotizing aspergillosis, which is related to the therapeutic use of corticosteroid.

Patients' consents have been obtained for images or other clinical information relating to the cases to be published.

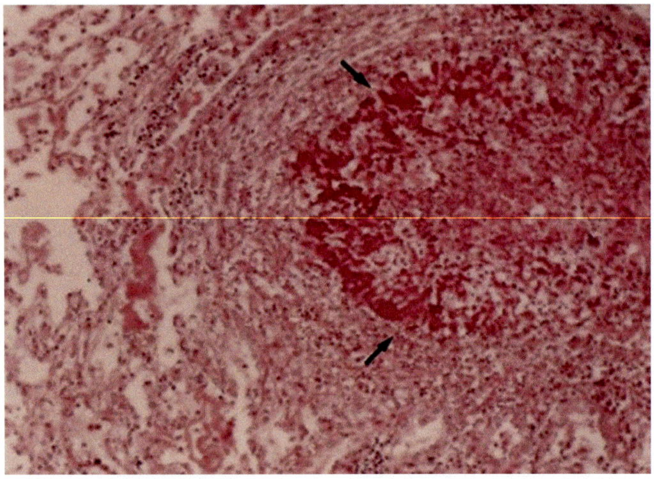

Fig. 4.3 Aspergillosis. Hemorrhagic lesion as the pathophysiological mechanism of halo sign

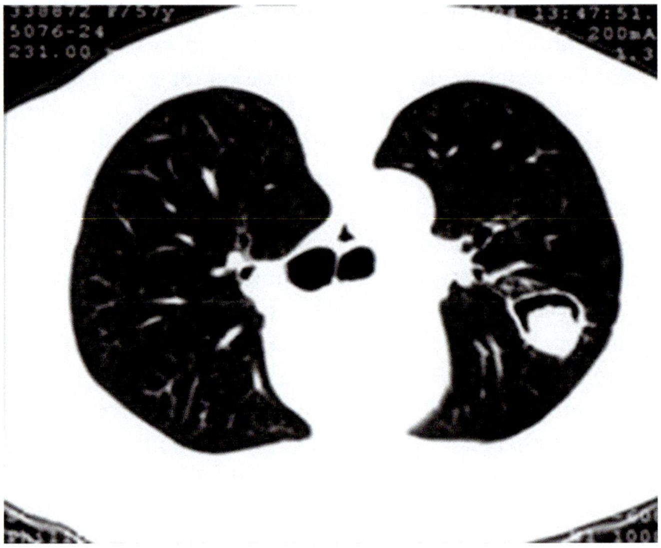

Fig. 4.4 Pulmonary aspergillosis. CT scan demonstration of air crescent sign

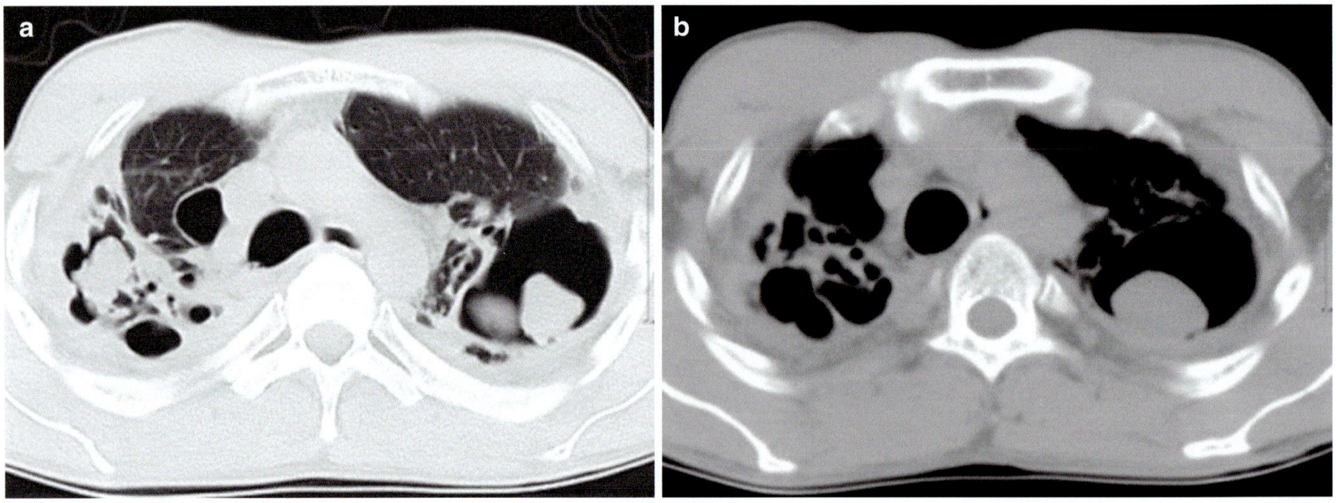

Fig. 4.5 (**a**–**d**) Chronic fibro-cavitary pulmonary tuberculosis complicated by aspergilloma

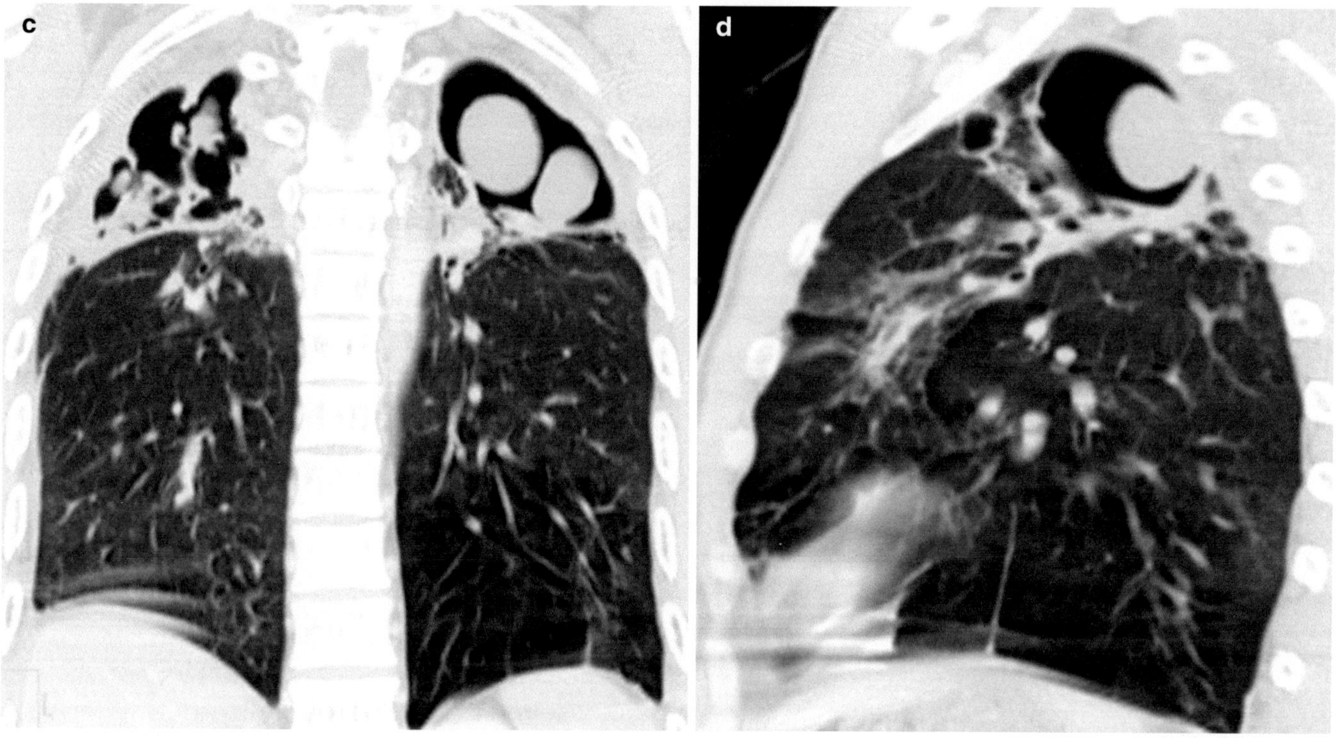

Fig. 4.5 (continued)

5 Clinical Manifestations of Pulmonary Aspergillosis

Dong-Na Su, Chen Qiu, Pu-Xuan Lu, Shi-Ping Wu, and Ying-Yun Fu

The lesion of invasive pulmonary aspergillosis rapidly spreads. With no timely appropriate treatment, progressive and finally fatal respiratory failure develops. Extrapulmonary diffuse aspergillosis may involve the liver, kidneys, brain, or other tissues, which commonly causes occurrence of death. Pulmonary allergic aspergillosis may induce inflammatory infiltration that is not related to fungal invasion of tissue.

5.1 Clinical Manifestations of Non-allergic Pulmonary Aspergillosis

5.1.1 Acute or Subacute Invasive Pulmonary Aspergillosis

Inhalation of a large quantity of aspergillus spores causes acute bronchitis. Invasion of the hyphae into the lung tissue further induces extensive infiltrative pneumonia or localized granuloma and, in some cases, necrosis, suppuration, and multiple small abscesses. The patients present with high fever or irregular fever, cough, breathlessness, and expectoration with greenish purulent sputum. In the cases with accompanying bleeding, the patients cough up coffee-colored sputum. The presenting symptoms also include chest pain, hemoptysis, dyspnea, and corresponding symptoms when aspergillus is disseminated to other organs. By physical examination, dye or moist rales of lungs are detected. In the early stage, chest X-ray demonstrates localized or multiple infiltrative/nodular opacity in both lungs. The lesions commonly enlarge and fuse into consolidation or necrosis to form cavities. In some cases, sudden occurrence of large wedge-shaped opacity may be demonstrated whose base is opposite to the pleura, which resembles to mild lung infarction. In rare cases, pleural effusion signs are demonstrated.

5.1.2 Chronic Pulmonary Aspergillosis

Chronic pulmonary aspergillosis includes aspergilloma, chronic cavitary pulmonary aspergillosis, chronic fibrotic pulmonary aspergillosis, and aspergillus nodules. Pulmonary aspergilloma commonly occurs on the basis of bronchiectasis, pulmonary tuberculosis, and other chronic lung diseases. The hyphae reproduce and aggregate in the intrapulmonary cavity to form spherical mass together with fibrin and mucous cells that does not invade other lung tissues. Most patients with pulmonary aspergilloma are asymptomatic or present symptoms of the basic lung disease. Some patients present symptoms of fever, cough, breathlessness, and expectoration of mucous-purulent sputum containing greenish or coffee-colored particles when the disease progresses. Due to the existence of abundant vascular network surrounding the aspergillus sphere, the patients may present recurrent hemoptysis. Chest X-ray demonstrates round aspergilloma hanging in the cavity to form a crescent-like translucent area, which has important diagnostic value. The patients with aspergillus nodules present slight symptoms. The disease is characteristic of nodules with a diameter of less than 3 cm, and the presenting symptoms resemble to cases of simplex aspergilloma. Chronic cavitary pulmonary aspergillosis is formerly nominated as complex aspergilloma, with complex symptoms and slow progression. As a constituent of asthenic syndrome, the symptoms include chronic pulmonary functional failure, long-term low-grade fever, cough, and expectoration of bloody sputum and purulent sputum. It commonly occurs in patients with bronchial or pulmonary structural disease that has caused formation of cavity with or with no aspergilloma. The lungs of the patients have multiple cavities due to the basic bronchial or pulmonary structural disease. Chronic fibrotic pulmonary aspergillosis presents as extensive pulmonary fibrosis that involves at least two lung lobes

D.-N. Su · C. Qiu · S.-P. Wu · Y.-Y. Fu (✉)
Second Clinical Medical College of Jinan University, Shenzhen, Guangdong, China

P.-X. Lu
Centre for Chronic Diseases Control of Shenzhen, Shenzhen, Guangdong, China

C. Qiu et al. (eds.), *Pulmonary Aspergillosis*, https://doi.org/10.1007/978-981-13-3435-1_5

with accompanying chronic cavitary aspergillosis. It severely impairs the functions of the lungs, and the symptoms resemble to those of chronic cavitary pulmonary aspergillosis, but with more serious pulmonary dysfunction.

5.2 Allergic Pulmonary Aspergillosis

Inhalation of a large quantity of dusts containing aspergillus spores by individuals with allergic constitution causes allergic rhinitis, bronchial asthma, and bronchitis. Several hours after inhalation, the patients present with wheezing, cough, and expectoration, possibly with accompanying fever. In most cases, the symptoms relieve within 3–4 days. And inhalation again causes relapse of these symptoms. By sputum test, large quantities of eosinophile granulocytes and hyphae can be detected. By sputum culture, growth of aspergillus can be observed. And by blood test, eosinophilia ($>1.0 \times 10^9$/L) can be detected with serum IgE above 1000 ng/mL.

Because aspergillus colonies are common in human daily life environment, sputum culture positive may be caused by contamination of air by aspergillus spores or colonization of aspergillus colonies in patients with chronic lung disease. Sputum culture in patients with aspergilloma commonly fails to detect the growth of aspergillus because of its separation from the airway by the cavity wall. The positive rate of sputum culture is low in patients with invasive pulmonary aspergillosis. However, sputum culture positive or bronchoalveolar lavage fluid culture positive in patients receiving corticosteroid or in patients with neutrophilic granulocytopenia or HIV/AIDS is strong evidence supporting the diagnosis of invasive pulmonary aspergillosis.

Patients' consents have been obtained for images or other clinical information relating to the cases to be published.

6 Diagnosis of Pulmonary Aspergillosis

Dong-Na Su, Chen Qiu, Pu-Xuan Lu, Shi-Ping Wu, and Wei-Dong Song

The basis for definite diagnosis of pulmonary aspergillosis is exposure to at least one risk factor, presenting one chief symptom or two associate symptoms plus one microbiological and/or histopathological evidence. The microbiological evidence should be based on exclusion of specimen contamination. The histopathological evidence is the golden standard for the diagnosis of pulmonary aspergillosis.

6.1 Risk Factor (Host Factor)

1. White blood cell count of peripheral blood is less than 0.5×10^9/L with neutropenia or deficient neutrophile granulocytes for at least 10 days.
2. When the body temperature is higher than 38 °C or lower than 36 °C, accompanied by one of the following conditions:
   (a) Within prior 60 days, neutropenia persisted for no less than 10 days.
   (b) Within prior 30 days, the patient received immunosuppressant therapy, or the patient is receiving immunosuppressant therapy.
   (c) The patient has a history of invasive fungal infection.
   (d) The patient has a diagnosis of HIV/AIDS.
   (e) The patient has a diagnosis of graft-versus-host disease.
   (f) The patient received or is receiving glucocorticoid for at least 3 weeks.
   (g) The patient has basic chronic disease.
   (h) The patient has one of the following conditions: trauma, major surgery, long-term stay in the ICU, long-term mechanical ventilation, intrapulmonary catheter dwell, total parenteral nutrition, or long-term use of broad-spectrum antibiotic.

6.2 Clinical Symptoms

6.2.1 Chief Clinical Symptoms

Chest X-ray and CT scan at the early stage of infection demonstrate subpleural, possibly with halo sign surrounding the lesion. At days 10–15 after onset, the lung consolidation is demonstrated with liquefaction and necrosis. Chest X-ray and CT scan demonstrate cavitary opacity or air crescent sign.

6.2.2 Associate Clinical Symptoms

1. Fever persists for at least 96 h and active antibiotic therapy shows no therapeutic effect.
2. The patient shows symptoms and signs of lung infection, including cough, expectoration, hemoptysis, chest pain, and dyspnea as well as lung rales or pleural rubs.
3. Diagnostic imaging demonstrates new non-specific lung infiltration opacity except for lesions corresponding to clinical symptoms.

6.3 Microbiological Examination

1. Hyphae are detected by direct microscopy in tracheal aspirates or qualified sputum specimen. The same species of fungus is isolated by at least two continuous cultures.
2. Hyphae are detected by direct microscopy in bronchoalveolar lavage fluid (BALF), and fungal culture shows positive.

D.-N. Su · C. Qiu · S.-P. Wu
Second Clinical Medical College of Jinan University, Shenzhen, Guangdong, China

P.-X. Lu
Centre for Chronic Diseases Control of Shenzhen, Shenzhen, Guangdong, China

W.-D. Song (✉)
Shenzhen Hospital of Beijing University, Shenzhen, Guangdong, China

C. Qiu et al. (eds.), *Pulmonary Aspergillosis*, https://doi.org/10.1007/978-981-13-3435-1_6

3. Latex agglutination shows *Cryptococcus neoformans* capsular polysaccharide antigen positive.
4. G-test shows serum 1,3-β-D-glucan antigen positive for two continuous times.
5. GM test shows serum galactomannan antigen positive for two continuous times.

6.4 Histopathological Examination

Histopathological examination refers to the harvest of lung tissue by percutaneous lung puncture, bronchoscopic biopsy, or surgical removal for pathological examination. By silver staining or PAS staining, pathological examination of lung tissue demonstrates aspergillus with Y-shaped septal hyphae that are uniform in size. Many patients with high risk of invasive aspergillosis suffer from thrombocytopenia, which is commonly accompanied by respiratory functional failure. Therefore, specimens for biopsy can be hardly harvested. In addition, due to insufficient tissue harvested for biopsy, the histopathological examination commonly shows negative results. And in most cases, the therapeutic decision-making is based on the inference of clinical evidence.

The diagnosis of pulmonary aspergillosis is recommended in the *Guidelines for the Diagnosis and Treatment of Aspergillosis* issued by the Infectious Diseases Society of America in 2016 as the following:

1. Sufficient tissue and body fluid specimens should be harvested for simultaneous examinations by histopathology/cytology and fungal culture. For the cases with atypical strain isolated or possible drug resistance, molecular biological test should be performed to identify the strain. This is strongly recommended but showing low-grade evidence.
2. The application of PCR of the peripheral blood for diagnosis of pulmonary aspergillosis still remains controversial [1, 2].
3. For patients with specific disease, such as patients with hematopoietic malignancies or hematopoietic stem cell transplant, serum test and bronchoalveolar lavage fluid (BALF) for GM level are recommended. It is believed to be the accurate marker of pulmonary aspergillosis. This is strongly recommended with high-grade evidence.
4. For high-risk patients, such as patients with hematopoietic stem cell transplant, serum test kit for 1-3-β-glucan is recommended for the diagnosis of aspergillosis. However, the test is non-specific to aspergillosis. This is strongly recommended showing moderate-grade evidence.
5. For clinically suspected cases of invasive pulmonary aspergillosis, whatever the chest X-ray shows, chest CT scan is recommended. This is strongly recommended showing moderate-grade evidence. Enhanced chest CT scan is not recommended, which is strongly recommended showing moderate-grade evidence. For the cases with the nodule or mass being adjacent to major blood vessels, enhanced chest CT scan is recommended. This is strongly recommended showing moderate-grade evidence.
6. For suspected cases of invasive pulmonary aspergillosis, bronchoscopy-assisted bronchoalveolar lavage is recommended. This is strongly recommended showing moderate-grade evidence.

References

1. Arwanitis M, Ziakas PD, Zacharioudakis IM, et al. PCR in diagnosis of invasive aspergillosis: a meta-analysis of diagnostic performance. J Clin Microbiol. 2014;52:3731–42.
2. Heng SC, Morrissey O, Chen SC, et al. Utility of bronchoalveolar lavage fluid galactomannan alone or in combination with PCR for the diagnosis of invasive aspergillosis in adult hematology patients: a systematic review and meta-analysis. Crit Rev Microbial. 2015;41:124–34.

7 Clinical Typing of Pulmonary Aspergillosis

Dong-Na Su, Chen Qiu, Pu-Xuan Lu, Shi-Ping Wu, and Guan-Xun Cheng

Conventionally, pulmonary aspergillosis is classified into three types, namely, invasive pulmonary aspergillosis, chronic and saprophytic pulmonary aspergillosis, and allergic bronchopulmonary aspergillosis. However, with the increase of knowledge about aspergillosis appreciated in the new editions of clinical guidelines, the clinical typing of pulmonary aspergillosis is increasingly improved [1].

7.1 Acute Invasive Aspergillosis

Acute invasive aspergillosis is common in patients with generalized immunosuppression. It develops rapidly, lasting for at least 1 month.

7.1.1 Acute Invasive Pulmonary Aspergillosis (AIPA)

AIPA is mainly the acute phase of inflammation, abscess, and necrosis. The two lungs are commonly demonstrated with diffuse consolidation opacity, cloud flocculation opacity, and patchy opacity. In some other cases, there are honeycomb-like multiple cavities with high-intensity opacity inside the cavity.

D.-N. Su · C. Qiu · S.-P. Wu
Second Clinical Medical College of Jinan University, Shenzhen, Guangdong, China

P.-X. Lu
Centre for Chronic Diseases Control of Shenzhen, Shenzhen, Guangdong, China

G.-X. Cheng (✉)
Shenzhen Hospital of Beijing University, Shenzhen, Guangdong, China

7.1.2 Invasive Tracheobronchial Aspergillosis (ITBA)

ITBA is a fairly rare aspergillus-related pulmonary disease. It occurs independently in a small quantity of patients or concurrent with invasive pulmonary aspergillosis. In some other cases, it occurs at the early stage of invasive pulmonary aspergillosis. Its diagnosis is based on deep invasion of aspergillus to involve the basilar membrane of the bronchus. The patients may show serious airway obstruction that rapidly develops into apnea and respiratory failure. Bronchoscopy should be ordered as early as possible to resolve airway obstruction.

7.2 Chronic Pulmonary Aspergillosis (CPA)

CPA induces no immunosuppression or slight generalized immunosuppression with formation of granuloma. The cases can be classified into chronic when the disease course lasts for more than 1 month. Therefore, chronic necrotizing pulmonary aspergillosis (CNPA) is categorized into CPA, commonly lasting for 1–3 months. And the other types of CPA last for more than 3 months. In recent years, along with the increase of patients with CPA, more researches have been conducted on the diagnosis and treatment of the disease, and the clinicians obtain more knowledge about the disease.

A research conducted in the year of 2013 reported that the total cases of sarcoidosis complicated by CPA was up to 71,907 and the cases in the USA and Arica account for 24% and 37% [2], respectively. A joint effort was made in the year 2015 by the European Congress of Clinical Microbiology and Infectious Diseases (ECCMID) and European Respiratory Society to summarize previous researches on CPA. The Clinical Guideline for Diagnosis and Treatment of CPA was then issued. According to the guideline, chronic

C. Qiu et al. (eds.), *Pulmonary Aspergillosis*, https://doi.org/10.1007/978-981-13-3435-1_7

pulmonary asperglosis (CPA) can be classified into the following types.

7.2.1 Single/Simple Pulmonary Aspergilloma

Single/simple pulmonary aspergilloma refers to the condition that one singular fungal sphere occurs in one pulmonary cavity. The serum test or biological test shows evidence of aspergillus infection. In patients with normal immunity, the patients show slight symptoms or are asymptomatic. Radiological follow-ups for at least 3 months demonstrate no progression of the disease.

Aspergilloma virtually consists of fungal hyphae and extracellular matrix, which is the most common type of CPA with characteristic radiological demonstrations. By chest CT scan, aspergilloma can usually be observed, which is commonly located in the lung cavity or dilated bronchus. Aspergilloma consists almost entirely of fungal hyphae and extracellular matrix. Air crescent sign is a characteristic radiological demonstration of aspergilloma. However, it is also demonstrated in the cases of invasive pulmonary aspergillosis. The substance within the cavity is the infracted lung tissue containing aspergilla or other fungi, which is more accurately known as mycotic lung sequestrum and is common in patients with compromised immunity.

7.2.2 Chronic Cavitary Pulmonary Aspergillosis (CCPA)

CCPA is the most common type of CPA, which is formerly known as complex aspergilloma. It is commonly radiologically demonstrated as singular or multiple lung cavities with thin or thick wall containing one or more aspergillomata. In some other cases, the cavity contains irregular substances indicating aspergillus infection by serum or biological test. The patients show obvious lung and/or systemic symptoms with increased inflammatory factors. Radiological follow-ups for 3 months demonstrate obvious progression of the disease, possibly with new cavities, enlarged area of infiltration surrounding the cavity, or increased lung fibrosis. With no appropriate treatment, these cavities increasingly enlarge with fusion within several years to infiltrate its surrounding tissue or to penetrate the pleura to form new aspergilloma.

7.2.3 Chronic Fibrotic Pulmonary Aspergillosis (CFPA)

With no treatment for CCPA, the disease gradually develops into CFPA. The extensive lung fibrosis involves at least two lung lobes with accompanying seriously impaired lung functions caused by CCPA. In the cases with serious lung fibrosis that involves one lung lobe with accompanying one cavity, this is known as CCPA with involvement of the lung lobe instead of CFPA.

7.2.4 Aspergillus Nodule

Aspergillus nodule is demonstrated as one or more nodules with a diameter of lower than 3 cm, which is a rarely found type of CPA. Resembling to tuberculoma, lung carcinoma, lung metastasis, *Cryptococcus* nodule, coccidioidomycosis, and other rarely found diseases, the pathogen can only be defined by histological examination. In the cases of aspergillus infection with the lesion larger than 3 cm and accompanying central necrosis, the diagnosis should be more accurately defined as mass-like change caused by aspergillus infection.

7.2.5 Subacute Invasive Pulmonary Aspergillosis (SAIA)

SAIA is formerly known as chronic necrotizing pulmonary aspergillosis (CNPA) or semi-invasive pulmonary aspergillosis. SAIA occurs in individuals with slightly compromised immunity or extremely weak individuals including patients with diabetes, malnutrition, alcoholism, chronic obstructive pulmonary disease (COPD), connective tissue diseases, non-tuberculosis mycobacteria infection, or HIV infection, the elderly, patients receiving long-term treatment of hormone or other immunosuppressants, and patients receiving radiotherapy. Compared to CCPA, SAIA has similar clinical and radiological demonstrations but with more rapid progression. The illness course of SAIA is usually 1–3 months. The radiological demonstrations include cavity, nodule, progressive consolidation, and accompanying formation of abscess. Histological biopsy demonstrates hyphae that invade lung tissue.

7.3 Allergic Bronchopulmonary Aspergillosis (ABPA)

ABPA is an allergic inflammatory response produced by the human body to fight against aspergillus that parasitizes in the bronchus. It commonly occurs in patients with a basic disease of chronic asthma or cystic fibrosis. And the disease occurs commonly in individuals with atopic constitution, and the symptoms include recurrent paroxysmal wheezing, fever, cough, expectoration of brown sputum bolt, and hemoptysis. By physical examination, diffuse wheezing can be heard on both lungs; fine and moist rales can be heard at the infiltration lesion in the lungs. Chest X-ray demonstrates infiltration lesions with lobar or segmental distribution that are commonly migratory, lung consolidation, and segmental or lobar atelectasis due to bronchial mucous obstruction with no interlobar fissure shift. In the cases with long-term recurrent attacks, the central bronchus may dilate, and the involved segmental or sub-segmental bronchus is then subject to cystic dilation which is distally normal. Chest X-ray also commonly demonstrates raillike, parallel lines-like, ringlike, strips-like, toothpaste-like, or fingertip-like opacity. By blood test, the eosinophile granulocyte count increases and serum IgE concentration increases. The intracutaneous test of aspergillus infiltrates shows double-phase reaction. In that, wheal reaction and flush reaction occur 15–20 min after the test that fade away within about 0.5–2 h (type I reaction), and local Arthus reaction can be observed within 4–10 h that fades away within about 24–36 h (type III reaction). Due to the presence of aspergillus-specific precipitin in the patients, the condensed serum specimen can be harvested for test, which has a positive rate of 92%.

References

1. Kosmidis C, Denning DW. The clinical spectrum of pulmonary aspergillosis. Thorax. 2015;70(3):270–7.
2. Denning DW, Alex P, Cole DC. Global burden of chronic pulmonary aspergillosis complicating sarcoidosis. Eur Respir J. 2013;41(3):621–6.

Treatment and Follow-Ups of Pulmonary Aspergillosis

8

Dong-Na Su, Chen Qiu, Pu-Xuan Lu, and Shi-Ping Wu

The following are recommended in the Clinical Guideline for Diagnosis and Treatment of Aspergillosis issued in the year 2016 by the Infectious Diseases Society of America (IDSA):

8.1 Medication for Treatment of Pulmonary Aspergillosis

8.1.1 Amphotericin B Deoxycholate and Its Lipid Derivatives

Amphotericin B deoxycholate and its lipid derivatives are an appropriate choice for initial treatment of aspergillus infection or when voriconazole cannot be administered. This is strongly recommended with moderate-grade evidence.

8.1.2 Aerosol of Amphotericin B

For patients with long-term neutropenia or recipients of lung transplantation, aerosol inhalation of amphotericin B can be prescribed for prophylactic treatment. This is weakly recommended with low-grade evidence.

8.1.3 Echinocandin

Echinocandin is an effective medication for remedial treatment of pulmonary aspergillosis. It can be prescribed for separate use or combined use. However, its routine separate use for treatment of IPA is not recommended. This is strongly recommended with moderate-grade evidence.

8.1.4 Triazole Drugs

For most patients, triazoles are a proximal choice for treatment and prevention of pulmonary aspergillosis. This is strongly recommended with high-grade evidence.

8.2 The Recommended Medication for IPA

8.2.1 Voriconazole

Voriconazole is recommended as the chief medication to treat aspergillosis, which is strongly recommended with high-grade evidence. The alternative medications include amphotericin B liposome which is strongly recommended with moderate-grade evidence, isavuconazole which is strongly recommended with moderate-grade evidence, or other amphotericin B lipid preparations which are weakly recommended with low-grade evidence. Echinocandin is not recommended as the chief medication to treat aspergillosis, which is strongly recommended with moderate-grade evidence. When the antifungal medications such as azoles and polyenes are contraindicated, echinocandins such as micafungin or caspofungin can be applied as the alternative, which are weakly recommended with moderate-grade evidence. For the patients with definitive diagnosis of IPA or for the cases with a serious condition, the combined use of voriconazole and echinocandin is recommended to fight against fungi, which is weakly recommended with moderate-grade evidence.

D.-N. Su · C. Qiu · S.-P. Wu (✉)
Second Clinical Medical College of Jinan University, Shenzhen, Guangdong, China

P.-X. Lu
Centre for Chronic Diseases Control of Shenzhen, Shenzhen, Guangdong, China

C. Qiu et al. (eds.), *Pulmonary Aspergillosis*, https://doi.org/10.1007/978-981-13-3435-1_8

8.2.2 Early Antifungal Medication

For the strongly suspected cases of IPA, antifungal medication should be administered as early as possible along with diagnostic assessment. This is strongly recommended with high-grade evidence.

8.2.3 Continuous Medication

Continuous medication for at least 6–12 weeks is recommended. The duration of medication largely depends on the severity and duration of immunosuppression, location of the lesions, and evidence of improvement. This is strongly recommended with low-grade evidence.

8.2.4 The Use of Immunosuppressant

If possible, a smaller dose of immunosuppressant should be administered along with anti-aspergillus medication, which is strongly recommended with low-grade evidence. For patients with definitive or suspected diagnosis of pulmonary aspergillosis, granulocyte-macrophage colony-stimulating factor GM-CSF can be selected for neutropenia, which is weakly recommended with low-grade evidence. For the cases of pulmonary aspergillosis with accompanying neutropenia, if the standard therapy shows no effects or the condition is predicted to last for more than 1 week, granulocyte infusion therapy can be administered, which is weakly recommended with low-grade evidence. For patients with chronic granuloma, recombinant gamma-interferon can be applied for prevention and treatment, which is strongly recommended with high-grade evidence.

8.2.5 Surgery

If the patient's lesion can be eliminated, surgery can be selected to treat pulmonary aspergillosis. This is strongly recommended with low-grade evidence.

8.2.6 Azoles

The clinicians should know about the serum minimal concentrations of azoles, such as itraconazole, voriconazole, posaconazole, and isavuconazole, and their possible cross-reactions with ciclosporin, tacrolimus, sirolimus, and other CYP3A4 substrates, such as tyrosine kinase inhibitor, to optimize the therapeutic efficacy and to avoid potential toxic effects. This is strongly recommended with moderate-grade evidence.

8.3 Therapies for Chronic Aspergillosis

8.3.1 Chronic Cavitary Pulmonary Aspergillosis (CCPA)

For the cases of CCPA with no following conditions, the patients should receive follow-ups every 3–6 months instead of antifungal therapy.

The condition is not complicated by lung symptoms, no weight loss or obvious fatigue, and no severely impaired lung function or progressively weak lung functions. This is weakly recommended with low-grade evidence. For the patients with CCPA and systemic or lung symptoms, progressively weak lung function, or progression of the condition demonstrated by radiology, antifungal therapy for at least 6 months should be administered. This is strongly recommended with low-grade evidence.

For oral medication, itraconazole and voriconazole should be the first choice [1]. This is strongly recommended with high-grade evidence. For those showing adverse effects or no favorable therapeutic responses, posaconazole can be selected as the third-line management medication. This is strongly recommended with moderate-grade evidence. For those showing no favorable therapeutic responses, resistance to azoles, and/or adverse effects, micafungin (weakly recommended with low-grade evidence), caspofungin (weakly recommended with low-grade evidence), or amphotericin B (weakly recommended with low-grade evidence) can be administered intravenously. But the therapeutic course may be prolonged.

For hemoptysis, oral medication of tranexamic acid (weakly recommended with low-grade evidence) or bronchial artery embolization (BAE) can be administered. If no favorable therapeutic responses, surgical removal should be performed, which is weakly recommended with moderate-grade evidence. For those with localized lesion and no favorable therapeutic response to medications, including aspergillus fumigatus infection resistant to most azoles or persistent hemoptysis after BAE, surgical removal of the lesions can be chosen. This is strongly recommended with moderate-grade evidence.

8.3.2 Aspergilloma

For asymptomatic patients with singular aspergilloma and no progression of cavity size in the past 6–24 months, the condition should only be observed. This is strongly recommended with moderate-grade evidence.

For symptomatic patients, especially serious hemoptysis, surgical removal, if no contraindication, should be performed. This is strongly recommended with moderate-grade evidence.

Perioperative or postoperative antifungal therapy is not routinely required. However, if aspergilloma is at risk of intraoperative rupture, voriconazole or echinocandin should be prescribed to prevent aspergillus empyema. This is weakly recommended with low-grade evidence.

8.4 Follow-Ups of Pulmonary Aspergillosis

8.4.1 Follow-Ups After Antifungal Therapy

Radiological follow-ups should be performed after antifungal therapy for CPA to assess the changes of the condition. After antifungal therapy, the patients should receive radiological follow-ups every 3–6 months, followed by lower frequency of radiological follow-ups. The signs signaling improvement in the cases of CPA include decreased pleural thickening, decreased substances in the cavity, more smooth inner wall of the cavity, smaller nodules, and smaller tissue consolidation around the cavity. The signs signaling therapeutic failure include enlarged cavity, emergence of new cavity, fusion of cavities, formation of aspergilloma, and enlarged consolidation area around the cavity. CT scan or other radiological techniques demonstrate the progression of the lesions via volume quantification in the respective software package.

8.4.2 Follow-Ups After Surgical Removal of Aspergillus Nodule

Except for those with compromised immunity, the patients cannot receive antifungal therapy after complete surgical removal of a singular aspergillus nodule. Serological quantification of aspergillus IgG antibody can be applied to monitor the relapse of an aspergillus nodule. However, no research conclusion supported by precise data has been reported. For the cases with incomplete surgical removal of the singular nodule, the progression of the lesions should be closely followed up. The follow-ups should be performed every 3 months, including serological quantification of aspergillus IgG antibody, inflammatory indices, and dynamic changes of the lesions by radiology. Based on these data, the necessity of antifungal therapy is assessed. For the patients with multiple nodules, when one nodule is surgically removed, antifungal therapy should be administered to treat other nodules. The radiological follow-ups, especially initial 3 months, should be performed for dynamic changes of the lesions. In all of the cases, glucocorticoid should be administered as less as possible.

8.5 Application of Bronchoscopy in the Diagnosis and Treatment of Aspergillosis

Concerning the application of bronchoscopy in the diagnosis and treatment of aspergillosis, the following are recommended in the *Clinical Guidelines for the Diagnosis and Treatment of Aspergillosis* issued in the year 2016 by IDSA:

8.5.1 The Standard for Definitive Diagnosis of Aspergillosis

The standard for definitive diagnosis of aspergillosis is defined to be histopathological fungal culture of the sterile tissue positive.

8.5.2 Accurate Biomarker for Diagnosis

For the patients with hematopoietic malignancies or receiving hematopoietic stem cell transplantation, GM in serum and alveolar lavage fluid is recommended as the accurate biomarker for the diagnosis of invasive aspergillosis.

8.5.3 Detection of GM

For patients receiving antifungal therapy or prophylactic therapy, routine screening of blood GM is not recommended. However, for these patients, bronchoscopic specimen can be harvested for detection of GM. This is strongly recommended with high-grade evidence.

8.5.4 Early Diagnosis

For early diagnosis, if possible, all the suspected cases of IPA should receive bronchoalveolar lavage (BAL). This is strongly recommended with moderate-grade evidence.

8.5.5 Bronchoalveolar Lavage (BAL)

Standardized procedures of BAL are recommended, and the harvested specimen should be routinely sent for fungal culture and cytological examination. Non-culture-based tests should also be performed, such as GM test. This is strongly recommended with moderate-grade evidence.

8.5.6 Invasive Tracheobronchial Aspergillosis (ITBA)

When fungal colonization occurs in patients with ITBA, antifungal therapy is not necessary. But for such patients with symptoms or compromised immunity, the therapies include antifungal therapy and bronchoscopic removal of mucous occlusion.

8.5.7 Breakthrough Aspergillosis

Breakthrough aspergillosis refers mainly to aspergillus infection during prophylactic antifungal therapy. In the guideline issued in the year 2016, active clinical examinations are recommended, including invasive examinations, to establish definitive diagnosis.

Reference

1. Liu X, Lu S. Diagnostic and therapeutic changes of aspergillosis: from the perspective of evidence based medicine. Chin J Tuberc Prev. 2017;39(1):16–21.

Part II

Typical Cases of Pulmonary Aspergillosis

9 Pulmonary Aspergillosis Resembling to Pulmonary Tuberculosis

Chen Qiu and Dong-Na Su

Pulmonary tuberculosis is still a common infectious disease that threatens human health. It is a public health issue and a social problem of human being. In China, it is one of the important diseases in the field of disease control. Since the 1980s, pulmonary tuberculosis has been globally deteriorating, and its prevalence has been obviously increasing in many developing countries including China. According to a report by WHO, about 550 million people were ever infected with Mycobacterium tuberculosis in China. A report by WHO in the year 2017 indicated that the cases of tuberculosis in seven countries account for 64% of the global total burden, with India ranking the first followed by Indonesia, China, the Philippines, Pakistan, Nigeria, and South Africa.

From an overall perspective, infection of *Mycobacterium tuberculosis* is the most common risk factor of pulmonary aspergillosis. A previous research in the UK indicated that the total cases of chronic pulmonary aspergillosis secondary to tuberculosis may be up to 1.2 million across the world. Therefore, pulmonary aspergillosis and tuberculosis may show concurrence or alternative occurrence.

The clinical manifestations of pulmonary aspergillosis are diverse that, along with radiological demonstrations, resembles to those of pulmonary tuberculosis. The symptoms of chronic pulmonary aspergillosis, such as weight loss, shortness of breath, fatigue, and hemoptysis, can be hardly differentiated from pulmonary tuberculosis. In some cases of chronic pulmonary aspergillosis, a past medical history of pulmonary tuberculosis is found. Their changing condition tends to be misdiagnosed as relapse of tuberculosis. Due to low positive rate of sputum aspergillus test, some cases of pulmonary aspergillus infection cannot be diagnosed timely, and the patients, therefore, cannot receive appropriate treatment. Because the clinical and radiological manifestations of pulmonary aspergillosis resemble to those of pulmonary tuberculosis and the two diseases even coexist, the diagnosis of pulmonary aspergillosis presents challenges to the clinicians. The misdiagnosis of pulmonary aspergillosis as pulmonary tuberculosis is overwhelmingly common. A comprehensive analysis of the case history, signs, radiological demonstrations, and microbiological and pathological findings is of great importance for an accurate diagnosis of pulmonary aspergillosis. For the cases with recurrent hemoptysis, unfavorable therapeutic responses to anti-tuberculosis therapy, characteristic chest X-ray, and CT scan demonstrations of aspergillus infection, pulmonary aspergillosis should be considered for the diagnosis.

A Bulletin of WHO Press indicated that more than one million cured patients of pulmonary tuberculosis are infected by aspergillus each year. They are usually misdiagnosed as relapse of tuberculosis and cannot receive appropriate treatment. Their condition gradually progresses with final occurrence of death. Therefore, for patients cured by

The corresponding author of section 9.1 is Songming Zhuo, Email: zsm68688@163.com.
The corresponding author of section 9.2 is Senquan Wu, Email: wusenquanpbl@qq.com.
The corresponding author of section 9.3 is Ruming Xie, Email: 13911320739@163.com.
The corresponding author of section 9.4 is Guofang Deng, Email: jxxk1035@yeah.net.
The corresponding author of section 9.5 is Zhijian Yu, Email: yuzhijiansmu@163.com.
The corresponding author of section 9.6 is Jing Yuan, Email: 13500054798@139.com.
The corresponding author of section 9.7 is Dong-Na Su, Email: sudona@qq.com.
The corresponding author of section 9.8 is Li Tu, Email: 258139501@qq.com.
The corresponding author of section 9.9 is Li Tu, Email: 258139501@qq.com.
The corresponding author of section 9.10 is Hui Zeng, Email: 24178743@qq.com.
The corresponding author of section 9.11 is Hongtao Chen, Email: 843139770@qq.com.

C. Qiu (✉) · D.-N. Su
Second Clinical Medical College of Jinan University, Shenzhen, Guangdong, China

C. Qiu et al. (eds.), *Pulmonary Aspergillosis*, https://doi.org/10.1007/978-981-13-3435-1_9

anti-tuberculosis therapy, follow-ups and appropriate tests are vitally important, especially microbiological tests including aspergillus smear test and culture as well as GM test, which are necessary for early diagnosis of aspergillus infection. Molecular biological examinations for nucleic acid of aspergillus, such as PCR, are more sensitive than aspergillus culture. Immunologic assays for antibody of aspergillus are also a tool for diagnosis of aspergillus infection. However, the golden standard for the definitive diagnosis of pulmonary aspergillosis is pathological examination of the lung tissue. In the *Clinical Guideline for the Diagnosis and Treatment of Chronic Pulmonary Aspergillosis* jointly issued by ESCMID and ERS in the year 2015, it was indicated that pulmonary tuberculosis may occur before, during, or after chronic pulmonary aspergillosis. The airway specimen smear, culture, and nucleic acid amplification of *Mycobacterium tuberculosis* are important ways for identification of pulmonary tuberculosis. Without sufficient evidence supporting tuberculosis, recurrence of pulmonary symptoms after anti-tuberculosis therapy cannot be defined as relapse of tuberculosis. Even for definitively diagnosed cases of *Mycobacterium tuberculosis* infection, concurrent pulmonary aspergillus infection cannot be excluded.

In this chapter, we present some typical cases of pulmonary aspergillosis that were misdiagnosed as pulmonary tuberculosis. The specialists comment on these cases to analyze the reasons of misdiagnosis, intending to help clinicians know more about pulmonary aspergillosis and therefore improve their ability in differentiating pulmonary aspergillosis and pulmonary tuberculosis. The objective is to decrease the misdiagnosis rate of pulmonary aspergillosis as pulmonary tuberculosis and to improve our diagnosis and treatment.

Patients' consents have been obtained for images or other clinical information relating to the cases to be published.

9.1 Case 1: Repeated hemoptysis for 1 year, aggrabated for 4 days

Songming Zhuo, Na Li, Chen Qiu, Dong-Na Su, Ying-Yun Fu, and Di Wu

9.1.1 Presenting Symptoms

Recurrent hemoptysis for 1 year which aggravated for 4 days.

9.1.2 Chief Case History

A 36-year-old male was hospitalized on August 19, 2012 with presenting symptoms of recurrent hemoptysis for 1 year that aggravated for 4 days. The patient experienced intermittent hemoptysis 1 year ago with no known reason. There was a little fresh red blood in the sputum once to several times in a week. The associate symptoms included slight cough and chest pain but no fever, night sweat, and emaciation. He seeked a doctor in a general hospital of Grade 2A, and the diagnosis was pulmonary tuberculosis with lesion at the right upper lung lobe. He then was transferred to a specialized hospital in chronic diseases for anti-tuberculosis therapy for about 1 year. After 1-month treatment, reexamination by chest X-ray demonstrated likely improvement of the lesion. But the patient still experienced hemoptysis that lasted for about 1 year. Four days prior to his admission to our hospital, he coughed up fresh red blood for about 50 ml, with accompanying dizziness, fatigue, chest distress, nausea, and abdominal distension. The specialist in the outpatient department arranged his admission due to hemoptysis of undefined reason. During the recent 1 year, his body weight decreased for about 5 kg.

9.1.3 Physical Examination

Normal development, good nutrition, shortness of breath with a respiration rate of 24times/min, no yellowish stain in systemic skin mucosa, no superficial lymphadenectasis, no lip cyanosis and reddish pharynx, slightly coarse breathing sounds at both lungs with no dry and moist rales, and no abnormalities detected in the heart and abdomen.

9.1.4 Radiological Investigation

Chest pain scan of HRCT on May 31, 2012, demonstrated quite favorable running course and distribution of lung markings in both lungs. The apical segment of the right upper lung was demonstrated with patches and spots of heterogeneous high-intensity opacity, and some were poorly defined. Other lung parenchyma was demonstrated with no definitive abnormality. The trachea and bronchi were demonstrated with no stenosis and obstruction. The mediastinum and both hilar areas were demonstrated with no enlarged lymph nodes. And the heart and major blood vessels were demonstrated with no obvious abnormalities (Fig. 9.1).

The initial diagnosis was that the reason of hemoptysis is to be defined. The diagnosis is likely to be infiltrative tuberculosis of the right lung or pulmonary aspergillosis.

9.1.5 Diagnosis and Treatment

After admission, the patient was improved the relevant examinations. On August 20, 2012, the routine blood test

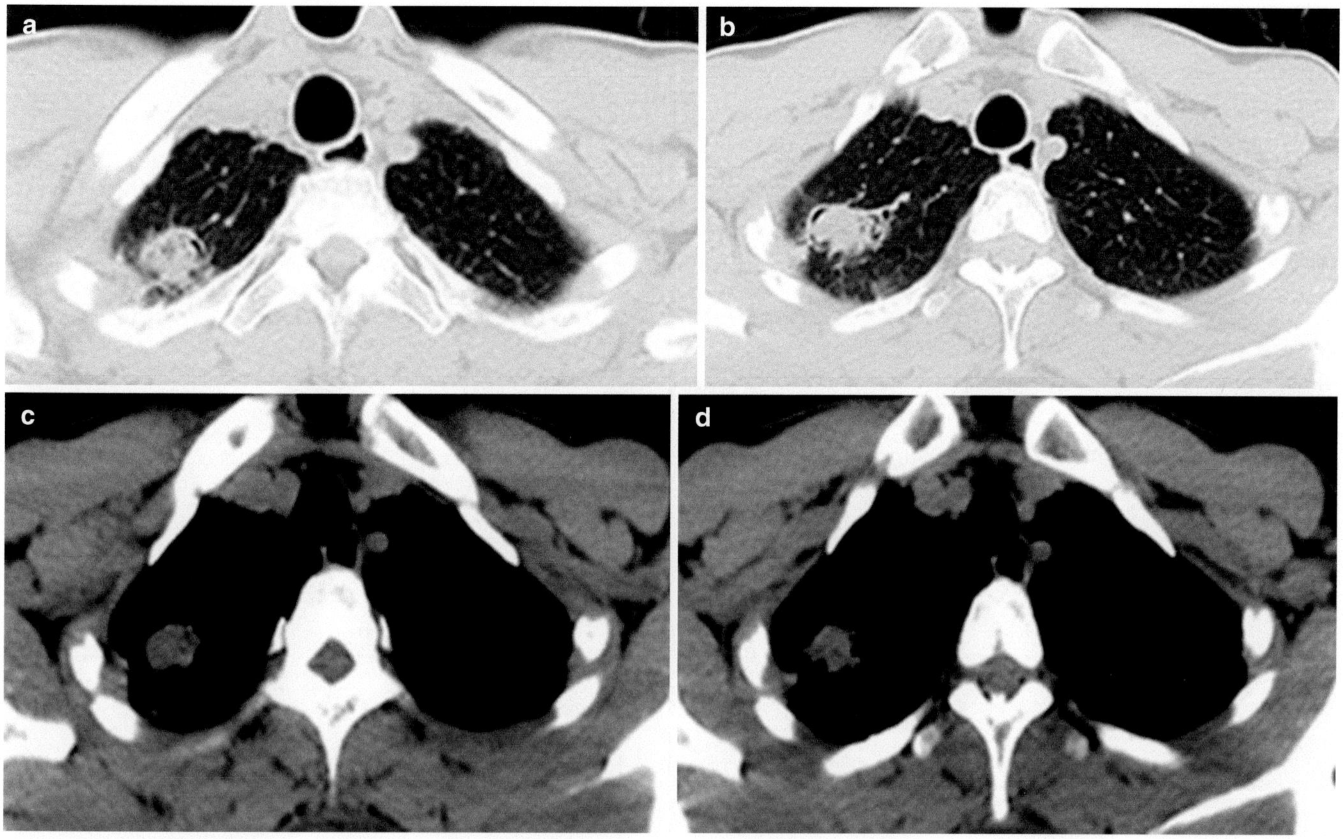

Fig. 9.1 (**a–d**) Chest pain scan of HRCT. (**a**) The apical segment of the right upper lung with high-intensity nodular opacity which connects with lateral pleura posterolaterally. (**b**) Air crescent sign in the high-intensity nodular opacity at the right upper lung. (**c**) Nodular opacity at the layer of the subclavicular vein. (**d**) Heterogeneous nodular opacity at the layer of the subclavicular vein

showed no abnormality; and 5-item biomarkers test for neoplasm showed CEA, CA125, CA19-9, NSE, and Cyfra 21-1 that were within normal limits. On August 21, 2012, and August 22, 2012, two sputum smear tests showed no acid-fast bacillus, fungal hyphae, and spores. On August 22, 2012, the sputum culture showed normal colonies of the upper respiratory tract.

On August 20, 2012, plain and enhanced CT scan demonstrated, compared to the previous scans on May 31, 2012, poorly defined patches and spots of heterogeneous high-intensity opacity at both lungs, crescent-shaped transparent opacity in the lesion of the right upper lung, and the long diameter of nodule inside being about 2.9 cm. Some segments of the right middle and lower lung were demonstrated with poorly defined small flakes of ground-glass opacity with slightly high intensity. The lateral segment of the right middle lung lobe and the lateral basilar segment of the left lower lung lobe were demonstrated with poorly defined small spot opacity with slightly high intensity. Several small oval transparent shadows were seen in the dorsal segment of the lower lobe of the right lung. An oval-shaped air cavity was demonstrated at the right paratracheal region. The mediastinum window demonstrated connection of the air cavity with the trachea. The trachea and bronchi were demonstrated with no stenosis and obstruction. And the mediastinal lymph nodes were demonstrated to be enlarged. By enhanced scan, the lesion at the right upper lung was demonstrated with heterogeneous slight enhancement. And the diagnosis was considered to be (1) both lung infection and progression of the lesion at the right middle lung lobe, which is most likely to be aspergillus infection; (2) bleeding of some segments at the right middle and lower lung lobes; (3) multiple bullae at the right lung; (4) slight enlargement of mediastinal lymph nodes; and (5) bilaterally local pleural thickening (Fig. 9.2).

After hospitalization, levofloxacin was administered for anti-infection and symptomatic treatment. To define the diagnosis, CT-guided puncture of the lesion at the right upper lung was performed on August 23, 2012. And postoperative reexamination by CT scan demonstrated pneumothorax, with about 50% shrinkage of the lung. Thoracic closed drainage was then performed. And the histopathological biopsy reported that microscopy of the tissue from the right upper lung showed a small quantity of alveolar tissue and a large quantity of degenerated mold hyphae, which

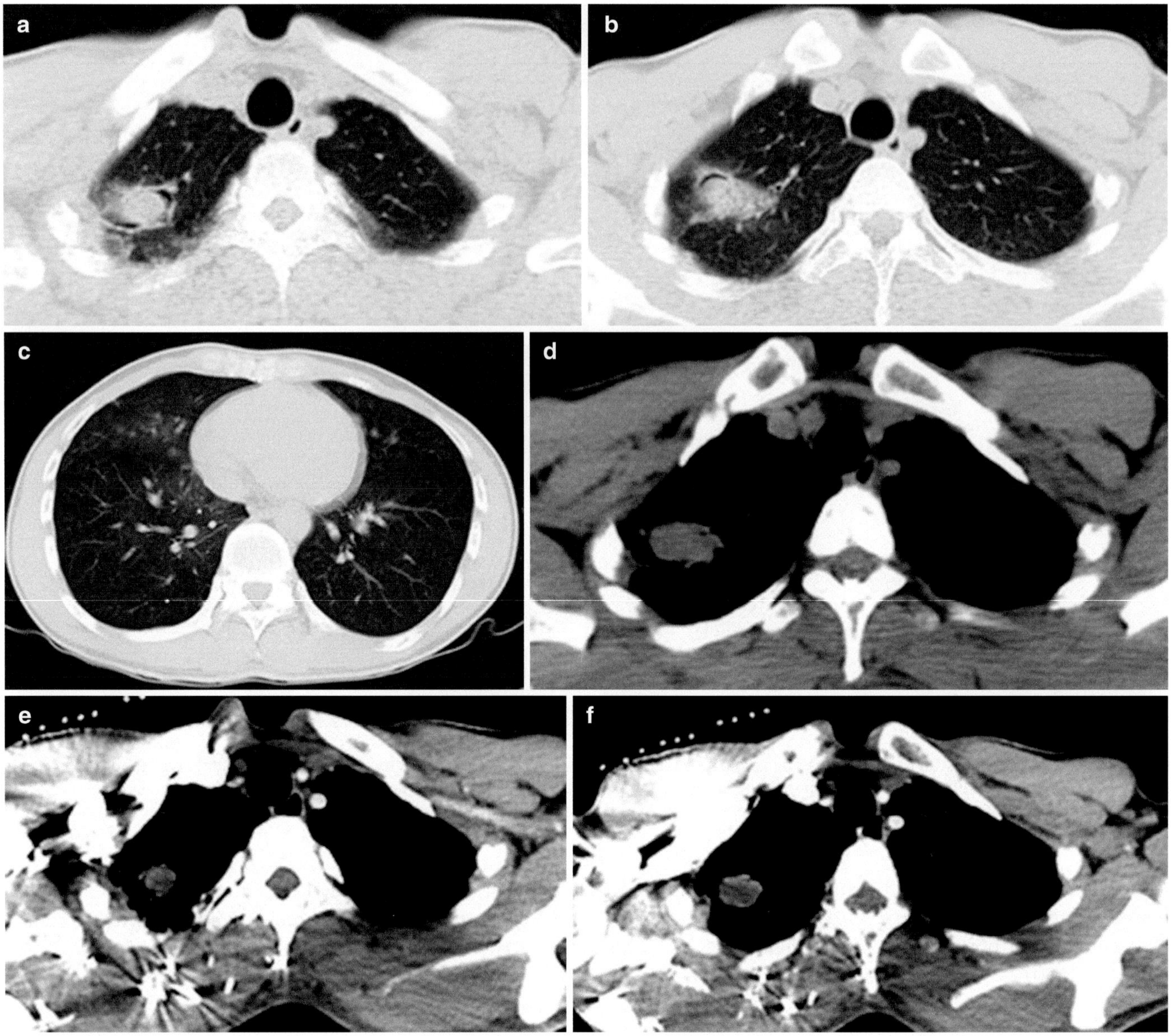

Fig. 9.2 (**a**–**f**) Plain and enhanced CT scan on August 20, 2012. (**a**) High-intensity nodular opacity at the layer of lung apex and air crescent sign around parenchymal nodule; (**b**) high-intensity opacity at the layer of lung apex with accompanying air crescent opacity; (**c**) ground-glass intensity opacity at the right middle and lower lung lobes; (**d**) heterogeneous dense opacity at the layer of the subclavicular vein and localized thickening of the lateral pleura; (**e**, **f**) heterogeneous enhancement of the lesion at the layer of the subclavicular vein by enhanced CT scan

is morphologically consistent to aspergillus. The diagnosis was clinically defined as pulmonary aspergilloma. On September 11, 2012, the patient received general anesthesia and thoracoscopic lesion removal from the right upper lung. By postoperative pathology, the removed lesion was reported to be a mass of lung tissue in size of 8.3 cm × 4.5 cm × 2.5 cm with mold infection, which was morphologically consistent to changes caused by aspergillus infection (Fig. 9.3). After the operation, cefotiam was administered as an anti-infection therapy, and fluconazole was administered as an anti-fungal therapy. Since September 14, 2012, fluconazole was discontinued, and voriconazole was given as anti-fungal therapy. The reexamination by chest X-ray indicated favorable expansion of the right lung, and the patient was discharged on September 27, 2012.

9.1.6 The Final Diagnosis

Final diagnosis: right upper lung aspergilloma.

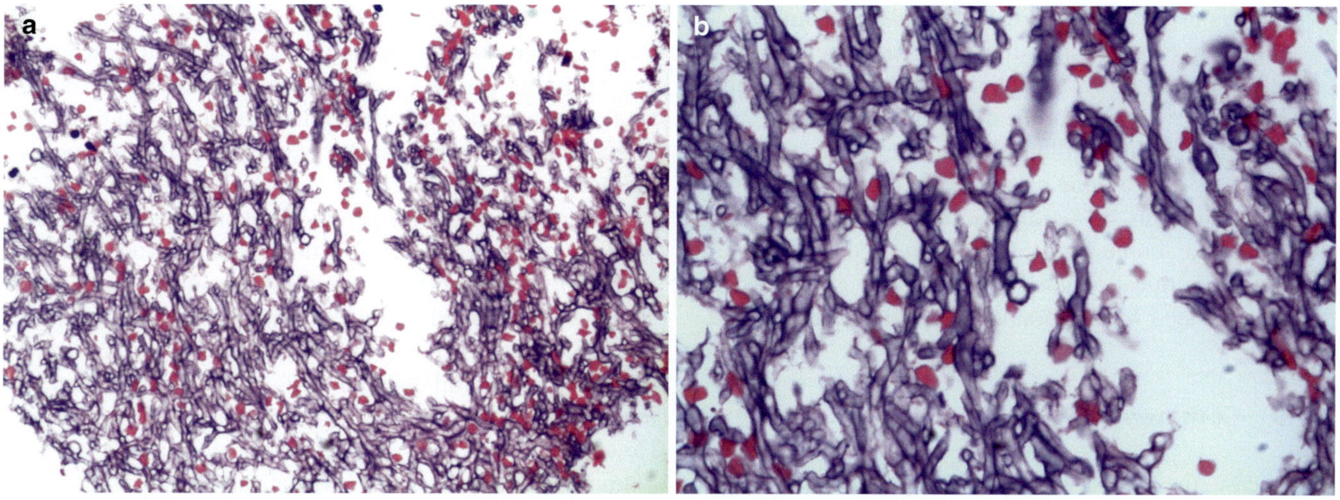

Fig. 9.3 (**a**, **b**) Pathology of the lung tissue, a large quantity of hyphae and spores detected. (**a**, **b**) By H&E staining

9.1.7 Prognosis

The patient was cured after the operation. Follow-ups after discharge showed no occurrence of hemoptysis.

9.1.8 Discussion

The patient was a middle-aged man who had been diagnosed with pulmonary tuberculosis due to recurrent hemoptysis for 1 year with accompanying polymorphous lesions at the right upper lung. And he was given anti-tuberculosis therapy for 1 year. However, during the treatment, he experienced intermittent hemoptysis in a small quantity and was transferred to a Grade 3 general hospital due to increased quantity of hemoptysis. By chest CT scan, puncture of the lesion at the right upper lung, surgical operation, and postoperative pathology, the diagnosis was defined to be aspergillus infection of the lung tissue, more accurately to be pulmonary aspergilloma.

The case was demonstrated by CT scan with mass-like lesion in the right upper lung and air crescent sign with no surrounding calcification and satellite lesions. The condition failed to improve after anti-tuberculosis therapy for 1 year but aggravated. In this case, the patient suffered from pulmonary aspergillosis but was misdiagnosed with tuberculosis. Therefore, for the cases with air crescent sign by chest CT scan, especially for those with a suspected diagnosis of tuberculosis but show unfavorable therapeutic efficacy by anti-tuberculosis therapy, pulmonary aspergillosis should be highly suspected. For the cases showing favorable therapeutic responses by anti-tuberculosis therapy but unfavorable absorption of the lesions, a diagnosis of pulmonary aspergillosis should still be suspected due to possible concurrence of the two diseases [1, 2].

After diagnosis and treatment of this case, we summarized the following knowledge about pulmonary aspergillosis:

1. Pulmonary aspergillosis may exist separately or concurrently with other diseases, and pulmonary tuberculosis is the most common basic disease of pulmonary aspergillosis. The other common diseases that are concurrent with pulmonary aspergillosis include carcinomatous cavity, sarcoidosis, pulmonary abscess cavity, and bronchiectasis [3]. The patients may be asymptomatic, and hemoptysis in a small quantity is the most common symptom. The underlying mechanism of hemoptysis caused by pulmonary aspergillus infection remains unknown. Based on literature reports, the possible mechanism includes the following: (a) the endotoxin of aspergillus and protease cause histolysis and necrosis of the tissue, which erode the vascular vessels to cause bleeding; (b) aspergillus infection impairs the vascular wall of its abundant surrounding vascular network and causes rupture of the angioma; and (c) the movement of aspergilloma in the cavity rubs the vascular network to impair the vascular wall. For patients with a small quantity of hemoptysis, palliative treatment of internal medicine should be administered. But for patients with a large quantity of hemoptysis, interventional embolization or surgical operation should be considered [4].
2. The characteristic CT scan demonstration of pulmonary aspergilloma is sphere-in-sphere sign [5], which is round or round-like dense opacity in pulmonary cavity or cavum with surrounding crescent or ring-shaped translucent opacity. In some cases, the translucent opacity moves along with changes of the posture. In the cases of carcinomatous cavity, no spherical content is demonstrated, and the translucent opacity does not move along with changes

of body posture. Tuberculous cavity is demonstrated with similar air crescent sign, but the inner sphere connects closely to the sphere of tuberculoma that is immobile. These are key points for the differential diagnosis.

3. The lesion of aspergilloma is located in the thick-wall cavity and has a poor blood perfusion. The anti-fungal medication can be hardly permeated into the lesion. Therefore, simple medication shows poor therapeutic efficacy. Surgical removal of pulmonary aspergilloma is recommended with favorable therapeutic efficacy.

9.1.9 Comments

In this case, the patient was a middle-aged man, with a disease course of 1 year. His condition had a chronic onset, with presenting symptom of hemoptysis, which had been diagnosed as pulmonary tuberculosis. However, the anti-tuberculosis therapy in a specialized hospital showed no favorable therapeutic efficacy. Lung CT scan demonstrated crescent translucent opacity in the right upper lung, with surrounding halo sign. Based on these findings, a clinical diagnosis of pulmonary aspergilloma can be established. It is obvious that pulmonary aspergillosis in this case was misdiagnosed as pulmonary tuberculosis.

According to the *2015 Clinical Guideline for Diagnosis and Treatment of Chronic Pulmonary Aspergillosis*, chronic pulmonary aspergillosis can be classified into singular aspergilloma, chronic cavitary pulmonary aspergillosis, chronic fibrotic pulmonary aspergillosis, aspergillus nodule, and subacute invasive pulmonary aspergillosis. In this case, the diagnosis should be singular aspergilloma. Singular aspergilloma refers to one fungal sphere in one pulmonary cavity, with serological or microbiological evidence of aspergillus infection and no progression in 3-month follow-ups. The patients with presenting symptom of hemoptysis tend to be misdiagnosed with pulmonary tuberculosis. For the cases with no favorable therapeutic responses to appropriate anti-tuberculosis therapy, especially the cases with crescent cavity opacity, relevant investigations should be ordered as early as possible to define the possibility of pulmonary aspergillosis. Currently, pulmonary aspergillosis-related investigations and examinations include sputum smear test, sputum fungal culture, G test, and GM test for microbiological evidence and bronchoscopy, percutaneous lung puncture, and lung lobectomy for pathological evidence. In this case, surgical removal of the lesion is the first choice. At day 2 after his admission, chest CT scan demonstrated typical crescent cavity opacity, which was considered to be pulmonary aspergillosis. In combination with the presenting symptom of hemoptysis, surgical removal of the lesion in the right upper lung is indicated. And postoperative pathology can define the diagnosis. With such a diagnostic and therapeutic plan, percutaneous lung puncture for biopsy can be skipped. Postoperative early medication of fluconazole to fight against aspergillus is inappropriate due to insensitivity of fluconazole to aspergillus. Several clinical guidelines indicate that voriconazole is the medication of choice for the treatment of pulmonary aspergillosis.

Surgical removal of aspergilloma is indicated for patients with sufficiently good lung functions. Actually, for all patients with serious hemoptysis, surgical removal of aspergilloma should be considered. Complete removal of the lesion and no leakage of aspergillus components into the pleural cavity indicate a successful operation. After a successful operation, the lesion of aspergilloma and hemoptysis rarely relapse. However, the success rate of operation for chronic cavitary pulmonary aspergillosis is comparatively low.

9.2 Case 2: Recurrent Hemoptysis for More Than 15 Months, Which Onset Again for 6 Days

Senquan Wu, Ping Zhang, Chen Qiu, Dong-Na Su, Shusong Peng, and Rong Huang

9.2.1 Presenting Symptoms

Recurrent hemoptysis for more than 15 months, with onset again for 6 days.

9.2.2 Brief Case History

A 31-year-old woman was admitted to our hospital on November 6, 2013 due to presenting symptom of recurrent hemoptysis for more than 15 months and onset again for 6 days. Since July 2012, the patient experienced hemoptysis of about 50 ml fresh red blood with no known causes. But she experienced no obvious cough, expectoration, fever, aversion to cold, chest distress, chest pain, and breathlessness. Chest X-ray in a local hospital demonstrated lesion at the right upper lung, which was then diagnosed as pulmonary tuberculosis. Appropriate anti-tuberculosis therapy was administered including medications of isoniazid, rifampin, pyrazinamide, and ethambutol. During the treatment, she still experienced cough up a small quantity of sputum with dark red blood streak, which indicated poor therapeutic responses. Since March 2013, she began anti-fungal therapy with medication of itraconazole, but she discontinued the medication after 2 months by herself and received traditional Chinese medicine. Six days ago, her hemoptysis onset again with about 30 ml fresh red blood, but no cause was known.

She also experienced chest distress and subjective fever, but the body temperature was not checked. No cough, expectoration, and breathlessness were reported. She then went to the outpatient department of our hospital for treatment. Chest CT scan demonstrated cavity or cavity-like lesion adjacent to the mediastinum at the apical segment of the right upper lung lobe, with mass-like lesion of soft tissue intensity inside. The patient was admitted to the hospital for further treatment. Since the onset of hemoptysis, the patient showed good spiritual state, fairly good appetite, and sleep. She reported no abnormality in bowel movement but showed slight weight loss.

The patient denied histories of hypertension and diabetes. She also denied histories of hepatitis and other infectious diseases. There was no history of surgery, trauma, and blood transfusion and no histories of drug or food allergy.

9.2.3 Physical Examination

She was well conscious, with no lip cyanosis. Bilateral respiration movements were symmetric and bilateral thoracic expansion no abnormality. The bilateral vocal fremitus was normal. Percussion of both lungs showed clear sounds, but auscultation showed coarse respiration sounds at both lungs with no dry and moist rales. The heartbeat was regular, with no murmur at valvular areas. The abdomen was soft, with no tenderness, rebound. And both lower limbs showed no edema.

9.2.4 Investigations

Chest CT scan in an outpatient department of a city's People's Hospital on November 4, 2013 demonstrated cavity or cavity-like lesion adjacent to the mediastinum at the apical segment of the right upper lung lobe, with mass-like lesion of soft tissue intensity inside. The diagnosis was considered to be congenital bronchiectasis or lung cavity secondary to tuberculosis that is complicated by aspergilloma. Chest CT scan also demonstrated surrounding alveolar hematocele of the lesion (Fig. 9.4).

The apical segment of the right upper lung lobe was demonstrated with a cyst-like translucent lesion adjacent to the mediastinum, with an irregular mass-like lesion of soft tissue intensity inside. Local fissures were demonstrated between the two lesions, which were visible at consecutive six layers from top down. At the layer with larger area of lesion, the involved area was up to about 2.2 cm × 1.8 cm, with small quantities of spots and small nodular calcification intensity opacities. Around the calcification intensity opacities, irregular round-like, column-like, and arch-shaped translucent areas were demonstrated. The lesion of soft tissue intensity was demonstrated with heterogeneous intensity, with a CT value of about 50–60 Hu. Around the soft tissue lesion, irregular patches of ground-glass-like high-intensity opacity were demonstrated with poorly defined edges.

9.2.5 Initial Diagnosis

The causes of hemoptysis were to be detected. The diagnosis was suspected to be infiltrative tuberculosis at the right upper lung or pulmonary aspergillosis.

9.2.6 Diagnosis and Treatment

After admission to our hospital, anti-infection therapy was administered with medication of ceftazidime. In addition, etamsylate and carbazochrome were given for hemostasis. The investigations and examinations, including routine blood test, neoplasm biomarker examination, ESR, CRP,

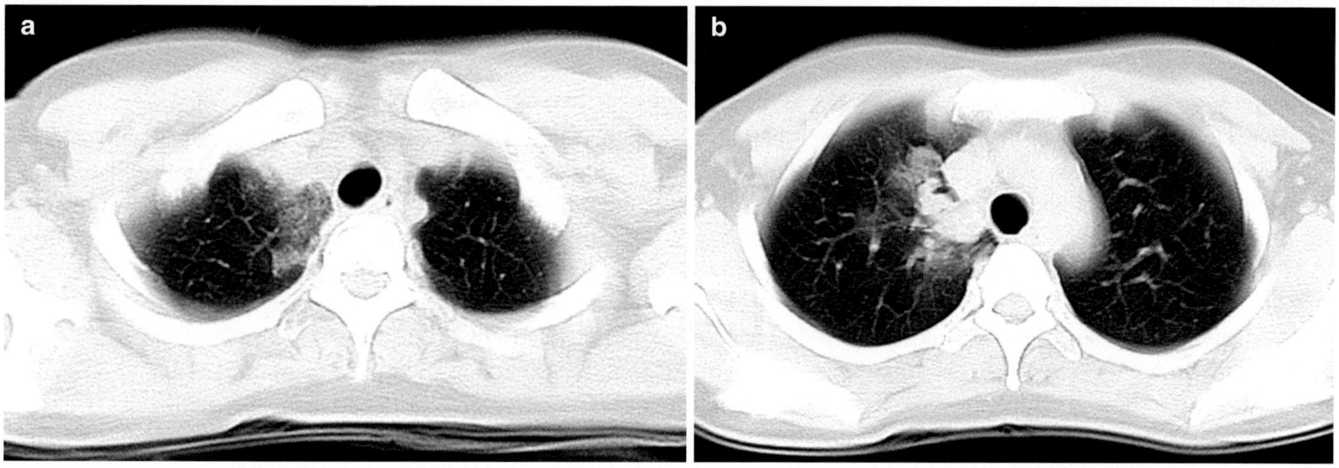

Fig. 9.4 (**a**, **b**) Chest CT scan

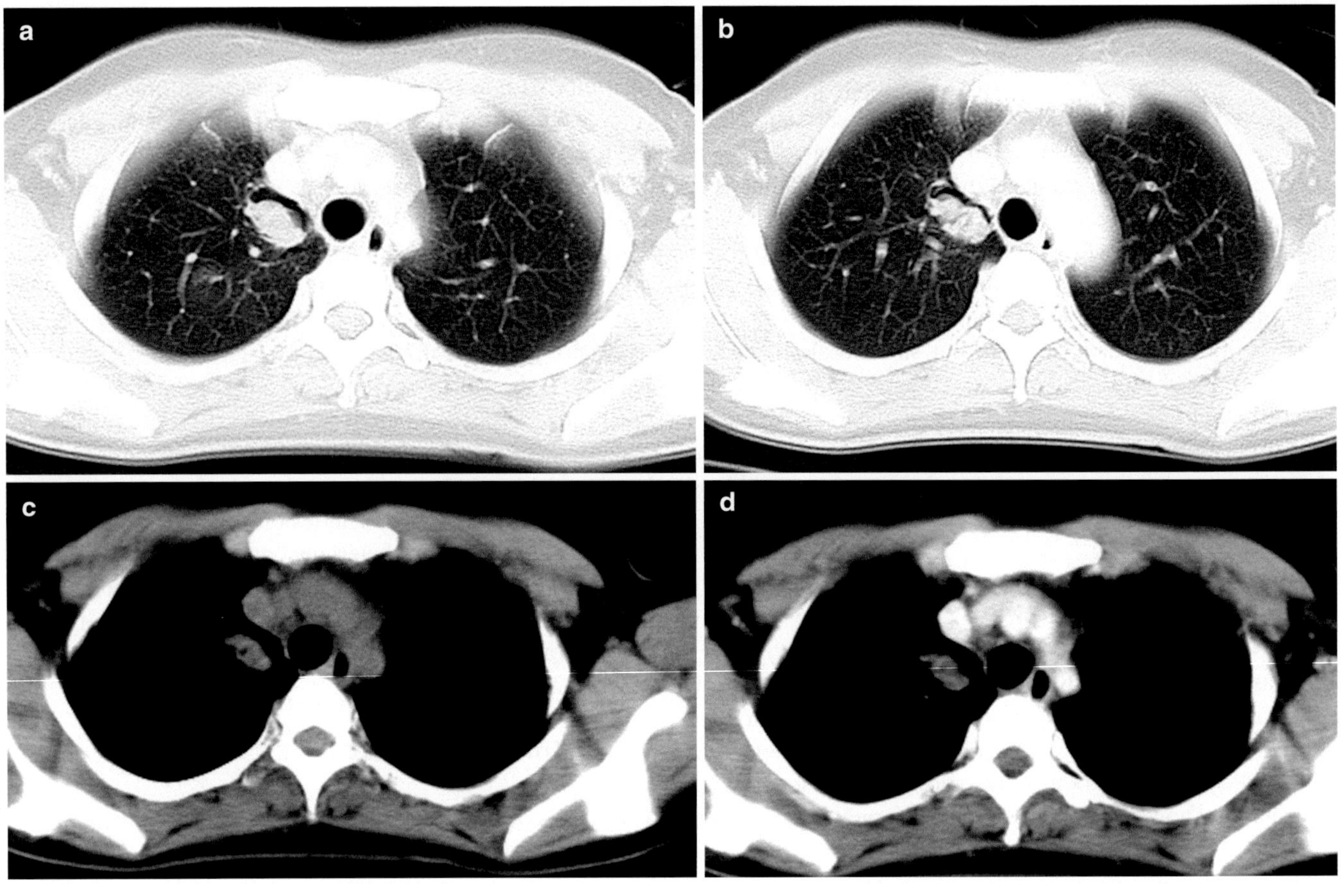

Fig. 9.5 (**a–d**) Chest CT scan. (**a**, **b**) A cyst-like translucent area adjacent to the mediastinum at the right upper lung lobe, with an irregular mass-like lesion of soft tissue intensity inside; local fissures between the two lesions in size of about 2.1 cm × 1.3 cm, with small quantities of spots and small nodular calcification intensity opacity inside. (**c**) Part of soft tissue lesion with heterogeneous intensity, with a CT value of about 43 Hu. (**d**) Slight enhancement by enhanced CT scan, with a CT value of about 60 Hu

sputum smear, sputum culture, and DNA examination for *Mycobacterium tuberculosis*, showed no abnormalities. On November 11, 2013, fibrobronchoscopy showed no abnormality of all levels of bronchi.

Reexamination of chest CT scan was performed on November 14, 2013 (Fig. 9.5).

Due to undefined lung lesion, specialist from the thoracic surgery department was consulted, and surgical removal of the right upper lung lobe was recommended. On November 20, 2013, surgical removal of the right upper lung lobe under a monitored thoracoscope was performed. The harvested lesion tissue was pathologically examined. And the pathological diagnosis was pulmonary aspergillosis (Fig. 9.6).

The pathological diagnosis was then defined as pulmonary aspergillosis.

After operation, itraconazole was administered at a dose of 0.2 g once a day for 3 months. The follow-ups in the following 3 months showed no hemoptysis. Reexamination by chest CT indicated postoperative changes of the right upper lung, and no abnormalities are detected at the other parts of the lungs.

The final diagnosis was aspergilloma at the right upper lung.

9.2.7 Discussion

Pulmonary aspergillosis is mainly caused by inhalation of aspergillus spores. Aspergillus is a conditional pathogenic fungus. Individuals with compromised immunity or using glucocorticoid or immunosuppressant are at high risk of infection. Especially when neutropenia occurs, its infection is the most likely. In this case, diagnostic imaging indicated formation of aspergilloma in cavity, which was then diagnosed as pulmonary aspergilloma.

In recent years, pulmonary aspergillosis with no host factors has been commonly reported [6, 7]. Aspergillus commonly colonized at the upper respiratory tract, and sputum culture positive cannot define it as the pathogen. Unless a large number of hyphae was found at the same time by microscopic examination, repeated cultures show the same strain or cultures of specimens from multiple body parts

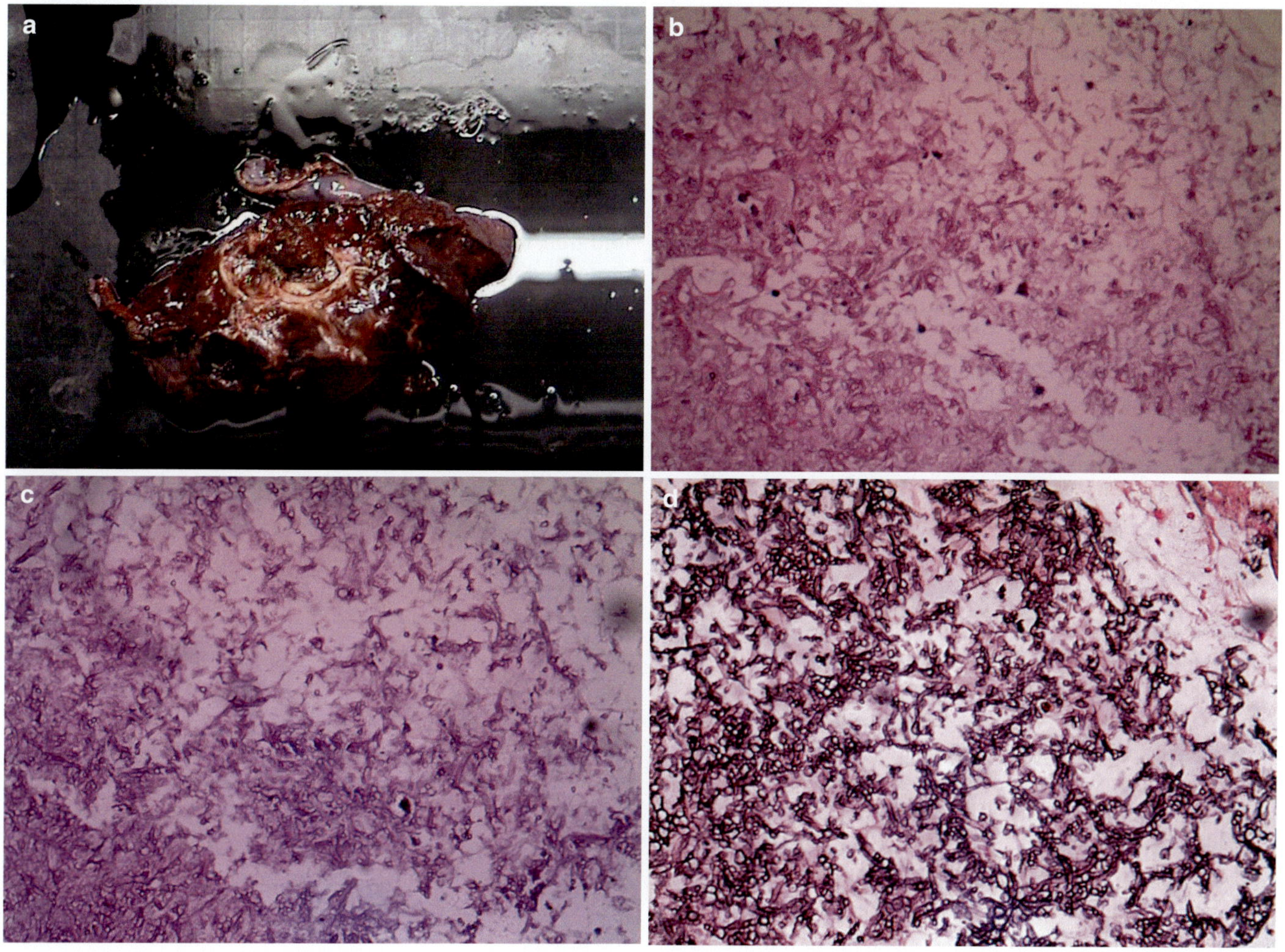

Fig. 9.6 (**a**–**d**) Pathology of pulmonary aspergillosis. (**a**) By naked eyes, a mass of lung tissue from the right upper lung in size of 11 cm × 8 cm × 3.5 cm was observed with a cavity of about 3.5 cm in diameter inside after incision near the incisal edge. The edge was surrounded by a cystic wall-like structure, with grayish red cotton wool-like substance. (**b**) By light microscopy, large quantities of hyphae and spores were observed. (**c**, **d**) By PAS staining and PASM staining, aspergillus was observed. And by immunohistochemistry, alveolar epithelial CK and TTF-1 positive, vimentin positive

show the same strain, it can be defined as the pathogen. Isolation of aspergillus from sterile specimens, such as blood, pleural effusion, or tissue for biopsy, is of clinical significance. However, contamination during operational procedures must be avoided. Therefore, specific radiological demonstrations are the basis for diagnosis, and histopathology is the basis for definitive diagnosis. In this case, radiological examinations indicated formation of aspergilloma in lung cavity, and microbiological test showed negative. The diagnosis was defined by postoperative pathology as pulmonary aspergillosis.

Aspergilloma commonly occurs secondary to pulmonary tuberculous cavity and bronchiectasis, which seldom invades the lung tissue. However, under certain condition, it may develop into invasive pulmonary aspergillosis. Hemoptysis is the most common symptom, and even life-threatening major hemoptysis may occur in some cases. In this case, the patient consulted the specialist in outpatient department of our hospital due to recurrent hemoptysis.

CT scan demonstrates typical aspergilloma as spherical content in lung cavity or cavitary lesion and crescent-shaped space between aspergilloma and the cavity. The crescent-shaped space is usually located at the upper or lateral part of the cavity. Aspergilloma is free in the cavity and can move along with body posture. Therefore, for clinically suspected cases of aspergilloma, supine and prone CT scan can be performed to compare the movement of aspergilloma. The shape of aspergilloma may be irregular with lobulation. But its edge and the inner wall of cavity are commonly smooth, which is caused by mechanical friction of movable aspergilloma with the inner wall of cavity. In this case, CT scan demonstrated irregular mass-like lesion of soft tissue intensity in a cavitary lesion and a crescent space between the two lesions. But supine and prone CT scans were not performed to compare the position of inner lesion. Spherical content in cavity and crescent-shaped space between the spherical content and the cavity are characteristic radiological demonstrations of aspergilloma. However, these demonstrations can also be found in other diseases, and differentiation is necessary. Spherical opacity in lung may also be demonstrated in the cases of tuberculoma, benign neoplasm, and pulmonary abscess, and differential diagnosis should be made based on other signs and clinical manifestations. The cases with crescent-shaped space should especially be differentiated from invasive pulmonary aspergillosis. The crescent sign in the cases of invasive pulmonary aspergillosis is a characteristic sign during the progression of cavity, which is formed by separation of infracted lung tissue from its surrounding normal lung tissue. It usually has irregular edge, commonly accompanied by infiltrative opacity around the cavity. However, aspergilloma is formed by parasite of aspergillus in cavity that is caused by other diseases, which is movable along with body posture. The inner wall of cavity is comparatively smooth due to mechanical friction of aspergilloma.

In 2008 guideline issued by Infectious Disease Society of America, no treatment or surgical operation is recommended for aspergilloma. In this case, the patient experienced recurrent hemoptysis, who was admitted to the hospital due to its onset again and aggravation. The possibility of its progression into life-threatening hemoptysis cannot be excluded. And the patient was comparatively young, with no chronic basic disease and good lung functions. Her conditions were well indicated to surgery, and surgical operation was then performed. Surgical removal is the only way to cure aspergilloma, which also provides chance for definitive diagnosis. Itraconazole was administered postoperatively to prevent relapse. Voriconazole is also a choice for postoperative medication for aspergilloma due to its favorable permeation into the cavity [8].

9.2.8 Comments

In this case, the patient was a young woman with chronic progression of the disease and hemoptysis as the initial symptom. CT scan demonstrated irregular mass-like lesion of soft tissue intensity in a cavity and crescent-shaped space between the mass-like lesion and the cavity. Radiologically, no definitive evidence was demonstrated to support tuberculosis, but typical crescent-shaped cavity opacity was demonstrated. But the case was misdiagnosed as pulmonary tuberculosis. Based on the *2015 Clinical Guideline for Diagnosis and Treatment of Chronic Pulmonary Aspergillosis*, this case should be categorized into singular aspergilloma. When early anti-tuberculosis therapy showed poor therapeutic responses, aspergillus infection should be considered. Anti-fungal therapy of itraconazole was administered in March 2013, but the patient showed a poor compliance. She discontinued the medication by herself 2 months later and received traditional Chinese medicine. Since then, her condition progressed with recurrence of hemoptysis. CT scan on November 4, 2013, demonstrated nodular opacity at the right upper lung lobe with surrounding halo sign and cystoid translucent area adjacent to the mediastinum. Based on these findings, aspergillus infection should be considered. CT scan on November 14, 2013, demonstrated typical crescent sign, which is consistent to the clinical progression of aspergillus infection.

Due to the symptom of hemoptysis, surgical removal of the lesion can be performed for treatment and postoperative pathology. Surgical removal is currently the main way for singular aspergilloma. For patients with serious hemoptysis, preoperative bronchial artery catheter embolism can save their life. However, embolization is rarely completely effective in controlling severe hemoptysis, so it can only be used as a early work before the final surgical treatment. When the lesion cannot be completely removed by surgery, anti-fungal therapy can be administered to prevent aspergillus empyema or to avoid relapse of the disease. The *2015 Clinical Guideline for Diagnosis and Treatment of Chronic Pulmonary Aspergillosis* issued by ESCMID/ERS indicates that close monitor is necessary after surgical removal of the lesion. Regular examinations for aspergillus antibody quantification, inflammatory markers, and lung radiology every 3 months should be performed to ensure no progression of the lesion.

9.3 Case 3: Recurrent Hemoptysisfor More Than 2 Years

Ruming Xie, Budong Chen, Pu-Xuan Lu, Jin Xu, Shi-Ping Wu, Hui Han, and Jiaxuan Zhou

9.3.1 Presenting Symptom

Recurrent hemoptysis for more than 2 years.

9.3.2 Brief Case History

A 51-year-old man was admitted to our hospital on November 28, 2014, due to presenting symptom of recurrent hemoptysis for more than 2 years. In February 2012, the patient experienced recurrent hemoptysis once or several times each week with no known causes. The blood he coughs up ranged from 10 to 200 ml. And he also experienced fatigue, breathlessness but no fever, chest pain, cough, expectoration, night sweat, and emaciation. He was then given anti-tuberculosis therapy of rifampin and ethambutol for about 1 year. Reexamination by chest X-ray demonstrated formation of cavity at the right upper lung. Hemoptysis occurred again on November 21, 2014. The volume was about 100 ml. Since the onset of symptom, he was in a good spiritual state, with good appetite and sleep. His body weight showed no obvious change, and bowel movements were normal.

He denied histories of diabetes and hypertension.

9.3.3 Physical Examination

The body temperature was 36.2 °C, pulse 84/min, respiration rate 20/min, and blood pressure 120/80 mmHg. He showed typical development, with average nourishment. And he was conscious and looked chronically ill. The patient showed an active position and compliance in physical examinations. The systemic superficial lymph nodes palpated no enlargement. The both lungs showed clear respiration sounds with no dry and moist rales. The heart was not enlarged, with a heart rate of 84/min that is regular. Auscultation showed no pathological murmur in valvular areas. The abdomen was soft with no palpable liver and spleen. Shifting dullness was negative and no percussion pain at the liver and kidney areas. Bowel sounds were normal.

9.3.4 Investigations

Routine blood test showed WBC 1.40 × 10^9/L, N 85.8%, L 5.0%, RBC 3.61 × 10^9/L, and PLT 295 × 10^9/L. CRP was detected 123.14 mg/L. Liver function test showed ALT 7.0 U/L and AST 20.0 U/L. The kidney function and blood electrolytes were normal.

9.3.5 Primary Diagnosis

Hemoptysis Unknown Origin: Right Upper Lung Cavity Tuberculosis.

9.3.6 Diagnosis and Treatment

After admission, the investigations and examinations were performed to find the reason of hemoptysis. Lung CT scan on December 2, 2014, demonstrated a thick-wall cavitary mass in the right upper lung lobe, with heterogeneous nodular lesion inside. The nodular lesion was demonstrated with surrounding air crescent sign, cotton wool-like opacity, and deranged cords opacity. The pleura that is adjacent to the lesion was demonstrated with thickening and adhesion (Fig. 9.7).

On December 3, 2014, his T-SPOT test of tuberculosis showed positive. On December 5, 2014, his fibrobronchoscopy demonstrated sharp tracheal protuberance, slight congestion of the bronchial mucosa at the right upper lung lobe, and unobstructed bronchial lumen with no neoplasm. After lavage and brushing biopsy, the smear was sent for pathology as well as bacterial and fungal culture. The endoscopic diagnosis was chronic bronchial inflammation of the right upper lung lobe (Fig. 9.8).

On December 9, 2014, bronchoalveolar lavage test showed no fungal growth. On the same day, bronchoscopic brushing biopsy and smear showed acid-fast staining negative. Due to recurrent hemoptysis of a large quantity of

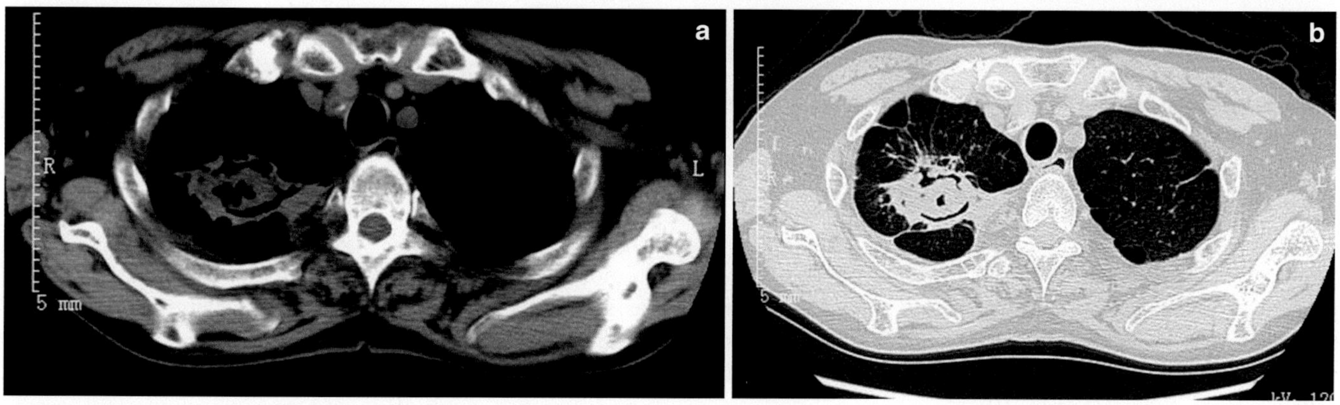

Fig. 9.7 (**a**, **b**) Lung CT scan. (**a**) A thick-wall cavity lesion at the apical segment of the right upper lung lobe by the soft tissue window. The cavity was demonstrated with a nodular lesion with heterogeneous intensity inside, which was surrounded by air crescent sign. The local pleural thickening was also demonstrated. (**b**) A thick-wall cavity lesion at the right upper lung lobe by the lung window. The cavity was demonstrated with a nodular lesion that had a high intensity, which was surrounded by air crescent sign. The inner edge of the lesion was demonstrated to be adhered with the pleura, and the adjacent lung parenchyma was demonstrated with deranged cords opacity. Both lungs were demonstrated with multiple air-containing spaces in different sizes with no wall and bubble opacity

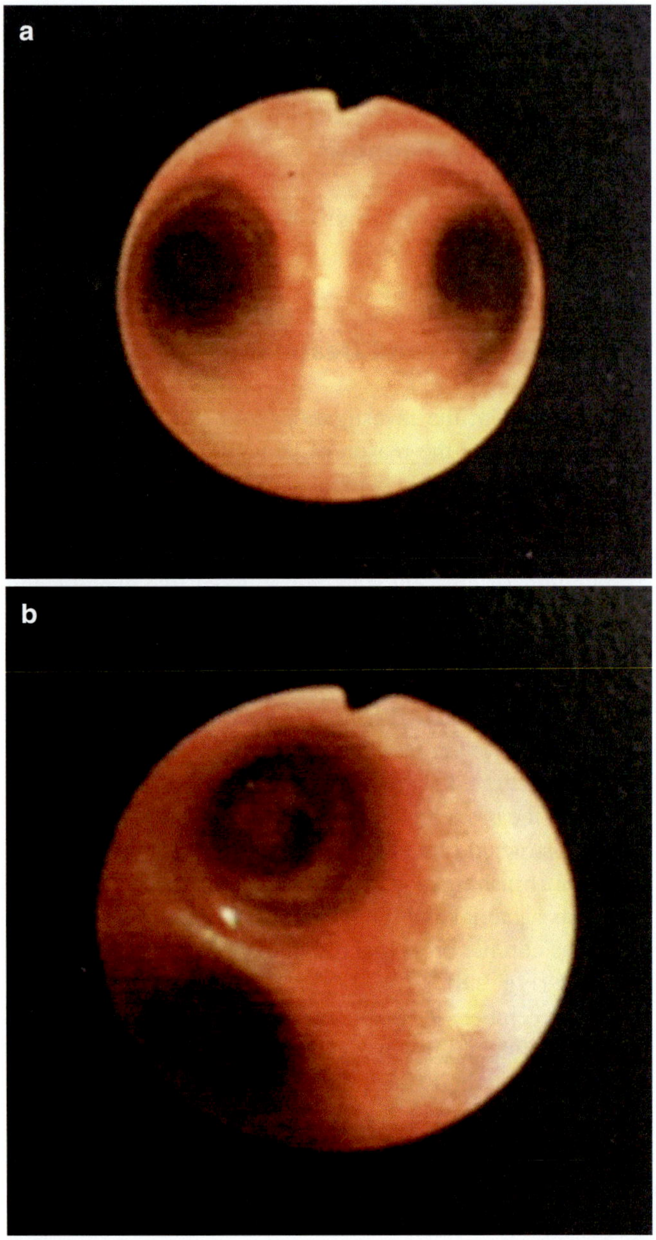

Fig. 9.8 (a, b) Findings by fibrobronchoscopy. (a) Smooth and sharp tracheal carina by bronchoscopy. (b) Slight congestion of the bronchial mucosa at the right upper lung lobe and unobstructed bronchial lumen with no neoplasm

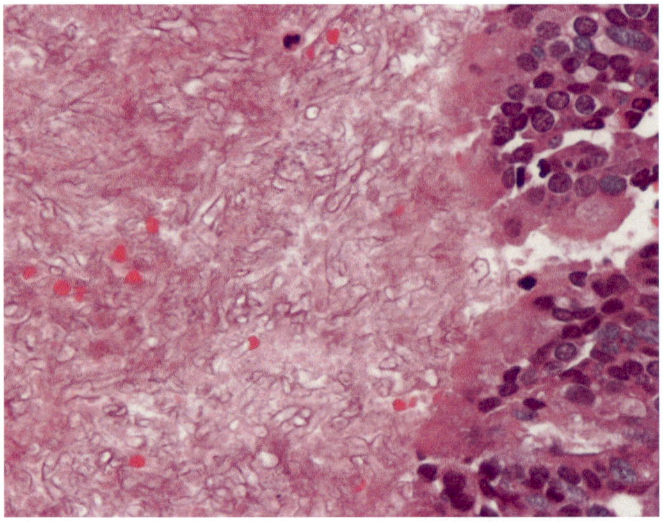

Fig. 9.9 Pathology of lung tissue. Dense distribution of aspergillus in the dilated bronchi and large thallus with acute angle branching and septum (H&E staining ×200)

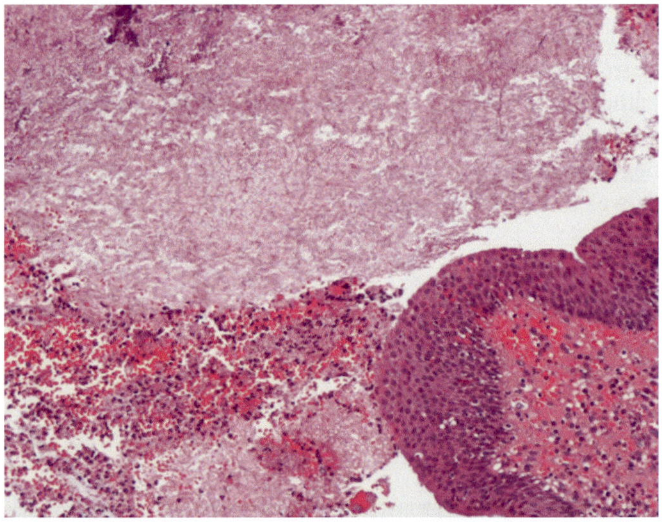

Fig. 9.10 Pathology of lung tissue. A large quantity of aspergillus in the dilated bronchi and chronic inflammation of bronchial mucosa with accompanying squamous metaplasia (H&E staining ×40)

blood, partial pneumonectomy of the right upper lung was performed under general anesthesia. The pathology of lung tissue showed bronchiectasis of the right upper lung lobe with accompanying aspergillus infection and purulent inflammation (Figs. 9.9 and 9.10).

9.3.7 Final Diagnosis

The final diagnosis was chronic cavitary pulmonary aspergillosis of the right upper lung.

9.3.8 Discussion

Pulmonary aspergillosis is commonly secondary to other basic diseases. In this case, pulmonary aspergillosis is related to the compromised immunity of the patient. Individuals of elderly and patients with hypoproteinemia, receiving long-term hormones, antibiotics, and immunosuppressant, are at high risk of pulmonary aspergillosis. Chotirmall et al. [9] believed that patients with compromised immunity are susceptible to pulmonary aspergillosis and neutropenia is positively related with the risk of pulmonary aspergillosis. Abnormal immunity is also related to pulmonary aspergillosis. Patients with allergic bronchopulmonary aspergillosis show increased level of serum aspergillus-specific IgE antibody, and the serum total IgE concentration usually exceeds 1000 ng/ml. Histopathology shows granuloma of eosinophile granulocytes and lymphocytes, which provide evidence for the role of abnormal immunity plays in the occurrence of pulmonary aspergillosis. Pulmonary aspergillosis commonly complicates COPD, bronchiectasis, pulmonary tuberculosis, and chronic pulmonary abscess cavity. The patients with these diseases show poor immunity and unsmooth bronchial drainage, which promote the growth of aspergillus in the cavity [10].

The radiological demonstrations of pulmonary aspergillosis are diversifying. These include nodule or mass in different sizes, exudative lesion of different sizes, formation of cavity with accompanying air crescent sign, and aspergilloma that complicates the basic disease, such as chronic pulmonary abscess, bronchiectasis, and bronchopulmonary cyst. Aspergilloma is the most common disease of chronic pulmonary aspergillosis. Dynamic chest X-ray demonstrates movable aspergilloma in pulmonary cavity. In this case, the final diagnosis was made by pathology as chronic cavitary pulmonary aspergillosis.

9.3.9 Comments

Pulmonary aspergillosis commonly occurs in patients with bronchopulmonary cyst, bronchiectasis, pulmonary abscess, and pulmonary tuberculosis. In this case, pulmonary aspergillosis occurred on the basis of bronchiectasis. The patient was a middle-aged man, with no other medical history. On admission, the peripheral white blood cell count was 1.40×10^9/L, which was obviously lower than normal level. The presence of granulocytopenia or deficient granulocytes deserved proving. As we know, granulocytic deficiency is the high-risk factor of aspergillus infection. It is to be regretted that relevant test data was absent. Obviously, the physician in charge failed to pay much attention on the granulocyte count.

The presenting symptom of pulmonary aspergillosis is commonly hemoptysis. In this case, the patient was admitted to the hospital due to recurrent hemoptysis for more than 2 years. According to literature report [11, 12], the incidence of hemoptysis in patient with aspergilloma ranges from 50% to 90%. The blood volume that is coughed up is also variable, from a small quantity to life-threatening large quantity. The cause of hemoptysis is also diverse, including mechanical friction of movable aspergilloma with blood vessels and imbalanced hemolyzation and anticoagulation induced by endotoxin of aspergillus.

Hemoptysis is the commonly encountered clinical acute symptom by physicians, especially physicians in respiratory department. Differential diagnosis should be made with caution. In this case, the patient had received anti-tuberculosis therapy for almost 1 year due to recurrent hemoptysis and lesion at the right upper lung. It was obviously a misdiagnosis that delayed appropriate treatment. The condition finally developed into pulmonary cavity. Clinicians should try to avoid such misdiagnosis.

In this case, the CT scan demonstrated thick-wall cavity at the apical segment of the right upper lung lobe, with a heterogeneous intensity nodule inside, which was surrounded by air crescent sign. In combination with his recurrent hemoptysis for more than 2 years and ineffective treatment by anti-tuberculosis therapy, pulmonary aspergillosis should be suspected. However, based only on radiological demonstrations, the basic disease underlying pulmonary aspergillosis cannot be defined. The basic diseases include chronic pulmonary abscess cavity, bronchiectasis, bronchopulmonary cyst, or tuberculosis. The differentiation should be based also on clinical manifestations. In this case, the diagnosis was finally defined by pathology, and the clinical typing was defined as chronic cavitary pulmonary aspergillosis.

9.4 Case 4: Intermittent Cough, Expectoration and Accompanying Hemoptysis for 1 Year

Guofang Deng, Peifen Chen, Pu-Xuan Lu, Shi-Ping Wu, Chen Qiu, and Guan-Xun Cheng

9.4.1 Presenting Symptoms

Intermittent cough, expectoration, and accompanying hemoptysis for 1 year.

9.4.2 Brief Case History

A 26-year-old young woman, a housewife, was admitted to our hospital on January 20, 2013, due to presenting symptoms of intermittent cough, expectoration, and accompanying hemoptysis for 1 year. Since January 2012, the patient had experienced cough, expectoration, sputum with a small quantity of blood but no fever, chest pain, breathlessness, night sweating, and emaciation. She then paid her clinic visit in a community health center and was diagnosed with acute bronchitis. Symptomatic therapy was administered (specifically not known), and no further treatment was given. In May 2012, she presented due to hemoptysis again of about 150 ml blood. After chest CT scan in a local hospital, the diagnosis was made as possible pulmonary tuberculosis and pulmonary aspergillus infection not excluded.

Since then, the patient had received anti-tuberculosis therapy with medications of isoniazid, rifampin, and ethambutol. During treatment, the patient showed intermittent cough, expectoration, and sputum with blood streak. On January 20, 2013, she presented again due to hemoptysis of about 20 ml blood with no known causes. The specialist in outpatient department admitted her due to the suspected diagnosis of pulmonary tuberculosis and hemoptysis. Since the initial onset of the disease, the patient had experienced an aversion to cold, fever, chest pain, and breathlessness. She had been in quite good spiritual state with quite good appetite and no obvious body weight loss.

The patient was always in good health. She denied histories of hepatitis and other infectious diseases. No history of surgical operation and trauma. No history of blood transfusion and drug allergy.

9.4.3 Physical Examination

Physical examination showed temperature of 36.3 °C, pulse rate of 94/min, respiration rate of 20/min, and blood pressure of 110/70 mmHg. She was in typical development and moderate nourishment. She was in voluntary posture and showed a good compliance to the physical examination. The superficial lymph nodes are not palpable, indicating no enlargement. The neck was soft, with the trachea at the midline. The thorax was symmetry, bilateral tactile tremor was symmetry too. Percussion showed clear sound at both lungs. Auscultation showed weak breathing sounds at the left upper lung and coarse breathing sounds at other parts of the lungs, with no dry and/or moist rales. The precordial region showed no eminence and the heartbeat at a rate of 94/min with a regular rhythm. Auscultation showed no murmur at the valvular areas. The abdomen was flat and soft, the liver and spleen can't be touched under the ribs. The movable dullness was negative and bowel sounds normal. The physiological reflexes were present, and pathological reflexes were not induced.

9.4.4 Auxiliary Investigations

9.4.4.1 Laboratory Tests

The routine blood test showed WBC 5.47 × 10^9/L, N 63.1%, L 27.9%, RBC 3.9 × 10^{12}/L, and PLT 182 × 10^9/L. The acid-fast staining of sputum showed negative. Sputum TB-DNA was negative. The common bacterial, fungal, and *Mycobacterium tuberculosis* cultures of sputum were all negative. G test showed negative. PPD showed 15 mm × 13 mm. The liver function, kidney function, electrolytes, ESR, CRP, and PCT were all normal. The blood CEA was negative, and biomarker of respiratory neoplasm was negative.

9.4.4.2 Radiology

Chest CT scan on May 31, 2012, demonstrated possible pulmonary tuberculosis, but pulmonary aspergillosis cannot be excluded (Fig. 9.11).

9.4.5 Initial Diagnosis

The initial diagnoses include secondary pulmonary tuberculosis that was treated with both upper lungs smear negative and suspected pulmonary tuberculoma at the left upper lung.

9.4.6 Diagnosis and Treatment

After admission, cefuroxime sodium was administered to fight against infection, hypophysin for hemostasis, and medications of isoniazid, rifampin, and ethambutol for tuberculosis. But the symptoms failed to be improved. Reexamination of chest CT scan indicated pulmonary tuberculosis and possible pulmonary aspergillus infection. The CT scan image is shown in Fig. 9.12.

To define the neoplasm in the lung, CT-guided lung puncture for biopsy was performed on January 28, 2013. The histopathological microscopy showed a small quantity of lung tissue, edema in alveolar cavity, infiltration of many lymphocytes and plasmocytes as well as less neutrophile granulocytes in alveolar cavity and lung septa, visible fungal mass that was positive by methenamine silver staining, no tuberculous nodule and caseous necrosis, and acid-fast staining negative (Fig. 9.13).

Due to the possibility of pulmonary aspergilloma and recurrent hemoptysis of the patient, surgical operation was considered to be indicated for the patient. Partial pneumonectomy of the left upper lung was then performed on February 18, 2013. Anti-fungal therapy by postoperative medication of voriconazole was given for 2 months. The condition was stabilized. The follow-ups showed no cough, expectoration, and hemoptysis.

9.4.7 Final Diagnosis

The final diagnosis was pulmonary aspergilloma and old pulmonary tuberculosis at the right upper lung.

9.4.8 Discussion

In recent years, along with the increasing incidence of pulmonary tuberculosis and the widespread use of immunosuppressants and hormones, the incidence of pulmonary aspergilloma has been increasing [13]. A review of literature

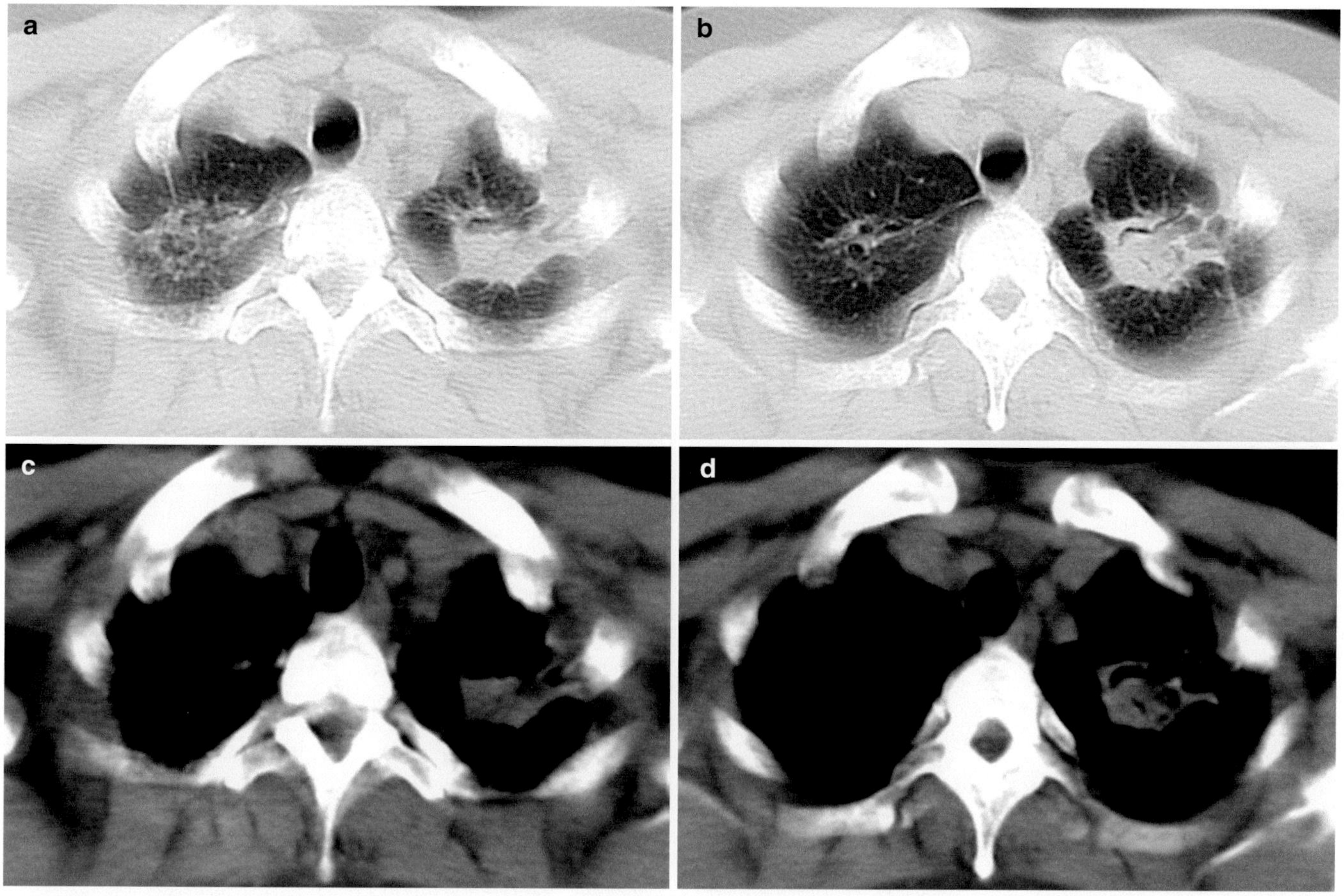

Fig. 9.11 (**a**–**d**) Chest CT scan. (**a**, **b**) In the lung window, a strip-like or nodular opacity at the posteroapical segment of the left upper lung lobe and small quantities of patches and cords like dense opacity at the apical area of the right lung. (**c**, **d**) In the mediastinum window, air-filled tube surrounding the edge of nodular opacity at the left upper lung, multiple spikes sign, peripheral air crescent sign, and marginal localized pleural adhesion

reports on tuberculosis complicated by chronic pulmonary aspergillosis by Denning et al. [14] has demonstrated that about 21–35% cases of pulmonary tuberculosis are complicated by pulmonary cavity, among which about 22% further develops into chronic pulmonary aspergillosis. Aspergilloma is a common type of chronic pulmonary aspergillosis, which can be categorized into parasitic/saprophytic type of aspergillosis. Therefore, tuberculosis complicated by pulmonary aspergilloma should be paid close attention by clinicians to avoid missed diagnosis and misdiagnosis. In this case, aspergillus infection occurred secondary to pulmonary tuberculosis. On her first admission, she was diagnosed with pulmonary tuberculosis and received routine anti-tuberculosis therapy for half a year, but the symptoms had not been improved, and the lesion at the right upper lung had showed no change. These indicated that the clinical symptoms were caused by pulmonary aspergilloma instead of pulmonary tuberculosis. The experience of such misdiagnosis should be analyzed and avoided.

The radiological demonstrations of pulmonary aspergillus infection resemble to those of pulmonary tuberculosis. Therefore, the diagnosis of pulmonary tuberculosis complicated by aspergillus infection presents challenges to the clinicians, which should be differentiated from pulmonary tuberculous cavity complicated by tuberculoma. Some specific radiological demonstrations are of great clinical significance. But the definitive diagnosis should be based on pathogenic examinations and pathology. In this case, the diagnosis was defined by lung puncture for biopsy after exclusion of tuberculoma of the left upper lung, which indicated that lung puncture for biopsy plays a critical role in the diagnosis. The therapeutic guideline for pulmonary tuberculosis complicated by pulmonary aspergilloma is still in disagreement. Surgical removal as a routine treatment for pulmonary aspergilloma remains controversial. No evidence so far has proved that anti-fungal medication is effective for aspergilloma. Generally speaking, for asymptomatic patients with aspergilloma, regular observation is necessary instead of treatment. Surgical removal should be considered only when the patient turns into symptomatic, which is usually hemoptysis, and most scholars believe that surgical removal is the optimal treatment for aspergilloma [15]. In this case,

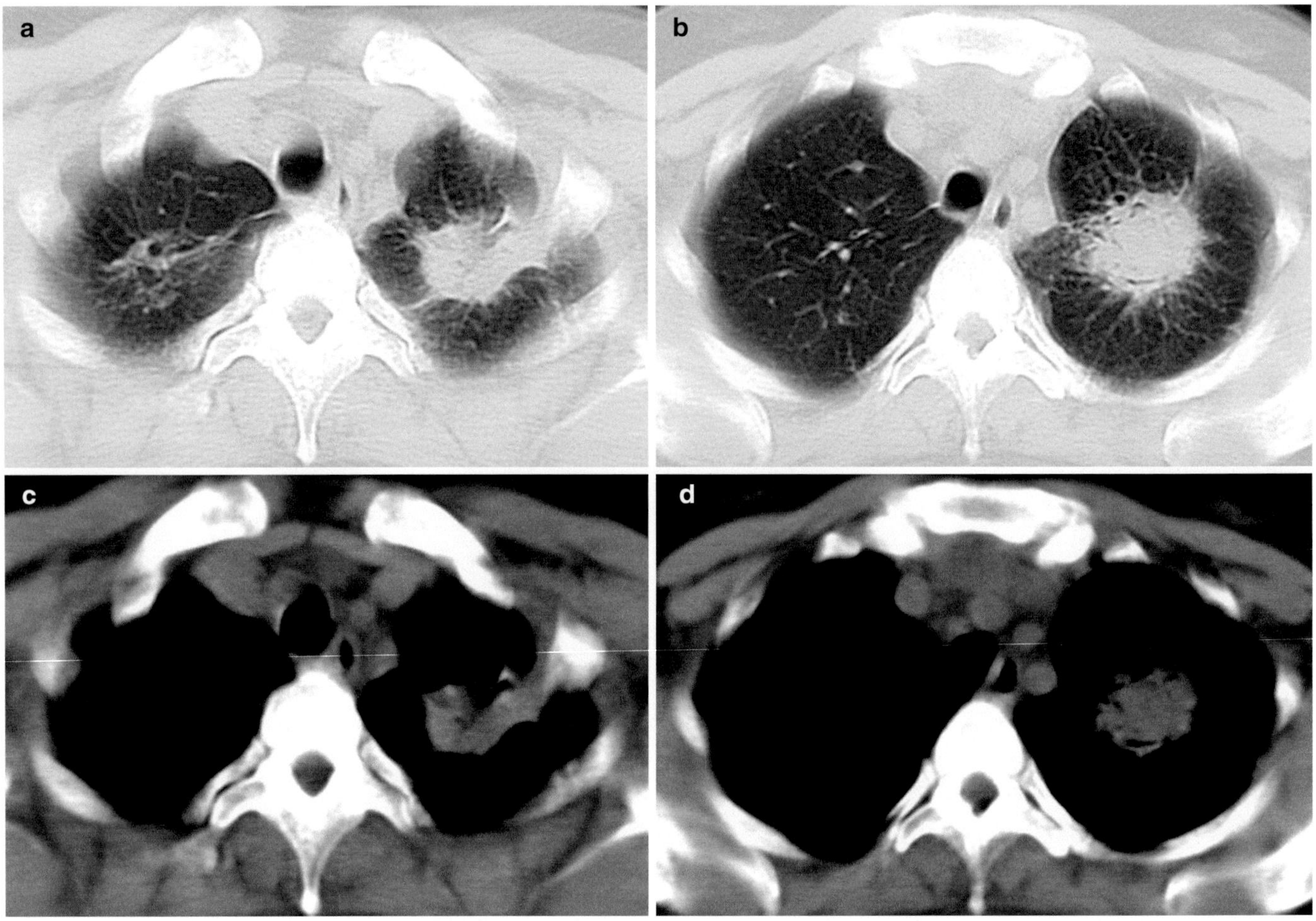

Fig. 9.12 (**a**–**d**) Chest CT scan. (**a**, **b**) In the lung window, a long strip-like or nodular lesion at the posteroapical segment of the left upper lung lobe, which extended from the lung apex to the left hilum, with the largest area of 28 mm × 26 mm. The right lung apical area was demonstrated with small quantities of patches and cords like dense opacity. (**c**, **d**) Air-filled tube surrounding the edge of nodular opacity at the left upper lung, multiple spikes sign, surrounding air crescent sign and accompanying localized pleural adhesion. Compared to the chest CT scan on May 31, 2012, the lesion showed no obvious change

the patient was cured by surgical removal. But anti-fungal medication is not indicated for postoperative patients [16]. In this case, voriconazole was administered for 2 months after the operation, and its clinical significance remains controversial. Actually, surgical operation for pulmonary tuberculosis complicated by pulmonary aspergilloma should be performed after considerate analysis of the tuberculosis lesion and the timing of surgery to outweigh its advantages. Only in such a way, the patient can be benefit from the surgical operation. In this case, the patient received the surgical operation in a stable condition, with a good timing of the surgery. From data of her follow-ups, the patient is optimally benefited, indicating a successful surgery. However, surgical operation is contraindicated for patients with poor cardiopulmonary functions and at a stage of active tuberculosis. In such cases, bronchial arterial embolization can be performed. Percutaneous injection of anti-fungal medication can also be considered, but with a low rate of successful treatment [17]. Clinical experience and data should be consistently summarized and analyzed to improve the therapeutic efficacy of the disease.

9.4.9 Comments

In this case, the outcome of the disease is favorable. We discussed and summarized the treatment for pulmonary tuberculosis complicated by aspergillus infection. The key points are the following for reference of the clinicians:

1. Pulmonary tuberculosis complicated by chronic pulmonary aspergillosis is not uncommon. According to literature report, about 22% of pulmonary tuberculous cavity is complicated by chronic pulmonary aspergillosis. Therefore, clinicians should pay close attention to pulmonary tuberculosis complicated by chronic pulmonary aspergillosis to avoid missed diagnosis and misdiagnosis.

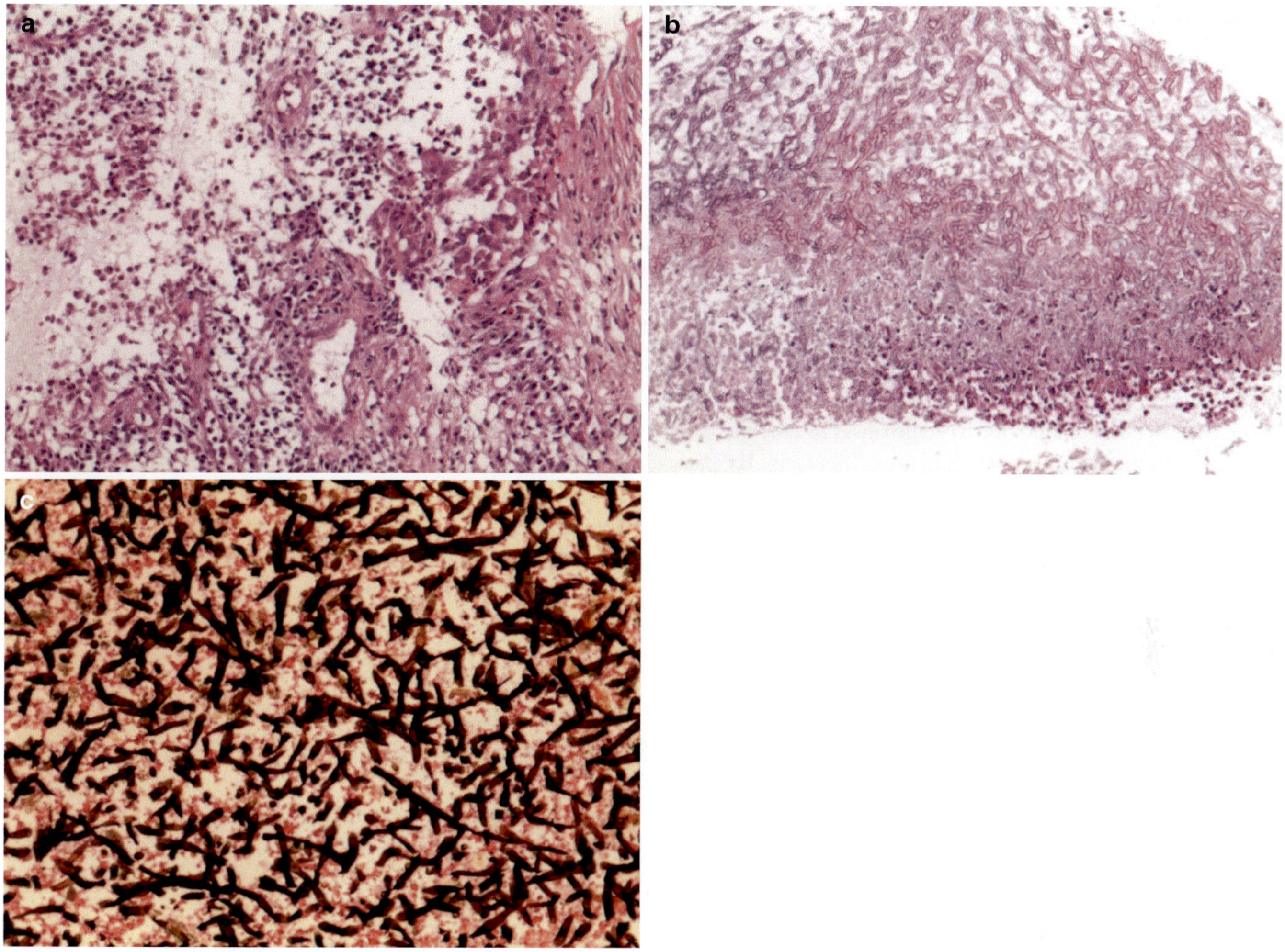

Fig. 9.13 (a–c) Pathology of lung tissue. (**a**) Edema fluid in the alveolar cavity, infiltration of many lymphocytes and plasmocytes, and less neutrophile granulocytes in the alveolar cavity and lung septa (H&E staining). (**b**) Aspergillus mass (H&E staining). (**c**) Branching of aspergillus hyphae (PASM staining)

2. The radiological demonstrations of pulmonary aspergillus infection resemble to those of pulmonary tuberculosis. The diagnosis itself is challenging. When pulmonary tuberculosis is complicated by aspergillus infection, the diagnosis is more difficult. Concerning the differentiation of pulmonary tuberculous cavity with accompanying aspergilloma from pulmonary tuberculous cavity complicated by aspergilloma needs more clinical experience.
3. The therapeutic planning for pulmonary aspergilloma is controversial. Generally, for asymptomatic patients with aspergilloma, clinical observation is necessary instead of treatment. Surgical removal is the optimal way for symptomatic patients with aspergilloma, commonly hemoptysis. No evidence so far has proved the therapeutic efficacy of anti-fungal medication. And the clinical significance of postoperative anti-fungal medication remains elusive.
4. The timing of surgery for symptomatic patients with pulmonary tuberculosis complicated by pulmonary aspergilloma should be chosen appropriately. It depends on the activeness of tuberculosis and the fatality of hemoptysis. We need more clinical experience on the diagnosis and treatment of the disease.

9.5 Case 5: Recurrent Breathlessness and Hemoptysis for More Than 6 Years

Zhijian Yu, Yanwei Chen, Qiwen Deng, Shi-Ping Wu, Hongtao Chen, and Ying-Yun Fu

9.5.1 Presenting Symptoms

Recurrent breathlessness and hemoptysis for more than 6 years.

9.5.2 Brief Case History

A 65-year-old man was admitted due to presenting symptoms of recurrent breathlessness and hemoptysis for more than 6 years. He had been admitted to hospitals for 17 times between the years of 2005 and 2011. In another hospital before his admission, he was diagnosed with secondary pulmonary tuberculosis complicated by hemoptysis in March 2004. By routine anti-tuberculosis therapy for 1 year, the symptom of hemoptysis was improved. Chest CT scan demonstrated absorption of the lesions. But he still experienced intermittent expectoration of a large quantity whitish foamy sputum and breathlessness after physical activities. In March 2005, he was hospitalized due to acute onset of chronic bronchitis, obstructive emphysema, and bronchiectasis. By physical examination, the patient was in good spiritual state and orthopneic position with breathlessness and slight cyanosis of lips. He had a barrel chest with weakened respiration movement of both lungs and weakened vocal fremitus. By percussion, hyperresonance was found. And by auscultation, the respiration sounds of both lungs were weakened with no dry and/or moist rales. After medications of antibiotics, aminophylline, and methylprednisolone, his condition was improved. Since then, he was hospitalized for four times till January 2007 due to similar presenting symptoms. During the remission period, the patient can manage his daily life by himself, with slight breathlessness after mild physical activities. In January 2007, chest CT scan during hospitalization indicated possible pulmonary aspergilloma. After 2-week medication of voriconazole, the patient discontinued it by himself. During January 2008 to September 2010, he was admitted to the hospital for several times due to hemoptysis. Reexaminations of chest CT scan demonstrated progressively enlarging pulmonary aspergilloma with gradual liquefaction. In September 2010, he was admitted again due to major hemoptysis, and the diagnosis was suspected to be pulmonary aspergilloma complicated by hemoptysis. Anti-infection therapy of voriconazole in combination with cefoperazone sodium, tazobactam, or imipenem was firstly administered for 1 month, followed by bronchoscopy due to unfavorable control of hemoptysis. The result showed endobronchial active bleeding at the posterior segment of the right upper lung lobe. Then bronchial arteriography and interventional embolization were performed, but with unfavorable therapeutic efficacy. In November 2010, right lobectomy and pleural adhesion lysis were performed, and postoperative pathology of lung tissue indicated a diagnosis of pulmonary aspergilloma and bronchiectasis. After the operation, hemoptysis was cured, and the patient was discharged. The following follow-ups till July 2011 showed that the patient was in a good health.

The patient was given intermittent oral medication of methylprednisolone, Celebrex, and *Tripterygium wilfordii* in the year 1995 due to a diagnosis of rheumatoid arthritis. In the year 2008, he was diagnosed with chronic kidney dysfunction (stage 2). He has a history of smoking for 20 years, smoking 2 packages per day.

9.5.3 Diagnosis and Treatment

9.5.3.1 Laboratory Test

Routine Blood Test and Biochemistry

The results of routine blood tests, C-reactive protein test, ESR, and serum albumin and kidney function test during 2008–2010 are shown in Table 9.1.

Sputum Smear and Bacterial Culture

Repeated multiple sputum smears and sputum cultures showed no growth of acid-fast bacteria. And repeated multiple sputum cultures showed growth of *Pseudomonas aeruginosa*.

Blood Bacterial Culture

Repeated multiple blood cultures showed no growth of pathogenic bacteria.

Blood Fungal (1,3)-β-D Glucan Test

Repeated multiple (1,3)-β-D Glugan tests showed negative.

9.5.3.2 Radiological Examinations

Chest X-Ray

Chest X-ray on May 16, 2008, demonstrated cavity-like lesion at the right upper lung (Fig. 9.14). Chest X-ray on April 14, 2010, demonstrated slightly enlarged lesion of aspergilloma at the right upper lung, with air crescent sign (Fig. 9.15).

Chest CT Scan

Chest CT scans since October 16, 2006, to June 23, 2011, are shown in Figs. 9.16, 9.17, 9.18, 9.19, and 9.20.

Based on the above findings, the diagnosis was made as possible aspergilloma at the right upper lung and chronic pulmonary emphysema complicated by bronchiectasis of the right upper lung.

9.5.3.3 Bronchoscopy

On October 26, 2010, bronchoscopy was performed, showing active bleeding at the posterior segment of the right upper lung lobe. The endoscopic diagnosis was endobronchial active bleeding at the right upper lung lobe.

On November 5, 2010, postoperative bronchoscopy indicated bronchial stump closure at the right upper lung lobe and clearly defined bronchial cartilage rings at the right

Table 9.1 Routine blood test and biochemistry during the hospitalizations

	Total WBC (10^9/L)	Percentage of neutrophiles (%)	Neutrophile count (10^9/L)	CRP (mg/L)	ESR (mm/h)	Albumin (g/L)	Creatinine (μmol/L)
January 10, 2008	8	78.4	6.3	88	140	24	185
May 1, 2008	6.4	73.9	4.71	52	105	26	193.5
July 23, 2008	5	65.9	3.31	71	108	24	145.9
January 24, 2009	12.4	87.6	10.88	83.5	93	25	144
February 2, 2009	8.6	73.1	6.25	22.6	90	25	117.7
June 7, 2009	6.5	76.5	4.3	53.9	95	25	125.3
December 24, 2009	6.8	78.5	5.3	79.2	90	27.4	118.1
January 5, 2010	4.5	65.2	2.97	54.1	65	29.1	113.5
March 20, 2010	4	63.2	2.53	58.4	140	29.1	121.4
April 13, 2010	7.5	77.4	5.77	45.2	110	30.6	89.8
June 4, 2010	6.2	74.8	4.61	26.3	55	33.5	79.6
August 23, 2010	7.8	80.4	6.25	60.8	60	33.9	259
September 7, 2010	4.4	55.1	2.42	17.6	35	31.8	103
October 26, 2010	4.8	51.8	2.46	54.8	70	30.9	95.1
November 23, 2010	4.4	54.2	2.37	51.2	67	32.1	93.1

Notes: The normal limits of total WBC count are (4–10) × 10^9/L. The normal limit of CRP is <5 mg/L. And the normal limit of ESR is <40 mm/h

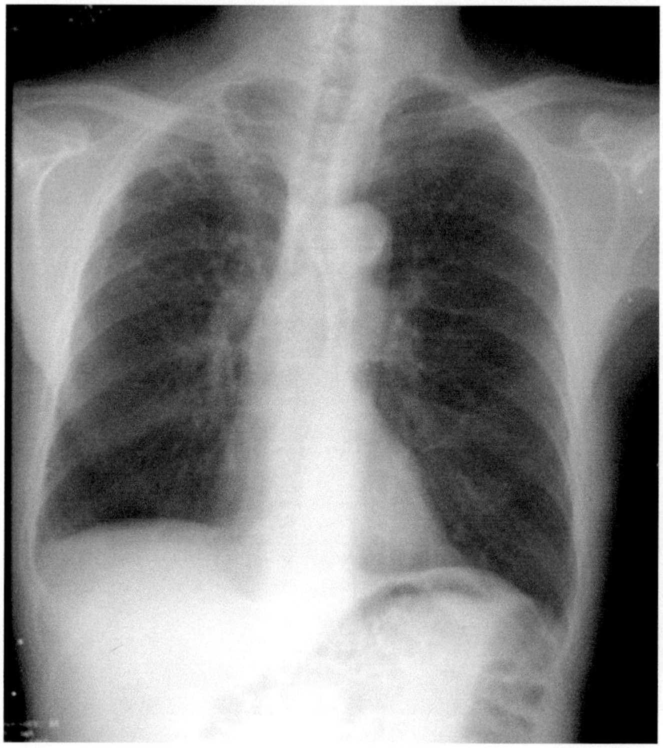

Fig. 9.14 Cavity-like lesion at the right upper lung with accompanying pleural thickening by anterior-posterior chest CT scan

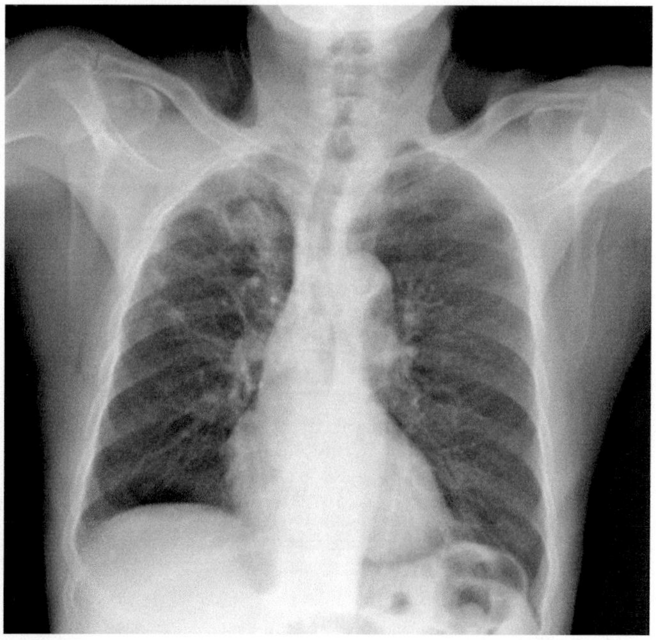

Fig. 9.15 Slightly enlarged lesion with increased air crescent sign at the right upper lung and more clearly defined boundary by anterior-posterior chest CT scan

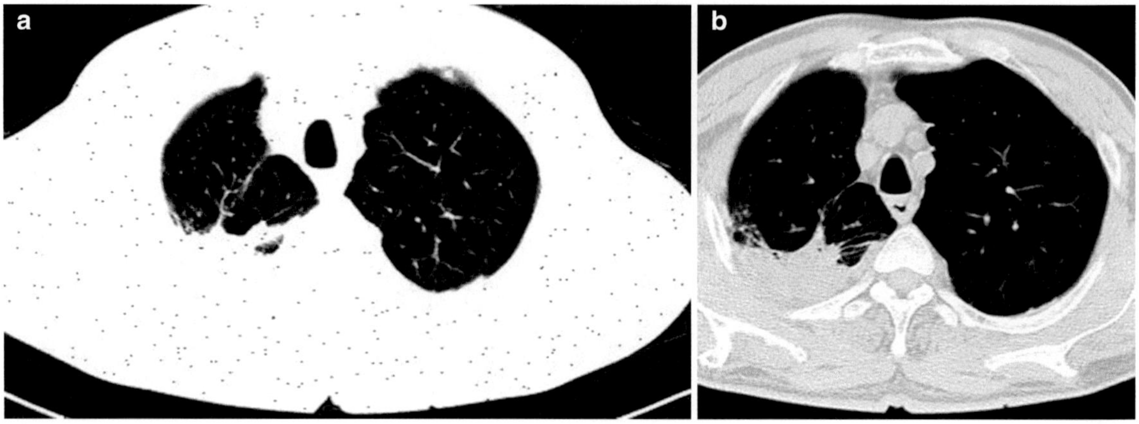

Fig. 9.16 (**a**, **b**) Large flakes of high-intensity opacity and surrounding cords like intensity opacity, irregular in shape by chest pain CT scan. The diagnosis is suspected to be old pulmonary tuberculosis of both lungs and slight bronchiectasis

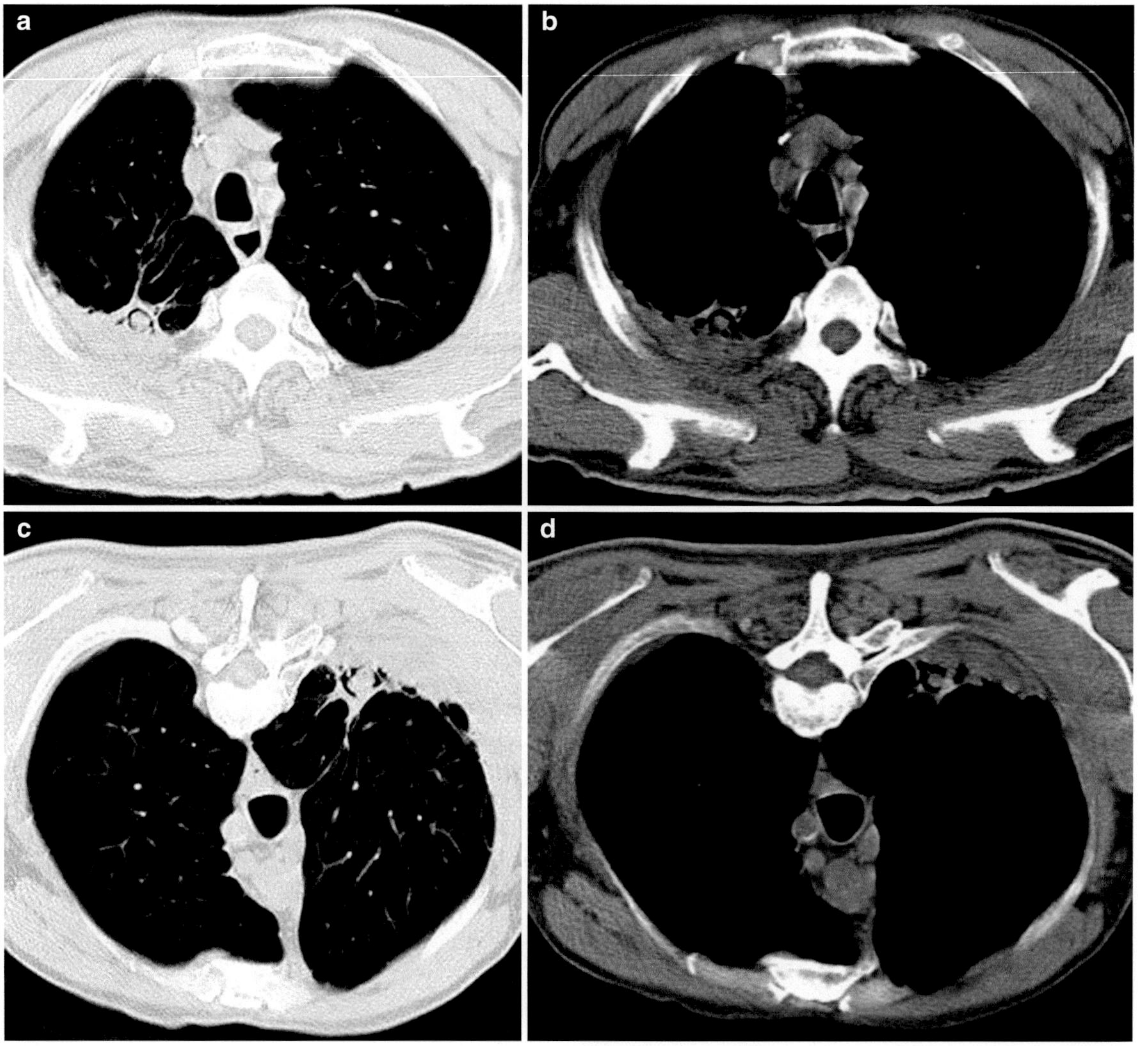

Fig. 9.17 (**a**–**d**) Chest CT scan. (**a**) The lung window of CT scan demonstrates cavity-like lesion at the posterior segment of the right upper lung, with central nodule that is surrounded by translucent ring. (**b**) The mediastinum window of CT scan demonstrates clearly defined nodule in the cavity at the right upper lung, with local pleural thickening. The posterior wall of the cavity is the thickened pleura. (**c**, **d**) The nodule shifts slightly forward at prone position

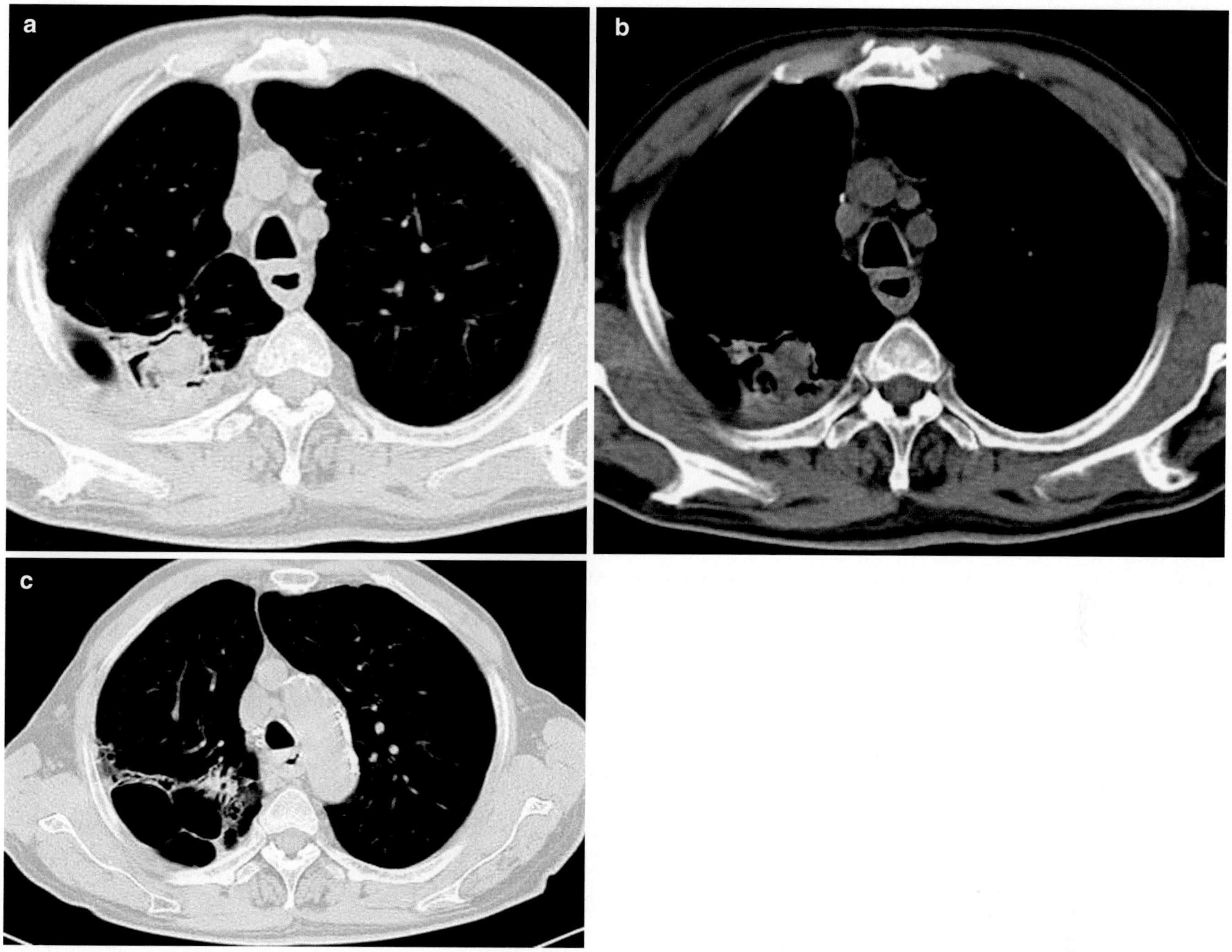

Fig. 9.18 (**a**–**c**) Chest CT scan. (**a**, **b**) Compared to CT scan on January 29, 2007, the nodule in cavity of the right upper lung lobe is demonstrated to be enlarged. (**c**) Multiple irregular translucent areas in the right upper lung lobe and the dorsal segment of the right lower lung lobe, lateral pleural thickening, and irregular patchy opacity in the lung near mediastinum

lower lung lobe with no neoplasm. The endoscopic diagnosis was postoperative change at the right upper lung lobe.

9.5.3.4 Bronchial Arteriography

On September 30, 2010, bronchography and embolization were performed (Fig. 9.21).

9.5.3.5 Pathology

On October 27, 2010, right upper lung lobectomy was performed under general anesthesia. Pathology demonstrated bronchiectasis of the right upper lung lobe, which was surrounded by infiltration of many chronic inflammatory cells and lymph follicle hyperplasia, cavity with aspergilloma at the right upper lung, and partial lung tissue necrosis with a large quantity of molds (Fig. 9.22).

9.5.3.6 Final Diagnosis

The final diagnosis was chronic cavitary pulmonary aspergillosis.

9.5.4 Discussion

Concerning the case history, the patient was at the following risks of aspergillus infection:

1. Infection of *Mycobacterium tuberculosis* induced destruction of the lung tissue. And bronchiectasis or occlusion induced unsmooth drainage of the secretions. These factors provided favorable circumstance for the colonization and growth of *Aspergillus*.

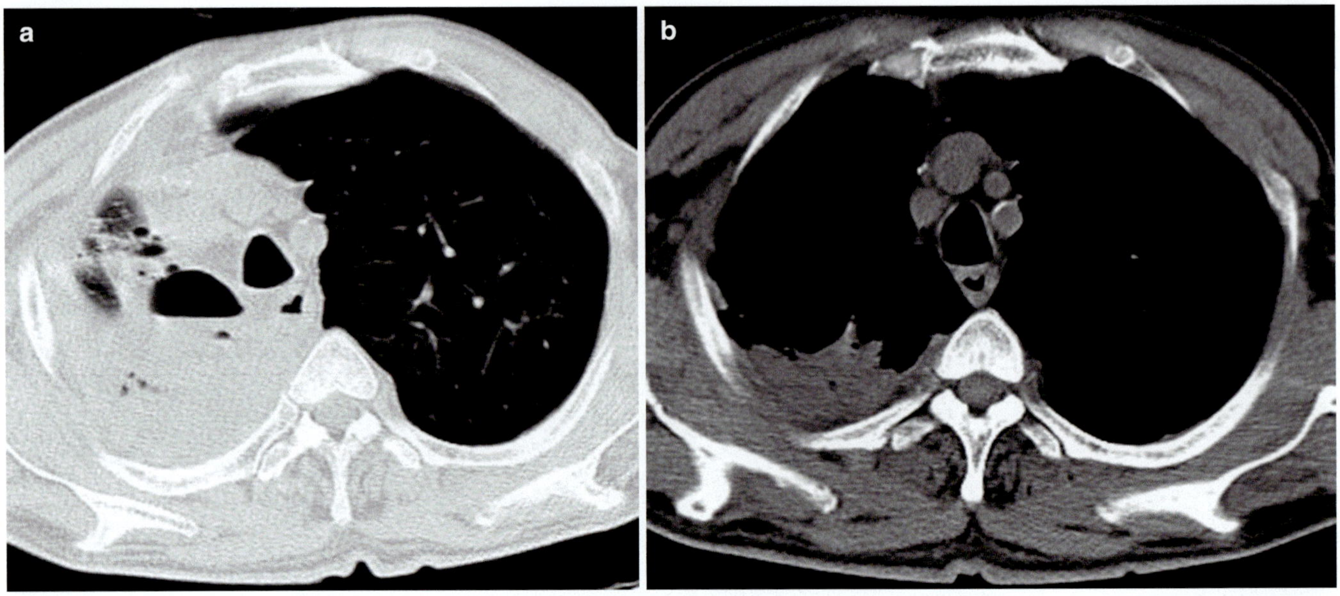

Fig. 9.19 (**a**, **b**) Chest CT scan. (**a**, **b**) Compared to CT scan on August 27, 2010, the lesion at the right upper lung lobe and the dorsal segment of the right lower lung lobe are enlarged, with liquid level in the cavity. The right pleural effusion and interlobular pleural effusion are demonstrated to be increased

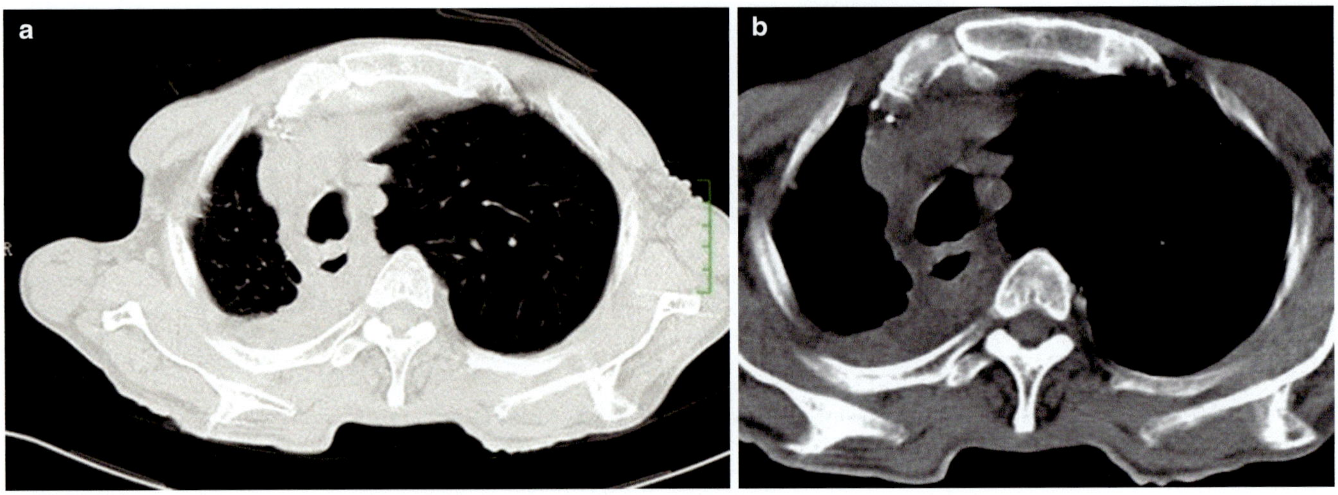

Fig. 9.20 (**a**, **b**) Plain chest CT scan. (**a**, **b**) After right lobectomy, the right thorax is narrowed, with shrinkage of the right lung. The right lung is demonstrated with scattering fibrous cords opacity

2. For acute onset of chronic obstructive lung disease and rheumatoid arthritis, intermittent anti-infection therapy and hormones were administered. This is also a risk factor inducing aspergillus infection. The occurrence of secondary pulmonary tuberculosis complicated by pulmonary aspergillosis exceeds 20% across the world, among which the cases of pulmonary cavitary tuberculosis complicated by chronic pulmonary aspergillosis account for up to 22% [14, 18]. In this case, during recurrent acute onset of chronic obstructive lung disease in 2006, multiple serological, imaging, and pathogenic investigations showed lung fungal infection negative. In January 2007, diagnostic imaging of the lungs demonstrated cavity-like lesion in the lung, which was suspected to be aspergilloma. Dynamic chest CT scan demonstrated large flakes of high-intensity opacity at the lung, followed by increased range of lesion as well as halo sign and air crescent sign. And the lesion finally developed into aspergilloma with liquefaction and necrosis. Therefore, dynamic monitoring of the lesion by radiology facilitates its early diagnosis [19, 20].

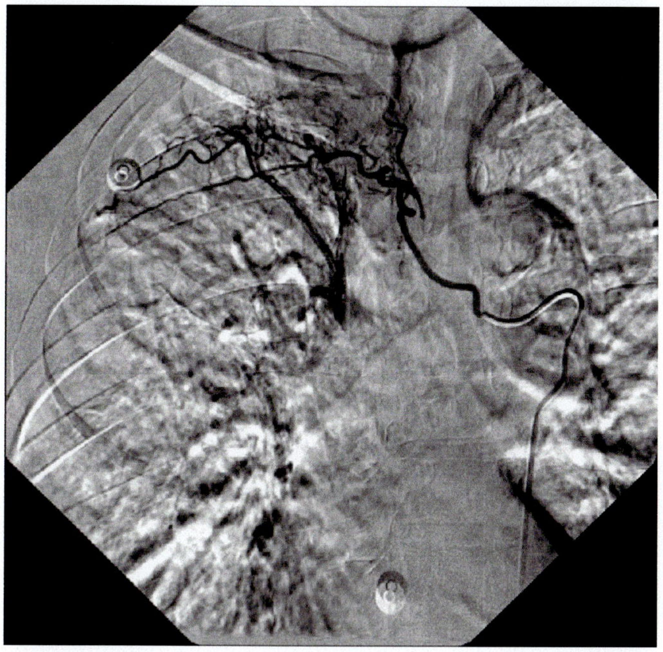

Fig. 9.21 Bronchial arteriography. Bronchial arteriography demonstrates well-defined right bronchial artery trunk and its branches as well as local thickening and twist of distal right bronchial artery with occlusion of the supplying area. The left bronchial artery trunk is well defined

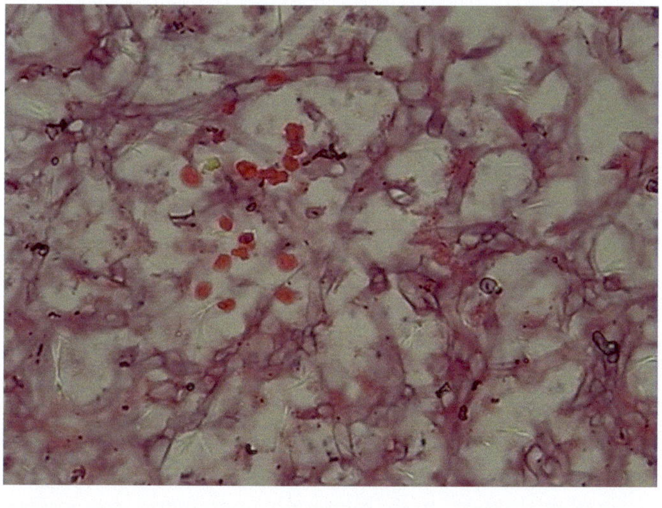

Fig. 9.22 Pathology of lung tissue. It is demonstrated with large quantities of aspergillus hyphae and spores (H&E staining)

Because anti-fungal medication can hardly permeate into the cavity and aspergilloma and aspergilloma can hardly be discharged via occluded or narrowed draining bronchus, simple administration of anti-fungal medication shows unfavorable therapeutic efficacy. In this case, interventional therapy was firstly chosen for the patient due to aspergilloma and hemoptysis. For some cases of aspergilloma, CT scan or MRI angiography can be applied. The demonstrations include abnormal increase of newly developed bronchial minor vessels into mass, dilation and twist of bronchial arteries, capillary stagnation, and local aneurysmal dilatation. For such patients, the effectiveness of embolization is uncertain due to complex lateral branches of bronchial artery. In this case, the symptom of hemoptysis failed to be relieved by interventional embolization, demonstrating its unfavorable therapeutic efficacy. At the early state of pulmonary aspergillosis, medications, such as voriconazole, can be administered. If the condition develops into pulmonary aspergilloma and no contraindication is shown, active surgical removal should be performed regardless of the severity of the symptoms [21, 22]. Surgical removal is mainly removal of affected lung lobe. Wedge-shaped removal or segmental removal can be performed for peripheral localized solitary lesion. The patient can be radically cured by early surgical removal of the lesion.

9.5.5 Comments

In this case, the patient suffered from basic diseases of chronic obstructive lung disease, bronchiectasis, and rheumatoid arthritis, with a long disease course. He was repeatedly hospitalized due to acute onset of chronic obstructive lung disease. And during his long disease course, new lesion emerged, and the patient experienced recurrent hemoptysis. Aspergilloma commonly occurs in the existing pulmonary cavity that may be induced by pulmonary tuberculosis, bronchiectasis, pulmonary cyst, and malignancies. Therefore, for patients with chronic obstructive lung disease and bronchiectasis and accompanying hemoptysis, close follow-ups should be performed. Dynamic monitoring of the lesion by radiology facilitates the early diagnosis of the secondary pulmonary aspergillus infection. In this case, the patient was intermittently administered methylprednisolone and other immunosuppressants for rheumatoid arthritis and acute onset of chronic bronchitis, which is also an important cause of pulmonary aspergillus infection.

The most common symptom of pulmonary aspergilloma is hemoptysis, with an incidence ranging from 50% to 90%. The volume of coughed blood may range from a small quantity to a large quantity that is fatal. The causes of hemoptysis include friction of aspergilloma to the vascular vessels when it moves along with respiration, hemolysis and anticoagulation induced by endotoxin of aspergillus, and local erosion of blood vessels at the cavity wall. Death occurs in about 5–10% of patients with aspergilloma due to major hemoptysis. In this case, the patient was repeatedly hospitalized during January 2008 to September 2010 due to recurrent hemoptysis.

In a small number of patients with pulmonary aspergilloma, the lesion can shrink or heal with no treatment. However, if immunosuppressant is applied, aspergilloma may develop into chronic necrotic (semi-invasive) pulmonary aspergilloma. In this case, multiple chest CT scans during January 2008 to September 2010 showed progressively enlarged pulmonary aspergilloma that was gradually liquefied, which is a typical course of lesion progression. Its relationship with long-term use of immunosuppressant needs further scholarly and clinical attention.

The management of aspergilloma remains controversial. Generally, patients with no or slight symptom should receive clinical observation. The symptomatic patients who are contraindicated to surgery or refuse surgery can try anti-fungal medication. However, no consistent evidence has been found to support the effectiveness of anti-fungal medication. Surgical removal is the only way for radical cure, which is indicated to patients with recurrent hemoptysis or fatal hemoptysis. Removal of aspergilloma under thoracoscopy is a new way for its treatment, with less complications and less hospitalization days. For patients with cardiopulmonary dysfunction that is contraindicated to surgery, bronchial artery embolization is a favorable way to control major hemoptysis. But due to abundant lateral branches of aspergilloma, hemoptysis may relapse after bronchial artery embolization. In this case, the patient received medication in the internal medicine department, followed by bronchial artery embolization but showing poor therapeutic efficacy. And the patient finally received surgical operation and following follow-ups. He has been, so far, in good health. The case demonstrates the advantages and disadvantages of the abovementioned therapies, which need further scholarly and clinical attention.

9.6 Case 6: Intermittent Cough, Expectoration and Sputum with Blood Streak for 9 Months

Jing Yuan, Xiaohe Li, Pu-Xuan Lu, Jin Xu,
Shi-Ping Wu, Qianqian Zhang, and Guan-Xun Cheng

9.6.1 Presenting Symptoms

Intermittent cough, expectoration, and sputum with blood streak for 9 months.

9.6.2 Brief Case History

A 67-year-old woman was admitted to our hospital on May 29, 2013, due to intermittent cough, expectoration, and sputum with blood streak for 9 months. She had experienced cough, expectoration, and sputum with blood streak 9 months before her admission. However, she had had no chest distress, breathlessness, chest pain, fever, flush, night sweat, dizziness, palpitation, abdominal pain, diarrhea, and melena. She had received anti-tuberculosis therapy (specific medication unknown) in a local hospital, and the symptoms had been relieved. But she had discontinued the medication by herself after 4 months. One month prior to her admission, she had experienced cough, expectoration of a large quantity, and sputum with blood streak. On May 6, 2013, chest CT scan in a district hospital of Shenzhen (Guangdong, China) demonstrated destructed left upper lung with cavity, aspergillus infection, and old pulmonary tuberculosis at the dorsal segments of the left and right lower lungs. On May 13, bronchoscopy in the Third People's Hospital of Shenzhen (Guangdong, China) demonstrated bronchial inflammatory change of the left upper lung lobe, but alveolar lavage smear demonstrated no sign of tuberculosis. Based on a diagnosis of aspergillus infection, she received oral medication of itraconazole but showed no obvious improvement. For further diagnosis and treatment, she was admitted to the surgery department of the hospital based on a diagnosis of pulmonary tuberculous cavity. Since the onset, she had been in good spiritual condition and had had average appetite and sleep.

She denied histories of diabetes, hypertension, and other diseases. And she denied any habitual smoking and drinking.

9.6.3 Physical Examination

By physical examination, she showed a temperature of 36.4 °C, pulse rate P 82/min, respiration rate 18/min, and blood pressure BP 130/65 mmHg. She was in a typical development with average nourishment. The patient was conscious with an appearance of chronic disease and active position. She showed favorable compliance during physical examination. The systemic skin showed no yellowish stain and no skin rash. Palpation for the systemic superficial lymph nodes showed no enlargement. No obvious positive sign at the eyes, ears, nose, and oral cavity. The thoracic cavity was bilaterally symmetric with no deformity. The respiration was in regular rhythm, with bilaterally symmetric respiration movement and vocal fremitus and no pleural rub. By percussion, the both lungs showed clear sounds, with clear respiration sounds and no obvious dry and/or moist rales. The both lungs showed voice conduction symmetry with no pleural rub. The precordial area showed no abnormal protrusion and pulse, and by percussion, the heart showed no enlargement. The heartbeat was 82/min, with regular rhythm, and the valvular areas showed no obvious pathological murmur. The abdomen was soft, with no tenderness and rebound. The liver and spleen were subcostally unpalpable. The hepatojugular reflux was negative, and the bowel sounds were 5/min. The both lower limbs showed no edema. And the nervous system showed no abnormalities.

9.6.4 Auxiliary Investigations

9.6.4.1 Laboratory Test

The alveolar lavage for bacterial culture on May 19, 2013, showed *Candida albicans* positive and filamentous fungi positive.

9.6.4.2 Radiology

Chest CT scan in a district hospital on May 5, 2013, demonstrated destructed left upper lung with cavity, aspergillus infection, and old tuberculosis lesion at the dorsal segments of the left lower and right lower lungs.

9.6.4.3 Bronchoscopy

Bronchoscopy on May 13, 2013, demonstrated bronchial inflammatory changes at the left upper lung lobe. The initial diagnosis was then made to be destruction of the left upper lung, with suspected pulmonary tuberculosis complicated by cavity and invasive pulmonary aspergillosis.

9.6.5 Diagnosis and Treatment

After admission, relevant examinations were performed. The routine peripheral blood test showed WBC 8.82×10^9/L, N 5.97×10^9/L, Hb 127 g/L, and PLT 218×10^9/L. The liver and kidney functions were normal. ESR was 26 mm/h and CRP 118 mg/L. The antibody of tuberculosis was weakly positive. And the sputum test showed TB-DNA lower than 5×10^2 copies/ml. The immunity to tuberculosis by Elispot showed negative. The sputum smear for *Mycobacterium tuberculosis* and culture showed negative. Chest X-ray demonstrated lesion at the left upper lung, which was considered to be tuberculosis complicated by cavity or bronchiectasis. Enhanced chest CT scan on May 30, 2013, demonstrated lesions at both lungs, which were considered to be secondary tuberculosis complicated by partial atelectasis or bronchiectasis at the left upper lung lobe (Fig. 9.23).

By group consultation with doctors from tuberculosis department and thoracic surgery department, it was believed that the patient may suffer from pulmonary tuberculosis and pulmonary aspergillus infection. In combination with the destruction of the left upper lung, levofloxacin, isoniazid, and rifapentine were recommended for tuberculosis and voriconazole for aspergillus infection. After her condition was stabilized, surgical removal of the destructed lung lobe should be performed. On June 6, 2013, thoracoscopy-assisted left lung lobectomy was smoothly performed. On July 6, 2013, the pus culture for *Mycobacterium tuberculosis* showed negative. Postoperative pathology indicated (Figs. 9.24, 9.25, and 9.26): The size of pulmonary resection specimens were 12.5 cm × 4 cm. Most of them are gray-brown and a few are gray. Section being grayish white or mousy; consolidation; and multiple soft cysts in diameters of 0.5–2.5 cm containing mousy substance. Microscopy demonstrated destruction of most lung tissue, partial bronchiectasis that contained fungal mass, interstitial congestion and bleeding of the bronchial wall and surrounding lung tissue, and accompanying infiltrations of lymphocytes and plasmocytes. Some alveolar cavities contained serous fluid, erythrocytes, and macrophages engulfing hemosiderin. No tuberculous nodules and caseous necrosis. The acid-fast staining was negative but methenamine silver staining positive. The pathological diagnosis was inflammatory lesion at the left upper lung, fungal infection which was considered to be pulmonary aspergillosis.

Reexamination of chest CT scan on June 11, 2013, demonstrated changes after left upper lung lobectomy, tuberculosis of the left lower lung complicated by left pleural effusion and pleural thickening. After the surgical operation, anti-tuberculosis medication and anti-fungal medication of voriconazole were continued. Reexamination of chest CT scan on July 11, 2013, demonstrated changes after left upper lung lobectomy, tuberculosis of the left lower lung complicated by left pleural effusion and pleural thickening. Compared to the CT scan on June 11, 2013, the exudative lesions at the left lung decreased and improved left pleural effusion. After treatment, the patient showed normal temperature, with no cough, expectoration, and hemoptysis. She was cured and discharged.

The diagnosis on discharge was chronic fibrotic pulmonary aspergillosis, destruction of the left upper lung, and tuberculosis of both lungs. The smear for tuberculosis was negative, and the anti-tuberculosis therapy was continued.

After discharge, the anti-fungal medication of voriconazole and anti-tuberculosis medication were continued. The condition was stabilized with no hemoptysis in follow-ups.

9.6.6 Discussion

Pulmonary aspergillus infection is commonly secondary to chronic lung disease, especially pulmonary tuberculosis. In China, the population with tuberculosis is large. According to a report in 2013 issued by Chinese Center for Tuberculosis Prevention and Control, the new cases of tuberculosis were 0.90–1 million each year in China. In recent years, the incidence of aspergillosis has been increasing. The incidence of systemic aspergillus infection proved by autopsy rose from 1.5% to 6% from 1978 to 1992 [23]. Therefore, patients with tuberculosis are at a high risk of pulmonary aspergillus infection.

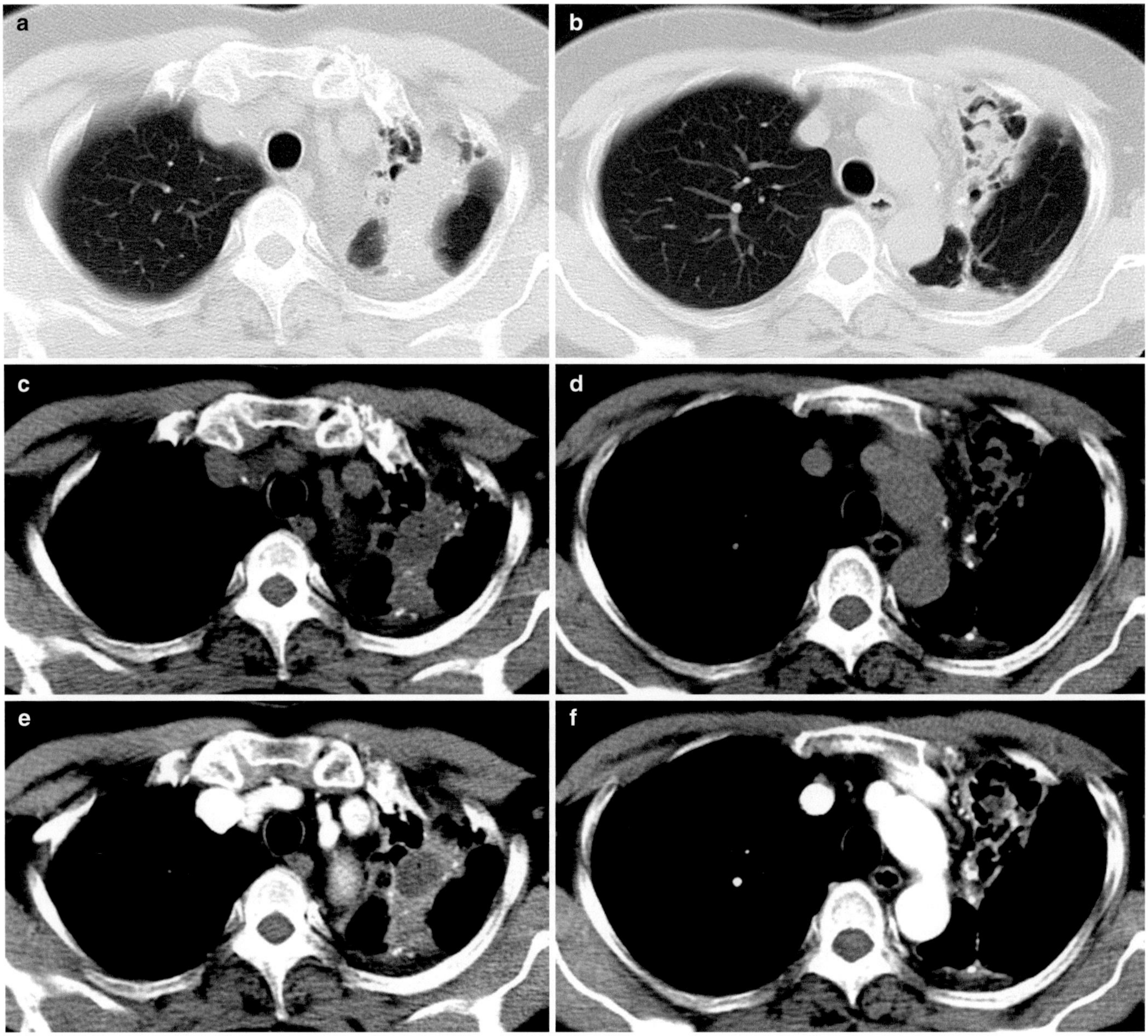

Fig. 9.23 (**a**–**f**) Enhanced chest CT scan. (**a**–**d**) The lung window of CT scan demonstrated slight collapse of the left thorax, shrinkage of the left upper lung lobe, and many irregular patches of opacity at the left upper lung lobe with heterogeneous high intensity. Some lesions were demonstrated with honeycomb-like change with many calcification lesions inside. And the left upper pleura was demonstrated to be thickened. (**e**, **f**) Enhanced scan demonstrated obvious irregular enhancement of the lesion at the left upper lung lobe, with a CT value of about 23 Hu

The pathogenesis of pulmonary tuberculosis with Aspergillus infection can be summarized as follows:

1. Pulmonary tuberculosis is a chronic lung disease, commonly with seriously destructed lung tissue. The pathological change impairs the cleanup effect of the airway, which renders the fungi at the oropharynx moving downward to invade the lung tissue [24]. In patients with pulmonary tuberculosis, formation of cavity and atelectasis due to bronchiectasis or bronchial occlusion are common, which further cause unsmooth drainage of secretions. All these changes construct a circumstance that is favorable for colonization and growth of aspergillus. A literature review by Denning et al. [25] estimated that the global incidence of chronic pulmonary aspergillosis following pulmonary tuberculosis is 21% (in the United States) to 35% (in Taiwan, China).
2. Pulmonary tuberculosis is a chronic consumptive disease. The patients show decreased T-cell count and/or dysfunc-

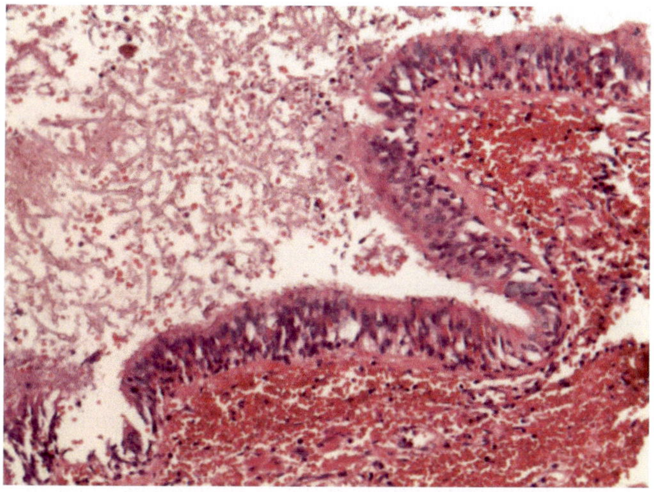

Fig. 9.24 Pathology of lung tissue. Partial lung tissue is destructed, with partial bronchiectasis which contains aspergillus mass (H&E staining)

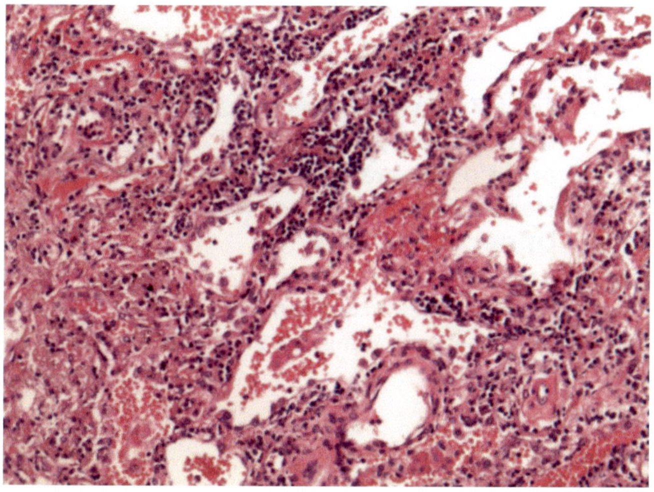

Fig. 9.25 Pathological microscopy of the lung tissue. Interstitial congestion and bleeding of lung tissue were demonstrated, with infiltrations of lymphocytes and plasmocytes. Some alveolar cavities contain exudative fluid, erythrocytes, and macrophages engulfing hemosiderin (H&E staining)

tional cellular immunity, which cause the increase of aspergillus infection rate [26].

3. The combination use of multiple anti-tuberculosis medications causes imbalanced microbial communities and the opportunistic pathogenic fungi thus invade [27].

The onset of pulmonary aspergillosis is insidious, with common symptoms of chronic cough, systemic upset, weight loss, and hemoptysis but non-specific. The condition therefore tends to be misdiagnosed as progression of tuberculosis, which presents challenges to the clinicians. The key points for the diagnosis of pulmonary aspergillosis are the following:

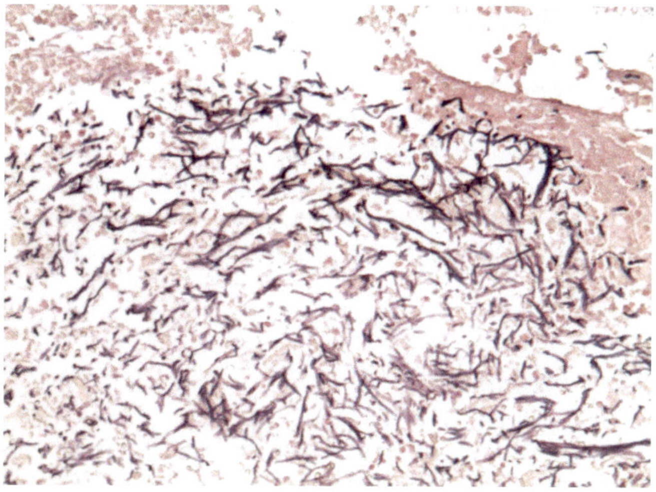

Fig. 9.26 PASM staining

1. For the cases with frequent hemoptysis or bloody sputum and uncontrollable condition by anti-tuberculosis therapy, pulmonary aspergillosis should be suspected.
2. Pulmonary aspergillosis is demonstrated with disappearance of most cavity lumen that is replaced by mass-like dense opacity.
3. By chest X-ray and CT scan, pulmonary aspergillosis is demonstrated with typical aspergilloma and air crescent sign [28].
4. Biopsy following fibrobronchoscopy demonstrates polyp-like or cauliflower-like proliferation of granulation tissue.
5. Sputum culture for molds shows a high positive rate, but sputum microscopy shows a low positive rate. Therefore, simple sputum microscopy is not sufficient for its diagnosis.
6. If necessary, bronchoalveolar lavage or biopsy should be performed for definitive diagnosis. In this case, the patient experienced the symptom of frequent hemoptysis. The condition was improved by anti-tuberculosis medication but failed to be controlled. The following bronchoalveolar lavage for culture and postoperative pathology finally defined the diagnosis.

Currently, most clinicians recommend surgery for major hemoptysis [29–31], serious hemoptysis, and moderate hemoptysis of pulmonary aspergillosis. The surgery radically eliminates the lesion and hemoptysis, which prolongs the survival period of the patients. It has been reported that patients with pulmonary aspergillosis can hardly benefit from anti-fungal therapy [32]. In addition, the anti-fungal medication is toxic, and few patients can tolerate their toxicity. Currently, most clinicians believed that asymptomatic patients should also receive active surgery when preoperative assessment shows tolerance to surgical operation because the benefits of surgery outweigh its risks. In this case, the patient suffered from pulmonary tuberculosis complicated by extensive aspergillosis that had destructed partial lung tissue with recurrent hemoptysis. For such patients, lung lobectomy is the most common way for treatment. Timely surgical removal of the lesion in combination with active anti-tuberculosis therapy and anti-fungal medication of voriconazole can achieve favorable therapeutic efficacy.

9.6.7 Comments

This is a case of pulmonary aspergillus infection based on pulmonary tuberculosis. The authors have made an intensive discussion on the incidence and pathomechanism of pulmonary tuberculosis complicated by pulmonary aspergillus infection. In addition, the authors have listed the key points on its diagnosis. Pulmonary tuberculosis complicated by pulmonary aspergillus infection is radiologically demonstrated as atypical, which presents challenges to the clinicians. In China, Qingfeng Li et al. summarized the radiological demonstrations of pulmonary tuberculosis complicated by fungal infection, which can be referred to as follows: (1) the lesion-affected area is enlarging; (2) the morphology of lesions is diverse with more poorly defined boundary, and the lesions commonly show multiple irregular patches of opacity, bronchial inflammatory change, and lobar infiltration; (3) bronchial dissemination of lesion is increasing; (4) there is increased incidence of pleural effusion with more volume of pleural effusion; (5) the cavity is enlarging and increasing in number, which is commonly multiple small cavities; and (6) specific signs of fungal infection are showing, such as fungal mass in cavity. These changes are non-specific radiological demonstrations of tuberculosis complicated by aspergillus infection. More clinical experience should be summarized.

Due to the challenges in the radiological differentiation, serological tests for aspergillus infection should be performed in the well-equipped hospitals, including serum precipitin antibody test and GM test. The *2015 Clinical Guideline for Diagnosis and Treatment of Chronic Pulmonary Aspergillosis* jointly issued by European Respiratory Society (ERS) and ECCMID indicated that above 90% patients with aspergillus infection show increased aspergillus antibody (precipitin). However, the test cannot be performed in most hospitals in China. GM test has great clinical value in the diagnosis of aspergillus infection. A meta-analysis published in an international journal has demonstrated that the sensitivity of GM test to aspergillus infection is up to 71% and the specificity up to 89%, and the GM test of bronchoalveolar lavage fluid (BALF) shows higher sensitivity. A meta-analysis showed that the sensitivity of GM test of BALF to invasive pulmonary aspergillosis is up to 90% and the specificity up to 94%. If no characteristic signs are radiologically demonstrated and no evidence from serum GM test, bronchoscopy for lung tissue biopsy and percutaneous puncture of lung tissue for microbiology and pathology should be performed to define the diagnosis as early as possible.

Along with increased knowledge about pulmonary aspergillosis, the spectrum of pulmonary aspergillosis is changing. Currently, pulmonary aspergillosis is commonly classified into invasive pulmonary aspergillosis, chronic necrotizing pulmonary aspergillosis, chronic pulmonary aspergillosis, allergic pulmonary aspergillosis, and overlapping syndrome. Chronic necrotizing pulmonary aspergillosis is also known as subacute invasive pulmonary aspergillosis or semi-invasive pulmonary aspergillosis. Chronic pulmonary aspergillosis is further classified into aspergillus nodule, singular aspergilloma, chronic cavitary pulmonary aspergillosis, and chronic fibrotic pulmonary aspergillosis. In this case, the patient experienced a long illness course. Based on the basic disease, radiology, and microscopy, the findings are consistent to chronic fibrotic pulmonary aspergillosis.

9.7 Case 7: Lesion Detected at the Right Upper Lung for 3 Years, and Postoperative Intermittent Hemoptysis for 1 Year After Right Upper Lobectomy

Dong-Na Su, Ling-Wei Wang, Hongtao Chen, Shi-Ping Wu, Guangsuo Wang, and Jian Zheng

9.7.1 Presenting Symptoms

Lesion detected at the right upper lung for 3 years and postoperative intermittent hemoptysis for 1 year after right upper lobectomy.

9.7.2 Brief Case History

A 22-year-old young man from Guilin (Guangxi, China) was admitted to our hospital on August 8, 2008, due to lesion detected at the right upper lung for 3 years and postoperative intermittent hemoptysis for 1 year after partial pneumonectomy of the right upper lung. In June 2005, the patient was detected with lesion at the right upper lung (specifically unknown) during his physical examination. He experienced no fever, cough, chest pain, chest distress, and other upsets. In a specialized hospital in chronic diseases, he was given anti-tuberculosis therapy (specifically unknown) for 1 year based on a diagnosis of tuberculosis. In June 2006, reexamination of chest CT scan demonstrated cavity at the right upper lung, which was considered to be aspergillus infection. In July 2007, he received partial pneumonectomy of the right upper lung in another hospital, and the postoperative pathology indicated benign lesion (specifically unknown). After the operation, he experienced intermittent cough, chest distress, and hemoptysis of a small quantity, which was commonly sputum with blood streak. He was then received several times reexaminations by chest CT scan, indicating cavity at the right upper lung. This time, he was admitted to our hospital due to cavity at the right upper lung to be detected. And he had experienced no fever, flush after noon, night sweat, and emaciation.

He was always in good health and denied histories of hepatitis and diabetes. His brother suffered from pulmonary tuberculosis.

9.7.3 Physical Examination

Physical examination showed a body temperature of 36.6 °C, pulse rate of 62/min, respiration rate of 20/min, and blood pressure of 118/85 mmHg. By palpation, his systemic superficial lymph nodes are not enlarged. The trachea was in the midline and the thorax bilaterally symmetric with no abnormality. An operation scar was at the anterolateral 7 cm to the fourth intercostal space. The respiration movement was bilaterally symmetric and vocal fremitus bilaterally symmetric. The pleural rubs were unpalpable. By percussion, the both lungs showed clear sounds with clear respiration sounds and no obvious dry and/or moist rales.

9.7.4 Auxiliary Investigations

Chest CT in June 2006 in another hospital demonstrated cavity at the right upper lung, which was suspected to be aspergilloma.

The initial diagnosis was cavity at the right upper lung to be detected. The diagnosis was suspected to be pulmonary aspergillosis or pulmonary tuberculosis.

9.7.5 Diagnosis and Treatment

After admission, the patient was further examined, with WBC 5.2 × 10^9/L, N 39.6%, L 48.3%, RBC 4.24 × 10^{12}/L, and PLT 121 × 10^9/L. His liver function was normal and ESR 8 mm/h. Chest CT scan on August 10, 2008, demonstrated thick-wall cavity at the posterior segment of the right upper lung lobe, which had smooth inner wall and inclusion in the cavity. Around the cavity, there were light flakes of ground-glass opacity and a small quantity of fibrous cords opacity. The right middle lung lobe and lingual segment of the left upper lung lobe were demonstrated with scattering patches of opacity. The radiological diagnosis was possible fungal infection at the right upper lung lobe and possible infection at the right middle lung lobe and the lingual segment of the left upper lung lobe (Fig. 9.27).

After admission, the tests and investigations were performed that showed no contraindications to surgical operation. To further define the diagnosis, the patient received right upper lobectomy on August 12, 2008, under general anesthesia. And the postoperative pathology demonstrated multiple fungal masses, with densely arranged hyphae and spores. The hyphae twined into mass and invaded surrounding lung tissue with poorly defined boundary. The surrounding tissues were demonstrated with infiltration of a large quantity of inflammatory cells. Microscopy after methenamine silver staining demonstrated brownish black hyphae, which are arranged into filiform or radial pattern with a diameter of about 7–10 μm. The hyphae were even in thickness with bilaterally parallel hypha walls and septa, which branched in 45° angle. The spores were scattering. By PASM staining, reddish purple hypha wall was demonstrated. The pathological diagnosis was mycosis at the right upper lung, and aspergillosis was highly possible (Figs. 9.28, 9.29, and 9.30).

After surgical operation, anti-fungal medications of fluconazole and voriconazole were firstly administered, together with pleural catheterization for persistent negative pressure drainage. The condition of the patient improved with favorable recovery. On September 2, 2008, reexamination of routine blood test showed WBC 5.7 × 10^9/L, N 49.2%, and L 31.1%, and chest X-ray demonstrated favorable lung recruitment. The patient was discharged on September 12, 2008.

The final diagnosis was chronic aspergillosis at the right upper lung.

After discharge, his condition was stable, with no hemoptysis in follow-ups.

9.7.6 Discussion

This case is characterized by a history of close contact to tuberculosis, anti-tuberculosis therapy for 1 year, cavity lesion at the lung after anti-tuberculosis therapy, and no tuberculosis toxic symptoms of afternoon low-grade fever, night sweat, and emaciation. Chest CT scan on June 2006 indicated possible aspergillus infection. In July 2007, right upper lung lobectomy was performed. And reexamination of chest CT scan 1 year after the surgical operation demonstrated cavity at the posterior segment of the right upper lung lobe, with inclusion inside. The diagnosis was then suspected to be fungal infection of the right upper lung lobe. Finally,

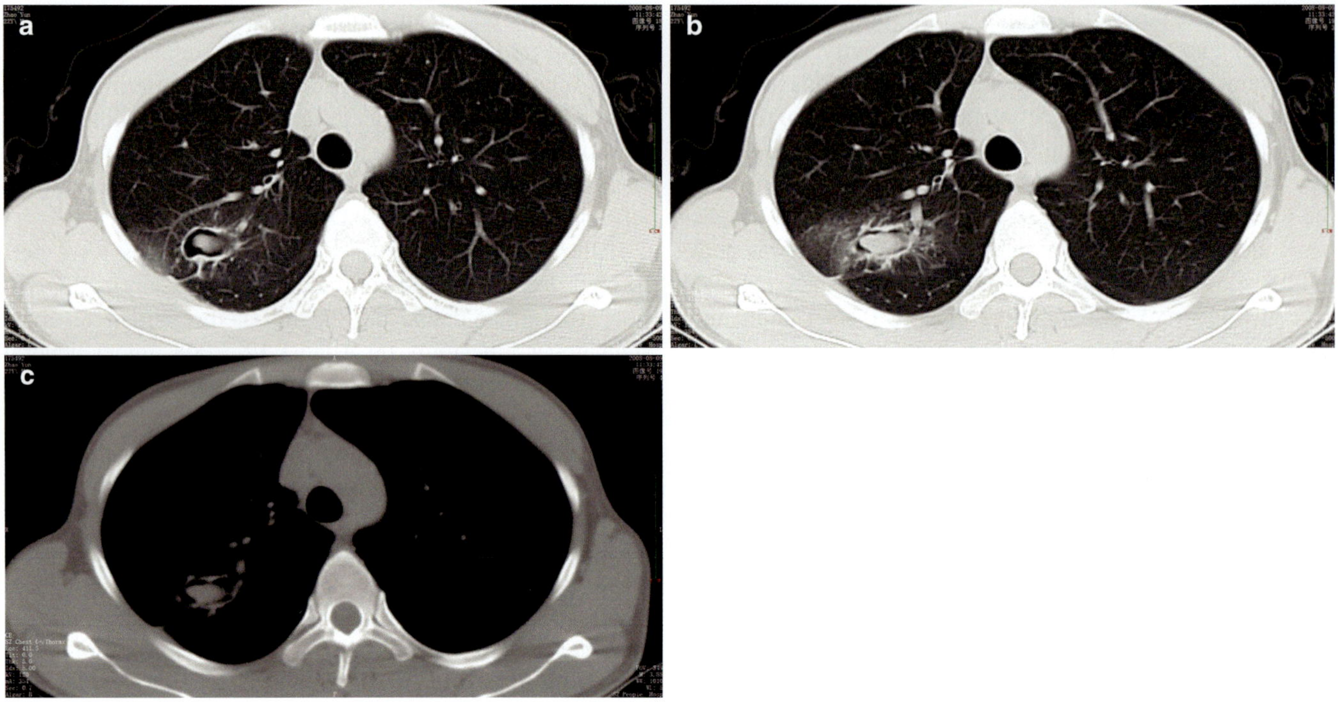

Fig. 9.27 Chest CT scan. (**a**) The lung window demonstrates a thick-wall cavity at the posterior segment of the right upper lung lobe, which has a smooth inner wall and inclusion in the cavity. The cavity is surrounded by light flakes of ground-glass opacity and a small quantity of fibrous cords opacity. (**b**) The lung window demonstrates a thick-wall cavity at the right upper lung lobe with inclusion inside. The cavity is surrounded by light flakes of ground-glass opacity. The fibrous cords opacity connects posterolaterally with the pleura. (**c**) The mediastinum window of CT scan demonstrates a thick-wall cavity at the posterior segment of the right upper lung lobe, which has smooth inner wall and inclusion inside

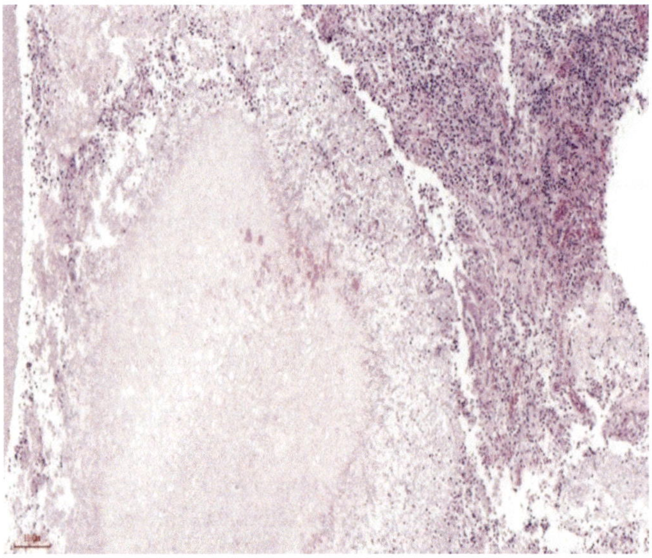

Fig. 9.28 Pathology of the lung tissue. Large quantities of hyphae and spores are demonstrated. The hyphae twine into mass, which is surrounded by infiltration of many inflammatory cells (H&E staining)

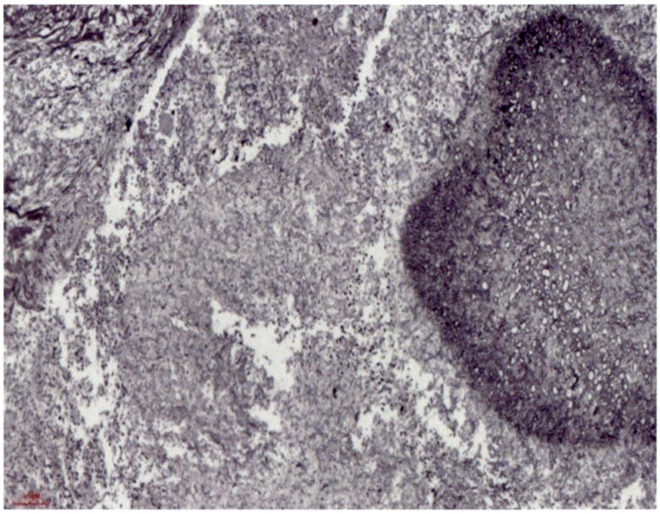

Fig. 9.29 Pathology of the lung tissue. The hyphae are brownish black in color and arranged in filiform or radial pattern. The hypha is even in thickness with septa, which branches into 45° angle. The spores are scattering (PASM staining)

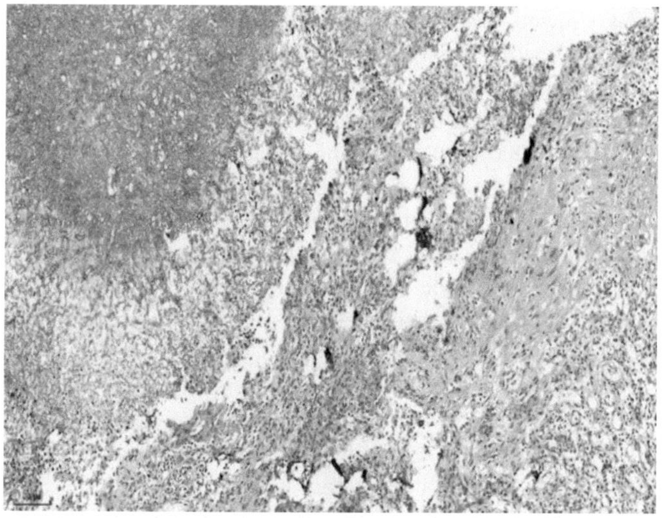

Fig. 9.30 Visible reddish purple hypha wall (PAS staining)

pathology confirmed the diagnosis of aspergilloma of the right upper lung. It is most likely to be postoperative relapse of aspergillosis of the right upper lung.

In this case, the patient was a young man, with an illness course of 3 years. His presenting symptoms include lesion at the right upper lung and hemoptysis. Anti-tuberculosis should poor therapeutic efficacy. Therefore, this case was chronic aspergillosis that was misdiagnosed as pulmonary tuberculosis. Clinically, the initial diagnosis was pulmonary tuberculosis. For the cases of pulmonary tuberculosis but with poor therapeutic efficacy, if the following conditions exist, aspergillosis should be suspected: (1) long-term recurrent hemoptysis, especially if coffee-colored particles were coughed up, and (2) chest X-ray demonstrating typical air crescent sign.

The pathological evidence by fibrobronchoscopic biopsy or percutaneous aspiration for biopsy is the golden standard for diagnosis. GM test has diagnostic value with specificity and sensitivity of up to above 80%. Especially, GM test of the alveolar lavage fluid can further increase the diagnostic positive rate. Serum precipitation test and aspergillus antigen intradermal test can provide reference for the diagnosis.

Cavity of pulmonary aspergillosis by radiology should be differentiated from the following diseases:

1. Tuberculosis. Liquefaction of tuberculoma is radiologically demonstrated as cavity with air crescent sign. It should be differentiated from cavity of pulmonary aspergillosis. Generally, the cavity after liquefaction of tuberculoma has comparatively thick wall, with satellite lesions.
2. Cancerous cavity. The cavity of lung carcinoma is commonly eccentric, irregular, and thick walled. During the follow-ups, the lesion shows rapid enlargement. Enhanced scan demonstrates obvious enhancement of the lesion.

The onset of chronic aspergillosis is insidious, and the clinical manifestations are non-specific, which present challenge to its diagnosis, with high rate of missed diagnosis and misdiagnosis. Radiology plays important role in its diagnosis. In this case, the radiological demonstrations resembled to those of simplex aspergilloma [33]. The sphere formed by aspergillus commonly parasitizes in the cavity induced by pulmonary tuberculosis, bronchial cyst, lung carcinoma, and sarcoidosis [8]. Chest X-ray, especially chest CT scan, can demonstrate characteristic signs that have diagnostic value.

1. When the spherical lesion is comparatively large, the cavity is only a narrow translucent area, namely, crescent sign. Spherical lesion with solitary crescent-shaped translucent area in the lung is the typical sign [34].
2. When the spherical lesion is at the center of the cavity, ring-shaped translucent area is demonstrated.
3. When the spherical lesion is small that adhere to the cavity wall, signet ring sign is demonstrated.
4. When the spherical lesion is connected with the cavity wall by pedicle and the spherical lesion is movable along with body postures, it is demonstrated as clock pendulum sign.
5. When the spherical lesion is free in the cavity and is movable along with body postures, it is demonstrated as ball rolling sign.

Singular aspergilloma is stable in nature, commonly with no progression in 3-month follow-ups. But in this case, it is postoperative relapse instead of simplex aspergilloma because the aspergillus invaded the lung tissue outside of the cavity. It should be clinically categorized into chronic necrotizing aspergillosis.

The differences of chronic necrotizing aspergillosis from simplex aspergilloma are the following:

1. The lesion of chronic necrotizing aspergillosis progresses rapidly, with an illness course of 1–3 months. However, the lesion of simplex aspergilloma progresses slowly, with an illness of more than 3 months.
2. In the cases of chronic necrotizing aspergillosis, the aspergillus invades the lung tissues outside of the cavity. But in the cases of simplex aspergilloma, the aspergillus mass is stable in nature with lesion within the cavity. It seldom invades the lung tissues outside of the cavity and shows no progression within 3-month follow-ups.
3. For simplex aspergilloma, treatment is mainly surgical removal, and postoperative relapse is rare, and anti-fungal

medication is unnecessary. But for the cases of chronic necrotizing aspergillosis, the aspergillus can invade the lung tissues outside of the cavity. Therefore, surgical operation cannot completely eliminate the lesion, and relapse commonly occurs.

In this case, the patient received surgical operation in October 2007. However, the administration of anti-fungal medication is unknown. Currently, no evidence has been found supporting surgical removal of singular aspergilloma followed by anti-fungal medication. For the cases receiving surgical removal of singular aspergilloma and no leakage of fungal substances, anti-fungal medication is unnecessary. But considering postoperative relapse, antibiotics that the patient is sensitive to should be administered, such as voriconazole and Itraconazole. For this case, the diagnosis was chronic necrotizing aspergillosis, and it is recommended that the treatment course should last for about 1–3 months. Aspergillus is not sensitive to fluconazole, and it should not be administered for aspergillus infection. In the clinical guideline, voriconazole is recommended as the medication of choice.

Hemoptysis is believed to be the most common symptom of aspergillus infection, with an incidence rate of 50–90%, and is the main cause of death [15]. The mechanism of hemoptysis is as follows: (1) friction of movable aspergilloma with abundant vascular network causes vascular rupture and bleeding; (2) endotoxin of aspergillus and protease cause necrosis and lysis of the tissue and the vascular vessels in the tissue are eroded; and (3) aneurysm occurs in the cavity wall during formation of the cavity, which ruptures to cause major hemoptysis when the lesion erodes the aneurysm or vascular pressure increases during severe coughs.

For the cases of serious hemoptysis, surgical operation should be considered. For the cases of major hemoptysis, acute bronchial arterial embolization can be performed in the early stage as emergency lifesaving measure. For the patients with accompanying multiple diseases or serious dysfunction of lungs, the surgical operation is contraindicated. Percutaneous injection of anti-fungal medication can be administered as an alternative, but with low success rate.

9.7.7 Comments

The authors well summarized the case in terms of the diagnosis, treatment, and clinical characteristics. In June 2005, the patient was detected with lesion at the right upper lung during his physical examination. In another hospital, the diagnosis was pulmonary tuberculosis, and anti-tuberculosis therapy was given. However, reexamination by chest CT scan showed unfavorable therapeutic efficacy. Instead of cure, the lesion progressed into cavity at the right upper lung. The initial diagnosis of pulmonary tuberculosis is obviously a misdiagnosis that delayed appropriate treatment.

In June 2006, chest CT scan indicated possible aspergillus infection, and in July 2007, the patient received right upper lung lobectomy. In August 2008, chest CT scan demonstrated again thick-wall cavity at the posterior segment of the right upper lung lobe with inclusion inside. Therefore, the diagnosis of postoperative relapse of aspergillus infection is reasonable.

The patient was a young man, with no chronic consumptive disease and other basic diseases. He received two operations for pulmonary aspergillus infection, which is rare. For the diagnosis, immunodeficiency and occupational diseases should be noted because some cases of pulmonary aspergillosis are associated with environmental exposure. If the first operation fails to completely eliminate the lesion and no anti-fungal medication is given after the operation, relapse may occur in some patients. The *2015 Clinical Guideline for the Diagnosis and Treatment of Chronic Pulmonary Aspergillosis* by ESCMID/ERS indicated that incomplete surgical removal of the lesion should be closely monitored. Regular aspergillus antibody quantification, inflammatory markers investigation, and chest radiology should be performed every 3 months to ensure no progression of the lesion.

According to the 2015 Clinical Guideline of Diagnosis and Treatment of Chronic Pulmonary Aspergillosis by ESCMID/ERS, chronic pulmonary aspergillosis can be classified into the following types: (1) chronic cavitary pulmonary aspergillosis (CCPA), (2) chronic fibrotic pulmonary aspergillosis (CFPA), (3) aspergillus nodule, (4) single/simple pulmonary aspergilloma, and (5) subacute invasive aspergillosis (SAIA). SAIA was formerly known as chronic necrotizing pulmonary aspergillosis (CNPA) or semi-invasive pulmonary aspergillosis. The radiological and pathological findings of this case are consistent to chronic necrotizing pulmonary aspergillosis.

The appropriateness of fluconazole in this case needs further discussion. Currently, the commonly applied anti-fungal medications for aspergillosis include polyene such as amphotericin; triazoles such as voriconazole, itraconazole, and posaconazole; and echinocandins such as caspofungin and micafungin. Amphotericin B and voriconazole are the medications of choice for invasive aspergillosis, and between the two medications, voriconazole is more convenient and safer. The remedial medications include AmBisome, posaconazole, itraconazole, caspofungin, or micafungin. In both foreign and domestic clinical guidelines, fluconazole is not recommended to treat aspergillus infection. The clinicians should have knowledge about these medications when choosing anti-fungal medications.

9.8 Case 8: Cough and Expectoration for 2 Years, Which Aggravated with Hemoptysis for 1 Month

Li Tu, Wei-Dong Song, Hui Yin, Ying-Yun Fu, Guan-Xun Cheng, and Jian Zheng

9.8.1 Presenting Symptoms

Cough and expectoration for 2 years, which aggravated with hemoptysis for 1 month.

9.8.2 Brief Case History

The patient was a 29-year-old young man from Guangxi, China. He was a staff member in a business company. The patient was admitted to our hospital on March 25, 2015, due to cough and expectoration for 2 years, which aggravated with accompanying hemoptysis for 1 month. Two years ago, the patient experienced cough, expectoration of no obvious inducement. The sputum was slightly yellow sticky, accompanied by breathlessness, and chest distress. The breathlessness and chest distress were obvious after physical activities, which were relieved by rest. He presented in a local hospital with a diagnosis of pulmonary tuberculosis. He then received anti-tuberculosis therapy (specifically unknown) in a specialized hospital of chronic diseases for more than 1 year. And the symptoms were obviously relieved. He discontinued the medications by himself. Since then, he experienced recurrent coughs and expectoration when weather changed. One month ago, he began to experience hemoptysis of a small quantity and took hemostatic medications, with poor therapeutic efficacy. For further diagnosis and treatment, he was hospitalized into our hospital. Since onset, his spiritual state, sleep, and appetite were quite good, with normal bowel movements and urinations but a weight loss of 5 kg.

He denied histories of hypertension, coronary heart disease, and diabetes. And he denied histories of trauma and operation.

9.8.3 Physical Examination

The physical examination showed a body temperature of 37.0 °C, pulse rate of 76/min, respiration rate of 19/min, and blood pressure of 130/74 mmHg. He was conscious. The left thorax slightly collapsed. Auscultation showed slightly weakened respiration sounds and a small quantity of moist rales at the left lung. The heart was not enlarged, with a heartbeat rate of 76/min and regular rhythm but no pathological murmurs. The abdomen was soft, with no palpable mass. The liver and spleen were subcostally unpalpable. The bowel sounds were normal. Clubbing fingers were not detected. And the neurological system showed no abnormalities.

9.8.4 Auxiliary Investigations

9.8.4.1 Routine Blood Test and Biochemistry

The routine blood test, liver and kidney function test, and electrolytes showed no abnormalities.

9.8.4.2 Sputum Test

Sputum smear showed acid-fast bacteria negative. And the sputum smear for fungi showed negative.

The initial diagnosis was hemoptysis possibly due to tuberculosis, bronchiectasis, and lung infection.

9.8.5 Diagnosis and Treatment

After admission, the examinations and tests were ordered. The routine blood test, routine urine test, blood gas analysis, coagulation function test, liver and kidney function test, two-item immune function test, and BNP showed no abnormalities. The sputum smear for fungi and the sputum smear for *Mycobacterium tuberculosis* showed negative. Chest CT scan on March 26, 2015, demonstrated a large cystic cavity at the apex of the left upper lung, with a range of about 5.5 cm × 5.3 cm and a round-like opacity of soft tissue intensity inside, which was movable along with body postures (Fig. 9.31).

After admission, chest CT scan indicated a large cystic cavity at the apex of the left lung with a mass inside that was movable along with body postures. The diagnosis was considered to be fungal infection. Voriconazole was then given for fungal infection, and cefoperazone and sulbactam were given for bacterial infection. The medications failed to relieve the symptom of hemoptysis. By consultation, all the specialists agreed that there were no contraindications to surgery. Then the patient was transferred to the thoracic surgery department. On April 2, 2015, left upper lung lobectomy, wedge removal of the left lower lung, and lung adhesion lysis were performed under general anesthesia. Postoperatively, anti-infection and hemostatic therapies were reinforced.

By postoperative pathology, the left upper lung lobe, neoplasm, and the left lower lung tissue were demonstrated with fungal mass, which was consistent to fungal infection. Based on the morphology of the hyphae, the fungus was considered to aspergillus. The left upper lung lobe and the neoplasm were demonstrated with a local pink stained necrosis and

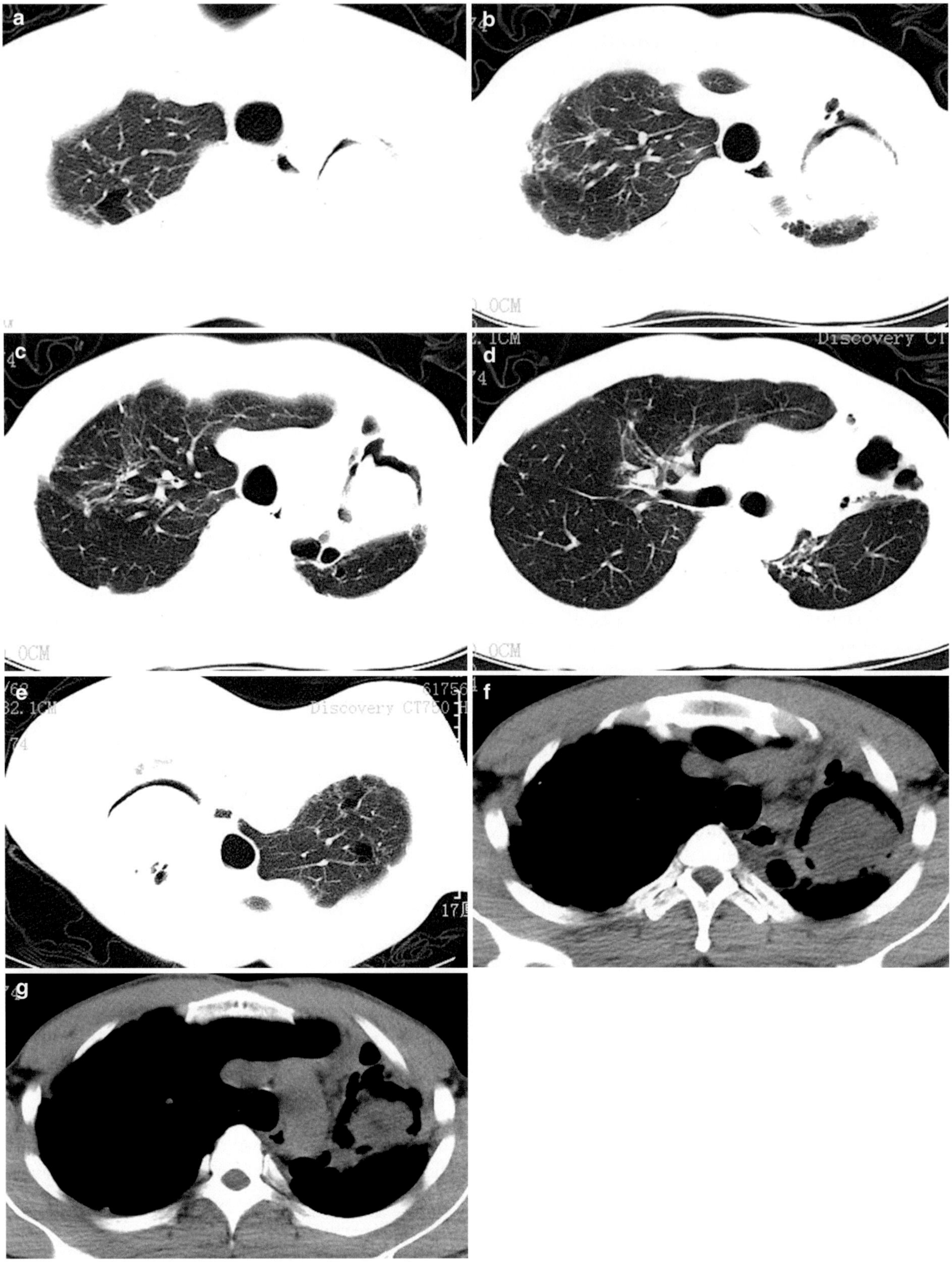

Fig. 9.31 (**a–g**) Chest CT scan. (**a–d**) The lung window demonstrates shrinkage of the left thorax, disappearance of the morphology of the left upper lung. The bronchi of the left upper lung lobe are demonstrated with irregular dilation, and some are demonstrated with column- or cyst-like change. The apex of the left lung is demonstrated with a large cystic cavity with a range of about 5.5 cm × 5.3 cm, and a round-like well-defined opacity of soft tissue intensity inside is demonstrated with a range of about 4.7 cm × 4.6 cm. (**e**) Prone CT scan demonstrates movable round-like mass opacity in the left upper lung. (**f, g**) The mediastinum window demonstrates cavity opacity in the left upper lung, with air crescent sign. The intensity of the round-like mass is homogeneous, with no calcification opacity

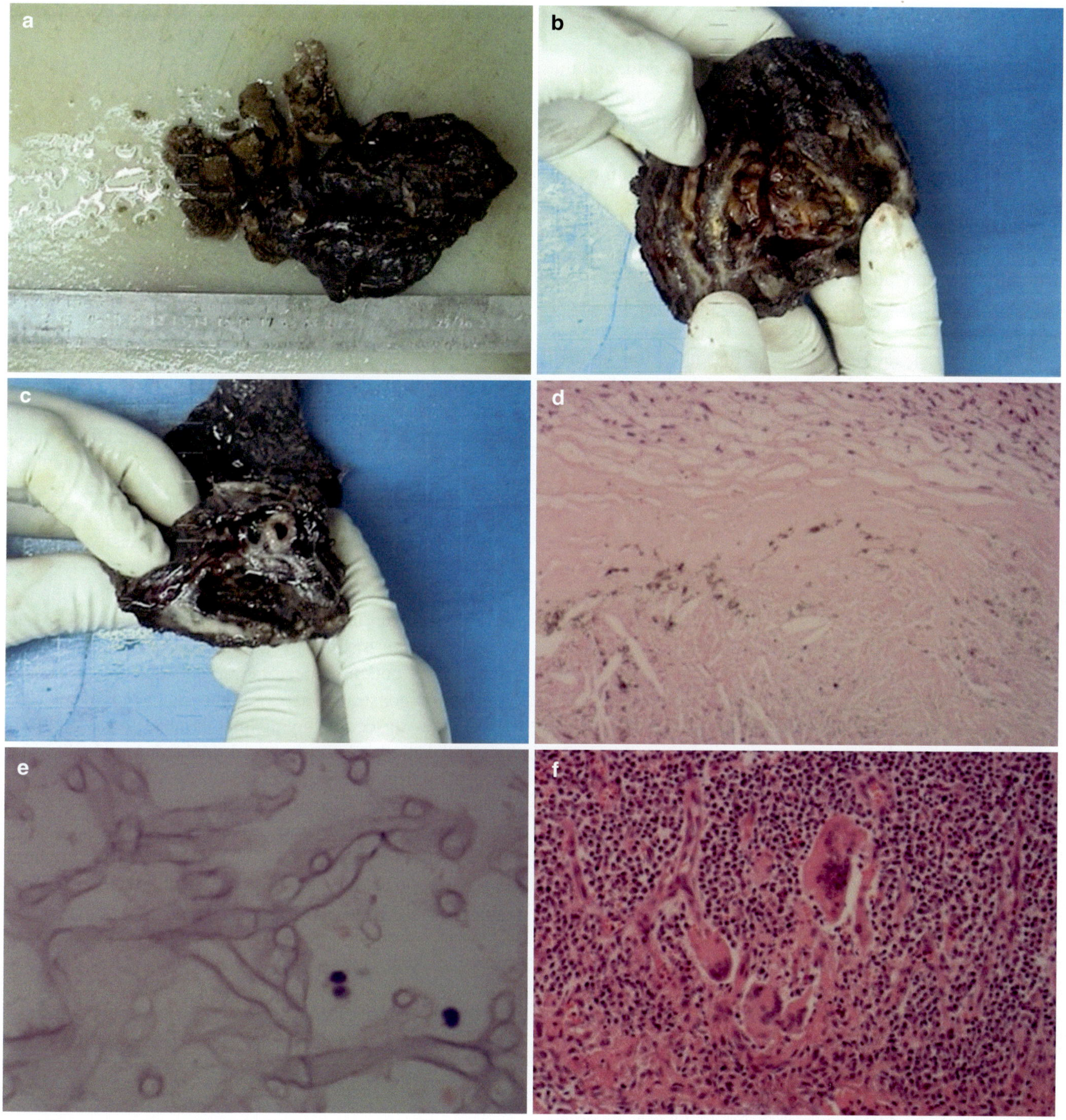

Fig. 9.32 (**a–f**) The left upper lung and the neoplasm that are visible by naked eyes. The left lower lung tissue is demonstrated with fungal mass. Based on the morphology of the hyphae, it is suspected to be aspergillus (H&E staining ×40, H&E staining ×400, H&E staining ×100)

accompanying calcification, which were surrounded by a small quantity of granulation tissue. Old tuberculosis lesion cannot be excluded (Fig. 9.32).

The final diagnosis was (1) chronic necrotizing pulmonary aspergillosis (subacute invasive pulmonary aspergillosis, (2) bronchiectasis complicated by lung infection, and (3) pulmonary tuberculosis.

After the operation, the patients showed favorable recovery and was discharged. Oral anti-fungal and anti-tuberculosis medications were continued after discharge.

9.8.6 Discussion

Aspergillus extensively exists in the natural world, and the pathogenic aspergillus includes *Aspergillus fumigatus*, *Aspergillus flavus*, *Aspergillus niger*, and *Aspergillus terreus*. Due to its direct communication with the external world, the lung is the most commonly involved. Pulmonary aspergillosis is a common clinical pulmonary invasive mycosis and can be clinically classified into three types, acute invasive pulmonary aspergillosis, chronic pulmonary aspergillosis, and allergic pulmonary aspergillosis [35]. And acute invasive pulmonary aspergillosis is the most serious type.

The main risk factors of aspergillus infection include neutropenia, long-term large dose of corticosteroid, organ transplantation (especially bone marrow transplantation), hematologic malignancy, and acquired immunodeficiency syndrome (AIDS) [36]. When the host has compromised immunity or flora imbalance, its invasive infection might be induced. In recent years, it has been found that the incidence of chronic lung diseases complicated by aspergillosis is high. Such chronic lung diseases include chronic obstructive lung disease, bronchiectasis, and pulmonary tuberculosis [37].

The CT demonstrations of pulmonary aspergillosis are characteristic. For instance, typical pulmonary aspergilloma is demonstrated as sphere or sphere-like opacity in lung cavity and crescent-shaped translucent area above the sphere (air crescent sign). Because aspergillus is free in the cavity, chest X-ray of some patients can demonstrate movable aspergillus mass along with body postures.

After aspergillus infection, the clinical symptoms are non-specific, and the positive rates of etiological detection in the sputum and bronchoalveolar lavage fluid are low, which present challenge to its diagnosis. If no early effective therapy, the mortality rate can be high [38]. In this case, the patient suffered from pulmonary tuberculosis complicated by aspergillus infection with clinical manifestations of cough, expectoration, and hemoptysis. Early anti-tuberculosis therapy showed unfavorable therapeutic efficacy, and the patient still showed recurrent hemoptysis. And radiological examinations demonstrated movable round-like soft tissue opacity. After comprehensive analysis, a diagnosis of mycosis can be clinically made. Due to long-term *Mycobacterium tuberculosis* infection, the patient showed a destructed change of the lung, and the lesions failed to be completely absorbed. Anti-fungal medication cannot permeate into the lesion of aspergillus infection that is secondary to tuberculosis. The medications are almost ineffective. Currently, surgical removal of the lesion is the most effective way for pulmonary tuberculosis complicated by pulmonary aspergillus infection [21, 39].

Invasive pulmonary aspergillosis can be further classified into three subtypes, acute invasive pulmonary aspergillosis, chronic necrotizing pulmonary aspergillosis or semi-invasive pulmonary aspergillosis, and airway invasive aspergillosis. In this case, the clinical typing was chronic necrotizing pulmonary aspergillosis. After surgical removal of the lesion, the symptoms were greatly improved, and the therapeutic efficacy was favorable.

9.8.7 Comments

The common risk factors of chronic necrotizing pulmonary aspergillosis include COPD, non-active pulmonary tuberculosis, lung cystic fibrosis, and lung nodules. And the clinical manifestations include cough, expectoration, and hemoptysis. Lung CT scan demonstrates lateral or bilateral round-shaped lung consolidation with or with no cavity and adjacent pleural thickening. Multiple nodular high-intensity opacities may be demonstrated, and the condition may slowly progress into aspergilloma in cavity with accompanying lung tissue destruction around the cavity. In this case, the patient had a past medical history of pulmonary tuberculosis, with symptoms of cough, expectoration, and hemoptysis. Chest CT scan demonstrated aspergilloma in cavity of the left upper lung with accompanying lung tissue lesions around the cavity as well as adjacent pleural thickening and adhesion. These demonstrations support the diagnosis of chronic necrotizing pulmonary aspergillosis. Based on the diagnosis and treatment experience of this patient, we know that pulmonary aspergillosis may also occur in patients with structural lung disease even though their immunity is not compromised.

Due to occurrence of aspergillus infection secondary to chronic cavitary lung disease, anti-fungal medication can hardly permeate into the lesion of aspergillosis. Medication therapy can hardly achieve favorable therapeutic efficacy. Surgical removal is a choice for treatment. In this case, the choice of surgery is successful.

9.9 Case 9: Recurrent Hemoptysis for More Than 4 Years and Aggravation for More Than 10 Days

Li Tu, Wei-Dong Song, Ping Xu, Xuemei Han, Chen Qiu, and Ying-Yun Fu

9.9.1 Presenting Symptoms

Recurrent hemoptysis for more than 4 years and aggravation for more than 10 days.

9.9.2 Brief Case History

A 49-year-old man from Sichuan, China, a security staff, was admitted to our hospital on December 30, 2012, due to presenting symptoms of recurrent hemoptysis for more than 4 years and aggravation for more than 10 days. The patient began to experience hemoptysis 4 years ago with no known causes. The blood that coughed up was fresh red in a volume of 20 ml per day, with no blood clot. The patient experienced no chest distress, chest pain, breathlessness, chills, fever, and night sweat. In another hospital, he was diagnosed with pulmonary tuberculosis, and anti-tuberculosis medication for 8 months (specifically unknown) showed favorable therapeutic responses. The symptoms were relieved. Since then, the patient suffered from recurrent hemoptysis and symptomatic therapy achieved improvement. About 10 days ago, hemoptysis slightly aggravated, and the blood coughed up was fresh red in a volume of 50 ml. In a local hospital, anti-infection and hemostatic therapies showed unfavorable therapeutic efficacy. Since onset of the symptoms, the patient had experienced breathlessness after physical activities but no fever, chill, headache, dizziness, chest pain, and night sweat. He was conscious, with quite good sleep and appetite. The bowel movements were normal, and the body weight was steady.

He reported a history of spontaneous pneumothorax 6 years ago.

9.9.3 Physical Examination

Physical examination showed a body temperature of 36.6 °C, a pulse rate of 92/min, respiration rate of 21/min, and blood pressure of 106/72 mmHg. The patient was conscious, and the superficial lymph nodes were unpalpable. The bilateral tonsils showed no enlargement. By auscultation, the respiration sounds of both lungs were slightly coarse with a small quantity of moist rales at the right lung but no dry rales heard. The heartbeat was regular in rhythm with no obvious murmur. The abdomen was soft, with no tenderness and rebound pain. The liver and spleen were subcostally unpalpable. The liver and kidney areas were not sensitive to percussion. The both lower limbs showed no edema. No clubbing finger was detected. The nervous system showed no abnormality.

9.9.4 Auxiliary Investigations

9.9.4.1 Blood Test

The routine blood test in the outpatient department showed no obvious abnormalities.

9.9.4.2 Microbiology

The sputum smear for *Mycobacterium tuberculosis* showed negative.

The initial diagnosis was hemoptysis due to pulmonary tuberculosis.

9.9.5 Diagnosis and Treatment

After admission, the examinations and tests were ordered. The routine blood test, ESR, electrolytes, liver function test, four-item coagulation function test, and five-item neoplasm test showed no abnormality. G test and GM test were positive. Sputum culture for 7 days showed no growth of fungi. And sputum culture for 7 days showed no growth of anaerobic bacteria. And sputum culture for bacteria showed growth of *Staphylococcus aureus*. On January 2, 2013, chest CT scan demonstrated cavity opacity at the right upper lung (Fig. 9.33).

After admission, chest CT scan demonstrated cavity opacity at the right upper lung and air crescent sign, which was considered to be possible fungal infection. Antifungal medication of voriconazole and hemostatic therapy were given, and hemoptysis was uncontrollable. By consultation with surgeon, it was believed that the patient was indicated to surgery. The patient was then transferred to the thoracic surgery department. On January 7, 2013, right upper lung lobectomy and pleural adhesion lysis were performed. Postoperative pathology findings suggest that: (1) cyst on the section and lining of the cystic wall on the stratified squamous epithelium, many plasmocytes surrounding the cystic wall, multifocal neutrophile granulocyte infiltration, and formation of fungal mass in the cystic cavity; (2) interstitial fiber hyperplasia of the lung and dilation and congestion of the vascular vessels; and (3) irregular dilation of some bronchioles with fungal mass in the dilated bronchiolar lumen and local slight congestion of the alveolar septa. Immunohistochemistry and methenamine silver staining showed fungal hyphae positive (Fig. 9.34).

The final diagnosis was pulmonary aspergilloma.

After surgical operation, the patient showed favorable recovery. Sequential therapy of oral voriconazole was continued after the operation.

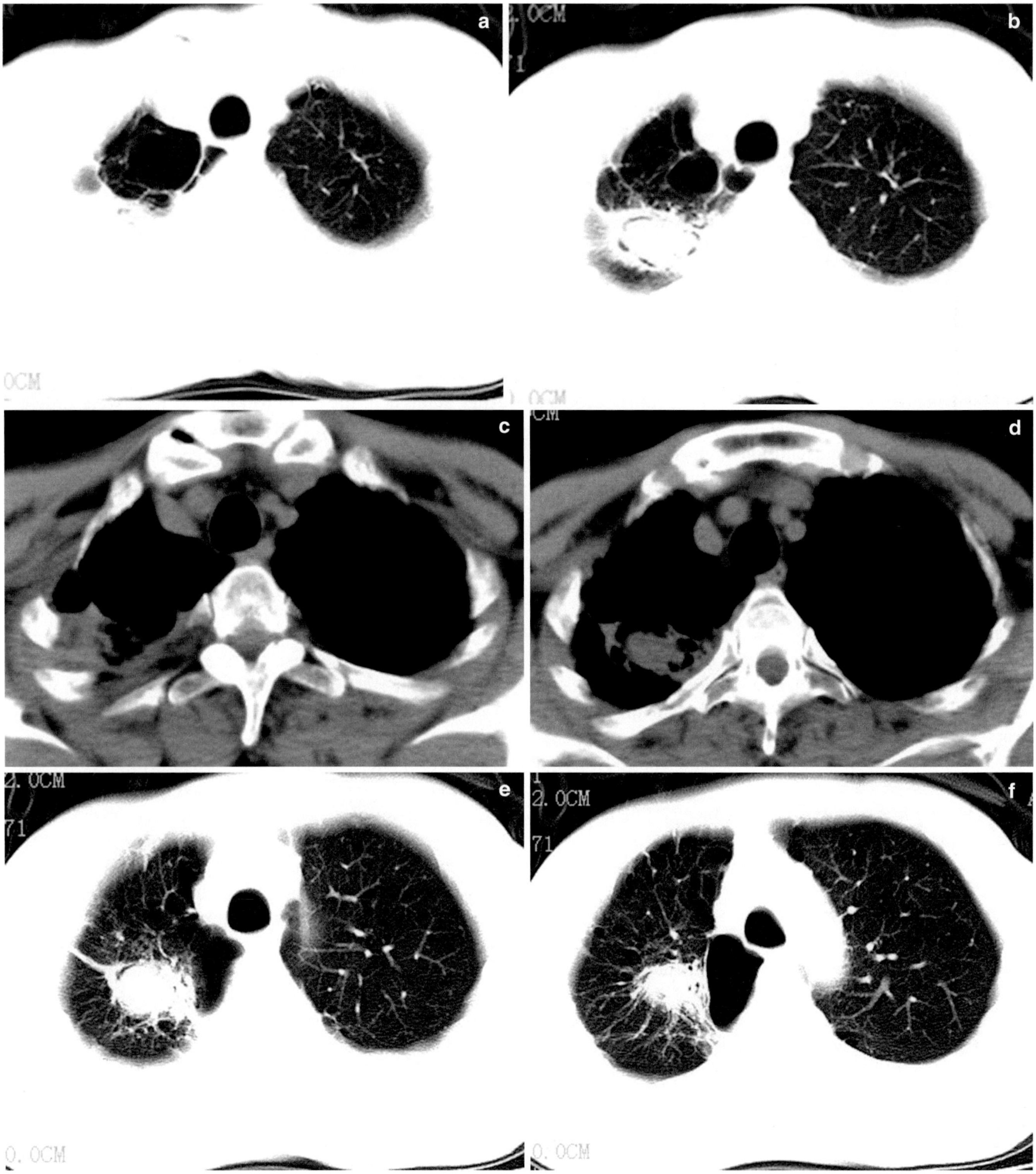

Fig. 9.33 (**a**–**j**) Chest CT scan. (**a**, **b**) The lung window demonstrates cavity opacity at the posteroapical segment of the right upper lung in size of about 2.6 cm × 3.5 cm, with large nodular opacity inside which is heterogeneous in intensity. The apex of right lung is demonstrated with bullae. (**c**, **d**) The mediastinum window demonstrates parenchymal nodular opacity in the cavity of the right upper lung, with homogeneous intensity and a CT value of about 21–44 Hu. (**e**, **f**) The lung window demonstrates cavity opacity in the right upper lung, with parenchymal mass-like opacity inside. The cavity is surrounded by irregular cords like opacity, some of which are connected with posteromedial pleura. Subpleural emphysema is demonstrated beside the trachea adjacent to the mediastinum. (**g**, **h**) The mediastinum window demonstrates cavity opacity at the right upper lung, with soft tissue opacity with homogeneous intensity inside. The cavity opacity is connected laterally and posteromedially with the pleura. (**i**–**k**) Enhanced chest CT scan demonstrates enhancement of the cavity wall but no obvious enhancement of the inner soft tissue opacity. The cavity is surrounded by many cords opacity, some of which are connected with the pleura

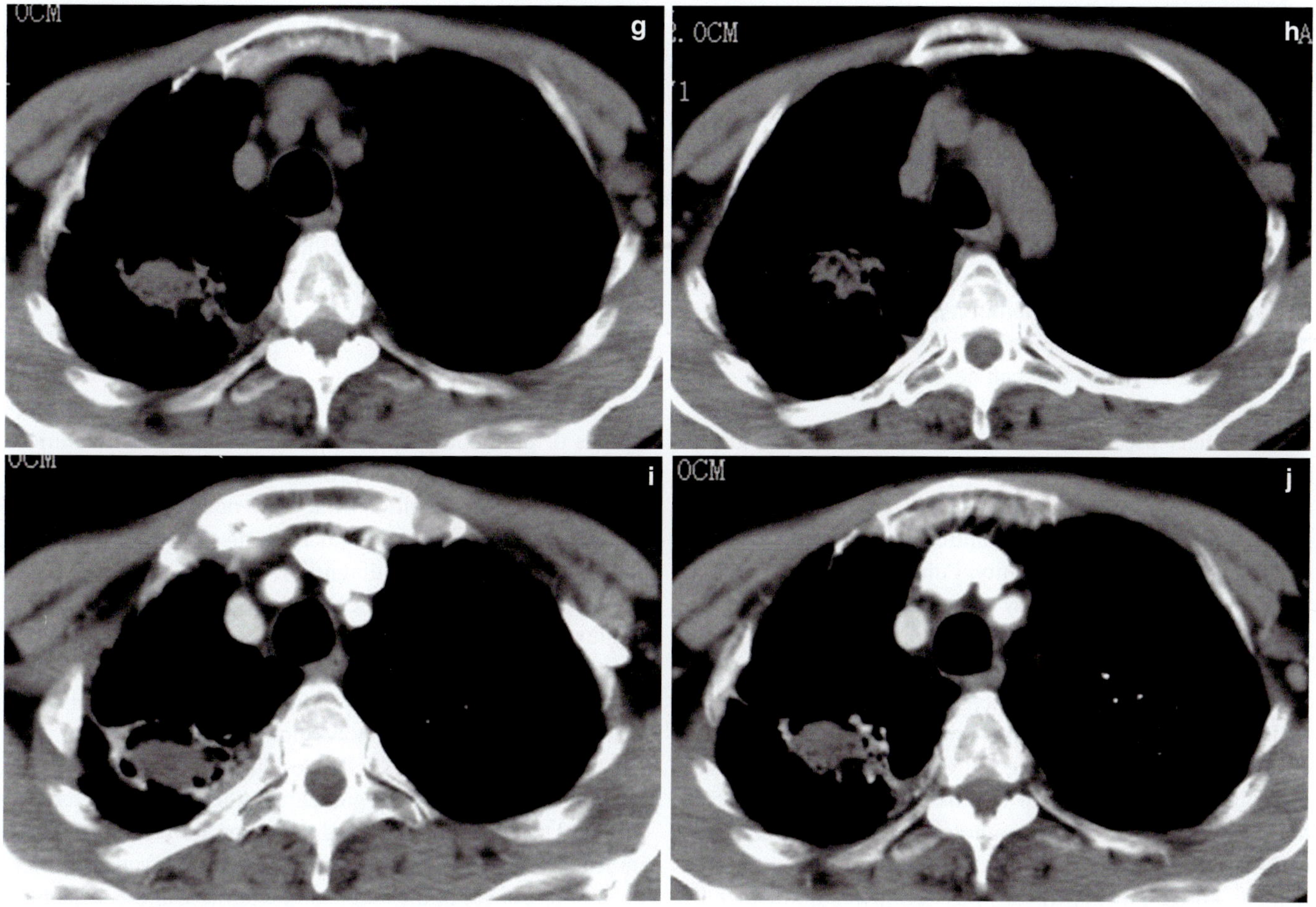

Fig. 9.33 (continued)

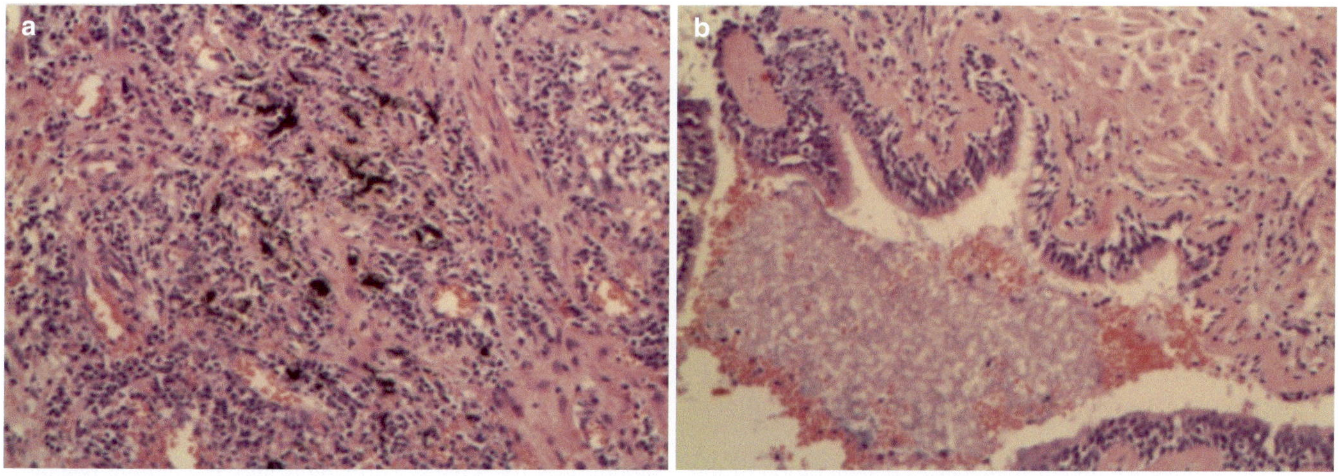

Fig. 9.34 (**a**, **b**) Pathology of the lung tissue. The cystic wall is lined by stratified squamous epithelium and is surrounded by infiltrations of many lymphocytes, plasmocytes, and neutrophile granulocytes. There is aspergillus mass in the cystic cavity (H&E staining)

9.9.6 Discussion

Aspergillus is a common pathogenic fungus that causes pulmonary mycosis, only less common than *Monilia albicans*. It extensively exists in the natural world. The factors that render their wide existence and spread include (1) simple need for metabolism (saprophyte provides optimal nourishment for its growth, and aspergillus can be always isolated from rotting plants); (2) good tolerance to temperature, humidity, and other environmental conditions; and (3) extensive distribution in the air. Each aspergillus drifts in the air in the form of thousands of spores that can be inhaled into human respiratory tract.

Pulmonary aspergillosis is commonly secondary to pulmonary tuberculosis, pulmonary cyst, and bronchiectasis. And it commonly occurs in patients receiving long-term medications of wide spectrum antibiotics and chemotherapy or with compromised immunity. Pulmonary aspergilloma is a common type of pulmonary aspergillosis, which is demonstrated as spherical aspergillus mass in the lung and is commonly secondary to chronic cavitary lung diseases, such as tuberculosis and bronchopulmonary cyst [40].

Pulmonary aspergillosis has no specific clinical manifestations. During its early stage, it tends to be misdiagnosed. Without timely appropriate treatment, the mortality rate is high. Therefore, its early diagnosis is of great importance. (1,3)-β-D glucan test (G test) and sera aspergillus galactomannan antigen test (GM test) have clinical significance for its diagnosis. Between the two investigations, GM test is superior to G test. GM test of bronchoalveolar lavage fluid shows higher specificity and sensitivity than serum GM test [41, 42].

In this case, the patient firstly experienced recurrent hemoptysis. In combination with the past medical history of pulmonary tuberculosis, typical air crescent sign by chest CT scan, and positive findings in G test and GM test, a clinical diagnosis of pulmonary aspergilloma can be made. The postoperative histopathology of the lesion supported the diagnosis.

Hemoptysis in the cases of pulmonary aspergilloma is possibly associated with the following factors:

1. Stimulated by surrounding inflammation, abundant vascular network and even aneurysm form around the aspergilloma. And the mechanic movement of the aspergilloma causes vascular rupture.
2. The inflammatory impairment causes degeneration of the cavitary lesion, which further causes bleeding.
3. The accompanying tracheal and/or bronchial inflammation.
4. The endotoxin and proteolytic enzyme produced by aspergillus cause necrosis and lysis of the tissue [43].

Due to parasitism of aspergillus secondary to chronic cavitary lung disease, anti-fungal medication can hardly permeate into the lesion of aspergillosis. Therefore, medication is almost ineffective [21, 42]. Currently, surgical operation is recommended by most scholars [44]. In this case, after surgical operation, sequential therapy of anti-fungal medication was given. The symptom of hemoptysis is relieved, and the treatment showed a favorable therapeutic efficacy.

9.9.7 Comments

Based on postoperative pathology, this is a case of bronchiectasis or pulmonary cyst complicated by aspergillus infection. We know from the diagnosis and treatment experience that pulmonary aspergillosis may also occur in immunocompetent patients with structural lung disease. The clinicians should be cautious in its diagnosis.

This case showed typical radiological demonstrations. For experienced clinicians and radiologists, a diagnosis of pulmonary aspergilloma is not challenging.

Medication by physicians for hemoptysis in patients with pulmonary aspergilloma shows unfavorable therapeutic efficacy. Surgical removal of the lesion is definitely effective. Based on the latest clinical guideline by IDSA, the disease can be cured by surgical removal of the lesion for patients who are indicated to surgery. In this case, the patient showed good therapeutic responses to the surgical operation. But the sequential therapy of anti-fungal medication has been arguable.

9.10 Case 10: Hemoptysis for 3 Days

Hui Zeng, Hui Wang, Jing Yuan, Ying-Yun Fu, Chen Qiu, and Pu-Xuan Lu

9.10.1 Presenting Complaint

Hemoptysis for 3 days.

9.10.2 Brief Case History

A 45-year-old man was admitted on April 26, 2013, due to hemoptysis for 3 days. Three days ago, the patient began to experience hemoptysis with no obvious known causes. He coughed up blood of about 20 ml each day, with accompanying dry cough and anterior chest upset. However, he experienced no symptoms of fever, aversion to cold, night sweat, chest pain, breathlessness, palpitation, and dizziness. Since the onset, he was in good spiritual condition, with good appetite and no weight loss.

9.10.2.1 Past Medical History

The patient had a medical history of pulmonary tuberculosis 28 years ago, which was treated by conventional anti-tuberculosis therapy. Four years ago, he was detected with opacity at the right upper lung during health examination. In a local hospital, he was diagnosed with old pulmonary tuberculosis. He also reported a history of hypertension for 4 years. And the blood pressure was controlled by medications of amlodipine, losartan potassium-hydrochlorothiazide, and metoprolol. And he was diagnosed with atrial fibrillation 4 years ago, and anticoagulation medication of Bayaspirin was long-term used. He denied histories of diabetes. And he had no habitual smoking and drinking.

9.10.2.2 Physical Examination

Physical examination showed a body temperature of 37.1 °C, a pulse rate of 98/min, a respiration rate of 20/min, and blood pressure of 127/90 mmHg. He was typically developed, with average nourishment. And he was conscious, with appearance of chronic disease. The patient was in an active position, with good compliance to the physical examination. The systemic superficial lymph nodes were unpalpable and not enlarged. By auscultation, the respiration sounds were clear with no dry and/or moist rales. The heart was not enlarged, with heartbeat rate of 105/min and irregular rhythm. The first heart sounds were in different strength, and the valvular areas showed no pathological murmur. The abdomen was soft, with the liver and spleen unpalpable. The shifting dullness was negative, and the liver and kidney areas were not sensitive to percussion. The bowel sounds were normal.

9.10.2.3 Auxiliary Investigation

Laboratory Test

Routine blood test showed WBC 8.94×10^9/L, N 69.4%, L 21.8%, RBC 5.24×10^{12}/L, and PLT 319×10^9/L. ESR was 14 mm/h and CRP 4.49 mg/L.

Radiology

On April 25, 2013, chest CT scan demonstrated shrinkage of the right upper lung and mass opacity at the right upper lung, which was considered to be old tuberculosis complicated by infection and inflammation at the right middle lung.

9.10.2.4 Initial Diagnosis

The initial diagnosis was (1) Right upper lung shadow unknown Origin: tuberculosis? Neoplasm? (2) lung infection; (3) bronchiectasis; (4) Grade 1 hypertension in high-risk group; (5) arrhythmia, and atrial fibrillation.

9.10.3 Diagnosis and Treatment

After admission, examinations and tests were ordered. The liver function test showed T-Bil 14.5 μmol/L, ALT 18 U/L, AST 13 U/L, TP 74.9 g/L, and ALB 44 g/L. The kidney function test showed BUN 5 mmol/L (normal range from 2.9 to 7.0 mmol/L) and Cr 77 μmmol/L (normal range from 44 to 115 μmmol). The 1–3-D gluten was lower than 10 pg/ml, and G-lipopolysaccharide was 54.68 pg/ml. The fibrinogen was 4.03 g/L. Tuberculosis antibody was weakly positive. CRP and ESR showed no obvious abnormalities.

After admission, aztreonam and ceftazidime were administered for infection, and batroxobin, aminomethylbenzoic acid, and carbazochrome sodium sulfonate were given for hemostasis. But the symptoms were not relieved. The patient still experienced hemoptysis of dark red sputum intermittently. From April 27 to May 15, 2013, sputum smear and acid-fast staining for three times showed no acid-fast bacillus. Sputum bacteria and fungi culture for two times showed negative. PPD test showed a hard nodule in size of 5 mm × 5 mm. To further define the cause of hemoptysis, enhanced chest CT scan was ordered on May 3, 2013, which indicated slight collapse of the right thorax, rightward shift of the mediastinum due to traction, small quantities of irregular patchy opacity, and cords opacity in the right upper, middle, and lower lung lobes with heterogeneous intensity and poorly defined boundary. Some of the lesions were demonstrated to be connected with the pleura, with less calcification opacity inside. The lesions were predominant in the right upper lung lobe. The other vascular markings of the lung coursed normally, and no other abnormal intensity opacity was demonstrated (Fig. 9.35).

To define the site and cause of persistent hemoptysis, fibrobronchoscopy was ordered on May 4, 2013, which had to be discontinued due to the patient's intolerance to it. The specialists from the thoracic surgery department and interventional department were then invited for consultation. It was believed that percutaneous lung puncture for biopsy was indicated for the patient. On May 8, 2013, CT-guided percutaneous lung puncture was performed under local anesthesia for biopsy. Postoperative pathology findings suggest that: many fungal hyphae and spores in the examined tissue, which were surrounded by infiltrations of acute and chronic inflammatory cells. The methenamine silver staining was positive, and acid-fast staining was negative. The pathological diagnosis was fungal infection, which was morphologically consistent to aspergillosis (Fig. 9.36).

After the operation, the patient showed a good recovery. Voriconazole was administered via intravenous infusion for 1 month, which was followed by oral medication of voriconazole tablets as sequential therapy. The patient was discharged on June 9, 2013.

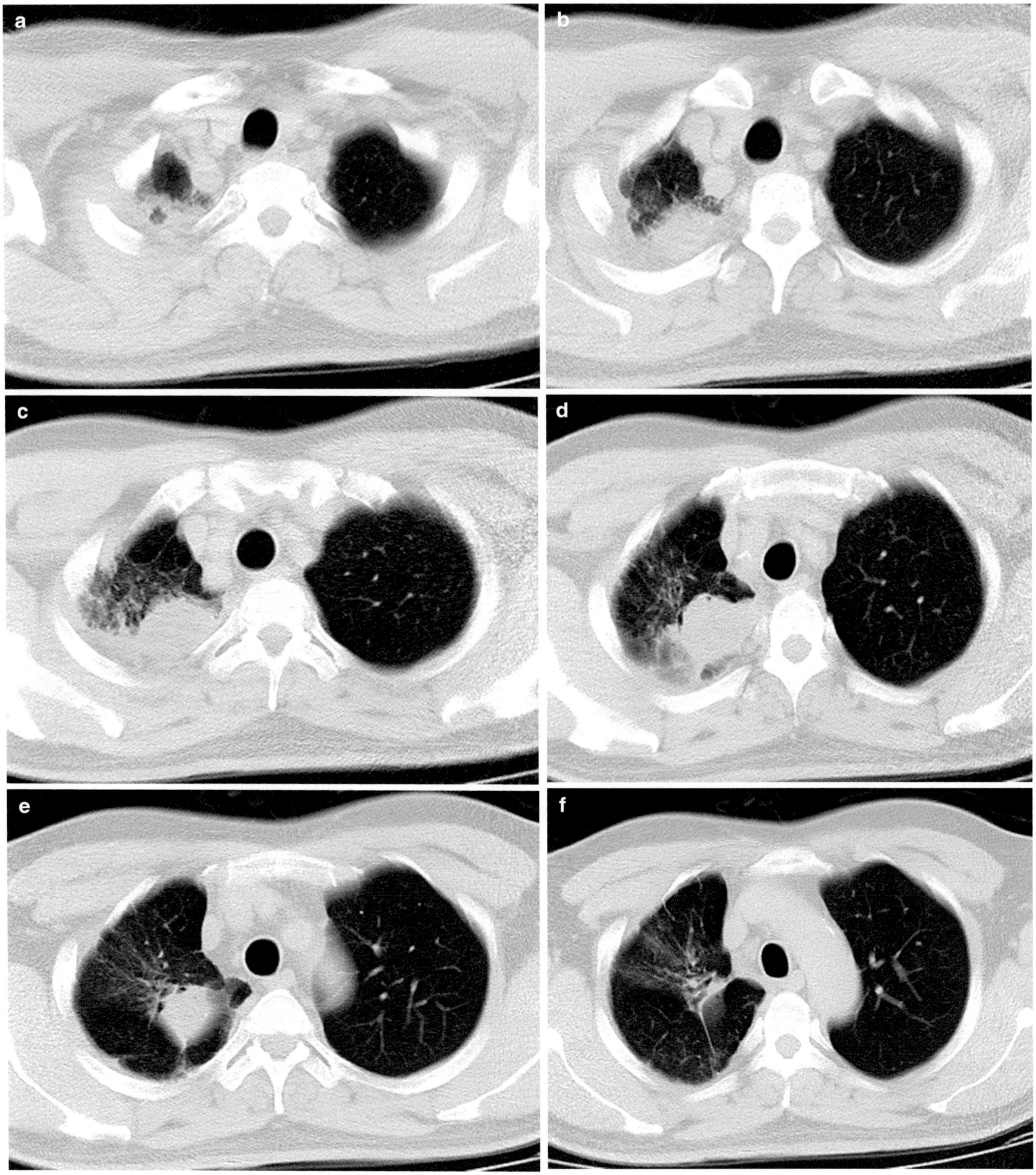

Fig. 9.35 (**a**–**j**) Chest CT scan. (**a**, **b**) The lung window demonstrates small quantities of irregular patchy opacity and cords opacity in the right upper lung lobe. (**c**, **d**) The lung window demonstrates mass opacity at the right upper lung lobe with heterogeneous intensity and poorly defined boundary. Some lesions are demonstrated to be connected with the pleura, with less calcification inside. (**e**, **f**) The lung window demonstrates slight collapse of the right thorax, rightward shift of the mediastinum due to traction, and irregular patchy opacity in the right middle lung lobe. (**g**, **h**) The mediastinum window demonstrates quite homogeneous round-like mass opacity at the right upper lung, which connects posteromedially with the pleura. (**i**, **j**) Enhanced scan demonstrates slight heterogeneous enhancement of the mass opacity at the right upper lung lobe

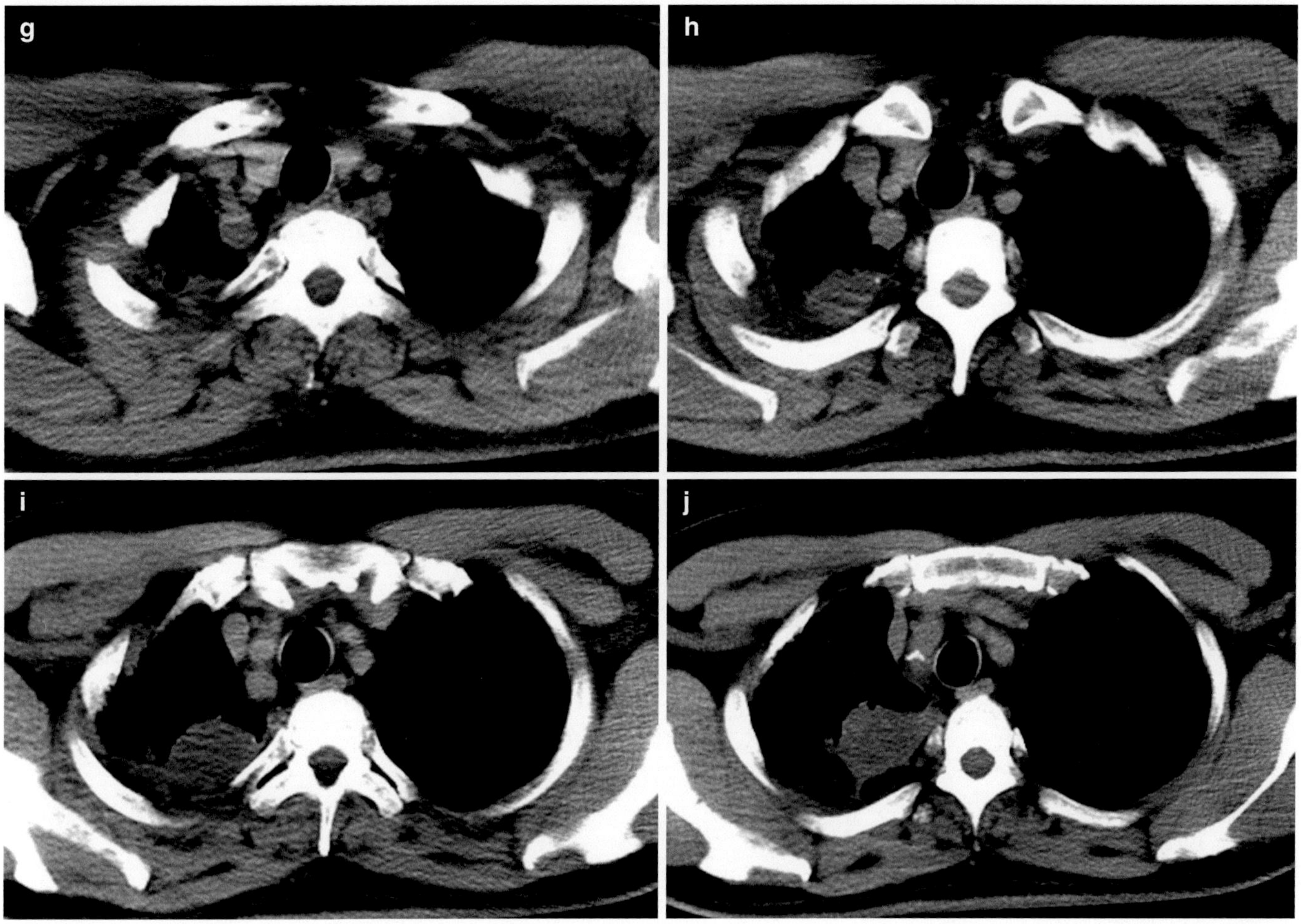

Fig. 9.35 (continued)

After treatment for 3 months, reexamination of chest CT scan on August 5, 2013, demonstrated slight collapse of the right thorax, rightward shift of the mediastinum due to traction, and small quantities of irregular patchy opacity and cords opacity at the right upper, middle, and lower lung lobes with heterogeneous intensity and poorly defined boundary. Some lesions were demonstrated to be connected with the pleura, with calcifications inside. The lesions were predominant at the right upper lung lobe. The vascular marking in the other lung lobes is normal, and no abnormal intensity opacity was demonstrated in the lungs. The bronchi above segments were unobstructed. The mediastinum was demonstrated with several small lymph nodes. The diagnosis was considered to be fungal infection of the right upper lung lobe (Fig. 9.37).

The final diagnosis was aspergillosis at the right upper lung.

9.10.4 Discussion

Pulmonary aspergillosis is mainly caused by *Aspergillus fumigatus* whose incidence ranks the second in the fungal pneumonia following pulmonary *Candidiasis albicans*. *Aspergillus*, with nonsexual dimorphism, is a filiform fungus which is coated by pigment. Under a microscope, hyphae and spores can be observed. Aspergillosis is pathologically characterized by extensive bronchitis, bronchiolitis as well as inflammation, erosion, ulceration, and necrosis of the lung tissues. The hyphae of germinating spores invade the bronchial endothelium to cause necrotizing bronchial pneumonia. After being invaded, the pulmonary vascular vessels show the following: (1) thrombosis, embolization, or infarction with accompanying tissue necrosis; (2) damage of the vascular vessels to cause hemoptysis; and (3) wide dissemination of the lesion to invade the heart, brain, kidney, and spleen. In some cases, extrapulmonary lesions can spread to the lungs along with blood circulation [45].

Based on the clinical manifestations, pulmonary aspergillosis can be classified into three types:

1. Invasive aspergillosis, which is the most common and the most serious type. The symptoms include dry cough, chest pain, and in some cases hemoptysis. In the serious cases, the patients may show breathlessness or even respi-

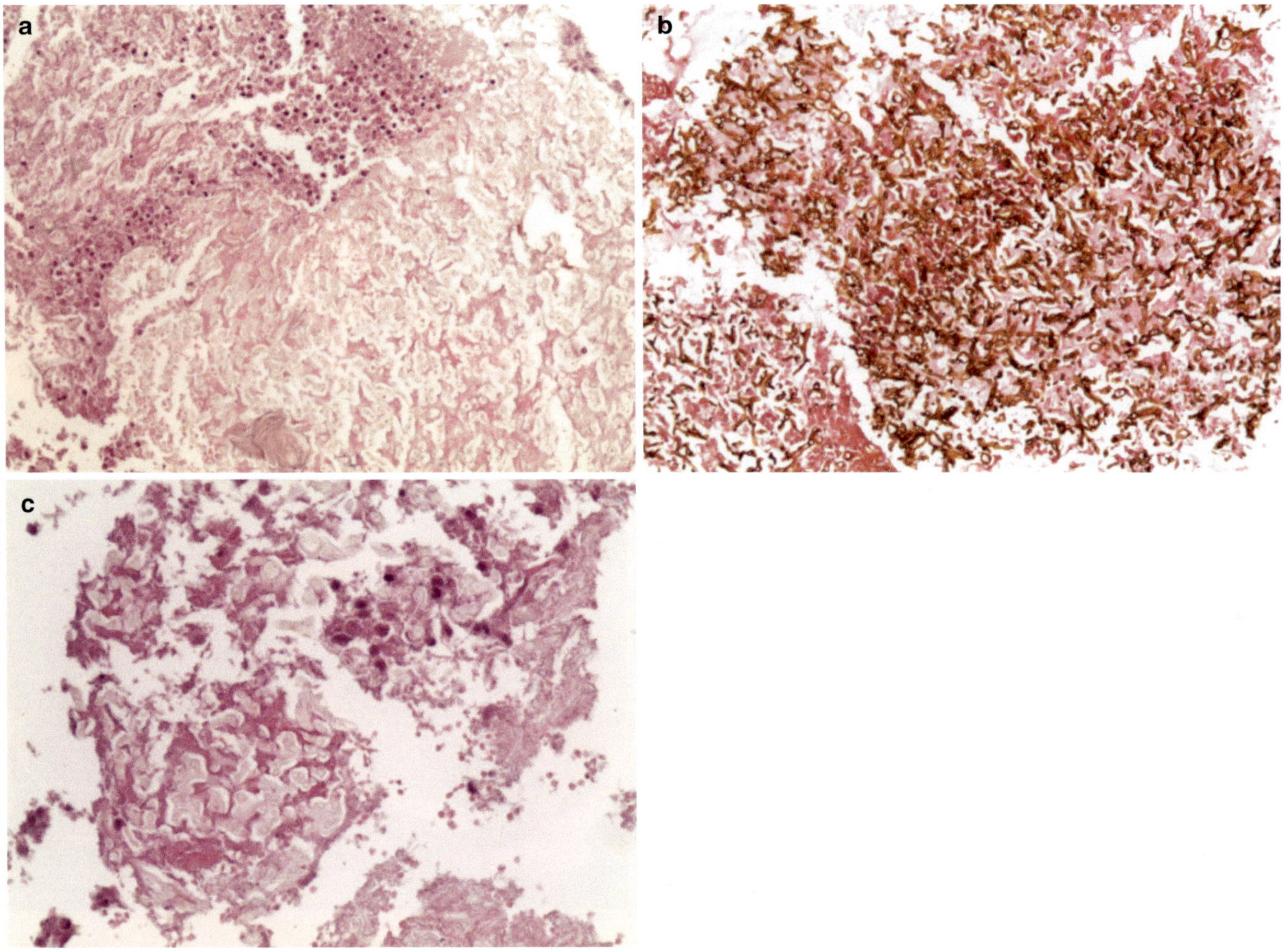

Fig. 9.36 (**a**–**c**) Pathology of lung tissue. (**a**) Many fungal hyphae and spores are demonstrated, with infiltrations of acute and chronic inflammatory cells in the surrounding tissue (H&E staining). (**b**) The special staining of PASM staining. (**c**) The special staining of acid-fast staining ×100

ratory failure, and some patients show symptoms of central nervous system infection.

2. Aspergilloma, which is commonly secondary to bronchial cyst, bronchiectasis, pulmonary abscess, and pulmonary tuberculous cavity. The common manifestations include recurrent hemoptysis or even major hemoptysis possibly with accompanying irritating dry cough.
3. Allergic bronchopulmonary aspergillosis, which is commonly an airway hyperreactivity disease caused by *Aspergillus fumigatus*. The common clinical manifestations include sudden onset of asthmatic episode, which cannot be relieved by common antiasthmatics [46].

In this case, based on radiology and pathology, chronic necrotizing pulmonary aspergillosis should be suspected. Despite the presenting complaint of hemoptysis for 3 days, opacity at the right upper lung had been detected for 4 years, which demonstrated a chronic illness course.

Chest CT scan has great clinical value for the diagnosis of pulmonary aspergillosis. The most valuable signs by chest CT scan include halo sign, crescent sign, or recent formation of cavity [47].

Amphotericin B is the medication of choice in management of invasive pulmonary aspergillosis. For patients with kidney dysfunctions, amphotericin B lipid complex can be prescribed for consecutive 1–3 months. Voriconazole is also a safe and effective medication for invasive pulmonary aspergillosis, with a cure rate and an effectiveness rate of 52.1% and 69.6% [45], respectively.

In this case, the patient was a middle-aged man with a past medical history of pulmonary tuberculosis. In the year 2009, he was detected with opacity at the right upper lung during health examinations. In a local hospital, he was diagnosed with old pulmonary tuberculosis. In our hospital, he was admitted due to hemoptysis. Chest CT scan in another hospital demonstrated mass opacity at the apicoposterior segment of the right upper lung lobe, which was larger than

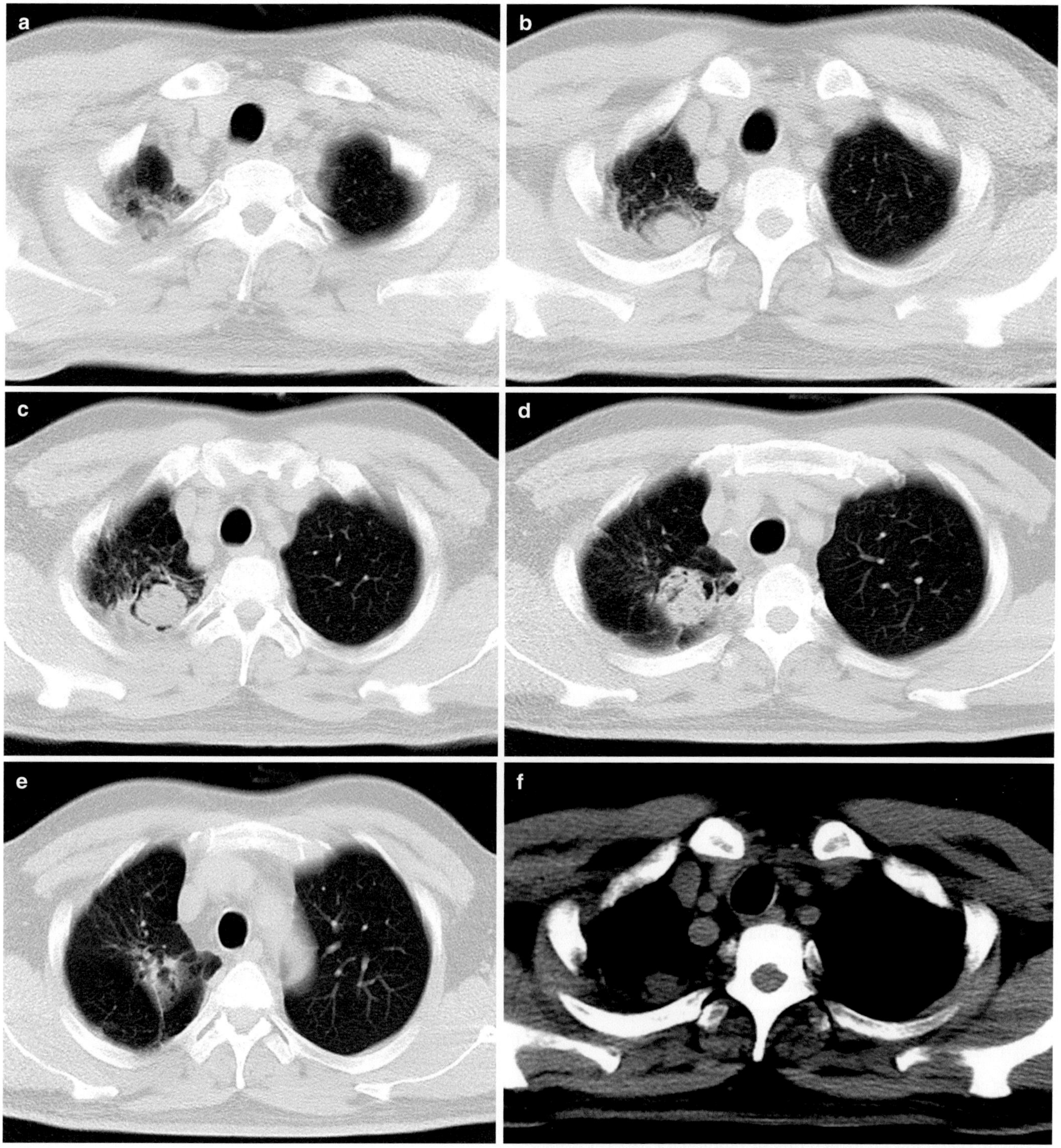

Fig. 9.37 (**a**–**g**) Chest CT scan. (**a**, **b**) The lung window demonstrates irregular nodular opacity and cords opacity at the right upper lung lobe, with heterogeneous intensity and poorly defined boundary. (**c**, **e**) The lung window demonstrates cavity opacity in the right upper lung lobe, crescent sign around the nodule, and connection of some lesions with the pleura. (**f**, **g**) The mediastinum window demonstrates heterogeneous irregular mass opacity and cords opacity at the right upper lung lobe, which connects posteromedially with the pleura

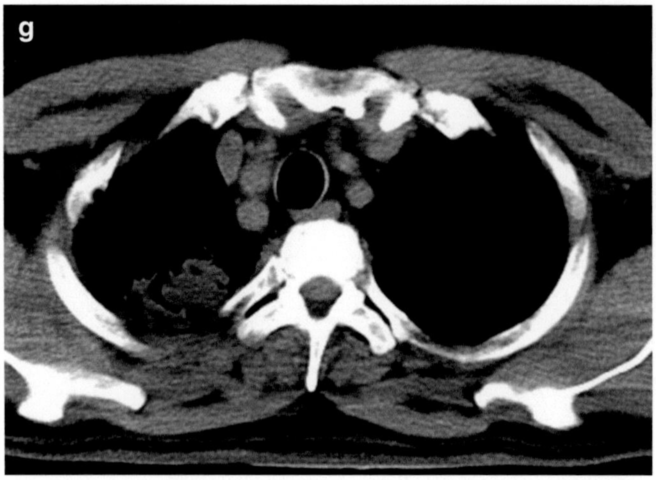

Fig. 9.37 (continued)

that demonstrated in 2009, and bronchiectasis. After admission, lung puncture for biopsy demonstrated fungal infection of the right upper lung. The patient suffered from aspergillus infection based on pulmonary tuberculosis but had no medication history of glucocorticoid, which indicated pulmonary aspergillosis may also occur in immunocompetent patients with structural lung disease. In this case, the patient received medication of voriconazole via intravenous infusion for 6 mg/kg body weight every 12 h and then 4 mg/kg body weight twice a day, followed by oral medication for 3 months. The symptoms of the patient were relieved, with shrinkage of the lesion and no adverse responses. Chest CT scan was of great clinical significance for its diagnosis. In this case, chest CT scan demonstrated recent emergence of dense mass opacity, which is one of the characteristic signs of pulmonary aspergillosis. But the patient suffered from pulmonary tuberculosis complicated by pulmonary aspergillosis, which presented challenge to its diagnosis. The diagnosis was finally defined by biopsy. Standard anti-fungal medication showed therapeutic efficacy. If the patient still experienced recurrent hemoptysis, surgical operation can be considered.

9.10.5 Comments

In recent years, the incidence rate of pulmonary aspergillosis complicating structural lung diseases, such as COPD, nonactive pulmonary tuberculosis, pulmonary cystic fibrosis, pulmonary sarcoidosis, and bronchiectasis, has been increasing. Hemoptysis is one of the most common clinical manifestations of pulmonary aspergillosis. However, hemoptysis in patients with a medical history of pulmonary tuberculosis is commonly believed to be relapse of pulmonary tuberculosis, and the possibility of pulmonary aspergillosis is commonly ignored. In the diagnosis and treatment of this patient, hemoptysis induced by tuberculosis was considered, but the possibility of pulmonary aspergillosis was ignored. Such experience should be avoided in the following clinical practice.

(1,3)-β-D Glucan test (G test) and aspergillus galactomannan antigen test (GM test) are the important tests for the diagnosis of fungal infection. Especially, the GM test is of great significance for the early diagnosis of pulmonary aspergillosis, which has a specificity of up to 70–90%. However, the cases of chronic pulmonary aspergillosis commonly show negative in both G test and GM test. But the sensitivity and specificity of GM test with bronchoalveolar lavage fluid can be up to 90%. Therefore, for the suspected cases of pulmonary aspergillosis, GM test of bronchoalveolar lavage fluid should be performed to improve the diagnosis of pulmonary aspergillosis.

The pathological biopsy is the golden standard for the diagnosis of pulmonary aspergillosis. In this case, the diagnosis was defined via biopsy following lung puncture. From the diagnosis and treatment of the patient, we learned that biopsy following lung puncture or fibrobronchoscopy can be considered if the condition of the patient is indicated.

The routine anti-fungal medication in this case showed favorable therapeutic efficacy. For the patients with recurrent hemoptysis, surgical operation can also be considered, which can prevent life-threatening major hemoptysis.

9.11 Case 11: Recurrent Cough, Expectoration and Hemoptysis for More Than 3 Years and Aggravation for 1 Month

Hongtao Chen, Dong-Na Su, Fuqiang Zhu, Wei-Dong Song, Ying-Yun Fu, and Guan-Xun Cheng

9.11.1 Presenting Complaint

Recurrent cough, expectoration, and hemoptysis for more than 3 years and aggravation for 1 month.

9.11.2 Brief Case History

A 42-year-old man was admitted to our hospital on November 13, 2007, due to recurrent cough, expectoration, and hemoptysis for more than 3 years and aggravation for 1 month. Three years ago, the patient began to experience recurrent cough, expectoration, and hemoptysis with no known causes. The sputum is commonly in a small quantity with blood streak, occasionally with dark red small clot. He showed no hemoptysis of a large quantity. And the patient experienced no fever, aversion to cold, night sweat, chest pain, chest distress, and breathlessness. In another hospital, he had been diagnosed with pulmonary tuberculosis and bronchial tuberculosis and had received anti-tuberculosis medications (specifically unknown) for 1 year. And he had been reported to be cured. After anti-tuberculosis therapy, the symptoms of cough, expectoration, and hemoptysis were relieved but relapsed when he was tired or caught a cold. In addition, his tolerance to physical activities decreased. In recent 1 month, the cough and expectoration deteriorated with a larger quantity of sputum of blood streak. He still experienced no fever, breathlessness, chest pain, lower limbs edema, and paroxysmal dyspnea at night. In another hospital, chest CT scan demonstrated tuberculosis at the right lung and lung destruction. For further diagnosis and treatment, he was transferred to our hospital and admitted to the thoracic surgery department of our hospital. Since the onset, he was in average spiritual state and appetite with poor physical strength. His sleep, urination, and bowel movements were normal, with a weight loss of about 5 kg.

9.11.2.1 Past Medical History

He reported a history of smoking for more than 20 years, 20 cigarettes per day. And he had quitted smoking for 3 years. He denied histories of diabetes, heart disease, and hypertension. And he reported no histories of chronic bronchitis, bronchial asthma, and bronchiectasis.

9.11.2.2 Physical Examination

Physical examination showed a body temperature of 36.1 °C, pulse rate 79/min, respiration rate 20/min, and blood pressure 125/77 mmHg. He was in active position and cooperative in physical examinations. The patient was thin. The respiration was smooth with coherent tone. No clubbing finger was detected. Superficial lymph nodes were unpalpable with no enlargement. The jugular vein showed no venous engorgement. The trachea was at the midline, the right thorax was slightly collapsed, and the right respiration were weakened. The bilateral vocal fremitus was symmetric with no palpable pleural rub. By percussion, the sounds of both lungs were clear. And by auscultation, the respiration sounds of the right upper lung were weakened, with no dry and/or moist rales at both lungs. The heart was no enlarged. The heart rate was 79/min, with clear heartbeat sound and regular rhythm. By auscultation, the valvular areas showed no pathological murmurs. The abdomen was soft, with no tenderness and rebound pain. The liver and spleen were unpalpable. The bowel sounds were normal.

9.11.2.3 Auxiliary Investigation

Laboratory Test

Routine blood test showed WBC 4.2 × 10^9/L, N 49%, L 41%, RBC 3.6 × 10^{12}/L, and PLT 117 × 10^9/L. ESR was 21 mm/h and CRP 6.2 mg/L. The coagulation function was normal. And the liver and kidney functions were normal. HIV antibody was negative.

Bronchoscopy

The findings in bronchoscopy are demonstrated in Fig. 9.38.

Radiology

In another hospital, chest CT scan on November 6, 2007, demonstrated tuberculosis at the right upper lung and destructed right upper lung.

9.11.2.4 Initial Diagnosis

The initial diagnosis was secondary tuberculosis at the right upper lung and destruction of the right upper lung.

9.11.3 Diagnosis and Treatment

After admission, sputum smear and sputum culture for many times showed acid-fast staining negative and no growth of mycobacteria. Chest X-ray on November 14, 2007, demonstrated small spots and fibrous cords opacity with high intensity at the right upper lung. The adjacent pleura was demonstrated to be thickened, and the other lung parts were demonstrated with slightly increased lung markings (Fig. 9.39).

Enhanced chest CT scan on November 14, 2007, demonstrated fibrous cords lesion and small nodular lesion at the right upper lung and slight adhesion of the adjacent pleura. The other parts of the lungs were demonstrated to be clear with no parenchymal lesion. Bilateral hila and mediastinum were demonstrated with no enlarged lymph nodes. The diagnosis was suspected to be tuberculosis at the right upper lung and slight bronchiectasis (Fig. 9.40).

On November 21, 2007, right upper lobectomy, cautery of pleural adhesion, and removal of right lung bullae were performed under general anesthesia. The postoperative pathology demonstrated pulmonary aspergillosis of the right upper lung, lung bullae, and lung destruction that was considered to be lesions after tuberculosis (Fig. 9.41).

9.11.4 Postoperative Treatment and Prognosis

After the operation, the patient showed good recovery. The symptoms of cough and expectoration were relieved, and hemoptysis was cured. The diagnosis on discharge was chronic pulmonary aspergillosis of the right upper lung, destruction of the right upper lung, and secondary tuberculosis of the right upper lung and bullae of both lungs.

9.11.5 Discussion

In 1952, Hinson [48] classified pulmonary aspergillosis into parasitic (aspergilloma), invasive, and allergic (or hypersensitive) bronchopulmonary aspergillosis. The typing has been

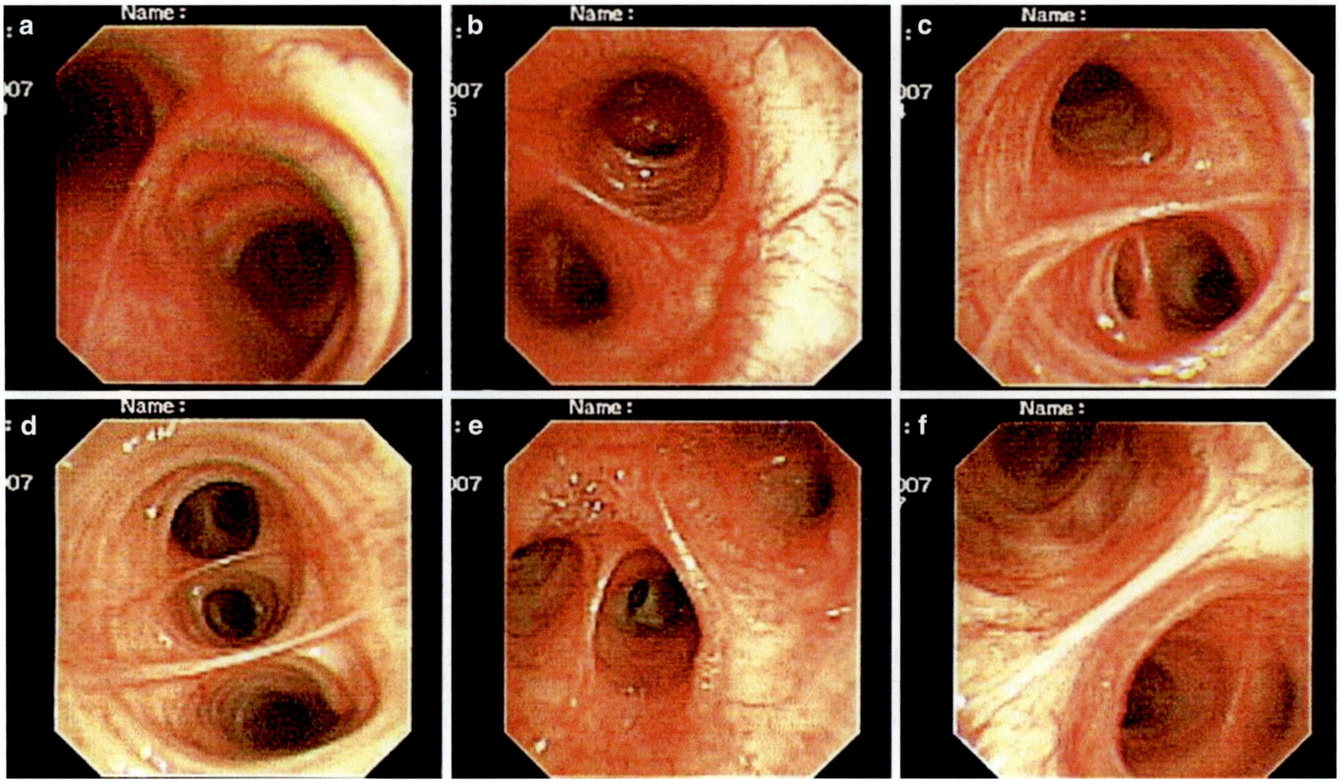

Fig. 9.38 (**a**–**f**) Bronchoscopy. Direct visual examination showed no abnormalities

Fig. 9.39 (**a**, **b**) Anterior-posterior and lateral chest X-rays. The right upper lung is demonstrated with small spots and fibrous cords opacity of high intensity. The adjacent pleura is demonstrated to be thickened

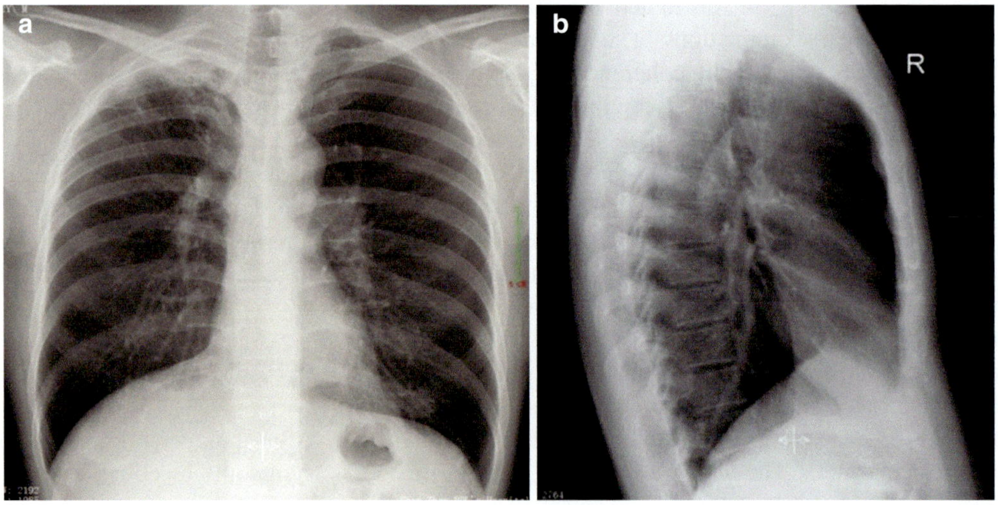

widely accepted and applied. About 80–90% cases of pulmonary aspergillosis are caused by *Aspergillus fumigatus* (*A. fumigatus*), which exist extensively in the natural world, especially in soil and rotting organisms. In manure mixture for fertilizing, *A. fumigatus* plays a fundamental role in carbon and nitrogen cycles. Since Fresenius discovered *A. fumigatus* 145 years ago, humans obtained the knowledge that *A. fumigatus* reproduces via gamogenesis in the year 2008. Due to airborne dissemination of its spores, hundreds of spores can be inhaled into the healthy human lungs each day. In immunocompetent hosts, the inhaled spores are rapidly eliminated by human immune system. However,

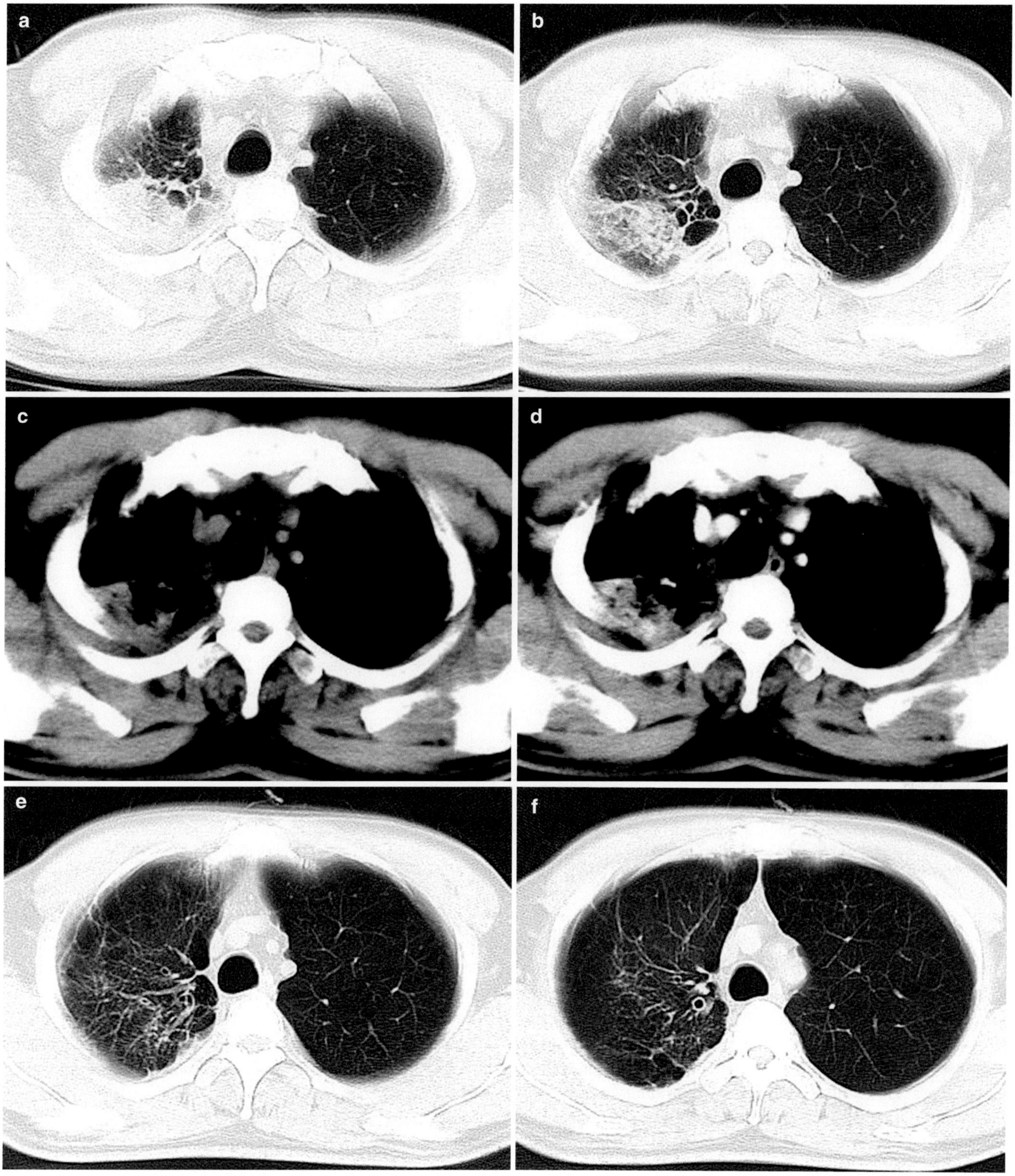

Fig. 9.40 (**a**–**f**) Enhanced chest CT scan. (**a**, **b**) The lung window demonstrates obvious fibrous tissue hyperplasia and formation of irregular cavity in the right upper lung above tracheal branching. The dorsal lesions are demonstrated to be adhered with the pleura. (**c**, **d**) Enhanced mediastinum CT scan demonstrates patchy opacity with slight enhancement at the right upper lung. (**e**, **f**) The right upper lung above tracheal branching is demonstrated with obvious fibrous tissue hyperplasia, formation of cavity, and pleural adhesion

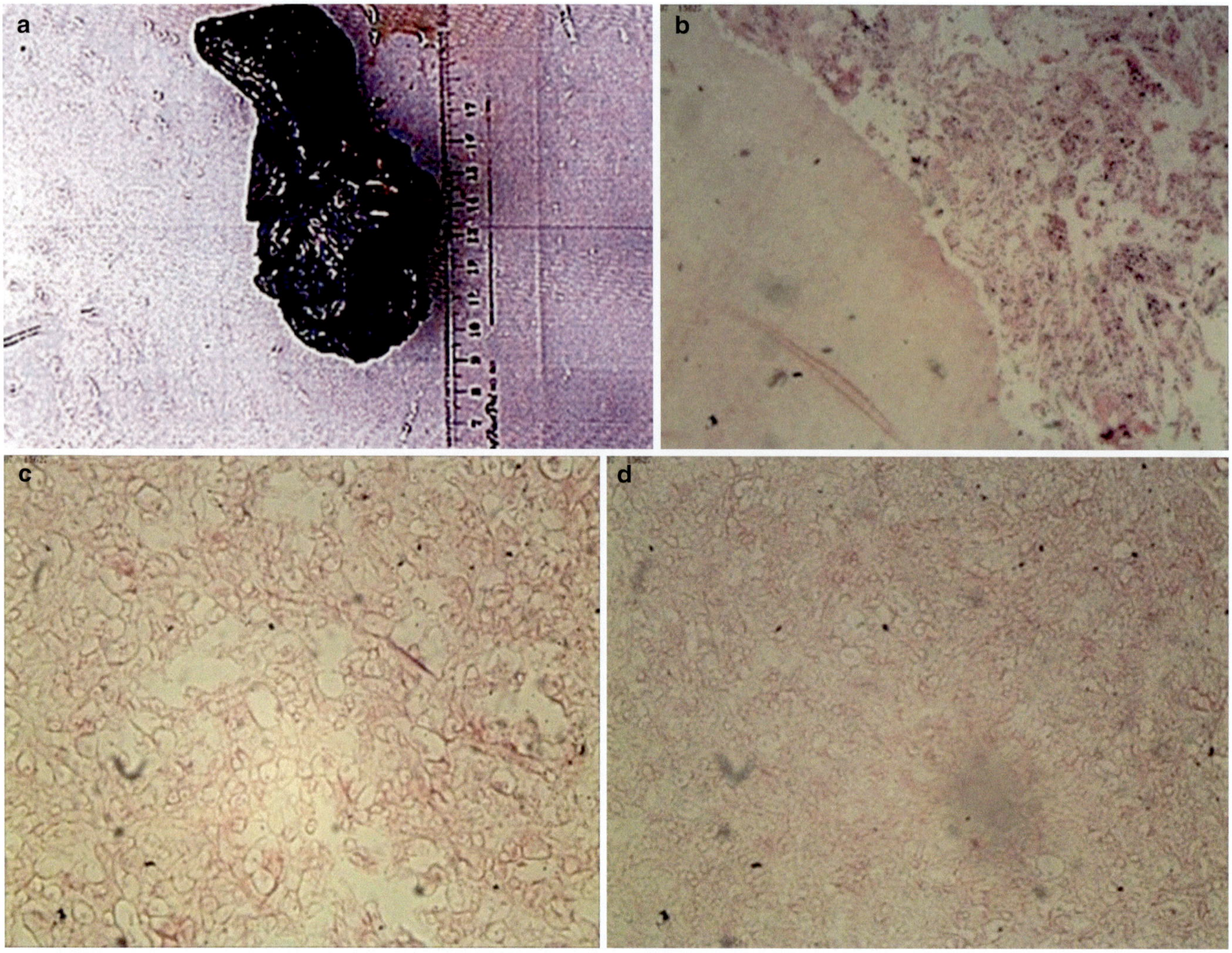

Fig. 9.41 (**a**–**d**) Pathology of lung tissue. (**a**) The gross tissue specimen by surgical removal. (**b**) Stained aspergillus hyphae in the lung tissue (H&E staining). (**c**) Stained aspergillus hyphae in the lung tissue (H&E staining). (**d**) Stained aspergillus in the lung tissue (H&E staining). The hyphae are in filiform arrangement with even thickness and septa. The hyphae are in sharp angle of 45°, and the spores can be observed

in immunocompromised hosts, such as recipients of organ transplantation and patients with HIV infection or leukemia, *A. fumigatus* constitutes pathogenic fungus. The clinical manifestations induced by *A. fumigatus* infection are diverse, which mainly depend on the type of abnormal immune response of the patients [8]. In patients with compromised immunity, acute or subacute invasive pulmonary aspergillosis occurs, while in patients with competent immunity but chronic lung impairment, such as bronchiectasis and pulmonary tuberculosis, chronic pulmonary aspergillosis or aspergilloma occurs. In patients with hyperactive immunity, allergic bronchial aspergillosis occurs [49]. Among all the types of pulmonary aspergillosis, invasive pulmonary aspergillosis has a mortality rate of above 50%. Under certain condition, the mortality rate can be up to 95%.

In this case, the patient suffered from the basic diseases of destruction of the right upper lung, bilateral lung bullae, and bronchial tuberculosis. Surgical removal of the right upper lung lobe provided an opportunity to detect the concurrent chronic pulmonary aspergillosis. Actually, statistical data indicated that almost all the patients with chronic pulmonary aspergillosis have concurrent chronic lung disease. In this case, a past medical history of tuberculosis is the highest risk factor. Other risk factors include non-tuberculous mycobacterial infection, COPD, bronchiectasis, sarcoidosis, lung carcinoma, and pneumothorax. According to literature report, in the patients receiving anti-tuberculosis therapy for 1 year and sputum conversing into negative, 14% suffers from pulmonary aspergillosis; and in the patients receiving anti-tuberculosis therapy for 4 years, 22% suffers from pulmonary aspergillosis. After anti-tuberculosis therapy, hemoptysis or bloody sputum is possibly the only symptom indicating pulmonary aspergillosis. Clinically, such patients tend to be misdiagnosed with complication of tuberculosis or relapse of tuberculosis [50].

Middle aged or elderly men are susceptible to pulmonary aspergillosis. And the patients commonly experience the systemic symptoms of weight loss, fatigue, sweating, and anorexia. The respiratory symptoms include chronic expectorating cough, dyspnea, chest upset, and hemoptysis. The positive findings by radiology include lung cavity, inflammatory infiltration, nodule, and lung or pleural fibrosis of different degrees. The laboratory tests with diagnostic significance include serum aspergillus-specific IgG (or precipitin) titer, sputum culture, PCR, and biopsy following lung puncture.

Despite of the more knowledge about pulmonary aspergillosis, its clinical diagnosis still presents challenges to the clinicians. The reasons are the following:

1. The clinical manifestations of chronic pulmonary aspergillosis are non-specific, which resemble to those of pulmonary tuberculosis and chronic bronchial lung disease.
2. The patients with aspergillus infection commonly have previous basic lung disease, and pulmonary tuberculosis is the most common basic disease of pulmonary aspergillosis (93%). Therefore, its overlapping with primary lung disease causes its missed diagnosis.
3. The common location of chronic pulmonary aspergillosis is almost the same as that of pulmonary tuberculosis, namely, the upper lung lobes and apical segment of the lower lung lobes.
4. The radiological demonstrations of pulmonary aspergillosis are nontypical [51].

During the early stage of invasive pulmonary aspergillosis, within 16 days after onset, radiology demonstrates characteristic nodule and halo sign. Radiology demonstrates other types of pulmonary aspergillosis as round-like nodule opacity, flakes of infiltrations with pleura as the base, and formation of cavity. In this case, the diagnosis was defined based on the finding of aspergillus hyphae by pathology of lung tissue. Therefore, the best evidence for the diagnosis of chronic pulmonary aspergillosis is detection of aspergillus hyphae in lung tissue specimen and aspergillus culture positive in the lung tissue specimen harvested at the same site. Sputum specimen positive for one time does not provide sufficient evidence for the diagnosis of pulmonary aspergillosis.

9.11.6 Comments

Along with improved diagnosis by CT scan, fibrobronchoscopy, and etiological techniques, we have been obtaining more knowledge about pulmonary aspergillosis. But it is still a lung disease that tends to be misdiagnosed.

In this case, the clinical typing is chronic necrotizing pulmonary aspergillosis (CNPA) whose clinical manifestations resemble to pulmonary aspergilloma. The differential diagnosis is necessary because the clinical management and prognosis are different between the two diseases. The common symptoms of CNPA include cough, expectoration, and hemoptysis, and the complicating systemic toxic symptoms occur in most cases, such as low-grade fever, weight loss, night sweating, and fatigue. The most common symptom of pulmonary aspergilloma is hemoptysis, which may be complicated by cough and expectoration, but systemic symptoms are rare. Compared to pulmonary aspergilloma, the symptoms of CNPA are complex, which tend to be complicated by systemic toxic symptoms. Such complex symptoms of CNPA are associated with its accompanying invasiveness.

The main therapy for CNPA is anti-fungal medication. However, surgical removal of the lesion is indicated for young patients with localized lesion and favorable lung reservoir, patients who are intolerant to anti-fungal medication and patients with active residual lesion after sufficient anti-fungal medication. Surgical operation is capable of complete removal of the lesion for postoperative pathology and for complete cure with no relapse. But the patients are more susceptible to postoperative complications than patients with pulmonary aspergilloma. Therefore, preoperative knowledge about the general condition of the patient, a past medical history of basic disease, and the cardiopulmonary functions of the patient is vitally important.

References

1. Chabi ML, Goracci A, Roche N. Pulmonary aspergillosis. Diagn Interv Imaging. 2015;96(5):435–42.
2. Tashiro T. Pathogenesis of chronic necrotizing pulmonary aspergillosis. Med Mycol J. 2015;56(1):3–13.

3. Warris A1. The biology of pulmonary aspergillus infections. J Infect. 2014;69(1):36–41.
4. Ruiz RL Jr, de Oliveira FHS, Piotto BLB, et al. Surgical treatment of pulmonary aspergilloma. J Bras Pneumol. 2010;36(6):779–83.
5. Blandin S, David G. Aspergillosis for the pulmonologist. Rev Pneumol Clin. 2008;64(4):202–10.
6. Yoon SH, Park CM, Goo JM, et al. Pulmonary aspergillosis in immunocompetent patients without air-meniscus sign and underlying lung disease: CT findings and histopathologic features. Acta Radiol. 2011;52:756–61.
7. Xu S, Dong X, Deng L, et al. Initial CT scan demonstration of invasive pulmonary aspergillosis. Chin J Emerg Med Crit Illn. 2013;25(4):229–32.
8. Walsh TJ, Anaissie EJ, Denning DW, et al. Treatment of aspergillosis: clinical practice guidelines of the Infectious Diseases Society of America. Clin Infect Dis. 2008;46(3):327–60.
9. Chotirmall SH, Al-Alwai M, Mirkovic B, et al. Aspergillus-associated airway disease, inflammation and the innate immune response. Biomed Res Int. 2013;2013:723129.
10. Patterson KC, Strek ME. Diagnosis and treatment of pulmonary aspergillosis syndromes. Chest. 2014;146(5):1358–68.
11. Schweer KE, Bangard C, Hekmat K, et al. Chronic pulmonary aspergillosis. Mycoses. 2014;57(5):257–70.
12. Ye Z, Cao Z, Pan J, et al. Clinical and CT scan manifestations of pulmonary aspergillosis: an analysis of 55 cases. J Med Imaging. 2015;25(6):998–1001.
13. Feng C, Shi Y. Diagnosis and treatment of pulmonary aspergilloma. Chin J Respir Intensive Care. 2014;13(4):427–9.
14. Denning DW, Pleuvry A, Cole DC. Global burden of chronic pulmonary aspergillosis as a sequence to pulmonary tuberculosis. Bull World Health Organ. 2011;89(12):864–72.
15. Limper AH, Knox KS, Sarosi GA, et al. American thoracic society fungal working group. An official American thoracic society statement: treatment of fungal infections in adult pulmonary and critical care patients. Am J Respir Crit Care Med. 2011;183:96–128.
16. Godet C, Philippe B, Laurent F, Cadranel J. Chronic pulmonary aspergillosis: an update on diagnosis and treatment. Respiration. 2014;88(2):162–74.
17. Marghli A, Zairi S, Osmen M, et al. Conservative surgery in pulmonary aspergilloma. Rev Mal Respir. 2012;29:384–90.
18. Koyama K, Ohshima N, Suzuki J, et al. Evaluation of clinical characteristics and prognosis of chronic pulmonary aspergillosis depending on the underlying lung diseases: emphysema vs prior tuberculosis. J Infect Chemother. 2015;21(11):795–801.
19. Gazzoni FF, Severo LC, Marchiori E, et al. Pulmonary diseases with imaging findings mimicking aspergilloma. Lung. 2014;192(3):347–57.
20. Sherif R, Segal BH. Pulmonary aspergillosis: clinical presentation, diagnostic tests, management and complications. Segal Curr Opin Pulm Med. 2010;16(3):242–50.
21. Ba PS, Ndiaye A, Diatta S, et al. Results of surgical treatment for pulmonary aspergilloma. Med Sante Trop. 2015;25(1):92–6.
22. Moodley L, Pillay J, Dheda K. Aspergilloma and the surgeon. J Thorac Dis. 2014;6(3):202–9.
23. Han J, Tang B. Old pulmonary tuberculosis complicated by pulmonary aspergillosis: a clinical analysis of 75 cases. J Henan Med Res. 2011;20(1):76–8.
24. Zhang L, Guo S, Zhai S. Pulmonary tuberculosis complicated by pulmonary fungal infection: a clinical analysis of 128 cases. J Med Innov China. 2013;10(19):92–3.
25. Denning DW, Pleuvry A, Cole DC. Global burden of chronic pulmonary aspergillosis as a sequel to pulmonary tuberculosis. Bull WHO. 2011;89(12):864–72.
26. Zeng D, Feng Y, Zheng Y, et al. Clinical pathology of pulmonary tuberculosis complicated by pulmonary aspergillus infection. Chin Clin Med. 2013;20(3):316–8.
27. Qian S, Gu H, Lu M, et al. Clinical diagnosis of pulmonary tuberculosis complicated by aspergillus infection by CT scan. J Chin Hosp Infect. 2014;24(2):418–20.
28. Chen J, Luan L, Wang W. CT demonstrations and differential diagnosis of pulmonary aspergillosis. J Integr Tradit Chin Med West Med. 2011;9(4):335–7.
29. Farid S, Mohamed S, Devbhandari M, et al. Results of surgery for chronic pulmonary aspergillosis, optimal antifungal therapy and proposed high risk factors for recurrence—a National Centre's experience. J Cardiothorac Surg. 2013;8(1):1–9.
30. Massard G, Olland A, Santelmo N, et al. Surgery for the sequelae of postprimary tuberculosis. Thorac Surg Clin. 2012;22(3):287–300.
31. Lazovic B, Stajic Z, Puthikovic B. Pulmonary aspergilloma. Med Arh. 2012;66(6):420–2.
32. Sagan D, Gozdziuk K. Surgery for pulmonary aspergilloma in immunocompetent patients: no benefit from adjuvant antifungal pharmacotherapy. Ann Thorac Surg. 2010;89(5):1603–10.
33. De Pauw B, Walsh TJ, Donnelly JP, et al. Revised definitions of invasive fungal disease from the European organization for research and treatment of cancer/invasive fungal infections cooperative group and the national institute of allergy and infectious diseases mycoses study group (EORTC/MSG)consensus group. Clin Infect Dis. 2008;46:1813–21.
34. Pappas PG, Kauffman CA, Andes D, et al. Clinical practice guidelines for the management of candidiasis: 2009 update by the Infectious Diseases Society of America. Clin Infect Dis. 2009;48:503–35.
35. Xu XY, Sun HM, Zhao BL, et al. Diagnosis of airway-invasive pulmonary aspergillosis by tree-in-bud sign in an immunocompetent patient: case report and literature review. J Mycol Med. 2013;23(1):64–9.
36. Guinea J, Torres-Narbona M, Gijon P, et al. Pulmonary aspergillosis in patients with chronic obstructive pulmonary disease:incidence, risk factors, and outcome. Clin Microbiol Infect. 2010;16(7):870–7.
37. Valerior A, Fabiano N, Huander FA, et al. The performance of real-time PCR, galactomannan, and fungal culture in the diagnosis of invasive aspergillosis in ventilated patients with chronic obstructive pulmonary disease (COPD). Mycopathologia. 2012;174(2):163–9.
38. Mikulska M, Raiola AM, Bruno B, et al. Risk factors for invasive aspergillosis and related mortality in recipients of allogeneic SCT from alternative donors: an analysis of 306 patients. Bone Marrow Transplant. 2009;44(6):361–70.
39. Infection Group of Respiratory Branch. Chinese Medical Society Consensus on diagnosis and treatment of lung mycosis., Chin J Tuberc Respir. 2007;30(11):821–34.
40. Patterson KC, Strek ME. Diagnosis and treatment of pulmonary aspergillosis syndromes. J Chest. 2014;146(5):1358–68.
41. Park SY, Lee SO, Choi SH, et al. Serum and bronchoalveolar lavage fluid galactomannan assays in patients with pulmonary aspergilloma. Clin Infect Dis. 2011;52(7):e149–52.
42. Zou M, Tang L, Zhao S, et al. Systematic review and meta-analysis of detecting galactomannan in bronchoalveolar lavage fluid for diagnosing invasive aspergillosis. PLoS One. 2012;7(8):e43347.

43. Zhang J, Qu J. Spectrum of pulmonary aspergillosis and its diagnostic strategy. Chin J Tuberc Respir. 2015;38(1):11–3.
44. Sagan D, Gozdziuk K. Surgery for pulmonary aspergilloma in immunocompetent patients: no benefit from adjuvant anti-fungal pharmacotherapy. Ann Thorac Surg. 2010;89(5):1603–10.
45. Editorial Committee of Chinese Journal of Internal Medicine. Diagnostic standards and management principles of invasive lung fungal infections. Chin J Intern Med. 2006;45(8):697–700.
46. Lee JK, Lee YJ, Park SS, et al. Clinical course and prognostic factors of pulmonary aspergilloma. Respirology. 2014;19(7):1066–72.
47. Li S, Zhang L, Wang X, et al. Early CT signs of invasive pulmonary aspergillosis and findings in its follow-ups. Chin J Clin Imaging. 2009;20(8):611–3.
48. Hinson KFW, Moon AJ, Plummer NS. Broncho-pulmonary aspergillosis: a review and a report of eight new cases. Thorax. 1952;7(4):317–33.
49. Kosmidis C, Denning DW. The clinical spectrum of pulmonary aspergillosis. Thorax. 2015;70(3):270–7.
50. Zhang H, Zhang H, Han Z, et al. Misdiagnosis of pulmonary aspergillosis as pulmonary tuberculosis: an analysis of 31 cases. Chin J Tuberc. 2005;27(3):143–7.
51. Li X, Xie H, Li S. Clinical typing and imaging diagnosis of pulmonary aspergillosis. Chin J Med Comput Imaging. 2010;16:384–8.

10 Pulmonary Aspergigehllosis with Presenting Symptoms of Chest Distress and Chest Pain

Ling-Wei Wang

Chest distress and chest pain are the common symptoms of invasive pulmonary aspergillosis. Research study has demonstrated that their incidence rates are 64.8% and 37.0%, respectively. About 34.3% of patients with COPD complicated by invasive pulmonary aspergillosis experience symptoms of chest distress and chest pain. Invasive tracheobronchial aspergillosis is a rare pulmonary aspergillosis, which may be accompanied by subacute onset of chest pain. In addition, statistical data indicated that the incidence rate of chest pain in patients with chronic pulmonary aspergillosis is about 17% and the incidence rates of chest distress and chest pain in patients with subacute invasive pulmonary aspergillosis are 27.8% and 16.7%, respectively.

In this section, we summarize five chronic pulmonary aspergillosis (CPA) cases with chest distress and chest pain as prominent manifestations. Their most common basic disease is old or active pulmonary tuberculosis, which is consistent with the literature reports. The chest pain induced by CPA is mostly pleuritis-like pain that is associated with respiration. The cause of chest pain is associated with pleural thickening and traction due to lesion site adjacent to the pleura, chronic non-specific inflammation, and even involvement of pleura by aspergillus infection. Clinically, the cases with presenting symptoms of chest distress and chest pain are not rare. In some cases, chest distress and chest pain are the only presenting complaints of the patients, which should be paid close attention by clinicians. Chest upset may also be associated with the concurrent basic disease, such as lung destruction and COPD.

From the clinical diagnosis and treatment of the five cases, we know that clinicians tend to miss diagnosed or misdiagnosed pulmonary aspergillosis because chest distress and chest pain are slight. The five cases in this section have an illness course ranging from 1 year to more than 30 years. Most of them received repeated antituberculosis therapy and radiological reexaminations. Until the emergence of air crescent sign or typical signs of aspergilloma, CPA was not considered by the clinicians. The reason is associated with the following factors: (1) CPA is commonly secondary to or concurrent with pulmonary tuberculosis, showing non-specific clinical manifestations. It resembles to pulmonary tuberculosis in terms of location, clinical manifestations, and radiological demonstrations. Due to the consideration of relapsed or drug-resistant tuberculosis by clinicians, the antituberculosis therapy is continued. (2) In some cases of CPA, the clinical manifestations are slight or absent. And the patients are reluctant for clinical consultations, which may also delay the diagnosis and treatment. (3) The clinicians and radiologists are insufficiently aware of CPA, which also causes its missed diagnosis and misdiagnosis.

Because pulmonary tuberculosis is a high-risk factor of CPA, we recommend CPA be listed into routine differential diagnosis of pulmonary tuberculosis with repeated sputum culture negative. And the patients who have been cured after routine antituberculosis therapy should also be paid close attention. Due to the low-positive rate of GM test to CPA, which is the most widely applied in clinical practice, serum GM test negative cannot exclude the possibility of CPA. Therefore, it is recommended in the clinical guideline by IDSA that GM test of alveolar lavage fluid, instead of serum, should be performed to diagnose or exclude CPA. Because the predictive value of anti-aspergillus IgG antibody positive is 100%, anti-aspergillus IgG antibody test

The corresponding author of section 10.1 is Peifen Chen, Email: drcpf@sohu.com.
The corresponding author of section 10.2 is Hui Han, Email: hanhui_boluo@126.com.
The corresponding author of section 10.3 is Mengjie Feng, Email: zwjfmj@163.com.
The corresponding author of section 10.4 is Yuemei Lu, Email: yuemeilu@126.com.
The corresponding author of section 10.5 is Jianfeng Zeng, Email: 452569057@qq.com.

L.-W. Wang (✉)
Second Clinical Medical College of Jinan University, Shenzhen, Guangdong, China

C. Qiu et al. (eds.), *Pulmonary Aspergillosis*, https://doi.org/10.1007/978-981-13-3435-1_10

or precipitin antibody test should be performed for all the suspected cases of CPA or subacute invasive pulmonary aspergillosis. In addition, histopathology following bronchoscopy, percutaneous puncture, or surgical thoracoscopy is also important for the diagnosis. The finding of typical aspergillus hyphae with septa in lung tissue is the golden standard for the diagnosis of invasive pulmonary aspergillosis. As a respiratory or infectious doctor who contacts most patients with CPA, it should be fully recognized that the immune status of these patients are different from patients with acute invasive pulmonary aspergillosis which faced by haematologists or oncologists. Most patients with CPA show deficient or slight immunosuppression, such as diabetes, COPD, NTM, elderly, and alcoholism.

Finally, we hope the case analysis and comments in this section could help the clinicians to know more about pulmonary aspergillosis with presenting symptoms of chest distress and chest pain. Such cases are not rare and we need to decrease missed diagnosis and misdiagnosis. This section is intended to improve the diagnosis and differential diagnosis of CPA and invasive pulmonary aspergillosis.

Patients' consents have been obtained for images or other clinical information relating to the cases to be published.

10.1 Case 1: Cough and sputum for more than 1 year, right chest pain for 3 months

Peifen Chen, Jianfeng Zeng, Qianqian Zhang, Dong-Na Su, Xueyan Liu, and Chang'e Jin

10.1.1 Presenting Complaint

Cough and expectoration for more than 1 year and right chest pain for 3 months.

10.1.2 Brief Case History

A 67-year-old man was admitted to our hospital on February 21, 2014, due to complaints of cough and expectoration for more than 1 year and right chest pain for 3 months. The patient began to experience cough with whitish thick sputum that aggravated during nights. But he experienced no fever, aversion to cold, headache, night sweat, hemoptysis, chest pain, chest distress, and breathlessness. And he paid no close attention to the symptoms and did not consult with the clinicians. About 3 months ago, he began to experience right chest pain and dull pain at his back, which was not regular and could be relieved by itself. The sputum showed a small quantity of fresh red blood streak. But he still experienced no flush, night sweat, and breathlessness. In a hospital specialized in traditional Chinese medicine, chest CT scan demonstrated patchy opacity at both upper lungs and accompanying cavity, which was suspected to be tuberculosis. He then was given routine antituberculosis therapy (HREZ) till now, and the symptoms of cough and expectoration were subjectively relieved. But the chest pain failed to be relieved. Reexamination of chest CT scan demonstrated patchy opacity at both upper lungs and accompanying cavity, based on which aspergillus infection cannot be excluded. The patient was then transferred to our hospital, a specialized hospital in Shenzhen (Guangdong, China), and was admitted to the department of tuberculosis on February 21, 2014. Since the onset of symptoms, he was in good spiritual state, with good appetite and sleep. The bowel movements were dry, one time per 1–2 days. In the recent 3 months, he had a weight loss of about 20 kg.

10.1.2.1 Past Medical History

He had a past medical history of diabetes for 2 years and was receiving insulin therapy. And he denied history of hypertension and denied habitual smoking and drinking.

10.1.2.2 Physical Examination

Physical examination showed a body temperature of 37.3 °C, pulse rate 102/min, respiration rate 20/min, and blood pressure 101/61 mmHg. He showed a typical development, average nourishment, and well consciousness, with appearance of chronic disease. The patient was in active position and well cooperative in physical examination. The systemic superficial lymph nodes were unpalpable with no enlargement. The respiration sounds of both lungs were clear, with no dry and/or moist rales. The heart was not enlarged, with a pulse rate of 102/min. The heartbeat was regular and the valvular areas showed no pathological murmur by auscultation. The abdomen was soft. The liver and spleen were unpalpable. The shifting dullness was negative. The liver and kidney areas were not sensitive to percussion. And the bowel sounds were normal.

10.1.2.3 Auxiliary Investigations

On November 10, 2013, chest CT scan in a specialized hospital of traditional Chinese medicine demonstrated patchy dense opacity at both upper lung lobes, some of which were poorly defined. Thin-wall cavity was demonstrated. The diagnosis was considered to be secondary tuberculosis at both upper lung lobes with predominant proliferation, small quantity of exudative lesion, and formation of cavity, emphysema.

On February 11, 2014, chest CT scan in a People's Hospital of Heyuan (Guangdong, China) demonstrated flakes and patchy opacity of high intensity at both upper lung lobes with poorly defined boundary and heterogeneous intensity. Both upper lung lobes were demonstrated with three irregular cavity opacities, with a diameter of 42 mm and adjacent pleural thickening. Nodular and patchy high density shadows were found in two of the cavities. The diagnosis was considered to be infiltrative pulmonary tuberculosis and multiple cavities of both upper lung lobes and suspected complication of aspergillus infection and emphysema.

10.1.2.4 Initial Diagnosis

The initial diagnosis was suspected aspergillosis and/or tuberculosis.

10.1.3 Diagnosis and Treatment

After admission, the tests and examinations were performed. The routine blood test showed WBC 7.46 × 10^9/L and neutrophile granulocytes 72.7%. ESR was 10 mm/h and CRP 9.95 mg/L (the normal value <8 mg/L). The Cyfra21-1 was 3.48 μg/L (normal limits of 0–3.3 μg/L), NSE 9.35 μg/L (normal limits of 0–16 μg/L), CEA 4.34 μg/L (normal limits of 0–5 μg/L), and PCT 0.05 ng/ml. The subgroups of T lymphocytes by flow cytometry were normal. The lymphocyte immunity for tuberculosis (FN1, IFN2, IFN3) was normal. HIV-Ab was negative. The liver and kidney functions were normal. The dynamic turbidity of 1–3-β-glucan was <10 pg/ml (negative <60 pg/ml, suspected 60–100 pg/ml, and positive >100 pg/ml). On February 21, 2014, the sputum smear demonstrated a small quantity of fungal spores. And the sputum smear for mycobacterium tuberculosis was negative. The sputum culture for common bacteria showed no growth of pathogenic bacteria. And the sputum culture for fungi showed no growth of fungi. Chest CT scan on February 21, 2014, demonstrated several cavities and spots of small nodular opacity at both upper lungs with larger cavity near the lung apex. The cavity at the right upper lung was demonstrated with a size of 43 mm × 25 mm, thin wall, generally intact inner wall, and no content. The cavity at the left upper lung was demonstrated with a size of 54 mm × 32 mm, with a wall thickness of 6 mm and strips of opacity inside. Pleural thickening was demonstrated adjacent to the lung apex. Enhanced scan demonstrated enhancement of the thick wall. The lateral subpleural nodule at the right upper lung was demonstrated with heterogeneous intensity and small cavity inside. The surrounding lung fields were demonstrated with ground glass opacity and cords opacity. Both upper lungs were demonstrated with multiple lesions and cavity. The diagnosis was suspected to be secondary tuberculosis possibly complicated by fungal infection (Fig. 10.1).

After admission, antituberculosis therapy (HRZE) was administered, and insulin was administered for blood sugar control. After 3 months of antituberculosis medication, radiology demonstrated no improvement. On February 27, 2014, fibrobronchoscopy was performed, showing sharp protuberance, whitish secretion adherence at the opening of bronchi of the left upper lung lobe with slight mucosal congestion and edema, and no abnormality at the other bronchi. Specimen was harvested from the left upper lung lobe for AFB, mycobacterium tuberculosis culture, fungi culture, and common bacteria culture. The endoscopic diagnosis was slight bronchial inflammation of both upper lung lobes (Fig. 10.2). Bronchial aspirates were harvested for common bacteria culture, fungi culture, and smear for tuberculosis, showing no growth of pathogenic bacteria, fungi, and mycobacterium tuberculosis. Gene amplification for DNA of mycobacterium tuberculosis was <5.0 × 10^2 copies/ml. And culture for mycobacterium tuberculosis showed negative.

Bronchoscopy showed no evidence of tuberculosis and the diagnosis was not defined. On March 1, 2014, percutaneous puncture was performed for biopsy. Pathology demonstrated proliferation of fibrous tissue around the necrotic tissue, epithelioid cells, and small flakes of fungal hyphae mass. The methenamine silver staining was positive and the acid-fast staining was negative. The pathological diagnosis was fungal infection of the left upper lung, which was suspected to be aspergillus infection (Fig. 10.3).

10.1.4 Final Diagnosis

The final diagnosis was chronic cavitary pulmonary aspergillosis.

10.1.5 Prognosis

After the diagnosis was defined, voriconazole was administered. The symptom of cough was gradually improved. Follow-ups showed no occurrence of chest pain and hemoptysis.

10.1.6 Discussion

In this case, the patient suffered from chronic basic disease of diabetes. Chest CT scan demonstrated cavity at

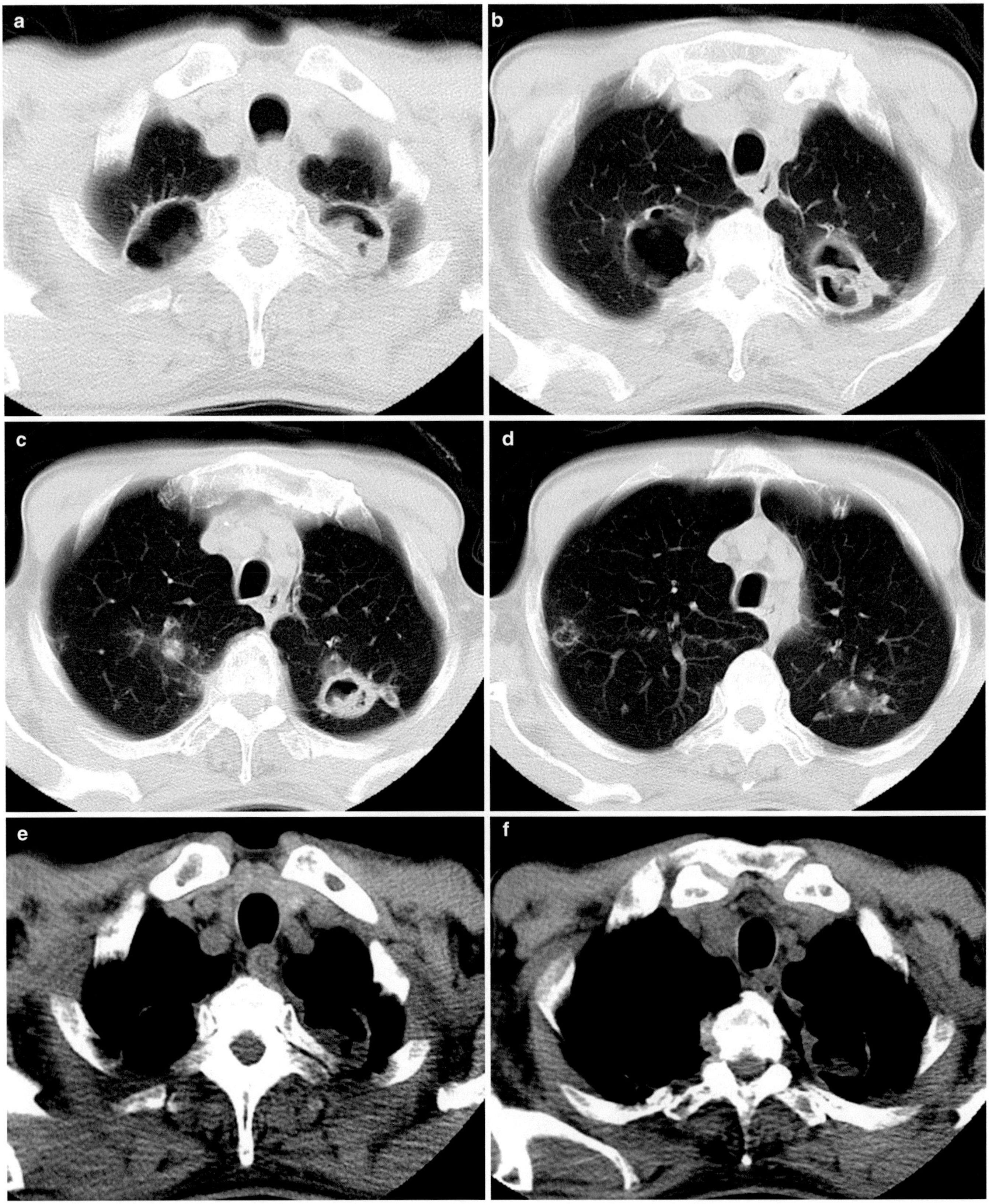

Fig. 10.1 (**a**–**h**) Chest CT scan. (**a**, **b**) The lung window demonstrates cavity opacity at both upper lungs. The cavity at the right upper lung is demonstrated with thin wall and no content. The cavity at the left upper lung is demonstrated with slightly thick wall and trips of opacity inside. (**e**–**h**) The mediastinum window demonstrates thin wall cavity at the right upper lung and slightly thick wall cavity at the left upper lung, which is predominantly posterolateral wall thickening

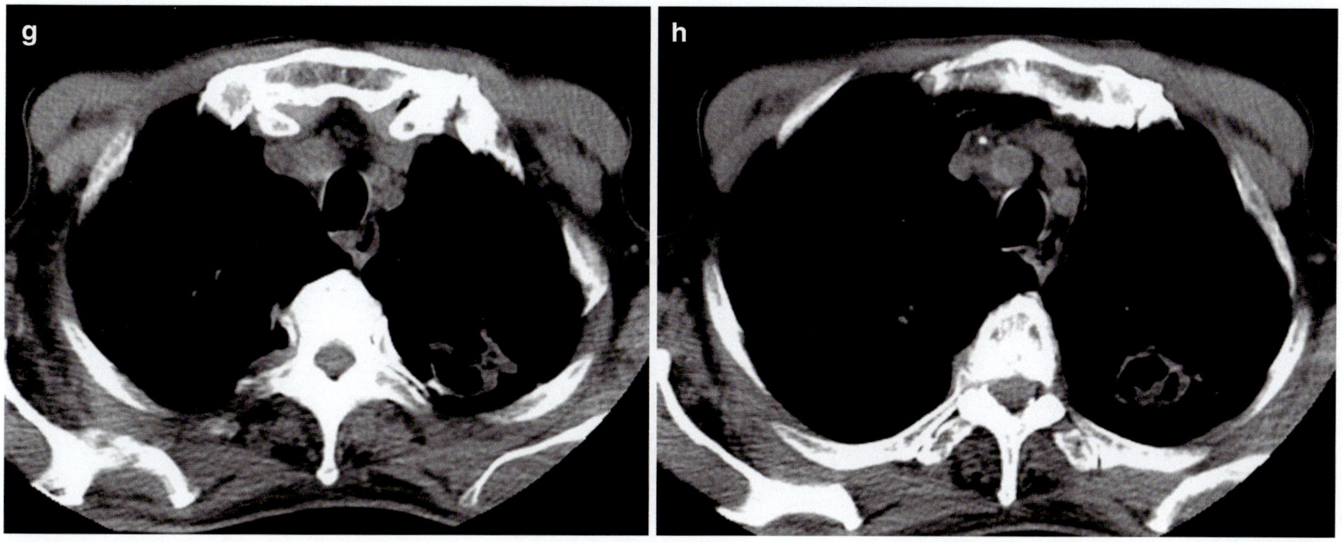

Fig. 10.1 (continued)

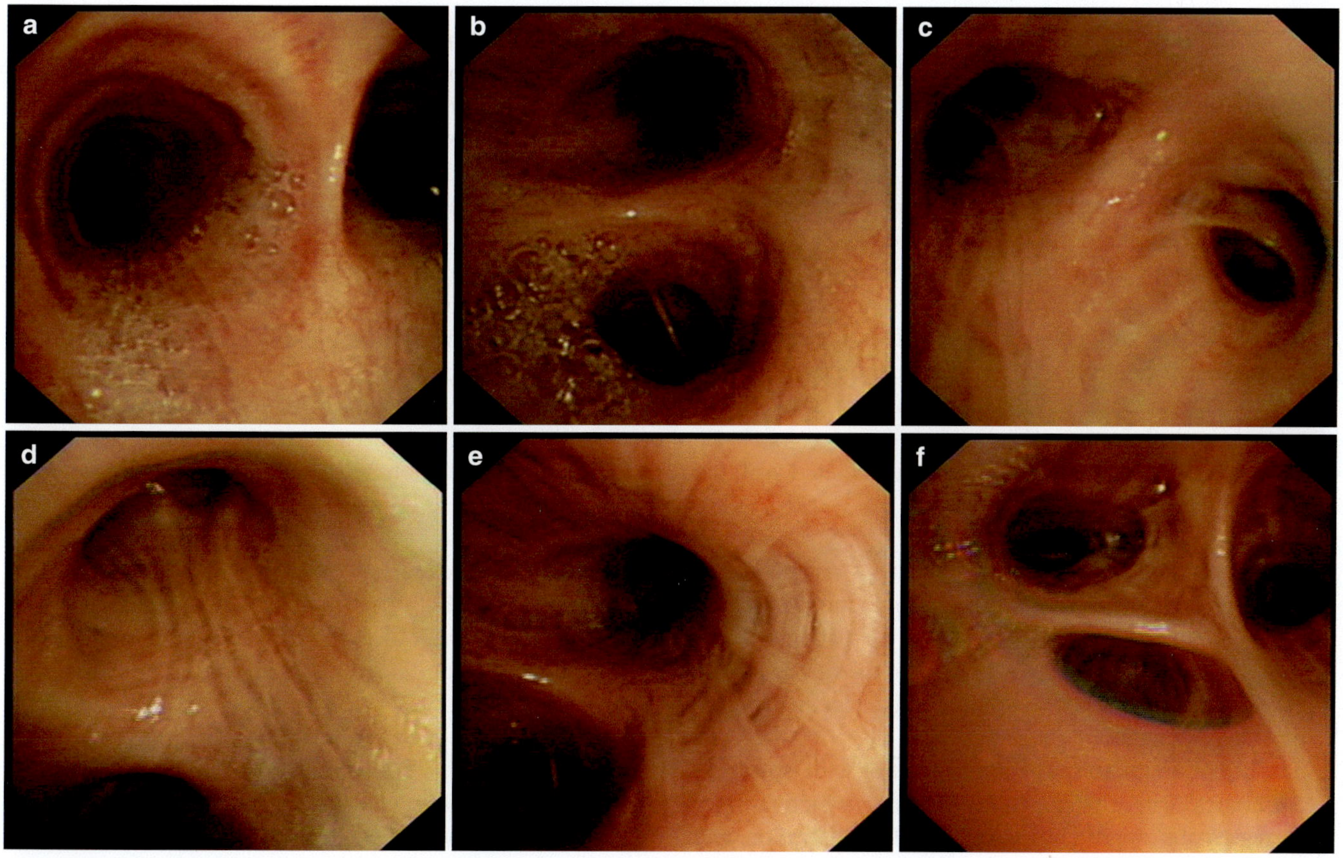

Fig. 10.2 (**a–f**) Fibrobronchoscopy. The bronchial opening at the right upper lung lobe is demonstrated with adherence of whitish thick secretions as well as slight mucosal congestion and edema

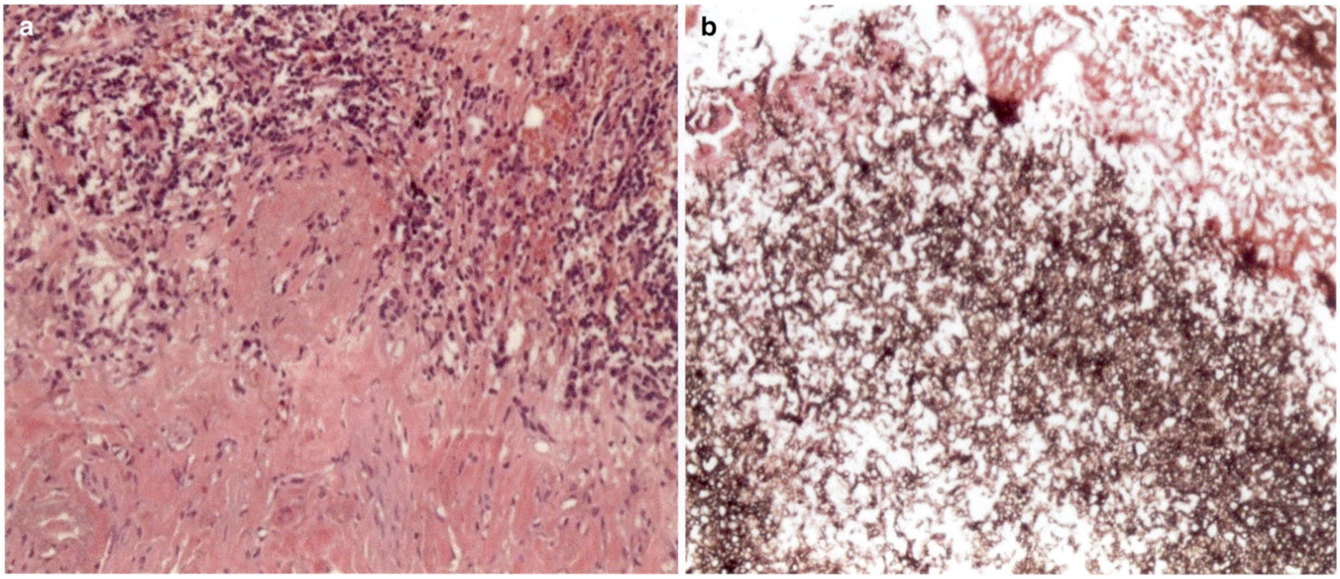

Fig. 10.3 (**a**, **b**) Pathology of the lung tissue. The lung tissue is demonstrated with proliferation of fibrous tissue, epithelioid cells, and small flakes of aspergillus hyphae mass. PASM staining is positive

both upper lungs with soft tissue intensity opacity. Pathology of the lung tissue demonstrated fungal hyphae mass with the methenamine silver staining positive. Based on these findings, the diagnosis can be defined as pulmonary aspergillosis.

The main risk factors of invasive pulmonary aspergillosis include serious immunosuppression, secondary neutropenia, bone marrow suppression, organ transplantation, and chronic granuloma. Patients with diabetes are susceptible to repeated infection of the respiratory system, and they need long-term use of multiple wide-spectrum antibiotics to control the inflammation after infection. And they are vulnerable to fungal infection. The occurrence of diabetes complicated by lung fungal infection is associated with the following factors:

1. The illness course. The longer the illness course is, the higher the incidence of lung fungal infection is. Along with the illness course of diabetes, the patients suffer from more complications with poorer resistance to diseases. They are susceptible to flora imbalance, which further causes fungal infection.
2. The use of antibiotics. The application of wide-spectrum antibiotics can change flora balance, which further increases the opportunities of fungal proliferation and invasion [1].

Although diabetes increases the chance of bacterial infection, patients with diabetes account for a small portion in the cases of invasive pulmonary aspergillosis, according to literature reports [2, 3]. So far, there have been two case reports on diabetes complicated by invasive pulmonary aspergillosis with no other risk factors [4, 5]. In this case, the patient suffered from diabetes for only 2 years and showed no exposure to other risk factors, indicating invasive pulmonary aspergillosis may occur in patients with a short illness course of diabetes and no exposure to other risk factors. Diabetes may also be complicated by tuberculosis. When lung disease occurs in patients with diabetes but inexplicable by tuberculosis showing unfavorable therapeutic responses to antituberculosis therapy, aspergillus infection should be considered. In this case, the patient received antituberculosis for more than 1 year, which delayed the therapy for aspergillus infection. The condition was initially diagnosed as tuberculosis instead of aspergillosis. And we should learn a lesson from the experience of diagnosis and treatment, especially diagnosis.

The insidious onset of pulmonary aspergillosis, its nonspecific clinical manifestations, and overlapping with the basic disease or primary symptom present challenges in its diagnosis. And the disease tends to be missed diagnosed or misdiagnosed. In this case, the patient had been diagnosed with pulmonary tuberculosis before his admission to our hospital and had been treated by routine antituberculosis therapy for 3 months. CT scan demonstrations are characteristic. During the early stage of invasive pulmonary aspergillosis, CT scan demonstrates singular or multiple poorly defined inflammatory nodules or mass with surrounding halo sign, which is highly specific in the diagnosis of pulmonary aspergillosis. Within 15–20 days, the nodule and consolidation are subject to necrosis and liquefaction, demonstrated as hollow cavity or crescent sign. CT demonstrations of halo sign and crescent sign highly indicate pulmonary aspergillosis [6]. In this case, CT scan demonstrated obvious hollow cavity sign with soft tissue intensity opacity inside, which is consistent to pulmonary aspergillosis.

Galactomannan (GM) is a polyantigen on the fungal cell wall, which shows up in human blood circulation about 1 week prior to clinical symptoms and radiological abnormalities. Consecutive serum GM tests facilitate the early diagnosis of invasive pulmonary aspergillosis [7]. However, the results of GM test are greatly variable [8, 9]. Although GM test of alveolar lavage fluid or blood shows high specificity, the positive rate remains to be about 40%, with less reliability. In addition to its high cost, its application value is negotiable. In this case, the patient did not receive the GM test.

Generally, we found that invasive pulmonary aspergillosis may occur in patients with a short illness course of diabetes and no exposure to the other risk factors. It should be paid close attention by clinicians.

10.1.7 Comments

In this case, the patient was an elderly man, who had comparatively long illness course and presenting symptoms of cough, expectoration, sputum with blood streak, and accompanying chest pain. Radiology demonstrated multiple lesions at both upper lungs, including several cavities and spots of small nodular lesions. In combination with the clinical data, the condition was considered to be chronic aspergillus infection based on pulmonary tuberculous cavity. And its clinical typing was chronic cavitary pulmonary aspergillosis (CCPA). Exudation, proliferation, caseous necrosis, cavity, and other intrapulmonary lesions induced by pulmonary tuberculosis provide chances for the growth and reproduction of aspergillus. Due to deficient immunologically active substances but appropriate temperature and humidity in tuberculous cavity, aspergillus tends to grow and reproduce inside it. Therefore, for patients with tuberculous cavity, if antituberculosis therapy shows unfavorable therapeutic responses, aspergillus infection should be considered. For such patients, G test, GM test, microbiological test, bronchoscopy, and puncture for biopsy should be performed as early as possible to obtain the evidence for diagnosis.

According to the 2016 Clinical Guideline for the Diagnosis and Treatment of Aspergillosis issued by IDSA, The patients with CCPA may not be treated, if no conditions such as lung symptoms, weight loss, obvious fatigue, serious lung dysfunction, or gradually weakened lung function. They are recommended for following up every 3-6 months instead of antifungal therapy. For patients with CCPA and systemic symptoms or lung symptoms, progressively weakened lung function, or lesion progression demonstrated by radiology, antifungal therapy should be administered for at least 6 months. The patients with CCPA commonly show slow responses to antifungal therapy. Most of them show therapeutic responses after treated for 6 months. Therefore, the therapeutic course of antifungal therapy should be more than 6 months. In this case, the patient showed obvious lung symptoms, and the routine antifungal therapy should be administered for sufficient therapeutic course.

For oral intake, itraconazole and voriconazole are medications of choice. For the patients who show adverse effects or failed treatment, posaconazole can be chosen as the third-line medication for treatment. For patients with failed treatment, resistance to triazoles, and/or adverse effects, intravenous infusion of micafungin, caspofungin, and amphotericin B can be administered, possibly with prolonged therapeutic course. If surgical removal for control of recurrent hemoptysis is contraindicated, perfusion of antifungal medication into the cavity can be performed in patients with no bleeding tendency. Several research studies have been reported that perfusion of antifungal medications into the cavity can be performed to treat aspergilloma when systemic antifungal medication shows no or adverse effects. Perfusion of antifungal medication into cavity containing aspergilloma can be performed via endotracheal intubation guided by fibrobronchoscopy, percutaneous transthoracic puncture, or catheterization.

10.2 Case 2: Intermittent Chest Distress and Cough for 3 Years

Hui Han, Yazhou Cai, Wei-Dong Song,
Ying-Yun Fu, Xuemei Han, and Xiongfei Sun

10.2.1 Presenting Complaint

Intermittent chest distress and cough for 3 years.

10.2.2 Brief Case History

A 34-year-old man from Guangdong, China, was admitted to our hospital on July 29, 2013, due to presenting complaints of intermittent chest distress and cough for 3 years. He began to experience chest distress and accompanying cough 3 years ago. But he experienced no expectoration, hemoptysis, and fever. In a local hospital, chest X-ray demonstrated opacity at lungs, and fibrobronchoscopy demonstrated no abnormalities. Since then, the symptoms onset intermittently, and he paid no attention to them and received no treatment. Six months ago, chest CT scan demonstrated honeycomb lung changes at the dorsal segment of the right lower lung. For further treatment, he consulted in our hospital and was admitted. Since the onset of the symptoms, the patient experienced no fever, emaciation, and night sweat. His spiritual state was quite good, with quite good appetite and sleep. His urination and bowel movements were normal.

10.2.2.1 Past Medical History

He had been in a good health. As a maintenance worker in an electronic workshop, he had a history of contacts to dusts. And he reported no habitual smoking and drinking.

10.2.2.2 Physical Examination

Physical examination showed a body temperature of 36.9 °C, pulse rate 74/min, respiration rate 18/min, and blood pressure 118/65 mmHg. He was conscious. The pharynx showed no congestion. The bilateral tonsils were not enlarged. The respiration sounds at both lungs were coarse, and the respiration sounds at the right lower lung were slightly low. The heartbeat was regular in rhythm with no obvious murmur. The abdomen was soft with no tenderness and rebound pain. The liver and spleen were subcostally unpalpable. The liver and kidney areas were not sensitive to percussion. Both lower limbs showed no edema. The fingertip blood oxygen was 98%, with no clubbing finger. The nervous system showed no abnormalities.

10.2.2.3 Auxiliary Investigations

Laboratory Test

The routine blood test, ESR, hs-CRP, liver and kidney functions tests, electrolytes, and antibodies of tuberculosis were normal. (1–3)-β-D Glucan was negative.

The sputum smear for fungi, the sputum smear for acid-fast bacillus, and sputum culture showed no abnormalities.

Radiology

The chest CT scan demonstrations on January 7, 2013; see Fig. 10.4.

The chest CT scan demonstrations on March 19, 2013; see Fig. 10.5.

10.2.3 Initial Diagnosis

The initial diagnosis was opacity at lungs and lung infection.

10.2.4 Diagnosis and Treatment

After admission, the routine blood test, liver function test, and kidney function test were performed. The sputum smears for consecutive 3 days for acid-fast bacillus and fungi showed negative. The sputum culture for 7 days showed negative. PPD test showed a hard nodule in size of 6 mm × 6 mm. Active anti-infection therapy was given. Reexamination by chest CT scan on July 31, 2013, demonstrated similar lung opacity to previous demonstrations by chest CT scan (Fig. 10.6).

After admission, anti-infection medication of moxifloxacin was administered for 1 week, but the symptoms showed no improvement. Reexamination of chest CT scan 6 months later demonstrated air crescent sign, which was considered to be aspergillus infection of the right lower lung lobe. Due to ineffective treatment by medications, thoracoscopic wedge removal of the right lower lung lobe and pleural adhesion lysis under general anesthesia were performed on August 7, 2013. Postoperative pathology (Fig. 10.7) demonstrated that the lesion at the right lower lung was consistent to aspergillus infection and accompanying infection.

10.2.5 Final Diagnosis

The final diagnosis was chronic cavitary pulmonary aspergillosis.

10.2.6 Prognosis

The condition was improved after surgical operation. The patient showed no symptoms of cough, expectoration, chest distress, and breathlessness. The operation wound healed. After discharge, oral intake of voriconazole was prescribed for sequential therapy.

10.2.7 Discussion

Pulmonary aspergillosis is mainly acute or chronic histopathological impairments induced by inhalation of aspergillus into the lung or bronchus. Its incidence ranks second in all types of fungal pneumonia, only following pulmonary candidiasis albicans. Aspergillus exists extensively in the natural world, which is a filiform fungus of nonsexual dimorphism. Under a microscope, its hyphae and spores can be observed. The group of conditional pathogenic aspergillus includes *Aspergillus fumigatus*, *Aspergillus flavus*, and *Aspergillus terreus*. The aspergillus parasitizing in human respiratory tract is mostly *Aspergillus fumigatus*. The conidiospores

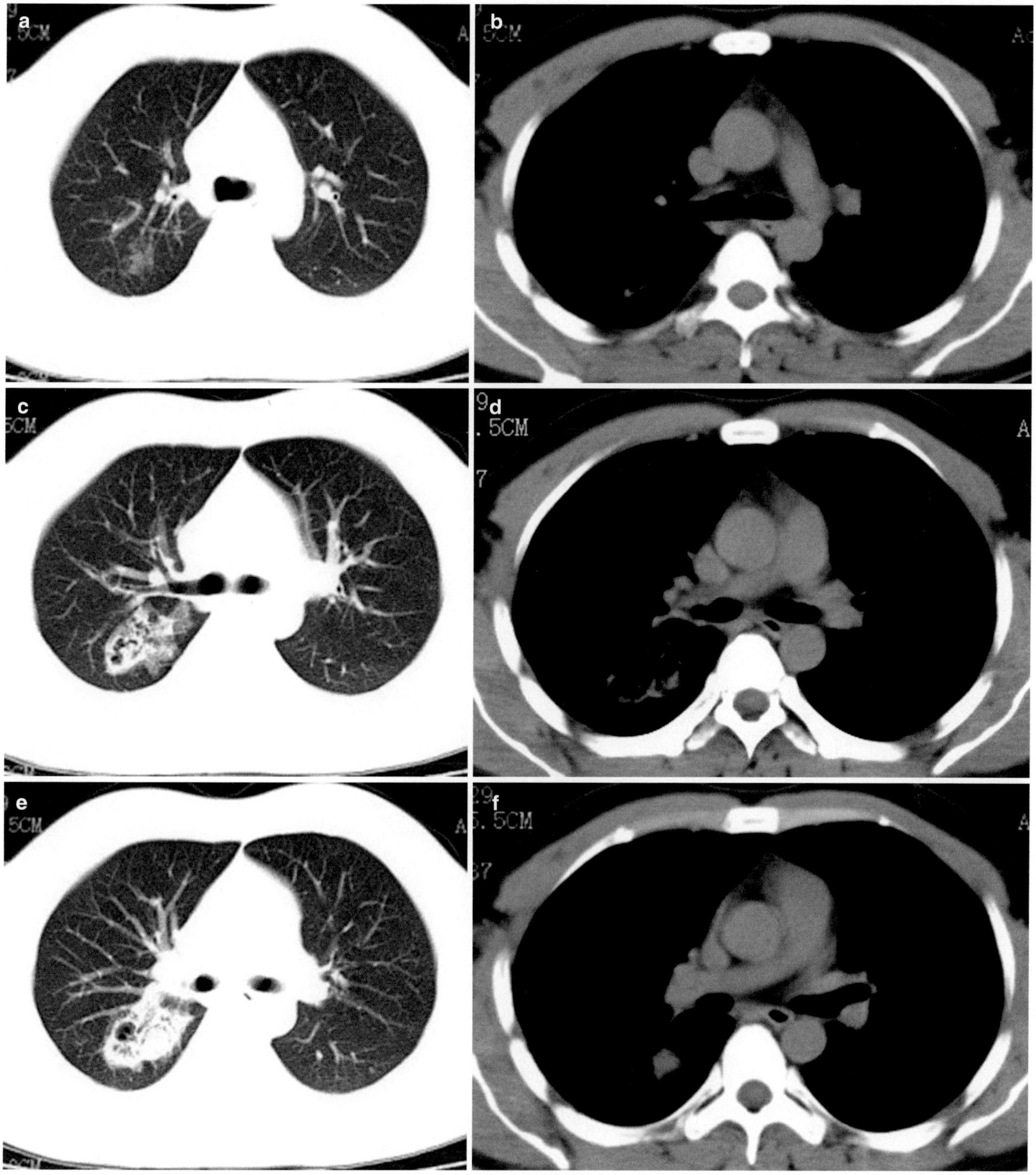

Fig. 10.4 (**a**–**f**) Chest CT scan. (**a**, **b**) The section of tracheal branching demonstrates mass and flakes of high-intensity opacity at the dorsal segment of the right lower lung lobe, which has heterogeneous inner intensity and cystic opacity with multiple septa. (**c**, **d**) The right major bronchus is demonstrated with an adjacent cystic translucent opacity with no lung markings and in a size of about 30 mm × 12 mm. The opacity is quite well-defined and connects with the mass and flakes of high-intensity opacity. (**e**, **f**) The dorsal segment of the right lower lung lobe is demonstrated with mass and flakes of high-intensity opacity, with cystic opacity of multiple septa. A well-defined spherical high-intensity opacity is demonstrated

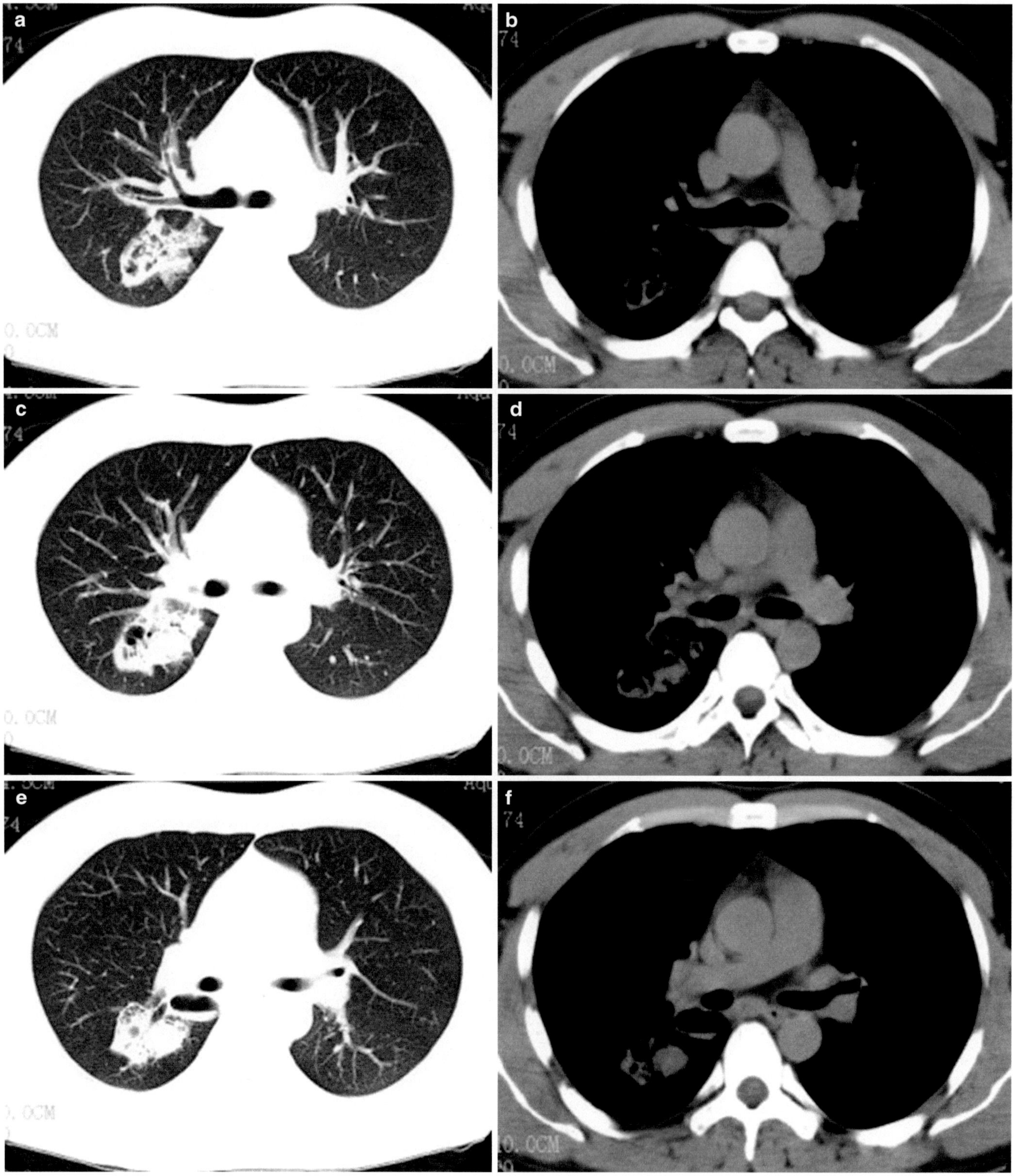

Fig. 10.5 (a–f) Chest CT scan. (**a**, **b**) The section of tracheal branching is demonstrated with mass and flake high-intensity opacity at the dorsal segment of the right lower lung lobe, with heterogeneous inner intensity and cystic opacity of multiple septa. The demonstrations are similar to those on January 7, 2013. (**c**, **d**) The right major bronchus is demonstrated with an adjacent cystic translucent opacity with no lung markings and in a size of about 30 mm × 12 mm. The opacity is well defined and connects to the mass and flake of high-intensity opacity. (**e**, **f**) The dorsal segment of the right lower lung lobe is demonstrated with mass and flake of high-intensity opacity, which has cystic opacity with multiple septa and spherical high-intensity opacities inside. The spherical high-intensity opacity is well defined

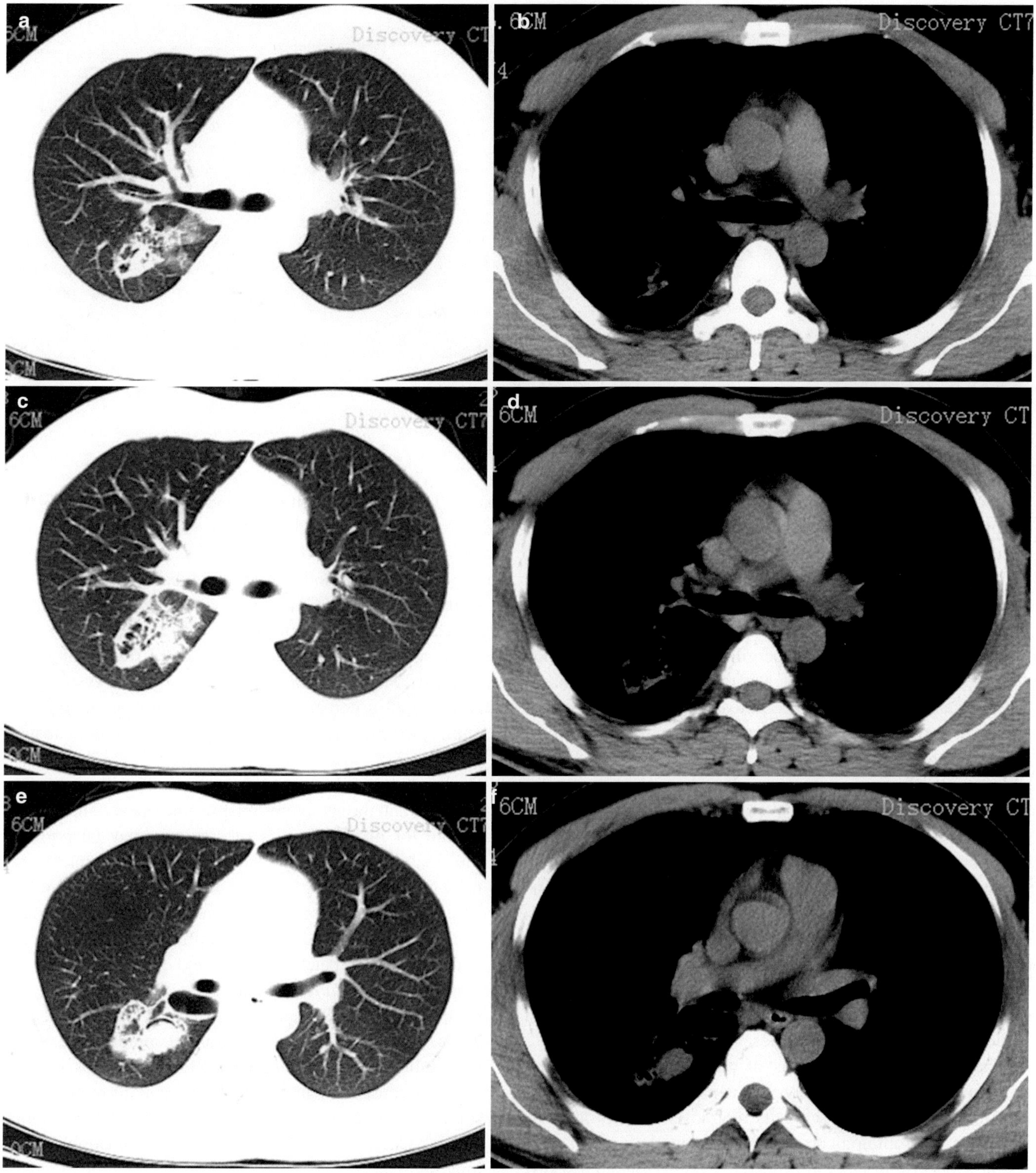

Fig. 10.6 (a–f) Chest CT scan. (**a**, **b**) The dorsal segment of the right lower lung lobe is demonstrated with mass and flake of high-intensity opacity, with heterogeneous inner intensity and cystic opacity of multiple septa. (**c**, **d**) The right major bronchus is demonstrated with an adjacent cystic translucent opacity with no lung markings and in a size of about 30 mm × 12 mm. The opacity is well defined and connects with the mass and flake of high-intensity opacity. (**e**, **f**) The dorsal segment of the right lower lung lobe is demonstrated with mass and flake of high-intensity opacity and cystic opacity with multiple septa. Air crescent sign is demonstrated

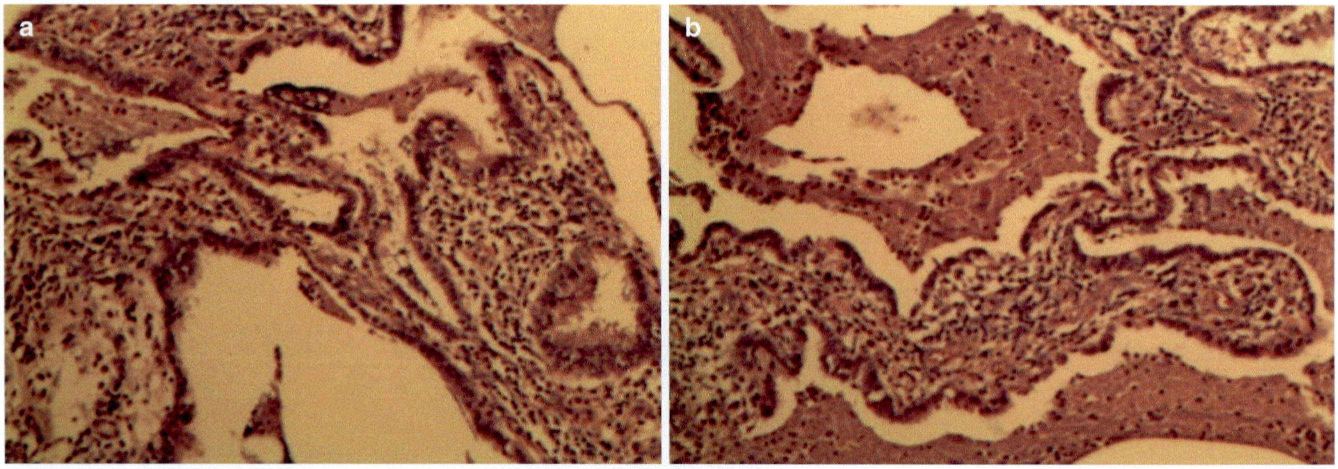

Fig. 10.7 (**a**, **b**) Pathology of lung tissue. The lung interstitium is demonstrated with slight fibrous hyperplasia and accompanying multifocal lymphoid follicles. Local aspergillus mass can be observed, with local lesion accompanied by necrosis and infiltration of neutrophile granulocytes (H&E staining)

produced by aspergillus disseminate along with airflow and temporarily parasitize in human respiratory tract after being inhaled. When a large quantity of conidiospores was inhaled or the host is immunocompromised, hyphae are developed to induce disease [10, 11].

Clinically, pulmonary aspergillosis is classified into three types: invasive pulmonary aspergillosis, aspergilloma, and allergic bronchial pulmonary aspergillosis. In these three types, invasive pulmonary aspergillosis is the most common and most serious type. The common symptoms of invasive pulmonary aspergillosis include cough, chest pain, and possible accompanying hemoptysis. In some serious cases, breathlessness, dyspnea, and even respiratory failure occur. Aspergilloma is commonly secondary to bronchial cyst, bronchiectasis, lung abscess, and tuberculous cavity. Recurrent hemoptysis is its main clinical manifestation. In some serious cases, there is even sudden onset of major hemoptysis. Allergic bronchial pulmonary aspergillosis is commonly airway hyperreactive disease caused by *Aspergillus fumigatus*. It is clinically characterized by sudden onset of asthma like symptoms but ineffective after medication of common antiasthmatics.

The clinical manifestations of pulmonary aspergillosis are non-specific, and its early diagnosis depends on laboratory test and chest CT scan. Its diagnosis can be defined based on microbiological test and histopathology of the lesion. Concerning laboratory test, (1, 3)-β-D glucan test (G test) and serum aspergillus galactomannan antigen test (GM test) show diagnostic significance. GM test is for early diagnosis of invasive fungal infection, which shows higher specificity and sensitivity than G test. By chest X-ray and chest CT scan, invasive pulmonary aspergillosis is demonstrated as subpleural nodular opacity of high intensity, possibly with surrounding halo sign and cavity opacity or crescent sign at its advanced stage. Aspergilloma is demonstrated as mass opacity in the primary chronic cavity, which is movable in the cavity along with body postures. Allergic bronchial pulmonary aspergillosis is demonstrated as transient consolidation or atelectasis of both upper lung lobes [12–14].

In this case, the patient was a young man with multiple cystic lesions at the right lower lung with accompanying nodule. The condition should be differentiated from pulmonary tuberculosis, *Staphylococcus aureus* pneumonia, cystic bronchiectasis with accompanying infection, and granulomatous vasculitis [15] (formerly known as Wegener granulomatosis).

1. Cavity due to pulmonary tuberculosis. The illness course prolongs and the symptoms relapse and relieve. The sputum culture for mycobacterium tuberculosis may be positive. The lesion is commonly located at the posteroapical segment of the upper lung lobe and dorsal segment of the lower lung lobe. Chest X-ray demonstrates cavity that infiltrates caseous lesion, fibroid cavity, and fibrous thick wall cavity, with surrounding patchy, nodular, and cords opacities.
2. *Staphylococcus aureus* pneumonia. The onset of the symptoms is sudden and acute. The symptoms include chills, high fever, chest pain, purulent sputum, and possible sputum with blood streak. Other symptoms include systemic muscular soreness, joint pain, and low spirits. In some serious cases, early peripheral circulation failure occurs. Chest X-ray demonstrates consolidation of the lung segment or lobe possibly with the formation of cavity or lobular infiltration with singular or multiple liquid-gas cysts. Another characteristic chest X-ray demonstration is variable lesion, which may be demonstrated as disappearance of inflammatory infiltration and emergence of new lesion at other sites. Otherwise the lesion is demonstrated to develop from small singular lesion into large opacity.
3. Cystic bronchiectasis with accompanying infection. The lung parenchyma is demonstrated with air-containing

cavity, and its branch is connected with the airway, with accompanying other airway abnormality, air trapping, thickening of the tracheal wall, and mucous plug of bronchioles. The lesion may be located unilaterally or bilaterally and mostly at the lower lung lobe. And most patients experience symptoms of chronic cough and expectoration. In some rare cases, the patients are asymptomatic or with unobvious initial symptoms.

4. Granulomatous vasculitis. It is an autoimmune disease, mainly involving the upper respiratory tract, the lower respiratory tract, and the kidney. The condition usually begins with localized granulomatous inflammation of the nasal mucosa and lung tissue, which further develops into diffuse necrotizing granulomatous inflammation of the vascular vessels. The lesions are intrapulmonary multiple nodules, which consist of granuloma and inflammation. Cavity occurs in large nodules that are in size of above 2 cm.

In this case, the patient was a maintenance worker in an electronic workshop, with a history of contact to dusts. It is possible that he inhaled a large quantity of spores but remained unknown to it. His G test showed negative, but fungal infection cannot be excluded due to its low sensitivity. GM test is applied for early diagnosis of invasive fungal infection, which has higher specificity and sensitivity than G test. But it cannot be performed in the hospital that he was admitted to. In combination with chest CT scan demonstrations, including honeycomb-like change and accompanying air crescent sign, a diagnosis of invasive pulmonary aspergillosis can be made. However, its definitive diagnosis should be based on histopathological evidence of the lesion and positive culture of normal sterile tissue [16].

In this case, the patient received bronchoscopy but was demonstrated with no abnormality. Finally, thoracoscopic wedge removal of the right lower lung and pleural adhesion lysis were performed. And the postoperative pathology indicated pulmonary aspergillosis, and the diagnosis was defined to be invasive pulmonary aspergillosis. Concerning the treatment, medication and surgery are recommended by IDSA. In this case, the symptoms were rapidly relieved after surgery, with favorable therapeutic efficacy.

10.2.8 Comments

Pulmonary aspergillosis is caused by acute or chronic histopathological lesion after inhalation of aspergillus into the lung or bronchus. Based on its clinical characteristics, it can be classified into invasive pulmonary aspergillosis, parasitic pulmonary aspergillosis, and allergic bronchial pulmonary aspergillosis. Chronic pulmonary aspergillosis is a clinical type of pulmonary aspergillosis, which is commonly asymptomatic or only with some non-specific respiratory symptoms such as chronic cough and hemoptysis. It commonly occurs in immunocompromised individuals. By chest CT scan, it is demonstrated as unilateral or bilateral consolidation, with singular or multiple thick wall cavities.

In this case, the patient only experienced chronic cough, with prolonged illness course. Clinically, it can be hardly differentiated from pulmonary tuberculosis. However, radiology demonstrated cystic opacity with multiple septa, mass, and flake of high-intensity opacity that gradually developed into cystic opacity with multiple septa and air crescent sign. These demonstrations are in consistent with chronic pulmonary aspergillosis. Radiologically, the condition should also be differentiated from bacterial pneumonia and cystic bronchiectasis with accompanying infection.

(1–3)-β-D-Glucan test (G test) and aspergillus galactomannan antigen test (GM test) are important tests for the diagnosis of fungal infection. Especially, GM test has clinical significance for the early diagnosis of pulmonary aspergillosis, which shows a specificity of up to 70–90%. However, serum G test and GM test show low-positive rate for chronic pulmonary aspergillosis because aspergillus antigen does not invade the vascular vessels into blood flow. GM test of the bronchoalveolar lavage fluid shows sensitivity and specificity of up to 90% in patients with chronic pulmonary aspergillosis. In this case, the patient showed negative in G test, based on which aspergillus infection cannot be excluded. For patients with suspected diagnosis of pulmonary aspergillosis, GM test of bronchoalveolar lavage fluid should be performed to improve its diagnosis.

10.3 Case 3: Chest Distress and Chest Pain for More Than 1 Year

Mengjie Feng, Dong-Na Su, Fei Shi, Xueyan Liu, Huaisheng Chen, and Xiongfei Sun

10.3.1 Presenting Complaint

Chest distress and chest pain for more than 1 year.

10.3.2 Brief Case History

A 42-year-old woman was admitted to our hospital on July 18, 2012, due to complaints of chest distress and chest pain for more than 1 year. One year ago, the patient began to experience symptoms of chest distress, chest pain, cough, expectoration, and whitish thick sputum of a small quantity. But she experienced no hemoptysis, fever, night sweat, fatigue, and breathlessness. She had received treatment (specifically unknown) in a local hospital but with unfavorable therapeutic efficacy. Chest CT scan in our hospital demonstrated lesions at both upper lung lobes and right lower lung lobe. The spherical lesion at the posterior segment of the right upper lung lobe is considered to be infection of acid-fast bacillus. The patient was then admitted due to a suspected diagnosis of pulmonary tuberculosis. Since the onset of symptoms, the patient was in a low spiritual state, with poor sleep, and appetite. The urinations and bowel movements were normal, with no obvious weight loss.

10.3.2.1 Past Medical History

She suffered from pulmonary tuberculosis 10 years ago, and she reported that the disease had been cured.

10.3.2.2 Physical Examination

Physical examination showed a body temperature of 36.5 °C, pulse rate 66/min, respiration rate 19/min, and blood pressure 120/76 mmHg. She was typically developed with moderate nourishment, and she was conscious with favorable compliance to the physical examination. Her skin showed no yellowish stain and no petechia and ecchymosis. The superficial lymph nodes were not palpable and enlarged. The trachea was at the midline. And the jugular vein showed no distension. The thorax was bilaterally symmetric, with no deformity. By palpation, the vocal fremitus is bilaterally symmetric. Both lungs showed clear percussion sounds, with no obvious dry and/or moist rales. The precordial region showed no bulge, and the apical heartbeat was strong, with a heart rate of 66/min that was regular in rhythm. By auscultation, the valvular areas showed no pathological murmur. The abdomen was soft, with no tenderness and rebound pain. The liver and spleen were subcostally unpalpable. The liver and kidney areas were not sensitive to percussion. The shifting dullness was negative. And the bowel sounds were 5/min. Both lower limbs showed no edema. No clubbing finger was detected. The nervous system showed no abnormalities.

10.3.2.3 Auxiliary Investigations

Laboratory Test

Routine blood test showed WBC of 4.1×10^9/L and neutrophile granulocytes 58.3%. The RBC, HGB, and PLT were within normal limits.

Routine urine test showed BLD 10/μl and LEU 25/μl.

The liver and kidney functions; myocardial enzymogram of AST, LDH, HBDH, CK, and CK-MB; blood lipid; and coagulation function were within normal limits. Procalcitonin (PCT), hs-CRP, and ESR were within normal limits. Immunologic assay for tuberculosis was negative. And the test for hepatitis B virus markers showed HBsAb positive, HBeAb positive, and HBcAb positive.

The culture of fibrobronchoscopic alveolar lavage fluid showed negative. Fibrobronchoscopic brushing showed no acid-fast bacillus.

Radiology

Chest CT scan on July 18, 2012, demonstrated lesions at both upper lung lobes and right lower lung lobe. The spherical lesion at the posterior segment of the right upper lung lobe was suspected to be infection of acid-fast mycobacteria. The bilateral pleura was demonstrated with thickening and adhesion. Bullae at the right upper lung lobe and dorsal segment of right lower lung lobe as well as traction bronchiectasis were demonstrated (Fig. 10.8).

10.3.2.4 Initial Diagnosis

The initial diagnosis was nodular cavity at the right lung, which was suspected to be pulmonary tuberculosis, old lesions at both lungs, and bullae at the right lung.

10.3.3 Diagnosis and Treatment

After her admission, the case was discussed and analyzed by a multispecialty team, and it was believed that surgery was indicated. On August 9, 2012, thoracoscopic removal of the right upper lung lobe, wedge removal of the right lower lung lobe, and closed thoracic drainage were performed under general anesthesia.

Postoperative pathology demonstrated chronic inflammation of the harvested tissue with accompanying emphysema and bullae, mycosis that was consistent to aspergillosis, and local formation of emphysema (Fig. 10.9).

After the operation, the body temperature of the patient was normal, with no cough and expectoration. Voriconazole was administered for 2 weeks, and then the medication was changed to oral liquid of itraconazole for sequential therapy. The patient was discharged then.

The diagnosis on admission was aspergilloma of the right lung, old lesion of tuberculosis at both lungs, and bullae of the right lung.

10.3.4 Discussion

Pulmonary aspergillosis is a common lung mycosis, and its pathogenic fungus is mainly *Aspergillus fumigatus*. The clinical manifestations and radiological demonstrations of pulmonary aspergillosis are diverse due to the different immunity of organisms to *Aspergillus fumigatus* [17]. Clinically, pulmonary aspergillosis is classified into aspergilloma, allergic bronchial pulmonary aspergillosis (ABPA), and invasive pulmonary aspergillosis (IPA). IPA mainly affects patients with seriously compromised immunity, such as patients receiving hematopoietic stem cell transplantation (HSCT), parenchymal organ transplantation, chemotherapy, and glucocorticoid therapy. Chronic pulmonary aspergillosis (CPA), simplex aspergilloma, and aspergillus bronchitis

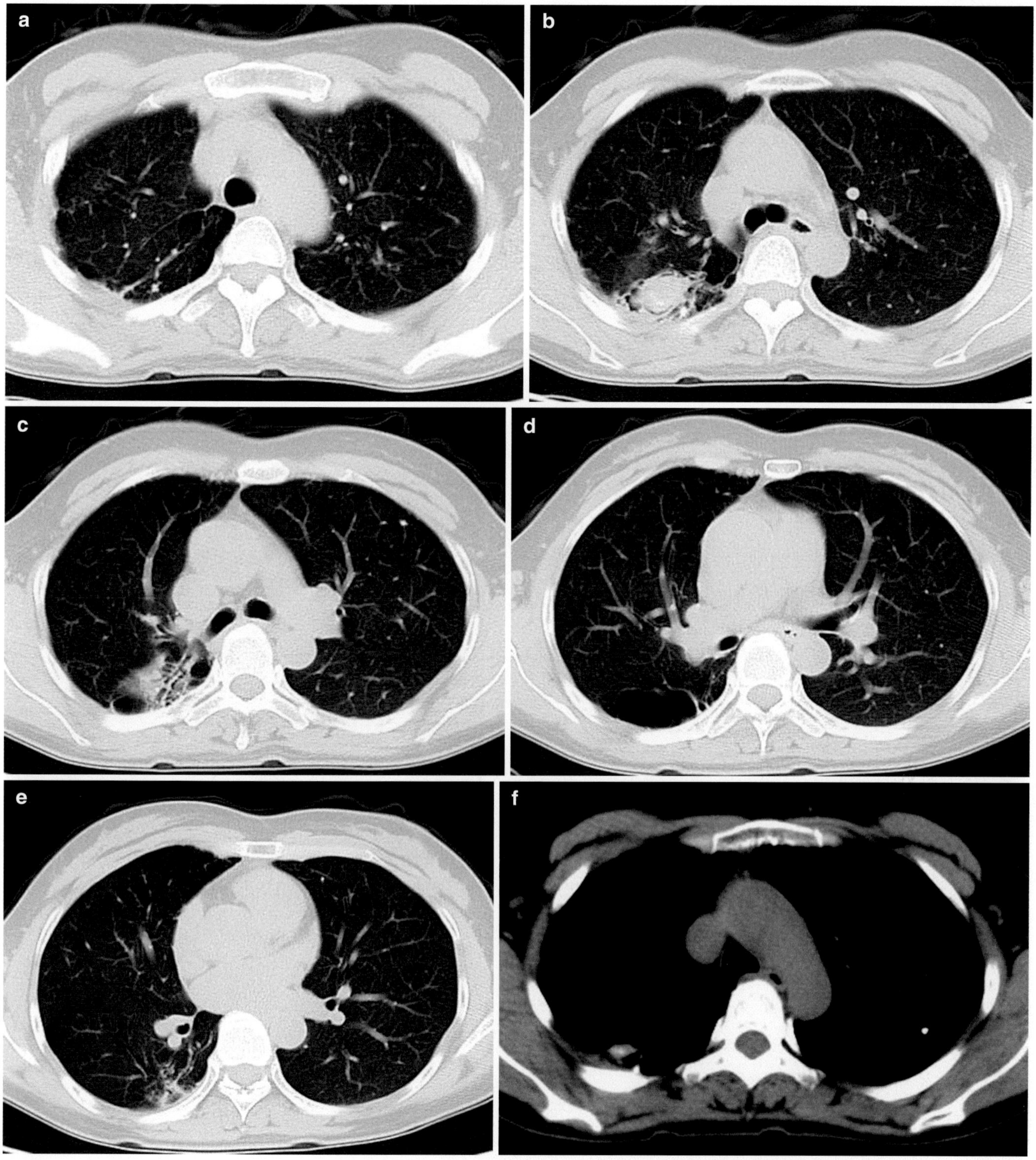

Fig. 10.8 (**a**–**g**) Chest CT scan. (**a**–**e**) The lung window demonstrates spots and cords opacity at both upper lung lobes, cavity opacity at the dorsal segment of the right lower lung lobe with nodular opacity, and crescent sign inside. Multiple small translucent areas inside the cavity are demonstrated. Local bronchiectasis and bilateral pleural thickening and adhesion are demonstrated. Bullae are demonstrated at the right upper lung lobe and dorsal segment of the right lower lung lobe. (**f**, **g**) The mediastinum window demonstrates dense nodular opacity at the right lung with spots of calcification inside, which is connected posteriorly with the pleura

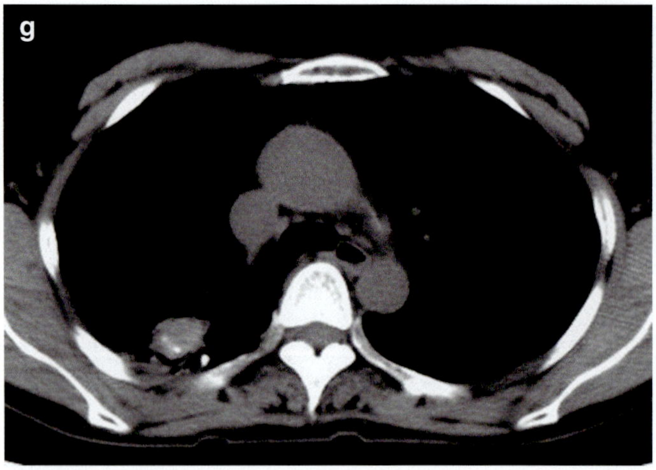

Fig. 10.8 (continued)

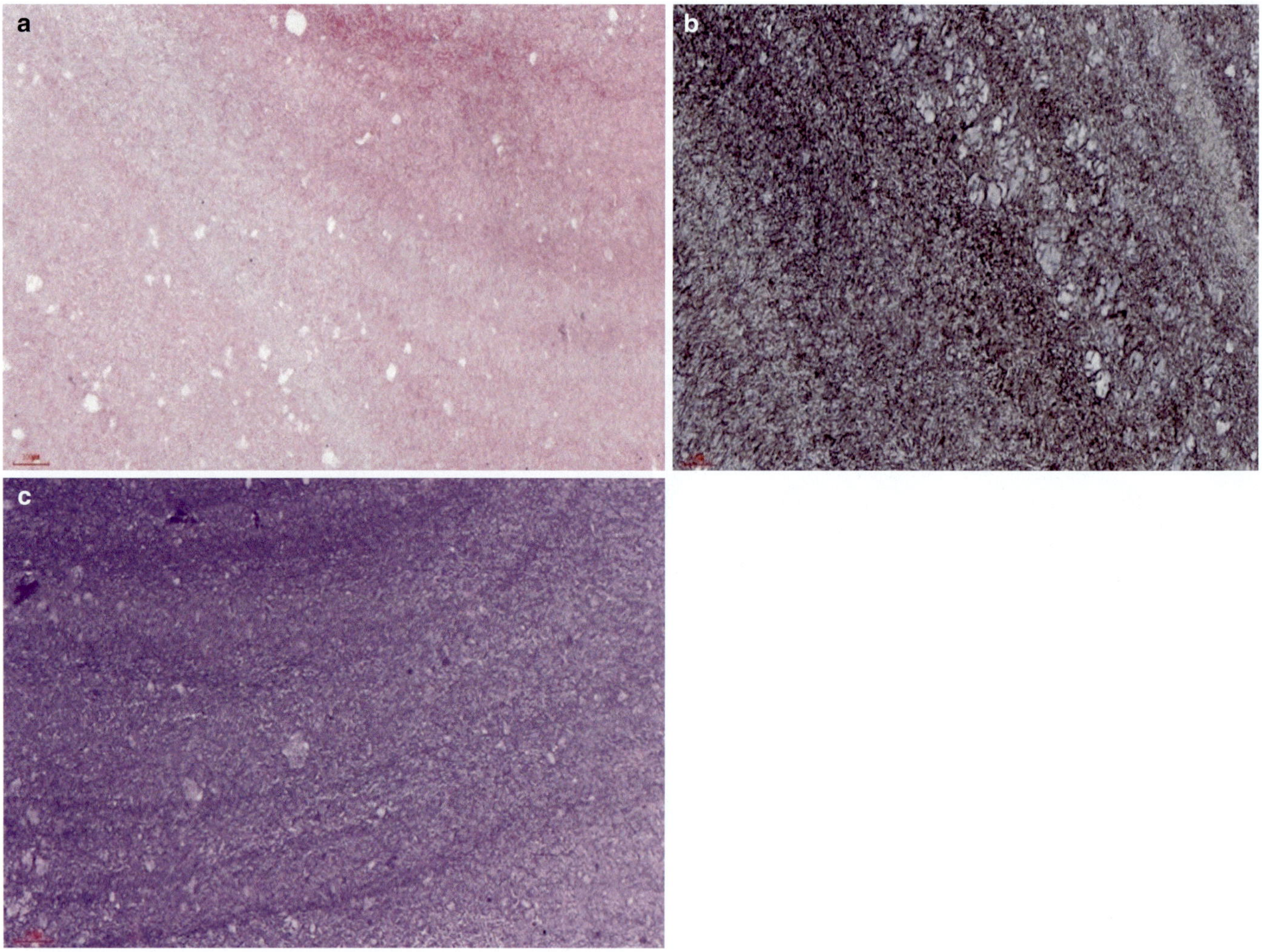

Fig. 10.9 (**a**–**c**) Pathology of lung tissue. (**a**) The hyphae wall of aspergillus is light purplish blue by H&E staining. (**b**) The hyphae wall and spores are brownish black by PASM staining. (**c**) The hyphae wall is in reddish purple by PAS staining

have a chronic progression, commonly affecting patients with potential lung disease. In patients with hyperactive immunity, the allergic reaction after inhalation of aspergillus can induce allergic bronchial pulmonary aspergillosis (ABPA) and serious fungal allergic asthma [18]. In this case, the patient had a past medical history of pulmonary tuberculosis. Chest CT scan on admission demonstrated lesions at both upper lung lobes and right lower lung lobe, among which spherical lesion at the posterior segment of the right upper lung lobe was demonstrated. Diagnosis on admission was suspected to be pulmonary tuberculosis. But postoperative pathology indicated pulmonary aspergilloma.

Pulmonary aspergilloma commonly occurs in cavity lesions of chronic lung diseases, such as bronchiectasis, purified cavity of pulmonary tuberculosis, or lung abscess. Pulmonary aspergilloma is a mixture of hyphae, cellular fragments, fibrin, and mucus. Its clinical manifestations include cough and expectoration. In some cases, hemoptysis occurs. The common affected sites include upper lung lobes and dorsal segment of lower lung lobes. Radiology demonstrates crescent-shaped translucent area due to space between aspergilloma and cavity wall, which is a characteristic radiological sign of pulmonary aspergillosis. Pulmonary aspergilloma should be differentiated from the following conditions: (1) tuberculoma, (2) cancerous cavity, (3) pulmonary hydatid cyst, (4) lung abscess, and (5) old blood clot in dilated bronchus.

In this case, the patient was initially diagnosed with pulmonary tuberculosis, which was mainly associated with the following factors: (1) her non-specific clinical manifestations of chronic cough, expectoration, chest distress, and chest pain, which resemble to those of pulmonary tuberculosis; (2) the same affected site as pulmonary tuberculosis, namely, the upper lung lobes; (3) formation of crescent sign after partial disappearance of caseous necrosis in the cases of pulmonary tuberculosis; (4) low-positive rates of sputum smear and culture for aspergillus and acid-fast bacillus and possible contamination of the specimens in the cases of sputum smear positive to aspergillus; and (5) a definitive past medical history of pulmonary tuberculosis and no basic disease that may compromise the immunity of the patient [19].

Surgery is indicated for patients with simplex aspergilloma and sufficient lung storage function. Lung lobectomy is the most common surgical procedure. In some cases, thoracoscopy can be performed to reduce hospitalization days. If thoracic adhesion occurs, complete thoracotomy is necessary. A previous research reported that the 10-year survival rate of simplex aspergilloma is 69–90% [20]. And the acknowledged surgical indications include the following: (1) The lesion of pulmonary aspergillosis is confined, the patient is symptomatic, and the condition is stable. (2) The diagnosis cannot be defined and carcinoma and other curable diseases cannot be excluded. (3) Surgical removal is predicted to improve the basic diseases of the patient. Lobectomy of the diseased lung is commonly performed, and segment removal or wedge removal is occasionally performed. Complete pneumonectomy should be avoided. In this case, the patient had a sufficient lung storage function. The nodular opacity at lungs cannot be differentiated from neoplasms, and lobectomy is indicated for her.

We summarized the diagnostic and therapeutic experience in this case as the following: (1) For patients with no obviously compromised immunity, pulmonary aspergillosis should be listed into differential diagnosis of common lung diseases. (2) For patients with cavity lesion, such as bronchiectasis, purified cavity of pulmonary tuberculosis, or lung abscess, the cavity is the site for formation of aspergillosis. The radiological data should be traced for differential diagnosis. (3) For the patients with sufficient lung storage function and local lesion that can hardly be differentiated from lung carcinoma and pulmonary tuberculosis, surgical operation can be considered. And the range of surgical removal should be decided based on the condition of the patient [21].

10.3.5 Comments

In this case, the patient was a young woman with her illness course prolonged for more than 1 year. CT scan in the outpatient department demonstrated spherical lesion at the posterior segment of the right upper lung lobe. The diagnosis was considered to be acid-fast mycobacteria infection. In addition to her past medical history of pulmonary tuberculosis, the patient was diagnosed with relapse of pulmonary tuberculosis. However, ESR, immunologic assay for tuberculosis, culture of alveolar lavage fluid, and fibrobronchoscopic brushing showed no evidence of pulmonary tuberculosis. For this case, the whole course of diagnosis and treatment was not unsmooth. And the finial diagnosis was defined to be pulmonary aspergilloma. We summarized the experience from the following key points:

1. The pathogenic aspergillus of pulmonary aspergillosis is mainly *Aspergillus fumigatus*, and its infection is mainly exogenous infection caused by inhalation of aspergillus spores into respiratory tract. Aspergillus is a conditional pathogenic fungus that fails to cause disease in immunocompetent individuals. However, when antituberculosis medication, hormones, and immunosuppressant are administered, human alveolar macrophages and neutrophile granulocytes show weakened ability to kill aspergillus spores and hyphae. At this time, aspergillus invades the cavity lesion at lungs or dilated cyst of the bronchus, where the hyphae reproduce to form mass. Their mixture with fibrin and mucous cells forms characteristic aspergilloma. In this case, the patient should be asked about

her housing for the possibility of inhaling aspergillus spores. An internationally published research reported that serum precipitin antibody is commonly positive in patients with aspergilloma, which constitutes an important basis for the diagnosis of aspergilloma. In well-equipped hospitals, the antibody assay should be performed.
2. For patients with a case history of chest distress and chest pain and radiological demonstrations of spherical lesion, rheumatic immune diseases, cancerous sarcoidosis, and parasitic cyst should also be considered. Relevant tests and examinations should be ordered.
3. Because the lesion is at the posterior segment of the upper lung lobe and bullae occur at the right upper lung lobe and dorsal segment of the right lower lung lobes, surgical removal of the spherical lesion and bullae should be considered for definitive diagnosis and treatment.
4. Currently, no consistent evidence has been found supporting the effectiveness of antifungal medication for aspergilloma. If singular aspergilloma is surgically removed, antifungal medication is unnecessary.

10.4 Case 4: Cough and Right Chest Pain for 5 Days

Yuemei Lu, Shusong Peng, Hongtao Jin, Jian Yang, Rong Huang, and Shi-Ping Wu

10.4.1 Presenting Complaint

Cough and right chest pain for 5 days.

10.4.2 Brief Case History

A 74-year-old man was admitted to our hospital due to complaints of cough and right chest pain for 5 days. Five days ago, the patient began to experience cough, expectoration with no sputum, and accompanying persistent right chest pain that aggravated when coughing or deep breathing. He also experienced palpitation, night sweat, and flush after noon. But he had no symptoms of aversion to cold, fever, breathlessness, and hemoptysis. He then took medication for inflammation (specifically unknown) by himself, but the symptoms were not improved. In another hospital, chest CT scan demonstrated space-occupying lesion at the posterior segment of the right upper lung lobe and possible complication of obstructive pneumonia. There were also mediastinal and the right hilar lymphadenectasis, pneumonia at the right middle lung lobe, and chronic bronchitis complicated by bullae at both upper lung lobes. For further diagnosis and treatment, he was admitted to the respiration department of our hospital on November 7, 2013.

10.4.2.1 Past Medical History

The patient had a past medical history of pulmonary tuberculosis in 1982 and was hospitalized to receive antituberculosis therapy for 6 months. After discharge, isoniazid, rifampicin, and ethambutol were administered for nearly 2 years. Since 1982, he had experienced hemoptysis of a small quantity for several times, but he paid no close attention to it.

10.4.2.2 Physical Examination

Physical examination showed a body temperature of 36.1 °C, respiration rate of 20/min, pulse rate of 64/min, and blood pressure of 174/84 mmHg. Both lungs showed bilaterally symmetric respiration movements, and vocal fremitus by palpation was bilaterally symmetric. By percussion, both lungs showed clear sounds. The respiration sounds were coarse, with wheezing sounds at the right upper lung lobe but no pleural rubs. The heart rate was 64/min, regular in rhythm. The valvular areas showed no pathological murmur by auscultation. The abdomen was soft, with no tenderness and rebound pain. Both lower limbs showed no edema.

10.4.2.3 Auxiliary Investigation

Laboratory Test

The routine blood test showed WBC 10.5×10^9/L, N 65.1%, and L 18.4%. The biomarkers for neoplasm were within normal limits. 1–3-β-D-Glucan test for fungus was 145.7 pg/ml, positive. The assays for antibodies of mycobacterium tuberculosis and mycoplasma pneumonia were negative. The sputum smear and culture showed no abnormalities. PPD skin test was positive. And the immunologic assay for tuberculosis was negative.

Radiology

Chest CT scan and enhanced chest CT scan were performed on November 14, 2013 (Fig. 10.10).

10.4.2.4 Initial Diagnosis

The initial diagnosis was nodule at the right lung, which was suspected to be tuberculosis, mycosis, or neoplasm.

10.4.3 Diagnosis and Treatment

After admission, ceftriaxone was administered via intravenous infusion for 1 week, but the symptoms were not improved. Bronchoscopy was performed on November 11, 2013, demonstrating granulation tissue and accompanying necrosis at the posterior segment of the bronchus of the right

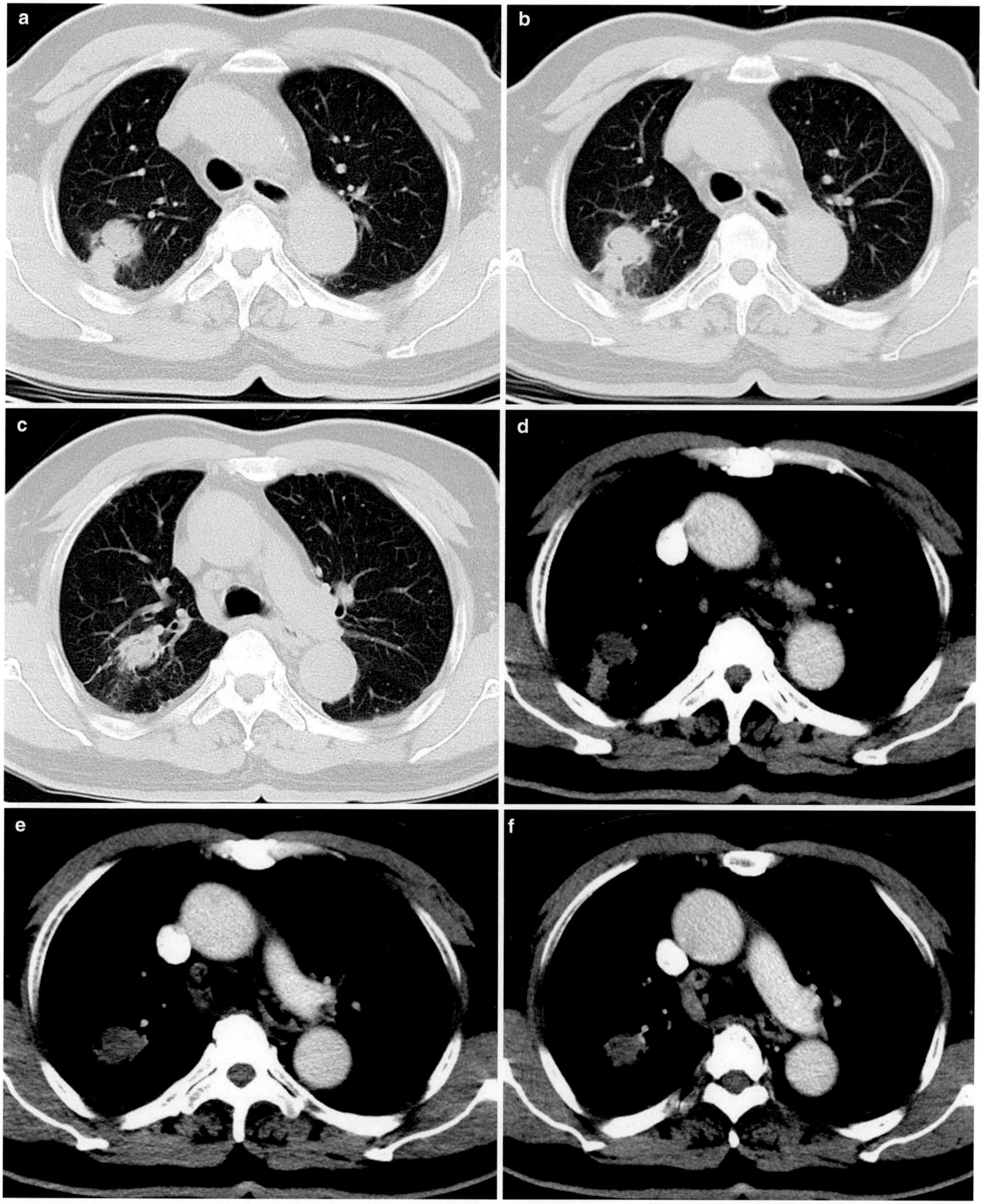

Fig. 10.10 (**a**–**f**) Chest CT scan. (**a**–**c**) The lung window demonstrates mass-like opacity at the right upper lung lobe with a size of about 3.2 cm × 2.5 cm. On its edge, patchy opacity and pleural adhesion are demonstrated. (**d**–**f**) Enhanced CT scan demonstrates mass-like opacity at the right upper lung with heterogeneous intensity and unobvious enhancement of the lesion

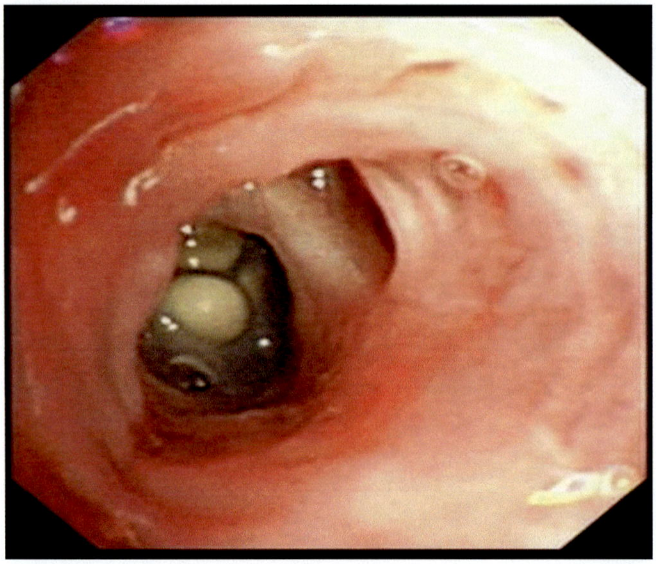

Fig. 10.11 Bronchoscopy. Granulation tissue and accompanying necrosis are demonstrated in the bronchus of the posterior segment at the right upper lung lobe

upper lung lobe (Fig. 10.11). Biopsy of the mucosa demonstrated well-differentiated bronchial mucosal epithelium, infiltration of many lymphocytes in interstitium, necrosis, and fungal mass (Fig. 10.12).

The final diagnosis was pulmonary aspergilloma.

Voriconazole was administered via intravenous infusion in a dose of 200 mg every 12 h for 1 week. The patient showed no symptoms of fever, cough, and chest pain. He was discharged on November 21, 2013. And oral intake of voriconazole was continued. Reexamination of chest CT scan on February 18, 2014, demonstrated mass-like opacity at the right upper lung lobe and crescent sign. Compared to the chest CT scan on November 17, 2013, the lesion was in almost the same size but with less surrounding exudation. The diagnosis was considered to be pulmonary aspergillus infection (Fig. 10.13). Due to unobvious absorption of the lesion, surgical operation was recommended. But the patient refused to receive surgical operation.

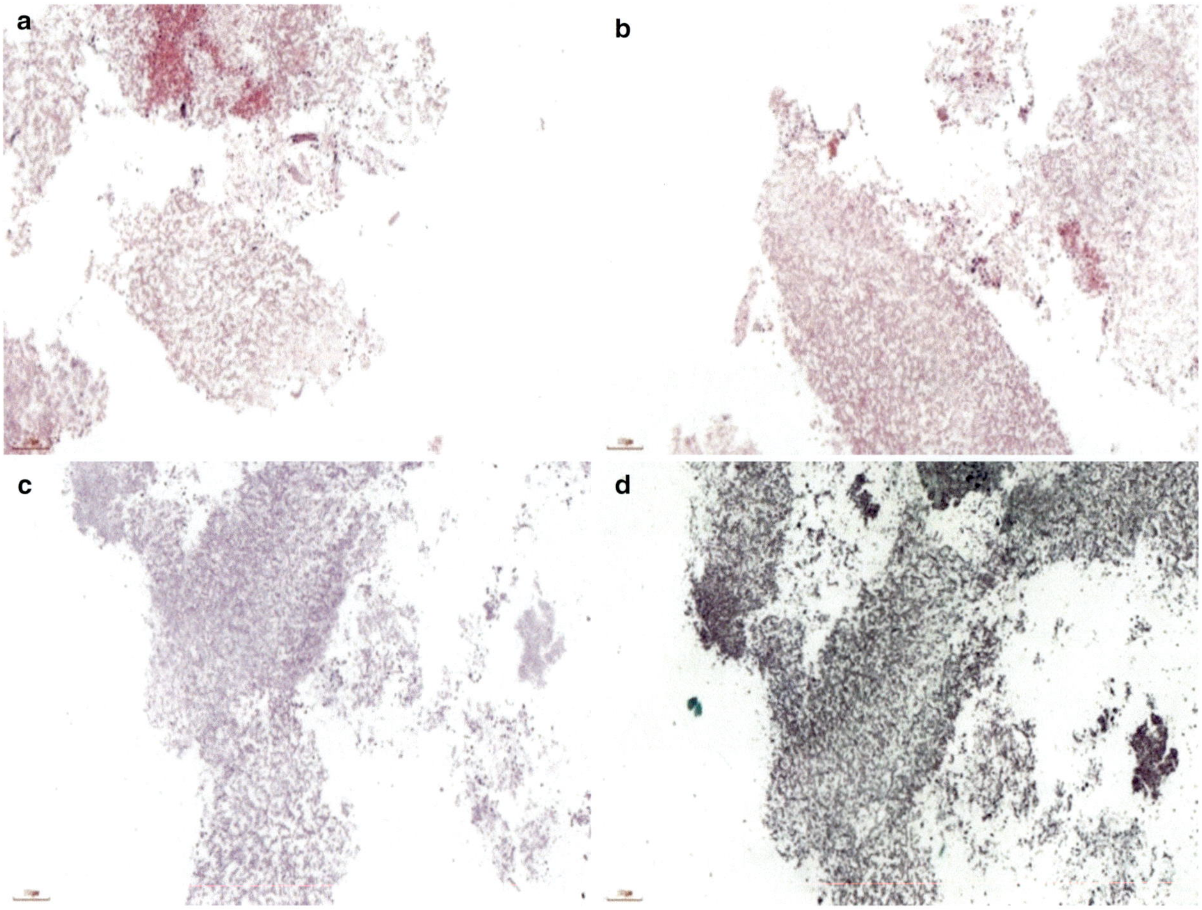

Fig. 10.12 (**a**–**d**) Pathology of the lung tissue. (**a**) Pathology demonstrates fungal hyphae at the bronchial mucosa (H&E staining). (**b**) Pathology demonstrates fungal hyphae at the bronchial mucosa (H&E staining). (**c**) PAS staining of the bronchial mucosa. (**d**) PASM staining of the bronchial mucosa

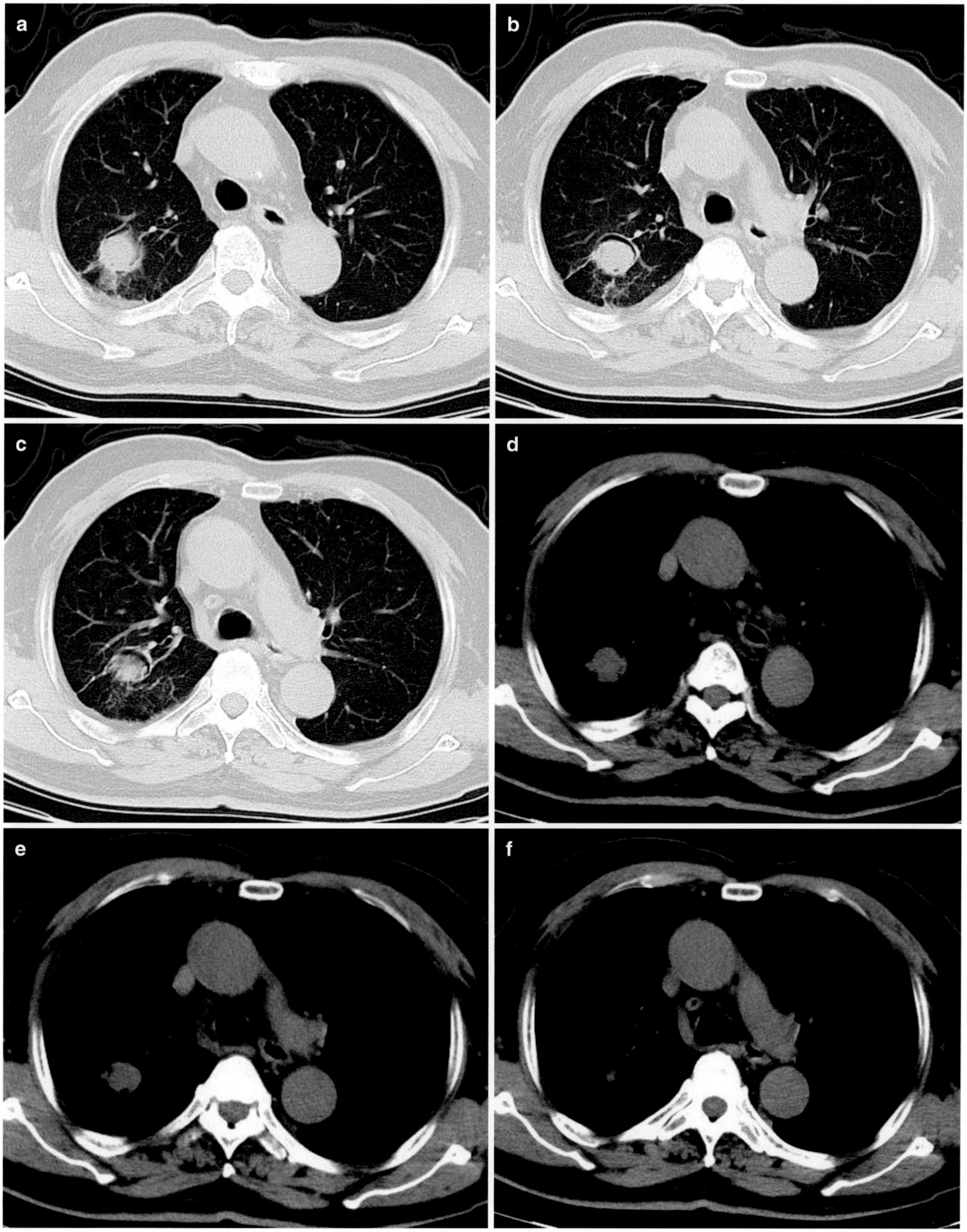

Fig. 10.13 (**a**–**f**) Chest CT scan. (**a**–**c**) The lung window demonstrates mass-like opacity at the right upper lung lobe and crescent sign. Compared to the chest CT scan on November 17, 2013, the lesion is in almost the same size but with less surrounding exudation. (**d**–**f**) The mediastinum window demonstrates lesion at the right upper lung with quite homogeneous intensity and quite well-defined boundary

10.4.4 Discussion

Along with extensive application of wide-spectrum antibiotics, hormones, and immunosuppressant, the incidence of aspergillus infection has been increasing [22]. So far, aspergillus has been the second common opportunistic fungus following candida and the top killer among various fungi. Aspergillus mainly parasitizes at the upper respiratory tract and is a conditional pathogenic fungus. It only causes aspergillus infection in individuals with compromised immunity or patients with long-term chronic basic disease. Based on the presence of basic disease and precipitating factor, aspergillosis is classified into primary aspergillosis and secondary aspergillosis.

Pulmonary aspergillosis is an acute or subacute and chronic inflammation of lung tissue caused by aspergillus. According to literature report, 96% of pulmonary aspergillosis is secondary aspergillosis, commonly secondary to chronic lung disease, such as pulmonary tuberculosis, lung abscess, lung neoplasm, and individuals with imbalanced flora or compromised immunity due to long-term use of antibiotics or antineoplasm. Denning et al. [23] systemically reviewed literature reports, and they found that 21% (Americans) to 35% (Chinese people of Taiwan) of patients with pulmonary tuberculosis shows lung cavity. And the patients of pulmonary aspergillosis account for about 22%. In this case, the patient suffered from aspergillus infection based on pulmonary tuberculosis. In combination with his repeated medication and a history of hemoptysis, it was believed that his pulmonary aspergillosis was related to compromised cellular immunity induced by pulmonary tuberculosis, imbalanced flora due to combined medications for tuberculosis, and structural change of the lung induced by pulmonary tuberculosis. Therefore, standard treatment for pulmonary tuberculosis is important.

The patients with pulmonary tuberculosis complicated by pulmonary aspergillus infection commonly experience no systemic symptoms. The common symptom is hemoptysis, and the other symptoms include fever, cough, expectoration, and chest pain. In this case, the patient had a past history of long-term hemoptysis, with recent symptoms of chest pain, cough, and night sweat. For its diagnosis, lung infection should be firstly considered, especially relapse of pulmonary tuberculosis. In addition, the patient was an elderly with weak immunity who belonged to high-risk population of fungal infection. Therefore, fungal infection should be considered for the diagnosis.

Currently, the diagnosis of pulmonary aspergillosis mainly depends on clinical symptoms, radiology, investigations for fungus, and pathology. The diagnosis can be defined by pathology. Chest X-ray and CT scan are the main ways for the diagnosis of pulmonary tuberculosis complicated by pulmonary aspergillosis. Clinically, patients with pulmonary tuberculosis complicated by pulmonary aspergillosis do not always show typical radiological demonstrations. And the atypical radiological demonstrations are diverse, which causes high rates of missed diagnosis and misdiagnosis. By chest CT scan and thin-layer CT scan, the definitive diagnostic rate of pulmonary tuberculosis complicated by pulmonary aspergillosis can be increased. G test is helpful in its diagnosis but false positive and false negative exist in clinical practice. In addition, the result of G test fails to differentiate aspergillus infection from candida infection. The sputum smear and culture for fungus are of clinical significance for its diagnosis. However, the positive rate of sputum investigations is low, and the specimen is susceptible to contamination. Positive findings for consecutive several times can define the diagnosis. By fibrobronchoscopy, the lesion can be directly observed, and the following pathology and etiological investigation facilitate its diagnosis. In this case, the diagnosis was defined by pathology following fibrobronchoscopy. Therefore, for patients with lung infection but with unfavorable therapeutic responses, fibrobronchoscopy should be routinely ordered.

The treatment of pulmonary aspergillosis remains controversial. The focus is the necessity of prophylactic surgery for asymptomatic patients and patients with slight symptoms. Currently, for patients with slight symptoms or occasional symptoms, conservative medications are recommended, including antifungal medication, hemostatic medication, and medication for primary disease. According to the reported clinical trials and medications, voriconazole is the medication of choice for pulmonary aspergillosis or disseminated pulmonary aspergillosis. The recommended dose is intravenous infusion of 6 mg/kg every 12 h twice, followed by intravenous infusion of 4 mg/kg every 12 h or oral intake of 4 mg/kg every 12 h [24, 25]. Amphotericin B and its liposomes, itraconazole, caspofungin, micafungin, and posaconazole can also be alternatives as initial or salvage therapy. In this case, voriconazole was administered after the diagnosis was defined to be pulmonary aspergillosis. The symptoms were then improved and the patient was discharged from the hospital.

10.4.5 Comments

Chronic pulmonary aspergillosis (CPA) is commonly secondary to chronic lung disease, such as pulmonary tuberculosis, lung abscess, bronchiectasis, and lung neoplasms. Mycobacterium tuberculosis infection may occur prior to or after CPA, or the two diseases may be concurrent. In this case, the patient had a past medical history of pulmonary tuberculosis. Prior to his admission to our hospital, chest CT scan demonstrated possible space-occupying lesion at the posterior segment of the right upper lung lobe. Reexamination of chest CT scan in our hospital demonstrated mass-like opacity at the right upper lung lobe in a size of about 3.2 cm × 2.5 cm. Clinically, the condition should be differentiated from pulmonary tuberculosis, lung neoplasm, and other pulmonary mycosis.

Aspergillus nodule is demonstrated as one or more nodules that are smaller than 3 cm with no cavity, which is a rare demonstration of CPA. Resembling to tuberculoma, lung carcinoma, lung metastasis, cryptococcus nodule, and coccidioidomycosis, it can only be defined by histopathology. In this case, the diagnosis was defined based on the findings of necrosis and fungus hyphae by bronchoscopy with following mucosa biopsy.

In this case, chest radiology demonstrated singular nodule at the lung during its early stage. Chest CT scan 3 months later demonstrated mass opacity at the right upper lung lobe and crescent sign. Therefore, in the cases of lung cavity or crescent sign based on the primary lesion, CPA should be suspected for the diagnosis.

Surgical removal of aspergilloma is the optimal treatment for pulmonary aspergilloma with accompanying hemoptysis. Complete removal of the aspergilloma and no leakage of fungal components into pleural cavity indicate a successful operation. Pulmonary aspergilloma rarely relapses after surgical removal of singular aspergilloma.

10.5 Case 5: Recurrent Cough for 4 Years and Breathlessness After Physical Activities for 1 Year That Aggravated for 1 Week

Jianfeng Zeng, Qunyi Deng, Jingjing Li, Chang'e Jin, Ying-Yun Fu, and Chen Qiu

10.5.1 Presenting Complaint

Recurrent cough for 4 years and breathlessness after physical activities for 1 year that aggravated for 1 week.

10.5.2 Brief Case History

A 61-year-old man was admitted to our hospital due to complaints of recurrent cough for 4 years and breathlessness after physical activities for 1 year that aggravated for 1 week. Four years ago, the patient began to experience paroxysmal cough, expectoration of yellowish green thick sputum, initially fever with the highest body temperature of 39 °C that was obvious after noon, and night sweat. But he experienced no aversion to cold, chill, chest pain, breathlessness, and hemoptysis. In another hospital, the sputum smear demonstrated acid-fast bacillus positive, and the diagnosis was secondary pulmonary tuberculosis. HRZE of antituberculosis therapy was given for 1 year. After the symptoms were improved, the patient discontinued the therapy. But he still experienced intermittent cough and expectoration of thick whitish sputum. One year ago, he began to experience chest distress and breathlessness that were obvious after physical activities. In a local hospital, intermittent anti-inflammatory therapy (specifically unknown) was given and the symptoms repeated. One week ago, the symptoms aggravated again, and he consulted in the outpatient department of our hospital and was hospitalized. Since the onset of the symptoms, he was in a generally good spiritual state, with quite good appetite and no obvious weight loss.

10.5.2.1 Past Medical History

Past physical fitness.

10.5.2.2 Physical Examination

Physical examination showed a body temperature of 36.2 °C, pulse rate 116/min, respiration rate 20/min, and blood pressure 109/72 mmHg. Barrel chest was present. The right lung showed slightly lower respiration sound, and the left lung showed coarse respiration sound. Both lungs showed no dry and/or moist rales by auscultation.

10.5.2.3 Auxiliary Investigations

Laboratory Test

In August 2011, the sputum smear for acid-fast bacillus showed (+++); TB-DNA showed positive; the sputum culture showed growth of mycobacteria, which was further identified to be human mycobacterium tuberculosis. The WBC was 7.32×10^9/L, neutrophile granulocytes 54.8%, lymphocytes 27%, hemoglobin concentration 139 g/L, and platelet count 323×10^9/L.

Radiology

Chest plain CT scan in July 2011 (Fig. 10.14) demonstrated shrinkage of the left upper lung lobe with honeycomb-like structure and patchy consolidation opacity inside. Some consolidation areas were demonstrated with air-filled bronchus opacity. And the other upper lung lobe and lower lung lobes were demonstrated with multiple scattering acinar nodules opacity as well as spots and flakes of opacity, which were heterogeneous in intensity and poorly defined. The medial segment of the right middle lung lobe was demonstrated with less cords opacity and spots of opacity.

Chest CT scan on February 11, 2012 (Fig. 10.15), demonstrated shrinkage of the left upper lung lobe with many patchy consolidation opacity, multiple cord opacities, and scattering acinar nodule opacity. The consolidation areas were demonstrated with air-filled bronchus opacity.

10.5.2.4 Initial Diagnosis

The initial diagnosis was pulmonary tuberculosis complicated by fungal infection.

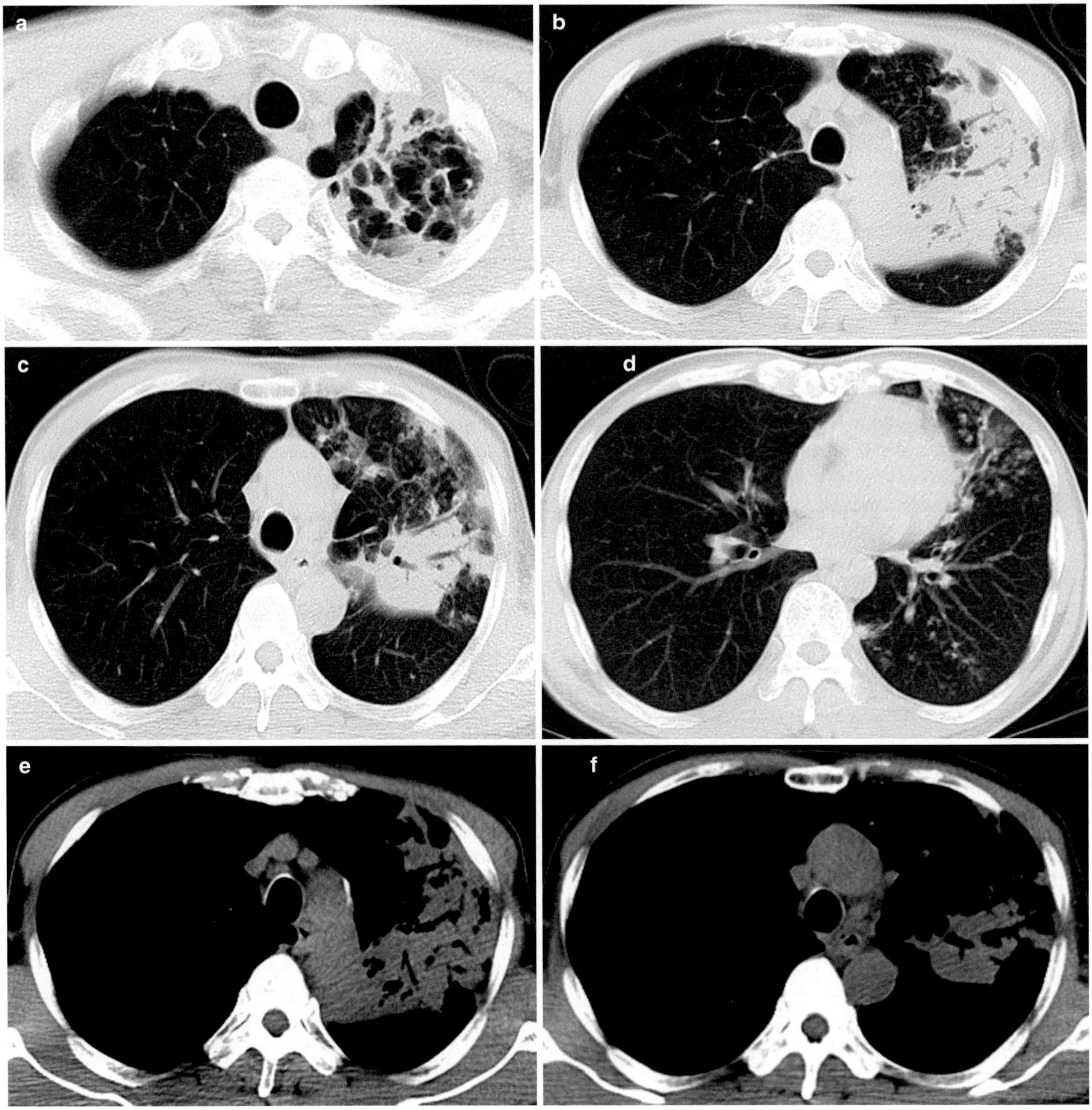

Fig. 10.14 (**a–f**) Chest CT scan. The left upper lung lobe is demonstrated with shrinkage with honeycomb-like structure and patchy consolidation. Some consolidation areas are demonstrated with air-filled bronchus opacity. The other upper lobes and lower lobes are demonstrated with multiple scattering acinar nodule opacities as well as spots and flakes of opacity, which are heterogeneous in intensity and poorly defined. The medial segment of the right middle lung lobe is demonstrated with less cords opacity and spots of opacity

10.5.3 Diagnosis and Treatment

After admission, cefamandole was administered for infection and mucosolvin for expectoration. However, the symptoms of cough and expectoration were not improved. During the hospitalization, 1–3-β-D Glucan was 88.14 pg/ml by the kinetic turbidimetric assay, and the ESR was 30 mm/h. Consecutive sputum smear for three times showed negative to acid-fast bacillus. TB-DNA for one time showed negative. The sputum cultures for common bacteria and fungi showed negative. Chest CT scan in February 2014 demonstrated patchy and nodular dense opacity at the left lung (Fig. 10.16).

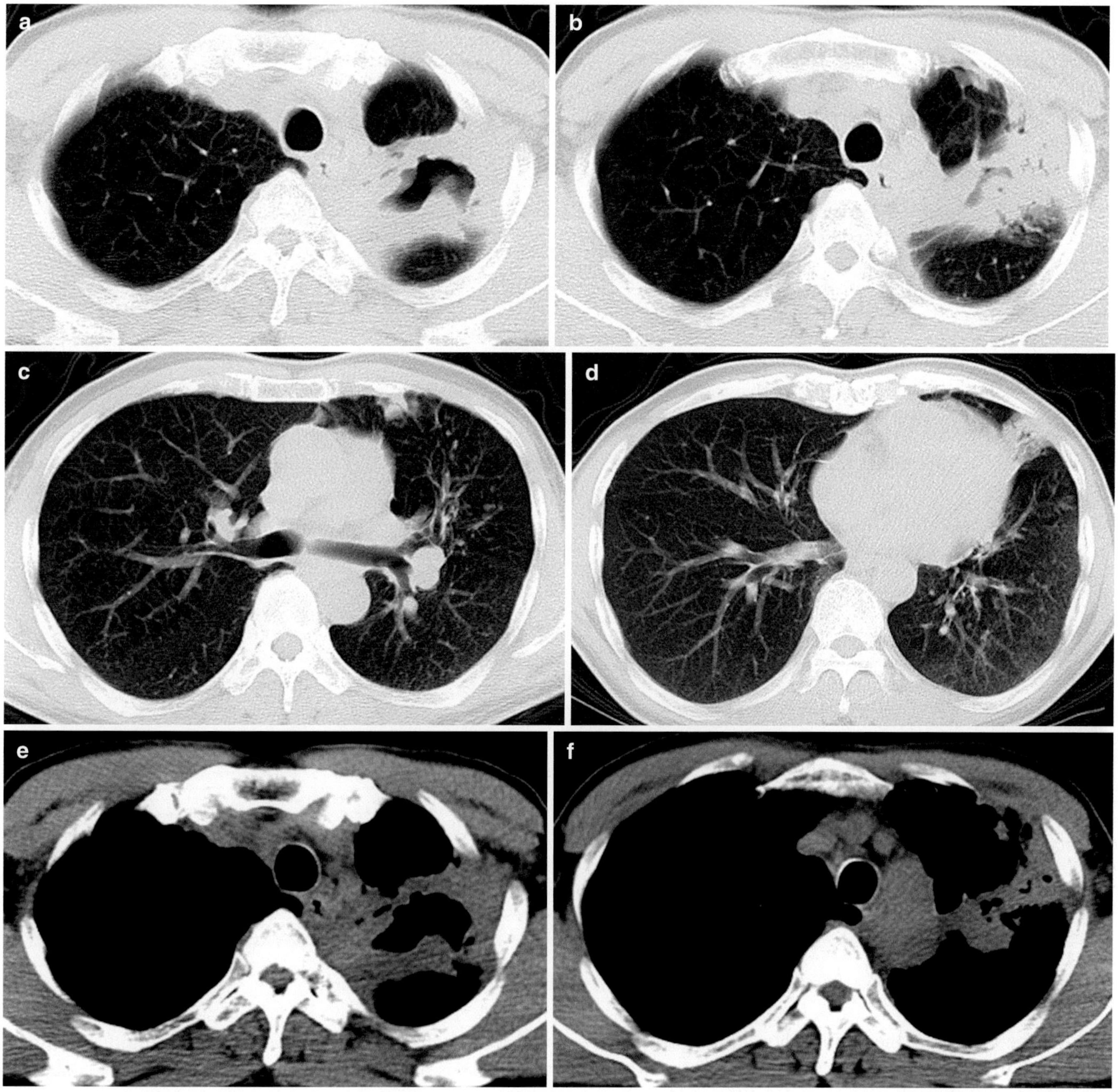

Fig. 10.15 (**a**–**f**) Chest CT scan. (**a**–**d**) The lung window demonstrates shrinkage of the left upper lung lobe with cavity opacity, multiple cords opacity, and scattering acinar nodule opacity inside. (**e**, **f**) The mediastinum window demonstrates cavity opacity at the left upper lung lobe, which connects with the mediastinum and lateral pleura

By the abovementioned medications, the symptoms were not improved. Due to insufficient evidence for active tuberculosis, secondary fungal infection cannot be excluded. After consultation with specialists from thoracic surgery department, aspergillus infection was considered, and surgical removal of the lesions was recommended. Thoracoscopy-assisted surgical removal of the left upper lung lobe was then performed under general anesthesia. The postoperative pathology demonstrated consolidation of most lung tissues, many caseous necrotic substances at the cavity wall, and surrounding scattering tuberculous nodules. Fungal mass was locally demonstrated that was negative by acid-fast staining and negative by methenamine silver staining (Fig. 10.17). The pathological diagnosis was pulmonary aspergillus infection and relapse of pulmonary tuberculosis.

The final diagnosis was pulmonary tuberculosis and aspergillus infection of the left upper lung.

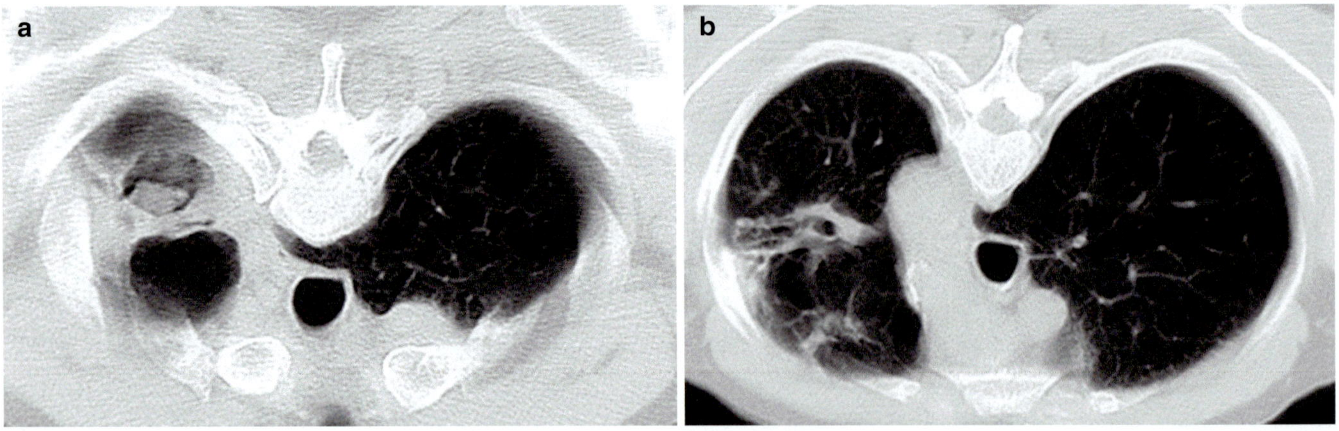

Fig. 10.16 (**a**, **b**) Chest CT scan. (**a**, **b**) Prone posterior-anterior scanning demonstrates patchy and nodular dense opacity at the left upper lung lobe. The patchy opacity is demonstrated with irregular translucent areas inside and the largest one in size of about 28 mm × 20 mm. At its medial dorsal part, a nodule is demonstrated with a size of about 18 mm × 12 mm that is adjacent to the anterolateral thorax. The left lower lung lobe is demonstrated with less scattering spots of nodular opacity

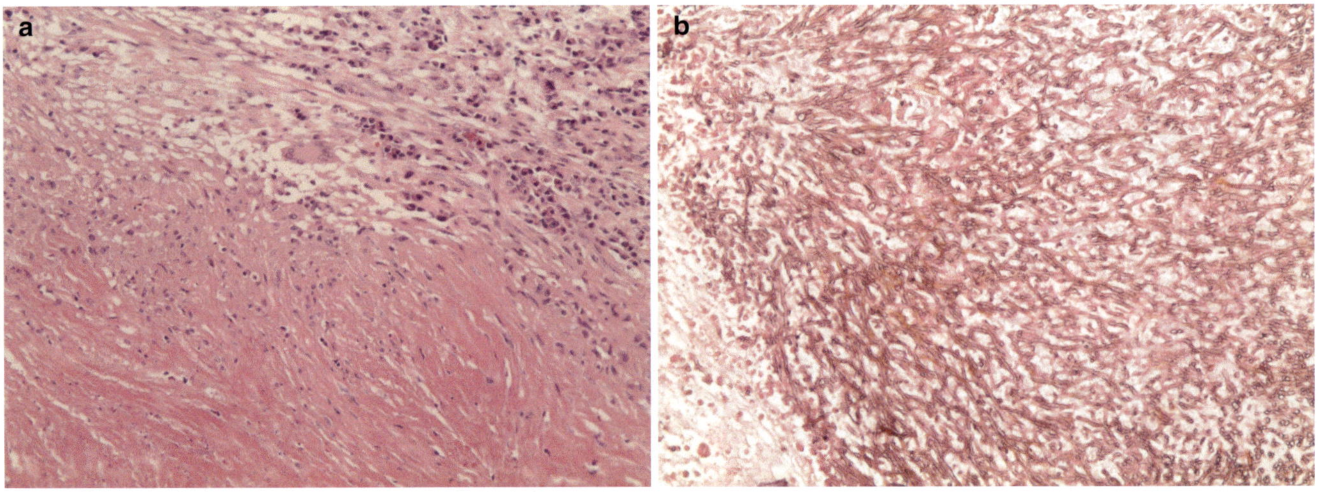

Fig. 10.17 (**a**, **b**) Pathology of the lung tissue. Many aspergillus mass at the cavity wall by H&E staining

After the operation, the patient showed favorable recovery. On May 24, he was discharged due to alleviated symptoms of cough and expectoration and stable condition.

10.5.4 Discussion

Aspergillus is one of the most common fungi in our living environment [26]. Aspergillus tends to infect open cavity, such as lung cavity induced by bronchiectasis, lung neoplasms, and pulmonary tuberculosis. Aspergillus infection secondary to these lung diseases mainly causes lesions of local invasive destruction. And in patients with compromised immunity, systemic infection occurs. In some cases, local infection may cause the formation of fungal sphere (aspergilloma), which is a characteristic mass of deranged hyphae, and accompanying fibrin exudation and infiltration of inflammatory cells in a small quantity that is commonly coated by fibrous tissue [27].

In this case, the patient experienced recurrent cough, expectoration, and hemoptysis. In the early stage of the disease, the sputum smear and culture demonstrated growth of mycobacteria tuberculosis. Chest CT scan demonstrated acinar nodular opacity and spots and flakes of opacity at the left upper lung with heterogeneous intensity. The medial segment of the right middle lung lobe was demonstrated with less cords opacity and spots of opacity. Along with antituberculosis therapy, the sputum smear and culture showed negative, with absorption of some lesions and formation of cavity at the left upper lung that had nodular opacity inside. Relapse of pulmonary tuberculosis, fungal infection, and even complicating neoplasm should be considered for the diagnosis. The cavity induced by tuberculosis is more common at the posteroapical segment of the upper lung and the dorsal segment of the lower lung. The cavity is commonly demonstrated as irregular thin wall cavity opacity with surrounding patchy and fibrous cords opacity. The edge of the cavity does not communicate with the bronchi. The lower lung is demonstrated with disseminating opacity of tuberculosis, and the mediastinum is demonstrated with calcified lymph nodes. In this case, reexamination of chest CT scan demonstrated newly emerged nodular opacity in the primary cavity induced by tuberculosis and crescent sign between nodular opacity and the inner wall of the cavity. The nodule in the cavity was movable along with posture change of the patient. The emergence of nodular opacity around the lesion of tuberculosis or small halo sign is radiologically consistent to pulmonary tuberculosis complicated by aspergillus infection. The following surgical removal of the left upper lung and the postoperative pathology demonstrated nodule of tuberculosis and aspergillus mass, supporting the diagnosis of pulmonary tuberculosis complicated by aspergillus infection.

When cough, expectoration, and hemoptysis recur in patients with a past medical history of pulmonary tuberculosis, it tends to be diagnosed as relapse of pulmonary tuberculosis. However, aspergillus infection also commonly occurs in the purified cavity after tuberculosis is stabled. In the cases with nodular opacity in the cavity and emergence of crescent-shaped translucent area, aspergillus infection should be highly suspected. Due to the low-positive rate of the sputum culture, being about 10–30%, characteristic signs by CT scanning such as halo sign, crescent sign, or newly emerged cavity are more significant for its early diagnosis. However, these radiological signs can be hardly differentiated from bronchiectasis and other lung cystic lesions. Surgical removal of the lesion should be considered for treatment and definitive diagnosis. In this case, the diagnosis was defined after surgical removal and postoperative pathology. The prognosis was favorable after the operation.

Active intravenous infusion of amphotericin B or voriconazole can be administered for pulmonary aspergillosis. Currently, voriconazole is believed to be the first-line medication for aspergillosis [28, 29], and surgical removal of the lesion facilitates the radical treatment of recurrent hemoptysis [30]. In this case, the patient was rapidly cured after operation, indicating successful treatment for him.

10.5.5 Comments

Pulmonary aspergillosis is commonly secondary to bronchopulmonary cyst, bronchiectasis, pulmonary abscess, or cavity induced by pulmonary tuberculosis. In this case, the patient suffered from pulmonary aspergilloma based on cavity induced by tuberculosis. The patient was a middle-aged man with no other medical histories of chronic diseases. Initially, he experienced cough, expectoration, and fever. The sputum smear and culture demonstrated positive to mycobacteria tuberculosis. In combination with the chest CT scan and the therapeutic efficacy, the diagnosis was defined to be secondary pulmonary tuberculosis. After the treatment, the patient still experienced cough and expectoration. Chest CT scanning in 2012 demonstrated cavitary pulmonary tuberculosis. By repeated sputum culture, mycobacteria tuberculosis infection resistant to medications was excluded. During the recent year, the patient experienced new symptoms, which was mainly breathlessness, and the condition was considered to be tuberculosis complicated by aspergillus infection. Due to non-specific symptoms, the condition may be misdiagnosed as relapse of pulmonary tuberculosis or other complicating bacterial infections.

Aspergillus tends to grow in cavities induced by chronic lung diseases, commonly chronic pulmonary tuberculosis, to form aspergilloma. A previous study from Britain has demonstrated that 14% of the patients with mycobacteria tuberculosis negative for 1 year by sputum smear or culture after antituberculosis therapy show aspergillus positive and 22% of the patients with mycobacteria tuberculosis negative for 4 years by sputum smear or culture after antituberculosis therapy show aspergillus positive. In this case, the patient received reexamination of chest CT scan in 2014, showing typical aspergilloma in cavity lesion. In combination with the results of pathology, the condition was diagnosed as chronic fibro-cavitary pulmonary tuberculosis complicated by aspergilloma. In the diagnosis and treatment of this case, we know that the condition of improved tuberculosis but new symptoms should be suspected to be aspergillus infection and chest CT scan and other investigations should be performed for the diagnosis.

Concerning the treatment, surgical removal of aspergilloma is the optimal choice for patients with sufficiently good pulmonary functions. This is a case of successful surgical operation for aspergilloma.

References

1. Sun Q. Diabetes complicated by lung infection in the elderly: an analysis of 42 cases. J Clin Respir. 2002;7(4):71.
2. Gallien S, Fournier S, Porcher R, et al. Therapeutic outcome and prognostic factors of invasive aspergillosis in an infectious infectious disease department: a review of 34 cases. Infection. 2008;36(6):533–8.
3. Garnacho-Montero J, Amaya-Villar R, Ortiz-Leyba C, et al. Isolation of Aspergillus spp. from the respiratory tract in critically ill patients: risk factors, clinical presentation and outcome. Crit Care. 2005;9(3):R191–9.

4. De Rosa FG, Terragni P, Pasero D, et al. Combination antifungal treatment of pseudomembranous tracheobronchial invasive: a case report. Intensive Care Med. 2009;35(9):1641–3.
5. Komase Y, Kunishima H, Yamaguchi H, et al. Rapidly progressive invasive pulmonary aspergillosis in a diabetic man. J Infect Chemother. 2007;13(1):46–50.
6. Limper AH, Knox KS, Sarosi GA, et al. An official American Thoracic Society Statement: treatment of fungal infections in adult pulmonary and critical care patients. Am J Respir Care Med. 2011;183(1):96–128.
7. Sarrafzadeh SA, Hoseinpoor RA, Ardanlan M, et al. The accuracy of serum galactomannan assay in diagnosing invasive pulmonary aspergillosis. Iran J Allergy Asthma Immunol. 2010;9(3):149–55.
8. Nguyen MH, Jaber R, Leather HL, et al. Use of bronchoalveolar lavage to detect galactomannan for diagnosis of pulmonary aspergillosis among nonimmunocompromised hosts. J Clin Microbiol. 2007;45(9):2787–92.
9. Sanguinetti M, Posteraro B, Pagano L, et al. Comparison of real-time PCR, conventional PCR, and galactomannan antigen detection by enzyme-linked immunosorbent assay using bronchoalveolar lavage fluid samples from hematology patients for diagnosis of invasive pulmonary aspergillosis. J Clin Microbiol. 2003;41(8):3922–5.
10. Infection Team of Respiration Branch, Chinese Medical Society and the Editorial Committee of Chinese Journal of Tuberculosis and Respiration. Consensus on clinical diagnosis and treatment of pulmonary mycosis. Chin J Tuberc Respir. 2007;11(30):821–34.
11. Qin Q. Clinical mycology. Shanghai: Fudan University Press; 2001. p. 401–30.
12. Leeflang MM, Debets-Ossenkopp YJ, Visser CE, et al. Galactomannan detection for invasive aspergillosis in immunocompromised patients. Cochrane Database Syst Rev. 2008;(4):CD007394.
13. Park SY, Lee SO, Choi SH, et al. Serum and bronchoalveolar lavage fluid galactomannan assays in patients with pulmonary aspergilloma. Clin Infect Dis. 2011;52(7):e149–52.
14. Zou M, Tang L, Zhao S, et al. Systematic review and meta-analysis of detecting galactomannan in bronchoalveolar lavage fluid for diagnosing invasive aspergillosis. PLoS One. 2012;7(8):e43347.
15. Hartman TE. CT of cystic diseases of the lung. Radiol Clin N Am. 2001;39(6):1231–43.
16. Limper AH, knox KS, Sarosi GA, et al. American thoracic society fungal working group. An official American thoracic society statement: treatment of fungal infections in adult pulmonary and critical care patients. Am J Respir Crit Care Med. 2011;183:96–128.
17. Lee JK, Lee YJ, Park SS, et al. Clinical course and prognostic factors of pulmonary aspergilloma. Respirology. 2014;19(7):1066–72.
18. Kosmidis C, Denning DW. The clinical spectrum of pulmonary aspergillosis. Thorax. 2015;70(3):270–27.
19. Zhang H, Zhang H, Han Z, et al. Misdiagnosis of pulmonary aspergillosis as pulmonary tuberculosis: an analysis of 31 cases. Chin J Tuberc Prev. 2005;27(3):143–7.
20. Muniappan A, Tapias LF, Butala P, et al. Surgical therapy of pulmonary aspergillomas: a 30-year North American experience. Ann Thorac Surg. 2014;97:432–8.
21. Ba PS, Ndiaye A, Diatta S, et al. Results of surgical treatment for pulmonary aspergilloma. Med Sante Trop. 2015;25(1):92–6.
22. Cen Y, Xu J, Lin J. Clinical pathology of pulmonary aspergillosis: an analysis of 30 cases. J Clin Misdiagn Ther Error. 2009;22(6):19–20.
23. Denning DW, Pleuvry A, Cole DC. Global burden of chronic pulmonary aspergillosis as a sequel to pulmonary tuberculosis. Bull WHO. 2011;89(12):864–72.
24. Working Group for Invasive Fungus Infection in China. The 2013 diagnostic standards and therapeutic principles for invasive mycosis complicating hematonosis/malignancies (the 4th edition). Chin J Intern Med. 2013;52(8):704–9.
25. Limper AH, Knox KS, Sarosi GA, et al. An official American Thoracic Society statement: treatment of fungal infections in adult pulmonary and critical care patients. Am J Respir Crit Care Med. 2011;183(1):96–128.
26. Zhu X. Rare CT signs of thoracic disease. Beijing: People's Medical Publishing House; 2007.
27. Zhang C, Sun C, Cui J. Surgical treatment of pulmonary aspergillosis: report of 31 cases. Chin J Hosp Infect. 2013;23(1):89–90.
28. Zeng W, Zhang X. Interpretations of the 2008 clinical guideline for diagnosis and treatment of aspergillosis by IDSA. Chin J Evid Based Med. 2015;15(7):767–71.
29. Tang S. Clinical tuberculosis. Beijing: People's Medical Publishing House; 2011.
30. Zhang Q, Kong J, Wu Y, et al. Clinical analysis of different types of pulmonary aspergillosis. Chin J Hosp Infect. 2013;23(24):5991–3.

Pulmonary Aspergillosis with Presenting Symptom of Fever

11

Pu-Xuan Lu and Ling-Wei Wang

In the clinical guideline for the diagnosis and treatment of aspergillosis issued by the IDSA, pulmonary aspergillosis is classified into three clinical types: chronic pulmonary aspergillosis (CPA) (including parasitic pulmonary aspergilloma), allergic pulmonary aspergillosis (APS), and invasive pulmonary aspergillosis (IPA). From the perspectives of incidence, mortality, and hazard, IPA is undoubtedly the most important type of pulmonary aspergillosis.

The consensus on diagnosis and treatment of pulmonary aspergillosis issued by Respiration Branch of Chinese Medical Society indicated that invasiveness refers to direct invasion of the fungi to the lung or bronchus to cause acute or chronic histopathological lesions with exclusion of lung lesions induced by fungal parasitism and allergy. That is to say, the definitive diagnosis of IPA depends on histopathological evidence of aspergillus hyphae or spores at the lung parenchyma or basilar membrane of the airway, which is also the basis for its differential diagnosis from other types of pulmonary aspergillosis.

IPA is commonly secondary to immunosuppression, for instance, in patients with or receiving persistent granular cell deficiency, allogeneic hematopoietic stem cell transplantation (HSCT), solid organ transplantation (SOT), primary or acquired immunodeficiency syndrome, large dosage of glucocorticoid, or other immunosuppressants. IPA also occurs in immunocompetent populations but the incidence is low. The occupational and environmental factors play important role in occurrence of IPA because IPA occurs after inhalation of a large quantity of aspergillus spores within a short period of time. Clinically, IPA is further classified into acute invasive tracheobronchitis, acute invasive pulmonary aspergillosis, and subacute invasive pulmonary aspergillosis (formerly known as chronic necrotizing pulmonary aspergillosis or semi-invasive pulmonary aspergillosis).

In this section, we introduce nine cases of pulmonary aspergillosis with presenting symptom of fever, all of which are acute IPA or subacute invasive pulmonary aspergillosis. From these cases, we know that fever is the main clinical manifestation of IPA. According to literature report, about 40% of the patients with IPA manifest only as fever and even no typical respiratory symptoms. The fever is high-grade fever or irregular fever, accompanied by different degrees of hemoptysis, cough, and expectoration of thick sputum. The pathological basis is that IPA induces infiltrative inflammation, localized granuloma, or tissue necrosis and suppuration which further develop into multiple small abscesses. In addition, fever in patients with IPA may be induced by aspergillus infection itself and concurrent bacterial or other pathogen infections. IPA should be suspected in the cases with or exposed to high-risk factors, fever, unfavorable therapeutic efficacy by wide-spectrum antibiotics, radiological halo sign, consolidation, buds-in-tree sign, and air crescent sign.

The corresponding author of section 11.1 is Jiaxuan Zhou, Email: 195137680@qq.com.
The corresponding author of section 11.2 is Lukun Zhang, Email: 271687978@qq.com.
The corresponding author of section 11.3 is Yulin He, Email: 33heyulin@163.com.
The corresponding author of section 11.4 is Budong Chen, Email: budongchen@sina.com.
The corresponding author of section 11.5 is Chengying Hong, Email: hcy2184with@hotmail.com.
The corresponding author of section 11.6 is Wei Gao, Email: gaomol@sina.com.
The corresponding author of section 11.7 is Mengjie Feng, Email: zwjfmj@163.com.
The corresponding author of section 11.8 is Zhengqiang He, Email: hzqxqyy@163.com.
The corresponding author of section 11.9 is Zhengqiang He, Email: hzqxqyy@163.com.

P.-X. Lu (✉)
Centre for Chronic Diseases Control of Shenzhen, Shenzhen, Guangdong, China

L.-W. Wang
Second Clinical Medical College of Jinan University, Shenzhen, Guangdong, China

C. Qiu et al. (eds.), *Pulmonary Aspergillosis*, https://doi.org/10.1007/978-981-13-3435-1_11

According to the diagnostic criteria and treatment principles of invasive pulmonary fungal infection, IPA should be diagnosed by grading diagnosis. Based on host (risk) factors, clinical manifestations, microbiology, and histopathology, the diagnosis of IPA is graded into suspected diagnosis, clinical diagnosis, and definitive diagnosis. It should be noted that the blood culture positive for aspergillus should exclude the possibility of specimen contamination. Concerning laboratory tests, the 2016 clinical guideline issued by the IDSA indicated that GM test of the serum and bronchoalveolar lavage fluid (BALF) is the accurate biomarker of IPA in specific populations, such as patients with or receiving hematopoietic malignancies and allogeneic HSCT. The serum GM test has a sensitivity of up to about 70%, and in patients with or receiving SOT, pulmonary aspergilloma, and chronic pulmonary aspergillosis, its sensitivity is 20%, 38%, and 23%, respectively. The sensitivity of BALF GM test in above populations exceeds 70%. Clinically, false positive and false negative should be excluded in serum or BALF GM test in combination with the clinical manifestations. (1,3)-β-ᴅ Glucan is the polysaccharide component of yeast and the cell wall of filiform fungus, accounting for above 50% of the fungus cell wall. G test is applicable for the diagnosis of various invasive mycoses excluding cryptococcosis and zygomycosis but incapable of their differentiation. Therefore, the G test has limited value in the diagnosis of IPA with presenting symptom of fever. It needs to be combined with GM test for the identification of invasive aspergillus infection. In general, a comprehensive analysis of clinical manifestations, radiological demonstrations, laboratory tests, microbiology, and histopathology should be performed for the diagnosis of IPA.

In this section, we analyze and comment on pulmonary aspergillosis with presenting symptom of fever. In the diagnosis and treatment of IPA, the clinicians should know the following two points: (1) IPA is an important infection in patients with hematologic malignancies and other populations at high risks. Fever with unfavorable therapeutic responses by wide-spectrum antibiotics in such populations should be high suspected as IPA. Serum or BALF GM test is the accurate biomarker for the diagnosis of IPA in populations with or receiving granular cell deficiency and HSCT. (2) Cases of primary IPA are increasingly reported in the community with no exposure to high risk factors. Its definitive diagnosis should be based on clinical manifestations, microbiology, and histopathology. In such patients serum GM test shows a low positive rate, but BALF GM test has a high diagnostic value. However, false positive should be noted. Presence of infection should not be based only on the diagnostic threshold value, and the clinicians should also consider the host (risk) factors and the clinical manifestations. For the cases with no clinical symptoms but GM value above 1.5 pg/ml, close observation and follow-ups can be performed. For the cases with or exposed to high risk factors or clinical symptoms but a GM value of 0.5 pg/ml, trial medication should be given as early as possible. Dynamic monitoring of GM value shows greater clinical significance.

Patients' consents have been obtained for images or other clinical information relating to the cases to be published.

11.1 Case 1: Cough, Expectoration, Fever and Accompanying Breathlessness for 20 Days

Jiaxuan Zhou, Qingsi Zeng, Jingjing Li, Xuemei Han, Mengjie Feng, and Shi-Ping Wu

11.1.1 Presenting Complaints

Cough, expectoration, fever, and accompanying breathlessness for 20 days.

11.1.2 Brief Case History

A 59-year-old woman was admitted to our hospital on August 14, 2012, due to chief complaints of cough, expectoration, fever, and accompanying breathlessness for 20 days. Twenty days ago, the patient began to experience running nose and sneezing due to catching a cold, followed by cough, expectoration of yellowish thick sputum in a large quantity, fever (with the highest body temperature of 39.7 °C), aversion to cold, and breathlessness after physical activities. She had been hospitalized in a local hospital and given medications (specifically unknown). During her hospitalization, she had experienced hemoptysis of fresh red blood in a large quantity. And the patient was transferred to our hospital due to unfavorable therapeutic efficacy. Since the onset of the symptoms, she was in quite good spiritual state, with normal appetite but a weight loss of about 1 kg during the recent 1 month.

11.1.2.1 Past Medical History

The patient had a medical history of hypertension for 4 years and had been receiving tablets of Double oxazine reserpine and nitrendipine for her hypertension. And she has a medical history of diabetes for 15 days, with the highest blood sugar of 21.3 μmol/L, and the treatment was unknown. She had no habitual smoking and drinking.

11.1.2.2 Physical Examination

Physical examination showed a body temperature of 38.7 °C, a pulse rate 119/min, respiration rate 22/min, and blood pressure 117/73 mmHg. She was typically developed with moderate nourishment. The patient was conscious, with smooth respirations and active position. She can answer the questions and well cooperated in the physical examinations. The skin mucosa showed no yellowish stain. And the systemic superficial lymph nodes were not palpable. By percussion, the middle and lower lungs showed dull resonance. By auscultation, the bilateral middle and lower lungs showed dry and moist rales. The heart was not enlarged, with regular heartbeat of 119/min and no pathological murmur. The abdomen was soft, with an unpalpable liver and spleen. The shifting dullness was negative. The liver and kidney areas were not sensitive to percussion. The bowel sounds were normal.

11.1.2.3 Auxiliary Investigations

Chest CT scan on July 22, 2012, in another hospital demonstrated infection of both lungs, which was considered to be fungal infection. And tuberculosis was to be differentiated.

11.1.2.4 Initial Diagnosis

The initial diagnosis was fungal infection of the lungs and/or pulmonary tuberculosis.

11.1.3 Diagnosis and Treatment

After admission, the investigations were performed. Routine blood test showed WBC 13.6 × 10^9/L and neutrophil granulocytes 83.5%. The ESR was 115 mm/h (normal range lower than 20 mm/h). The serum procalcitonin was 0.43 ng/ml (normal range lower than 0.05 ng/ml). Cryptococcal antigen was negative. And quantification of fungal 1-3-β-D glucan was lower than 10 pg/ml. The *Mycoplasma hyopneumoniae* antibody was negative; *Mycobacterium tuberculosis* antibody was negative by golden standard method.

Chest anterior-posterior X-ray on August 15, 2012, demonstrated poorly defined patchy and large flake of high-intensity opacity at the right middle and lower lung fields and the left lower lung field. Both lower lung fields were demonstrated with multiple thick wall cavity, some of which had gas liquid level. The right costophrenic angle was absent (Fig. 11.1). The diagnosis was suspected to be cystoid bronchiectasis, pulmonary abscess, or pulmonary cyst complicated by infection.

After admission, the patient was given medication for infection and blood sugar control and symptomatic medications for cough and expectoration. Chest CT scanning on August 16, 2012, demonstrated multiple thick wall cavities at both lungs, and the thickness of cavity wall was about 9 mm. Some cavities were demonstrated with liquid level and some cavities with irregular inner wall and linear septa. The parenchyma of the other parts of the lungs was demonstrated with scattering poorly defined patchy and small nodular opacity, most of which showed halo sign. The hila of both lungs were demonstrated with no enlarged lymph nodes and the mediastinum with multiple lymph nodes whose short diameter of the larger ones was 1.2 cm. Both inferior pleura were demonstrated to be slightly thickened with less opacity of liquid intensity (Fig. 11.2). The diagnosis was considered to be invasive pulmonary aspergillosis.

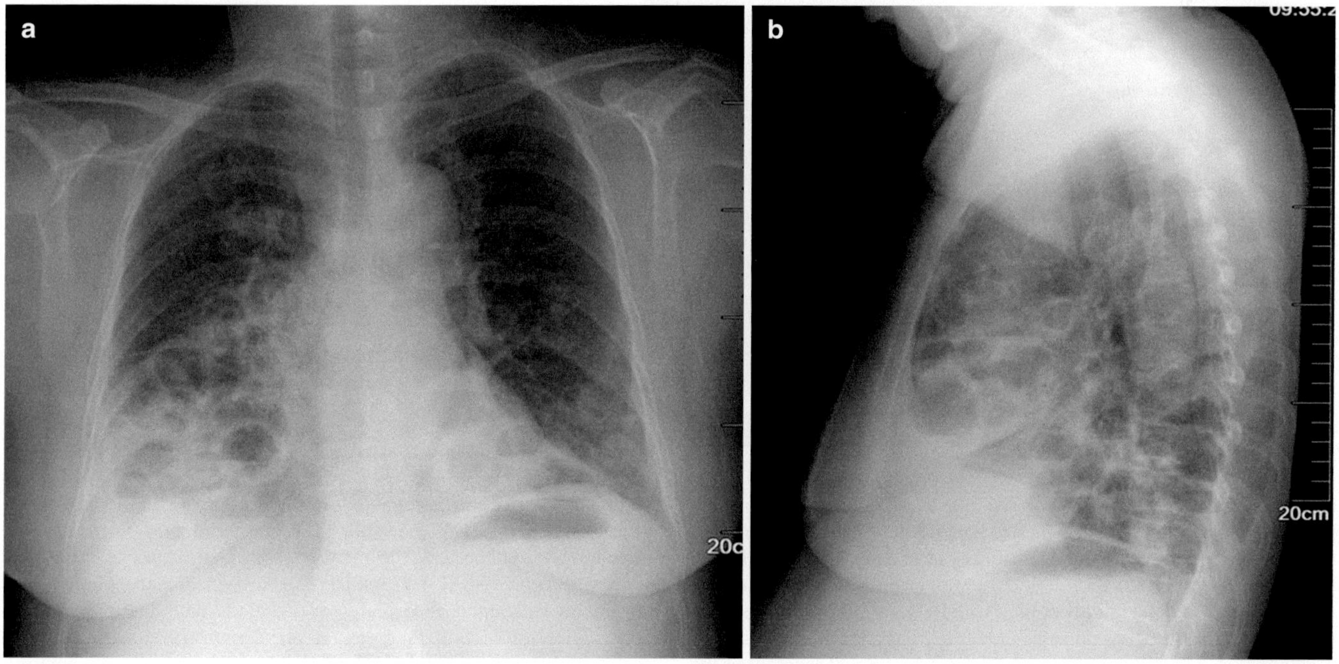

Fig. 11.1 (**a**, **b**) Chest anterior-posterior and lateral CT scan. (**a**, **b**) The right middle and lower lung fields and the left lower lung field are demonstrated with poorly defined patchy and large flakes of opacity. Both lungs are demonstrated with multiple thick wall cavities, some of which showed liquid level. The right costophrenic angle is absent

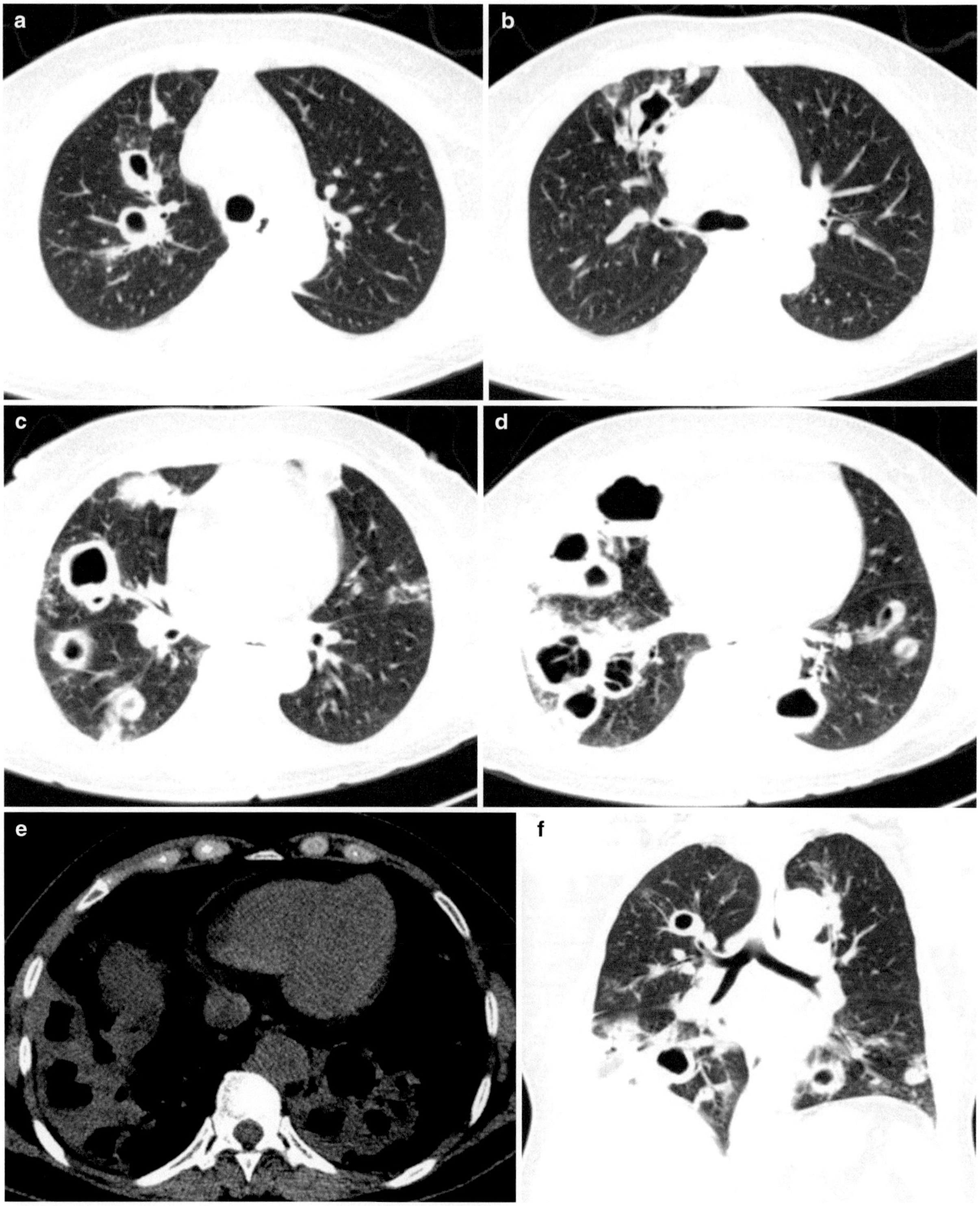

Fig. 11.2 (**a**–**f**) Chest CT scan. (**a**) The lung window demonstrates thick wall cavity at the right upper lung with smooth inner wall. The anterior segment is demonstrated with small flakes of consolidation. (**b**–**d**) The lung window demonstrates multiple thick wall cavities at the right middle and lower lung and the left lower lung with irregular inner wall, some of which show fine linear septum and liquid level. The edge of some cavities is demonstrated to be poorly defined. The inferior lingual segment of the left upper lung and the basilar segment of both lower lungs are demonstrated with nodular opacity, some of which show accompanying halo sign. (**e**) The mediastinum window of plain scanning demonstrates multiple thick wall cavities at both lower lungs. The right lesions are connected with the posterolateral thoracic wall, and the lesions at the left lower lung are connected with medial mediastinal pleura. (**f**) The lung window of coronal MPR demonstrates the basilar segments of both lower lungs with subpleural flakes of consolidations and multiple cavities inside. The surrounding lung tissues are demonstrated with multiple small nodular opacities and poorly defined patchy opacity. The anterior medial basilar segment of the left lower lung is demonstrated with nodules and small cavities inside

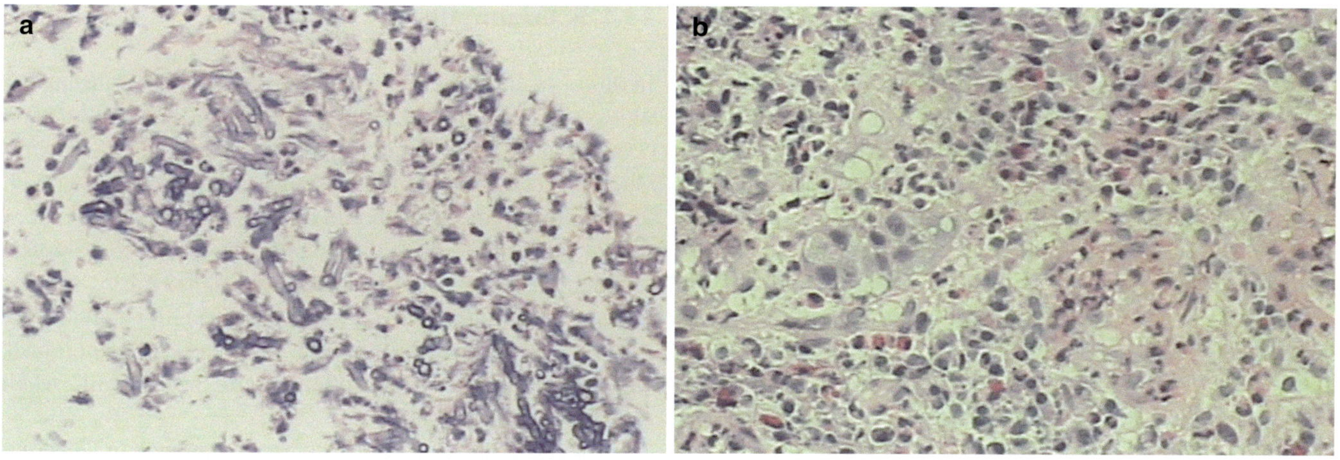

Fig. 11.3 (**a**, **b**) Histopathology of the lung tissue

To further define the diagnosis, bronchoscopy was ordered for biopsy. And the pathology demonstrated large quantities of hyphae and spores at the bronchial mucosa, even thickness of the hyphae with branches in sharp angle and septa, and submucosal infiltration of lymphocytes, neutrophil granulocytes, and eosinophile granulocytes. By special staining, acid fast staining showed negative, methenamine silver staining positive, AB staining negative, and PAS staining positive. Histologically, the diagnosis should be pulmonary aspergillosis (Fig. 11.3).

Large quantities of aspergillus hyphae and spores are demonstrated at the bronchial mucosa. The hyphae are in even thickness with branching in sharp angle and septa. There are also infiltrations of large quantities of neutrophil granulocytes, lymphocytes, and eosinophile granulocytes (H&E staining).

The final diagnosis was pulmonary aspergillosis.

After the diagnosis of IPA was defined, voriconazole and caspofungin were administered. Medication was also given for blood sugar control. Reexamination of routine blood test showed WBC 9.19×10^9/L, neutrophil granulocytes 76.4%, hemoglobin 91 g/L, and platelets 578×109/L. Biochemistry showed glutamic-pyruvic transaminase 62 U/L, total protein 59.6 g/L, and albumin 15.1 g/L. The blood albumin was low and human blood albumin was administered for hypoproteinemia. After treatment, the condition of the patient was greatly improved, and her family members required transfer to a local hospital for further treatment.

11.1.4 Discussion

IPA is the most common opportunistic infection in fungal infections, which is one of the main reasons of increasing incidence and mortality in immunosuppressed patients [1]. In this case, the patient suffered from the basic disease of diabetes with low cellular and humoral immunity, and the condition tended to be complicated by lung infection including fungal infection. The lung infection may then aggravate diabetes and the compromised immunity [2, 3].

According to literature report [4], IPA can be radiologically classified into:

1. Vascular invasion type, whose CT scanning demonstrations are consistent to the following at least two items: halo sign; infarction-shaped consolidation; inner low intensity, cavity, or crescent sign; and mass-shaped opacity.
2. Airway invasion type, whose CT scanning demonstrations are consistent to the following at least two items: small airway lesions, consolidation around the airway, bronchiectasis or wall thickening, consolidation of the airway, and accompanying ground-glass opacity.
3. Mixture invasion type, whose CT scanning demonstrations are consistent to both the vascular invasion type and the airway invasion type.

In this case, the radiological demonstrations included multiple nodular or mass-like opacities in both lungs and subpleural consolidation opacity with multiple cavities inside. These are the main demonstrations of vascular invasion type and also demonstrations of middle-stage or advanced IPA. Huai Chen et al. reported nine cases of IPA with cavity. They found that most cavities show fine linear septa opacity, which might be formed by hyphae and necrotic tissue in the cavity. The linear septa opacity in the cavity is known as cavity septa sign, which has been believed as the characteristic radiological demonstration of IPA. In this case, the cavity was shown with thick wall. Some cavities had smooth inner wall with liquid level inside, and some cavities had irregular inner wall with linear septa. The edge of some cavities was poorly defined with accompanying halo sign. The surrounding lung tissue was demonstrated with poorly defined patchy opacity, ground-glass opacity, and multiple small nodular opacities. These are typical radiological demonstrations of IPA [5, 6]. The underlying pathological basis is that the invasion of aspergillus hyphae destroys minor vascular vessels of the lungs. The lung parenchyma is then subject to bleeding and infarction, and surrounding alveolus is also subject to bleeding. The lesion is then surrounded by bleeding areas. Along with progression of the disease, the halo sign gradually decreases.

In the cases with multiple cavities in both lungs, the diagnosis of IPA should be differentiated from the following conditions:

1. Tuberculous cavity, which commonly occurs at the posteroapical segment of both upper lung lobes and the dorsal segment of the lower lung lobes. The tuberculous cavities are in varying sizes with thick or thin wall. The cavities are surrounded by arch-shaped, ring-shaped, and satellite lesions. However, the edge of IPA cavities is accompanied by halo sign. The cavity is demonstrated with septa sign or air crescent sign. The changes of IPA cavity are radiologically more rapid than those of tuberculous cavity.
2. Multiple lung abscesses, whose cavities are in varying sizes with thick wall and liquid level. The condition of the lungs is complicated by multiple poorly defined patchy and nodular opacities but rarely with cavity septa. The patients show obvious symptoms, with acute onset, of aversion to cold, high fever, and expectoration of purulent stinky sputum.
3. Lung metastasis, whose multiple cavities in the lungs are commonly complicated by multiple nodules. The cavities are commonly located at the middle and lower lung fields and marginal areas of the lung tissue. The cavities and nodules are well marginated, with primary lesion. However, the cavities in the cases of IPA are poorly defined with halo sign. The cavities show liquid level and cavity septa.
4. Wegener granulomatosis of the lung, whose radiological demonstrations also include multiple nodules and cavities in the lungs. The cavities may show liquid level with surrounding exudation opacity and fine and long spikes. Pleural indentation sign may be demonstrated adjacent to the pleura. However, the cavities in the cases of IPA rarely show spikes and pleural indentation sign. Wegener granulomatosis is a systemic disease, and the patients commonly experience nasal hemorrhage, kidney dysfunction, and multiple subcutaneous small nodules. The systemic symptoms are serious but the respiratory symptoms are slight. Laboratory test shows increased level of leukocyte cytoplasmic antibody.

11.1.5 Comments

In this case, the patient was detected with diabetes during the illness course, with high blood sugar level, which indicated occurrence of lung infection based on untreated diabetes. Due to existence of hemoptysis and multiple cavities at both lungs, clinical attention should be focused on the differentiation of pulmonary tuberculosis and IPA. In this case, radiology demonstrated some characteristic signs of IPA, such as linear septa in some cavities (cavity septa sign) and halo sign of some lesions, which indicated possible IPA. Radiologists and clinicians should pay attention to these details when reading radiological images.

Bronchoscopy is an extremely important way in detecting IPA and is relatively contraindicated to the symptom of hemoptysis. The patients with IPA experience different degrees of hemoptysis, which affects the clinical application of bronchoscopy in the diagnosis of IPA. However, bronchoscopy can be actively applied based on the symptomatic therapy for hemostasis. Although biopsy is contraindicated to hemoptysis, microbiology with secretions can greatly improve the definitive diagnosis rate.

Combined use of collaborative antifungal medications is an important way in the treatment of serious IPA. But due to their high-cost and prolonged therapeutic course, the combined use of collaborative antifungal medications increases the economic burden of the patients. For some patients, antifungal medications may be withdrawn early due to economic reason, which may cause relapse of symptoms.

11.2 Case 2: Fever and Cough for 1 Week and Hemoptysis for 2 Days

Lukun Zhang, Hui Wang, Jingjing Li, Dong-Na Su, Shi-Ping Wu, and Pu-Xuan Lu

11.2.1 Presenting Complaint

Fever and cough for 1 week and hemoptysis for 2 days.

11.2.2 Brief Case History

A 49-year-old woman from Guangdong (China), a housewife, was hospitalized on February 4, 2015, due to presenting complaints of fever and cough for 1 week and hemoptysis for 2 days. One week prior to her admission, she began to experience fever with no known causes which had no obvious regularity, and the highest body temperature was 39 °C. Associated symptoms include aversion to cold, no chill, paroxysmal cough, and expectoration of yellowish white purulent sputum. In a local community clinic, cephamycin was given intravenously for 2 days, and her body temperature returned to normal, with relieved cough and expectoration of whitish mucous sputum. Two days ago, she began to experience hemoptysis of 1–2 ml each time for 3–4 times a day. And she consulted in our hospital. Since the onset of symptoms, she experienced no dizziness, chest distress, breathlessness, chest pain, night sweat, and nasal and gingival hemorrhage. Her spiritual state was poor with poor appetite. But her bowel movements were normal, with no obvious weight loss.

11.2.2.1 Past Medical History

On March 19, 2004, she was confirmed HIV positive by the city CDC, and since April 2004, she had been receiving highly active antiretroviral therapy (HAART). The treatment plan was combined use of tenofovir, lamivudine, and lopinavir/ritonavir. During treatment by HAART, her CD4+ T-cell count fluctuated between 240 and 300/μl. In the year of 2004, she was diagnosed with pulmonary tuberculosis and chronic viral hepatitis C. From February 2004 to March 2005, standard antituberculosis therapy was given for 1 year. In the year of 2006 and 2009, she received combined use of ribavirin with long-acting interferon for viral hepatitis C, but the treatment failed.

11.2.2.2 Epidemiological History

She received blood transfusion in 1995 due to cesarean section.

11.2.2.3 Physical Examination

Physical examination showed a body temperature of 36.5 °C, pulse rate 66/min, respiration rate 19/min, and blood pressure 120/76 mmHg. She was typically developed with moderate nourishment. The patient was conscious with average spiritual state, active position, and well cooperation during the physical examination. The skin showed no yellowish stain and liver palm positive. The systemic superficial lymph nodes were not palpable and not enlarged. The sclera was slightly yellowish stained. The lips showed no cyanosis and oral mucosa showed no cheese-like white spot. The pharynx was not congested and the bilateral tonsils were not enlarged. The neck was soft, with no distention of the jugular vein and trachea at the midline. The thorax was bilaterally symmetric with no abnormality. By palpation, the vocal fremitus was bilaterally symmetric. By percussion, both lungs showed clear sounds. By auscultation, both lungs showed clear respiration sounds, with no dry and/or moist rales. The precordial area showed no protrusion and fibrillation was unpalpable. The heart was not enlarged, with heartbeat rate of 66/min, regular. The heart sounds were normal, and the valvular areas showed no pathological murmur by auscultation. The abdomen was soft, with no tenderness and rebound pain. The liver and spleen were subcostally unpalpable. The liver and kidney areas were not sensitive to percussion. The shifting dullness was negative. The bowel sounds were 5/min. Both lower limbs showed no edema. No clubbing finger was detected. And the nervous system showed no abnormalities.

11.2.2.4 Auxiliary Investigation

Laboratory Test

On February 4, 2015, routine blood test in the outpatient department showed WBC 5.95 × 10^9/L, N 3.49 × 10^9/L, L 2.01 × 10^9/L, EO 0.05 × 10^9/L, RBC 4.48 × 10^{12}/L, HB 150 g/L, and PLT 93 × 10^9/L.

Radiology

On February 4, 2015, chest CT scan in the outpatient department demonstrated multiple lesions at both lungs and more obvious lesions in the right lung, which was considered to be lung infection. The posterior segment of the right upper lung lobe and the right lower lung lobe was demonstrated with multiple lobular and segmental atelectasis, which was considered to be bronchial involvement (Fig. 11.4).

11.2.2.5 Initial Diagnosis

Hemoptysis possibly induced by infection or neoplasm, AIDS of Stage IV, and chronic viral hepatitis C.

11.2.3 Diagnosis and Treatment

After admission, HAART was continued. And hemostatic therapy and liver protection therapy were given. Chest CT scan demonstrated lesions at both lungs. Based on chest CT demonstrations, differential diagnosis of pneumonia, pulmonary tuberculosis, and bronchial carcinoma should be paid focused attention. Other investigations for infection and fibrobronchoscopy were ordered to define the diagnosis.

The blood biochemistry after admission showed Alb 33.3 g/L, TB 27.2 μmol/L, DB 10.7 μmol/L, ALT 115 U/L, AST 81 U/L, and γ-GTT 45 U/L. CRP was 0.41 mg/L. Procalcitonin (PCT) was 0.08 ng/ml. ESR was 11 mm/h. Both G test and GM test showed negative. The blood coagulation function was normal. The absolute auxiliary CD4+ T-cell count was 287/μl. The blood HIV-RNA was lower than 500 copies/ml. The blood HCV-RNA was 3230 copies/ml. The blood immunological assay for tuberculosis showed negative. Repeated sputum tests by acid fast staining for three times showed negative. The repeated sputum TB-DNA for two times showed negative. The culture of common bacteria, fungi and tuberculosis in sputum was negative.

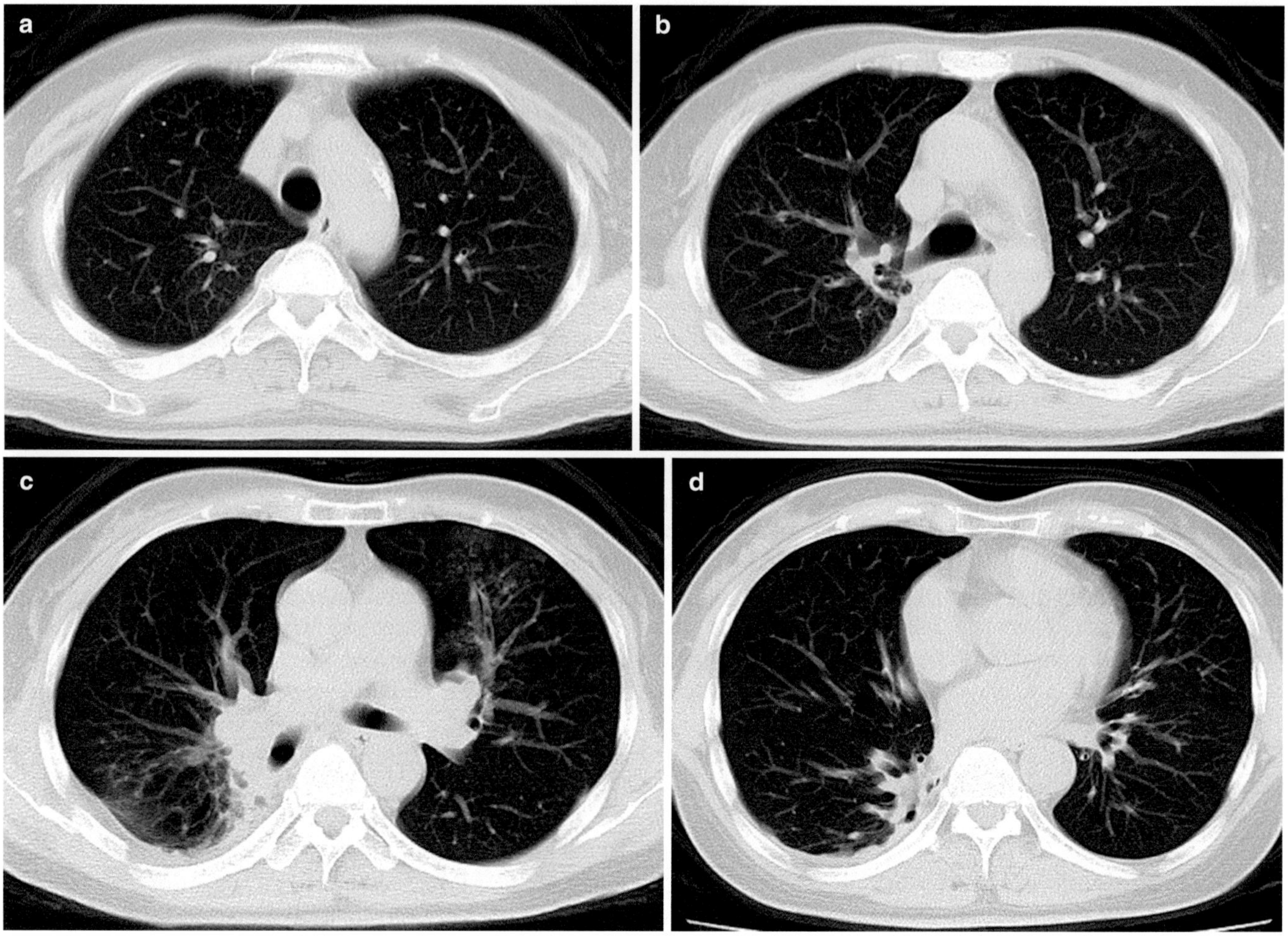

Fig. 11.4 (**a–d**) Chest CT scan. (**a, b**) The left upper lung lobe is demonstrated with scattering spots of light opacity. And both lungs are demonstrated with scattering nodular opacities. (**c, d**) The dorsal segment, medial base, and posterior basilar segment are demonstrated with shrinkage, with local cord opacity

On February 6, 2015, fibrobronchoscopy demonstrated multiple neoplasms and accompanying infection at the trachea and the posterior segment of right upper lung lobe and active bleeding at the anterior segment of the left upper lung lobe and the medial segment of the right middle lung lobe (Fig. 11.5).

The BALF showed acid fast staining negative and TB-DNA negative. The culture of BALF showed growth of aspergillus (Fig. 11.6).

Based on the results of BALF culture, the diagnosis can be defined as pulmonary aspergillus infection. Voriconazole was administered for aspergillus infection. To avoid adverse reactions between medications, the HAART was changed into combined use of tenofovir, lamivudine, and raltegravir. After the treatment, her body temperature returned to normal, with no cough, expectoration, and hemoptysis. After injection of voriconazole for 2 weeks, the medication was changed to oral liquid of itraconazole for sequential therapy, and the patient was discharged.

The diagnosis on discharge was acute invasive pulmonary aspergillosis, AIDS of Stage IV, and chronic viral hepatitis C.

On April 3, 2015, reexamination of chest CT scan demonstrated absorption of the lesions at the right middle lung lobe and the lingual segment of left upper lung lobe and almost the same lesions at the other parts of the lungs (Fig. 11.7).

On April 7, 2015, fibrobronchoscopy demonstrated decreased number of local neoplasms at the right upper lung lobe, with no lesion of hemorrhage (Fig. 11.8). Reexamination of BALF culture for fungi showed negative.

11.2.4 Discussion

IPA commonly occurs in patients with compromised immunity, which is known as secondary IPA. Its diagnosis is challenging and its mortality rate is up to 85% [7]. The clinical manifestations of pulmonary aspergillosis include cough,

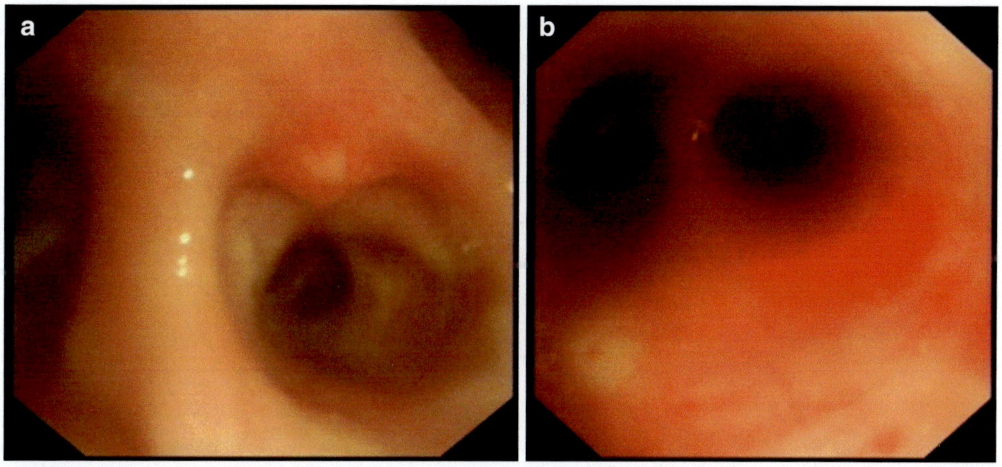

Fig. 11.5 (**a**, **b**) Pathology of the lung tissue. (**a**) The bronchial mucosa at the posterior segment of right upper lung lobe is demonstrated with granulomatous neoplasm. (**b**) The medial segment of right middle lung lobe is demonstrated with active bleeding

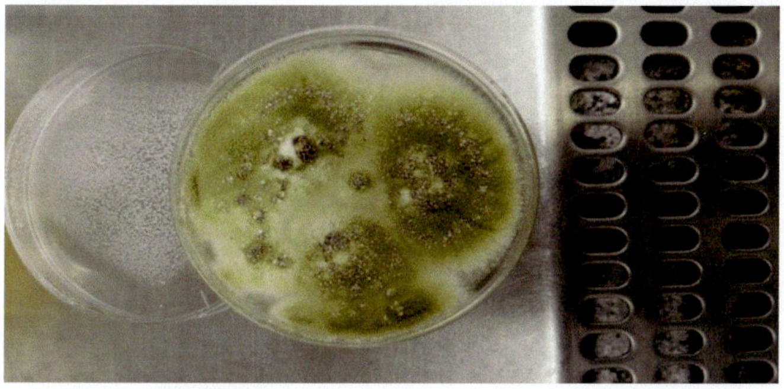

Fig. 11.6 Colonies by BALF culture

expectoration, hemoptysis, chest pain, and other respiratory symptoms as well as fever, fatigue, night sweat, and other systemic symptoms. About 40% of patients with IPA show no respiratory symptoms and only fever [8]. The symptoms of IPA resemble to those of pulmonary tuberculosis, bacterial pneumonia, lung carcinoma, and other lung diseases. The radiological demonstrations of IPA are diverse, based on which IPA has been classified into vascular invasion type and airway invasion type. The radiological demonstrations of the vascular invasion type include halo sign, wedge-shaped consolidation, low-intensity necrosis in consolidations, and cavities with air crescent sign. The radiological demonstrations of the airway invasion type include linear thickening of the lobular septa, nodules and exudations along minor airway, linear opacity of the tracheal wall, and bud-in-tree sign [9]. IPA tends to be miss diagnosed or misdiagnosed due to its non-specific clinical manifestations.

In this case, the initial symptoms of the patient include fever, cough, and expectoration of yellowish purulent sputum. In another hospital, the antibacterial therapy had been given, and her body temperature returned to normal, with relieved cough and expectoration. The condition then may be misdiagnosed as bacterial pneumonia. However, the patient experienced hemoptysis after the body temperature returned to normal, and cough and expectoration were relieved. And G test and GM test showed negative when she consulted in our hospital. Chest CT scan demonstrated multiple nodular lesions at both lungs. The patient had a past medical history of tuberculosis. The manifestation of hemoptysis and radiological demonstrations of nodular opacity in the lungs may indicate relapse of pulmonary tuberculosis. Therefore, for this case, pathogenic diagnosis was especially important. The BALF culture for fungi showed growth of aspergillus, which provided pathogenic evidence for the clinical diagnosis. Without the results from BALF culture for fungi, the diagnosis would be challenging.

In 2008, the Infectious Diseases Society of America (IDSA) issued the clinical guideline for diagnosis and treatment of aspergillosis. In the guideline, voriconazole is recommended as the medication of choice for IPA, and the alternative medications include amphotericin B, caspofungin, micafungin, and itraconazole [10]. The therapeutic course of IPA lasts at least for 6–12 weeks. For patients with compromised immunity, the medication should be continued till all the clinical manifestations and radiological demonstrations are stabled. If immunosuppression is predicted, antifungal medication should be administered again to present its relapse. In this case, the respiratory symptoms rapidly disappeared, and some lesions in the lungs were absorbed after voriconazole was administered. But reexamination of chest CT scan after treatment for 2 months showed incomplete absorption of the lesions in the lungs, indicating a prolonged period of time in treatment of aspergillosis. We summarized the case as the following:

1. In patients with compromised immunity, the lungs may be infected by multiple microorganisms to show multiple nodules and inflammation-like changes. In such cases, fungal infection should also be considered in addition to bacterial infection and *Mycobacterium tuberculosis* infection. Especially when common antibacterial therapy

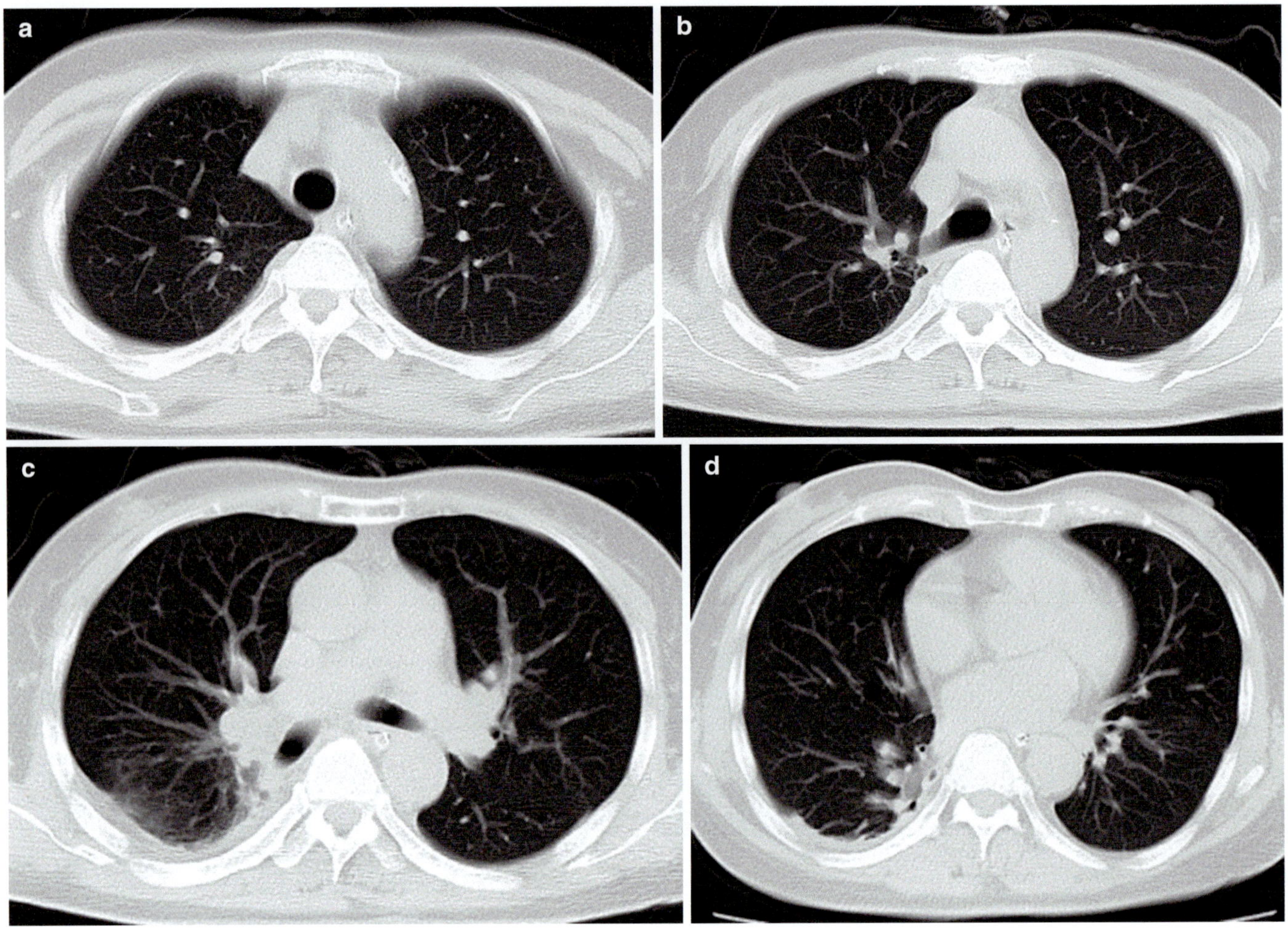

Fig. 11.7 (**a–d**) Chest CT scan. (**a**, **b**) Multiple nodules at the left lung apex and at the lingual segment of left upper lung lobe near the heart border are demonstrated. (**c**, **d**) Absorption of the lesions at the right lung lobe is demonstrated

Fig. 11.8 (**a**, **b**) Fibrobronchoscopy. (**a**) Neoplasms are demonstrated at the bronchial mucosa of right upper lung lobe. (**b**) The bronchi at the right middle lung lobe are demonstrated with no hemorrhage

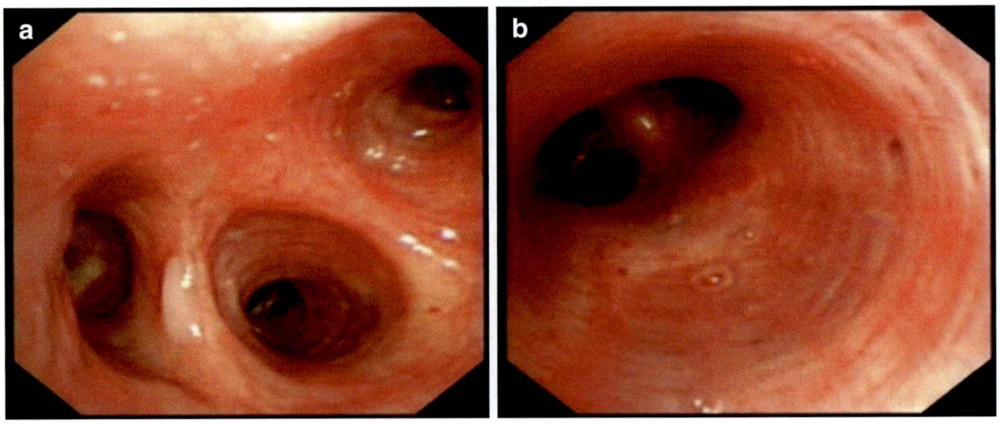

is ineffective, BALF culture should be further ordered for pathogen or biopsy for definitive diagnosis.

2. Pulmonary aspergillosis in patients with compromised immunity shows atypical CT demonstrations, such as different types of nodules or consolidation, surrounding halo sign, and crescent sign. Therefore, in patients with compromised immunity, CT scan has limited value in the diagnosis of aspergillus infection.
3. In patients with compromised immunity, pulmonary aspergillosis can be treated with medication of voriconazole and/or itraconazole, whose therapeutic efficacy is favorable. But the therapeutic course is prolonged.

Withdrawal of the medication should be based on the absorption of lesions in the lungs.

11.2.5 Comments

In this case, the patient was a middle-aged woman and the onset of symptoms was acute. The patient had a past medical history of definitively diagnosed AIDS and had been receiving long-term HAART. The typical symptoms include fever, cough, and hemoptysis, and chest CT scan demonstrated multiple infection lesions of both lungs. By bronchoscopic harvest of BALF and flowing culture, growth of aspergillus was demonstrated. In combination with case history and radiological data, the diagnosis was defined as acute invasive pulmonary aspergillosis (AIPA). AIDS complicated by pulmonary aspergillosis is characterized by the following manifestations: (1) commonly invasive lesions in the alveolar wall, bronchial wall, and vascular wall; (2) bilateral lesions that involve bronchi and even lung parenchyma to cause luminal obstruction as well as intrapulmonary purulent and necrotic lesions; and (3) mixed infections at the lungs with more complex radiological demonstrations. In clinical practice, these manifestations should be paid close attention by radiologists and clinicians.

In this case, voriconazole was injected for anti-aspergillus treatment, and the medication was changed to oral liquid of itraconazole as the sequential therapy. Her condition was improved and the patient was discharged. Currently, voriconazole is the medication of choice in the treatment of IPA. Itraconazole and posaconazole can also treat IPA effectively. However, a recent research has demonstrated that in patients receiving the same antifungal medication for more than 1 year, posaconazole shows the most favorable therapeutic efficacy, followed by voriconazole, and the condition of many patients deteriorates after medication of itraconazole, which may be due to side effects of long-term medication. For patients who show no therapeutic response to azoles or are intolerant to azoles, echinocandins or amphotericin B can be considered for treatment. In the serious cases of aspergillus infection, the combined use of voriconazole and echinocandins is recommended to fight against infection. It should be noted that the therapeutic course of antifungal therapy lasting for 6–12 weeks is not enough for patients with AIDS complicated by IPA; the medication should be administered for a prolonged period or even lifelong period.

11.3 Case 3: A Diagnosis of Partial Maturation Type of Acute Myelocytic Leukemia for 6 Months

Yulin He, Wanling Qi, Wei Ma, Xuemei Han, Ying-Yun Fu, and Xiongfei Sun

11.3.1 Presenting Complaint

A diagnosis of partial maturation type of acute myelocytic leukemia for 6 months.

11.3.2 Brief Case History

An 8-year-old girl was admitted to our hospital for chemotherapy on August 18, 2014, due to the diagnosis of partial maturation type of acute myelocytic leukemia for 6 months. The girl was diagnosed with acute myeloid leukemia (M2) on February 3, 2014, and began to receive chemotherapy (DAE, TAE, MA, HA) on March 4, 2014. And she was admitted again to our hospital for further chemotherapy.

11.3.2.1 Physical Examination

Physical examination showed a body temperature of 36.5 °C, pulse rate 92/min, respiration rate 19/min, and blood pressure 120/76 mmHg. She was typically developed with moderate nourishment. The patient was conscious with stable respirations. The systemic skin showed no yellowish stain and no bleeding spots. The neck showed no palpable enlarged lymph nodes. The skull was detected with no deformity and the sclera showed no yellowish stain. The lips were less ruddy. The oral mucosa showed no cheese-like white spots. The pharynx was not congested and the bilateral tonsils were not enlarged. The neck was soft with no distension of the jugular vein. The trachea was at the midline. The thorax was bilaterally symmetric with no deformity. The vocal fremitus was bilaterally symmetric. No three depression signs were detected. By percussion, both lungs showed clear sounds. By auscultation, both lungs showed clear respiration sounds, with no dry and/or moist rales. The precordial area showed no protrusion with no palpable fibrillation. The heart border was not enlarged, with a heartbeat rate of 92/min, regular. The heart sounds were normal and the valvular areas showed no pathological murmur. The abdomen was soft, with no tenderness and rebound pain. The liver and spleen were subcostally unpalpable. The liver and kidney areas were not sensitive to percussion. The shifting dullness was negative and the bowel sounds were 5/min. The joints of the four limbs showed no deformity, redness, and swelling. Clubbing finger was not detected. The nervous system showed no abnormalities.

11.3.2.2 Auxiliary Investigation

Routine blood test showed WBC 0.08×10^9/L, RBC 3.24×10^{12}/L, HB 92 g/L, PLT 22 × 109/L, and C-reactive protein 124 mg/L. The procalcitonin was 0.14 ng/ml. The plasma bacterial endotoxin was lower than 0.01 EU/ml.

11.3.2.3 Initial Diagnosis

The initial diagnosis was acute myeloid leukemia.

11.3.3 Diagnosis and Treatment

On August 31, 2014, the day 10 after withdrawal of chemotherapy IA, the patient showed high fever with the highest body temperature of 40 °C. Associate symptoms included aversion to cold, chills, and palpable bean-sized mass at the right mandible. Meropenem was administered for infection and the body temperature returned to normal. On September 4, 2014, the patient experienced high fever again and accompanying cough. Due to possible fungal infection, G test was performed on September 5, 2014, that showed negative. On September 6, the patient began to experience breathlessness, and chest CT scan demonstrated no obvious abnormality. On September 8, she suddenly showed inspiratory dyspnea, cyanosis around lips, hoarseness, chest distress, and anxiety. The three depression signs were obvious and the oxygen saturation of blood was low. Emergency neck and chest CT scan demonstrated narrowed upper airway (under the glottis) and narrowed right major bronchus (Fig. 11.9).

To further define the diagnosis, fibrobronchoscopy was ordered in the emergency department on September 9, 2014. The bronchoscope could not be further inserted at the opening of the trachea, indicating obvious stenosis at the initial part of the trachea. The tracheal wall was demonstrated to be adhered by many moss-like milky white substances that caused narrowness of the tracheal lumen. A small quantity of tissues were harvested for biopsy. The pathology indicated hyphae and spores of aspergillus in the harvested tissues (Fig. 11.10).

On September 16, 2014, microscopy demonstrated large quantities of hyphae and spores of mold in red-stained unstructured substance of the granulation tissue from the airway. Reexamination of chest CT scan on September 17, 2014, demonstrated bronchial narrowness of the right lower lung (Fig. 11.11). Repeated two times sputum smears for fungi on September 19, 2014, demonstrated fungal hyphae and spores. The acid fast staining of the sputum showed negative. And the sputum smear for common bacteria showed negative. The blood cultures for fungi, aerobic bacteria, and anaerobic bacteria showed negative. G test on September 20, 2014, showed positive. On September 22, 2014, microscopy demonstrated the neoplasm on airway wall to be bronchial soft tissue and interstitium, with large quantities of fungal hyphae and spores as well as necrotic substances inside. After admission, the tests and investigations were ordered, and symptomatic supports were applied including respirator for ventilation, blood transfusion, and WBC elevation. Fluconazol and caspofungin were consecutively administered as antifungal therapy. Reexamination of chest CT scan on September 29, 2014, demonstrated poorly defined small nodules at both lungs and subpleural flakes of opacity, with halo sign (Fig. 11.12). On October 15, 2014, electronic endoscopy demonstrated pharyngeal congestion, swelling, and stenosis of the vocal cords and subglottis and restricted abduction of the vocal cords.

After intravenous infusion of caspofungin, aerosol inhalation of amphotericin B, and symptomatic support therapies, her condition was greatly improved. On October 30, 2014,

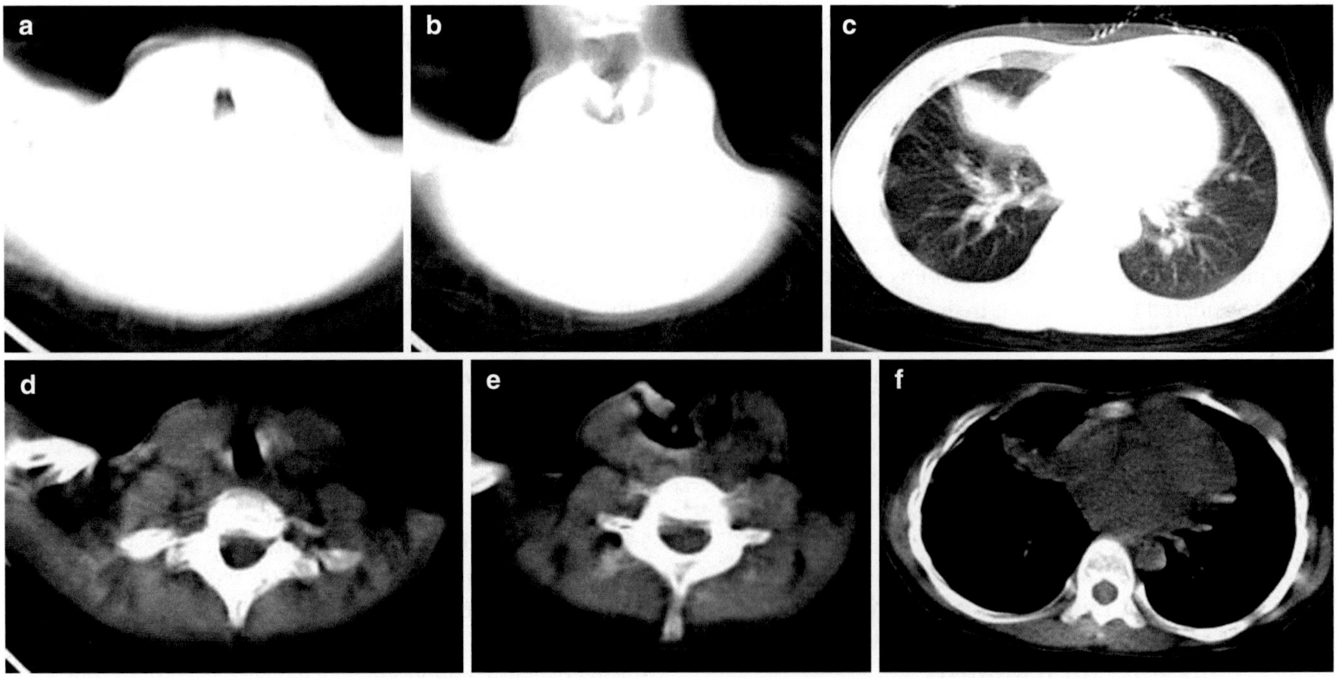

Fig. 11.9 (**a**–**f**) Chest CT scan. (**a**, **b**) Narrow initial trachea of the upper airway is demonstrated. (**c**) Atelectasis of the right middle lung lobe is demonstrated. (**d**–**f**) The mediastinum window demonstrates narrowed airway and segmental atelectasis of the right middle lung lobe

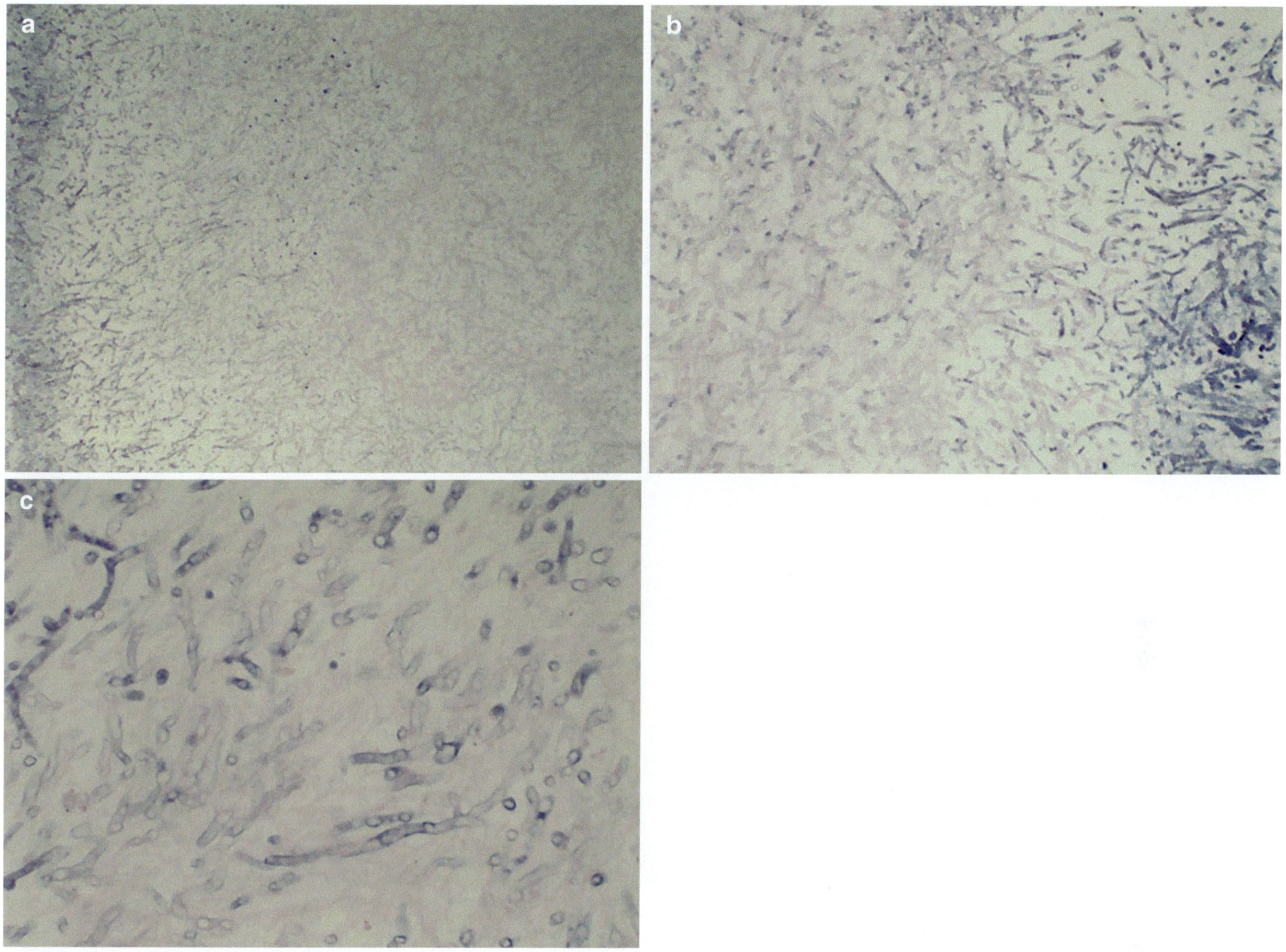

Fig. 11.10 (**a**–**c**) Pathology of the lung tissue. (**a**–**c**) Bronchoscopy and the following biopsy demonstrate hyphae and spores of aspergillus (H&E staining)

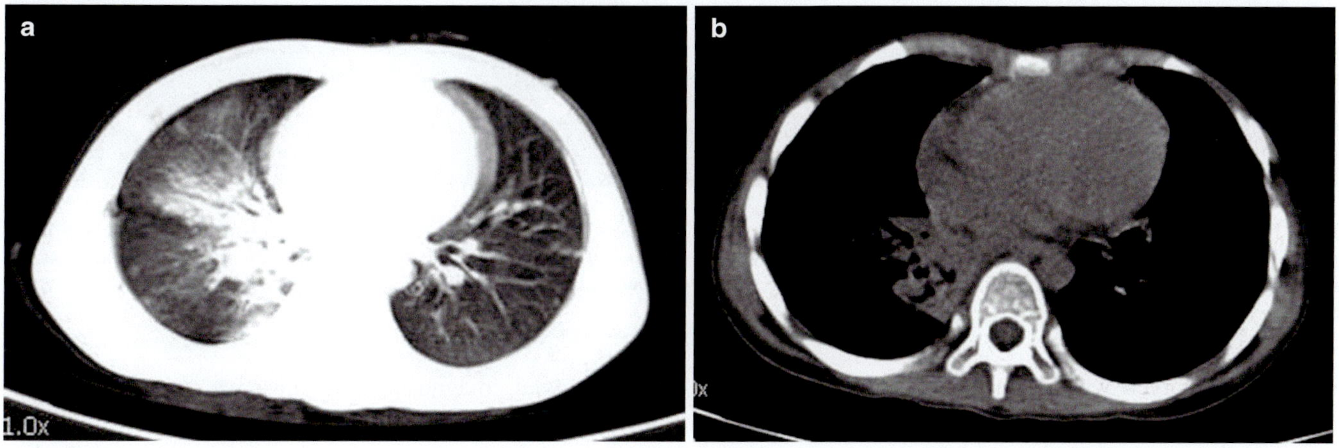

Fig. 11.11 (**a**, **b**) Chest CT scan. (**a**, **b**) The lung window and the mediastinum window demonstrate decreased air volume in the right lower lung and incomplete inflation, which indicate bronchostenosis of the right lower lung

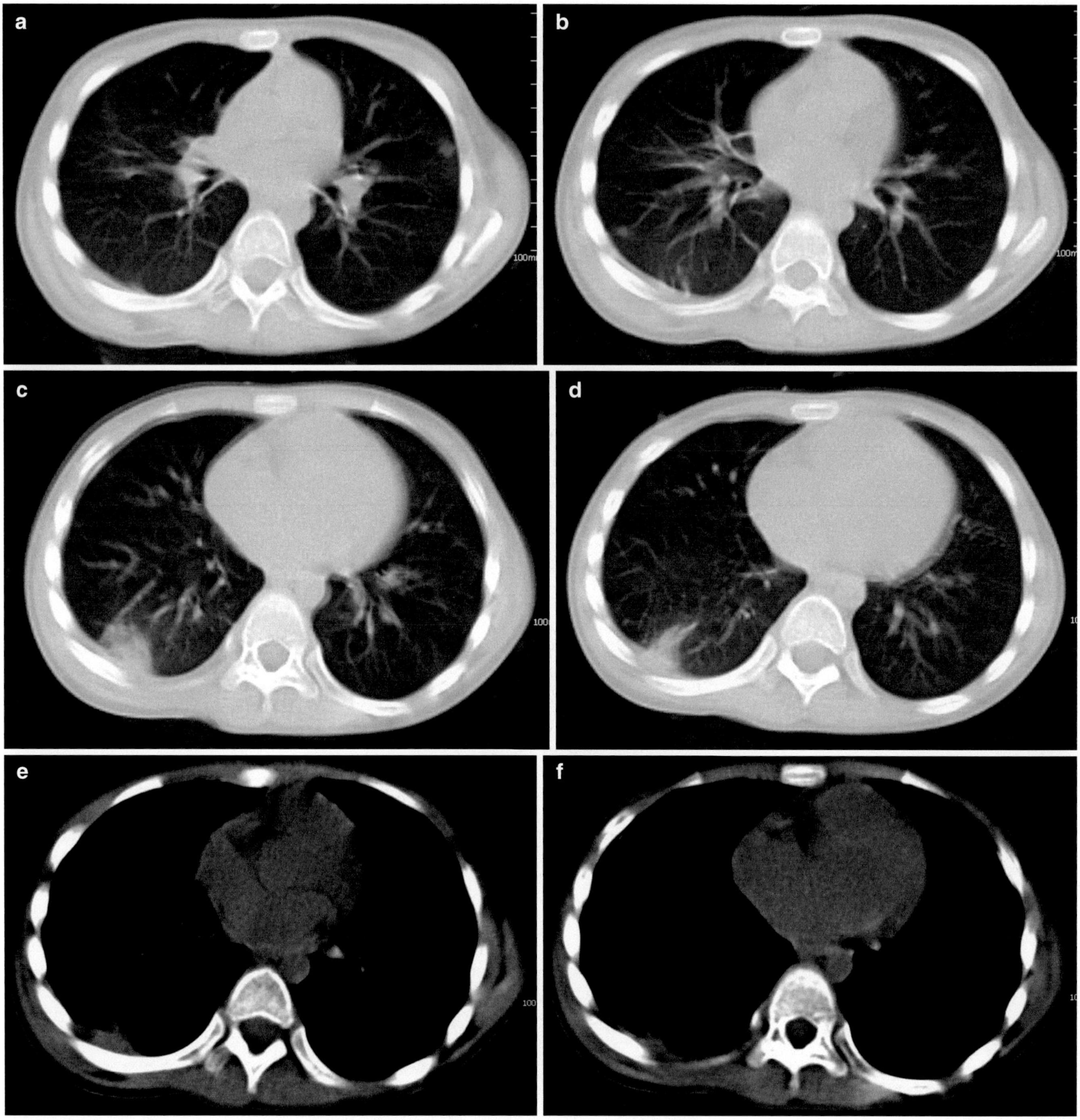

Fig. 11.12 (**a**–**f**) Chest CT scan. (**a**, **b**) The lung window demonstrates poorly defined small nodular opacity at both upper lungs. (**c**, **d**) The lung window demonstrates poorly defined nodular and patchy opacity at both lower lungs and superolingual segment of the left upper lung, some of which show halo sign. (**e**, **f**) The mediastinum window at the ventricular level demonstrates subpleural patchy opacity

she was discharged with catheter. Oral intake of voriconazole was continued. And reexamination of chest CT scan on the same day demonstrated cured bronchostenosis and atelectasis as well as absorption of most nodular and patchy opacities in the lungs (Fig. 11.13).

The final diagnosis was invasive tracheobronchial aspergillosis.

The condition was improved and the patient was discharged with catheter. Antifungal medication was continued after discharge.

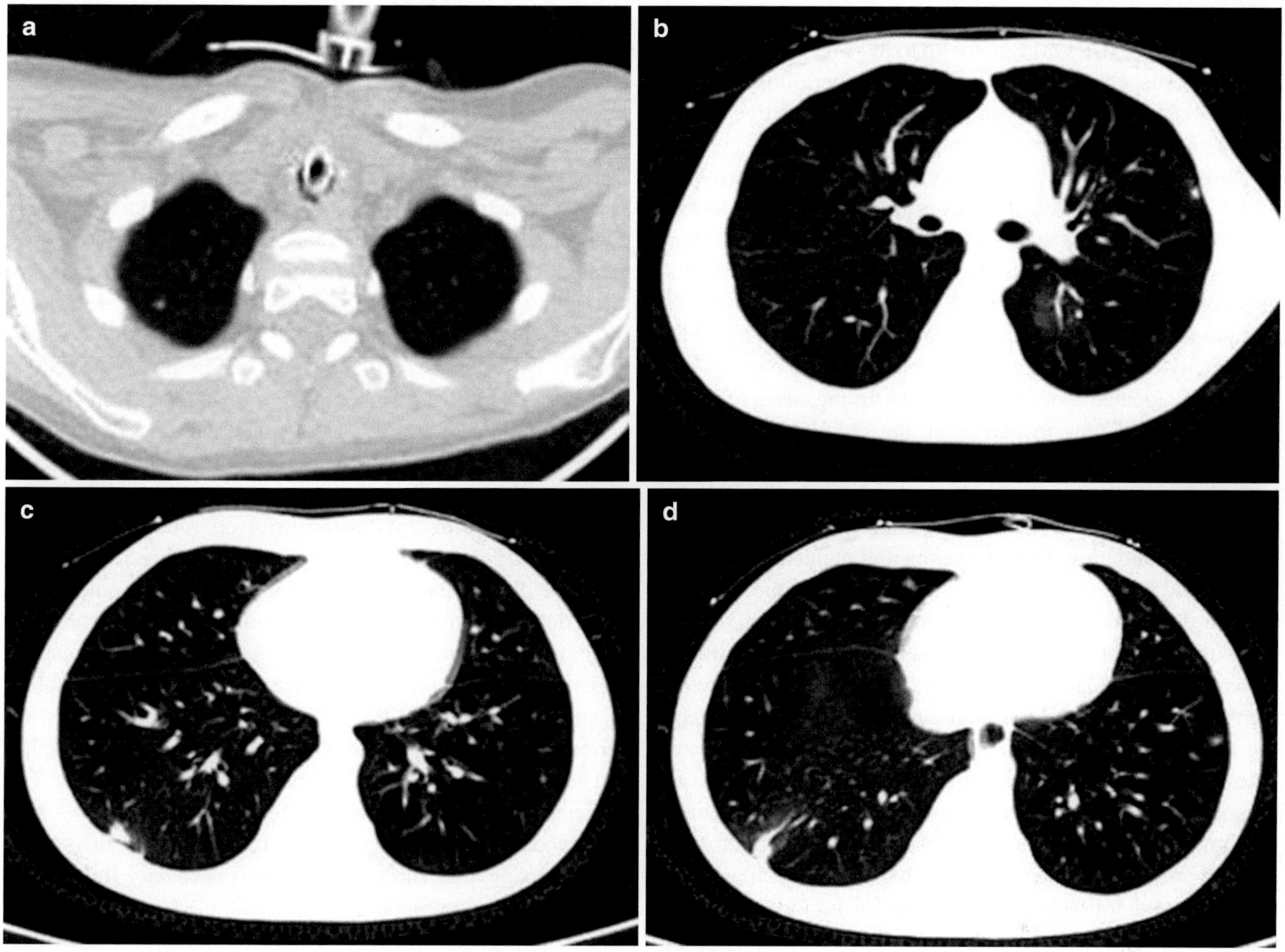

Fig. 11.13 (**a–d**) Chest CT scan. (**a**) The lung window at the lung apex level demonstrates indwelling catheter in the trachea as well as obvious absorption of nodular and patchy opacities in the lungs. (**b–d**) High-resolution CT scan demonstrates subpleural patchy opacity in the right lower lung and surrounding ground-glass opacity. Compared to the CT scan on September 27, 2014, the lesions in the right lower lung are absorbed and improved

11.3.4 Discussion

Invasive tracheobronchial aspergillosis (ITBA) is a rare type of aspergillosis. It independently occurs in a small number of patients. Otherwise, it concurs with or occurs in the early stage of invasive pulmonary aspergillosis (IPA) [11]. ITBA commonly occurs in patients with serious immunosuppression and long-term neutropenia, such as patients with various malignancies, diabetes, chronic obstructive pulmonary disease (COPD), systemic lupus erythematosus (SLE), AIDS, respiratory tract stricture after alcoholism or tuberculosis, and other chronic diseases. ITBA may also occur in patients with chronic disease but no immunosuppression and even in immunocompetent individuals [12]. The clinical symptoms of ITBA include cough, wheezing, expectoration of mucous plug, hemoptysis, and fever. One third of patients with ITBA develop respiratory distress and even respiratory failure. And about 15.1% of patients with ITBA are asymptomatic when diagnosed [13]. The main pathological changes include necrosis of bronchial mucosa. In addition, there is pseudomembrane formed by adherence of moss-like agglutination containing abundant fibrin after mixture of hyphae and spores of aspergillus as well as airway secretions to the tracheal inner wall that further induces tracheal luminal stricture and atelectasis. The condition rapidly develops. And the induced atelectasis is different from chronic atelectasis induced by endobronchial tuberculosis.

In this case, the patient received serum GM test, which showed positive. GM test has great diagnostic value for pulmonary aspergillosis. A meta-analysis of 30 original studies by Zou et al. [14] has demonstrated that the sensitivity and specificity of BALF GM test are up to 87% and 89%, respectively. For suspected cases of pulmonary aspergillosis, BALF GM test should be performed to improve the positive rate in the diagnosis of pulmonary aspergillosis.

Chest X-ray and chest CT scan may show no abnormality in the lungs in the cases of ITBA with trachea and bronchus involved. In the early stage of ITBA, the tracheal and bronchial wall may be subject to thickening [15]. Along with progression of the disease, local consolidation or multiple nodular and cavity opacities can be observed [16]. The nodular opacity may be singular. The nodules and cavities are commonly located around the bronchi. In the cases of ITBA with concurrent lung involvement, the radiological demonstrations of the lungs are diverse and non-specific. The radiological demonstrations include poorly defined centrilobular nodule opacity around the bronchi, namely, bud-in-tree sign, patchy consolidation, lobar or segmental atelectasis or infiltration, and large areas of consolidation around the bronchi. Bronchoscopy is the most important investigation for the early diagnosis of ITBA. Due to absence of lung exudation in the early stage of ITBA, radiology commonly fails to detect signs of infection, while bronchoscopy is capable of detecting the signs of infection. CT scan of the lungs facilitates assessing involvement of the other lung tissue. The definitive diagnosis of ITBA is based on invasion and involvement of respiratory basilar membrane by aspergillus. The pathological and microbiological evidence harvested by fibrobronchoscopy and following biopsy is quite important for the diagnosis of ITBA. In this case, the diagnosis was defined based on fibrobronchoscopy and following biopsy.

ITBA should be firstly differentiated from foreign body in the airway. In this case, the condition was initially misdiagnosed as foreign body in the airway. The following chest CT scan indicated tracheobronchial aspergillosis, and the diagnosis was defined after emergency fibrobronchoscopy and following biopsy. Then, ITBA should be differentiated from endobronchial tuberculosis and airway neoplasm. Endobronchial tuberculosis and airway neoplasm show chronic onset. Patients with tuberculosis commonly experience associate symptoms of cough, hemoptysis, and emaciation, while patients with neoplasm are commonly elderly, and its diagnosis can be defined by radiological demonstration of airway mass.

The treatment of ITBA is challenging, and collaboration of long-term systemic anti-aspergillus therapy and interventional therapy under a bronchoscope is necessary. For patients with highly suspected IPA, such as patients with persistent fever and neutropenia, trial antifungal therapy should be administered early along with diagnostic assessment. The medications include voriconazole, itraconazole, caspofungin, and amphotericin B. In the clinical guideline issued by the IDSA, voriconazole is recommended as the first choice medication for ITBA. It is also recommended that the therapeutic course should be individualized depending on the immunity and prognosis of the primary disease of the patients.

11.3.5 Comments

ITBA is a rare disease and the condition is subject to miss diagnosis or delayed diagnosis. In this case, the girl suffered from agranulocytosis after chemotherapy for acute myeloid leukemia, with symptoms of chill and high fever. About 1 week later, she suddenly showed inspiratory dyspnea, indicating obstruction of major airway. Clinically, ITBA should be suspected. This rare aspergillus-related lung disease independently occurs or is complicated by IPA in a small number of patients. Otherwise, it occurs in the early stage of IPA. The radiological demonstrations are diverse and non-specific. Especially in the cases of ITBA with only trachea involved, routine chest X-ray and chest CT scan demonstrate no abnormalities. Thus clinically, the disease tends to be miss diagnosed with outcome of death due to airway obstruction and suffocation. Bronchoscopy is the most important investigation for the early diagnosis of ITBA. It helps for timely definitive diagnosis and elimination of airway obstruction. But for patients in myelosuppression period, bronchoscopy commonly induces secondary infection and hemorrhage due to agranulocytosis and thrombopenia. The clinicians are commonly cautious for the use of bronchoscopy. The successful experience in this case indicated that active bronchoscopy after strict sterilization is necessary for patients with immunosuppression.

The treatment in this case needs open discussion. Firstly, for patient with persistent fever due to agranulocytosis, trial antifungal therapy should be administered early along with diagnostic assessment. Secondly, fluconazol is ineffective in the treatment of aspergillosis. Invasive pulmonary aspergillosis should be suspected based on the findings of moss-like milky white substance on the tracheal wall by emergency bronchoscopy. Antifungal medication of voriconazole, caspofungin, and amphotericin B instead of fluconazole can be administered.

11.4 Case 4: Recurrent Cough, Expectoration and Accompanying Fever for 6 Months

Budong Chen, Ruming Xie, Dong-Na Su, Shi-Ping Wu, Huaisheng Chen, and Pu-Xuan Lu

11.4.1 Presenting Complaint

Recurrent cough, expectoration, and accompanying fever for 6 months.

11.4.2 Brief Case History

A 31-year-old woman was admitted to our hospital on September 10, 2013, due to presenting complaint of recurrent cough, expectoration, and accompanying fever. Half a year ago, the patient began to experience paroxysmal cough, expectoration of yellowish white mucous sputum occasionally with fishy smell, and fever mainly at afternoons and nights. Her body temperature fluctuated around 38 °C and showed decrease with no treatment. She also experienced chest distress and breathlessness that was more obvious after physical activities. There were also symptoms of general fatigue, night sweat, and weight loss. Chest X-ray in a local hospital indicated pulmonary tuberculosis. And antituberculosis therapy was administered (specifically unknown) for more than 3 months. After treatment, the symptoms were relieved, but the patient began to experience intermittent hemoptysis of a small quantity. Reexamination of chest CT scan demonstrated no exclusion of lung abscess. Antituberculosis medication was then withdrawn, and penicillin was given for half a month to fight against infection. Fever was then relieved. Reexamination of chest X-ray demonstrated absorption of lesions. CT scan of the lungs in a hospital of PLA demonstrated space-occupying lesion at the right lower lung lobe, which is possibly peripheral lung carcinoma. The anti-infection therapy, cough and expectoration relieving therapy, and other symptomatic support were then administered. But the symptoms were not relieved. The patient still experienced cough, expectoration of sputum occasionally with blood, occasional low-grade fever, dizziness, headache, and ache of elbow, knee, and wrist. For further diagnosis and treatment, the patient presented in our hospital and was admitted due to opacity at the right lung. Since the onset of symptoms, the patient showed poor spiritual state with poor appetite and sleep. Her urinations and bowel movements were normal, and she reported a weight loss of about 5 kg.

11.4.2.1 Past Medical History

The patient denied histories of hepatitis, tuberculosis, and malaria. In addition, she denied histories of hypertension, heart disease, and diabetes.

11.4.2.2 Physical Examination

Physical examination showed a body temperature of 36.5 °C, pulse rate 88/min, respiration rate 22/min, and blood pressure 130/100 mmHg. She was typically developed, with good nourishment and healthy appearance. The patient was in active position, consciousness, and good cooperation in physical examination. The systemic skin mucosa showed no yellowish stain, with no skin rash, liver palm, and spider. The systemic superficial lymph nodes were unpalpable and not enlarged. The thorax was normal and the sternum showed no tenderness. The respiratory movements were normal with no pleural rubs. By percussion, both lungs showed clear sounds. The respiration sounds at the right lower lung were coarse, with rare moist rales. The beat of heart apex was normal, with no pericardial rub. And the border of cardiac dullness was normal. The heartbeat was 88/min, regular with no murmur, no pericardial rubs, and no peripheral vascular sign. The abdomen was soft, with no tenderness, rebound pain, and mass. The liver and spleen were unpalpable. The Murphy's sign was negative. The kidney area was not sensitive to percussion. Shifting dullness was negative. And the bowel sounds were normal.

11.4.2.3 Auxiliary Investigation

Laboratory Test

Routine blood test showed WBC 5.48 × 10^9/L, N 57.3%, L 33.9%, RBC 4.41 × 10^{12}/L, and PLT 333 × 10^9/L. ESR was 50 mm/h and CRP 33.91 mg/L. The liver function test showed T-Bil 10.8 μmol/L, ALT 119.0 U/L, AST 47.0 U/L, TP 64.0 g/L, and ALB 33.8 g/L. The kidney function test showed BUN 3.64 mmol/L (normal limites 1.7–8.3 mmol/L) and Cr 37.2 μmmol/L (normal limits 22.1–106 μmmol/L).

Radiology

Chest CT scan on August 18, 2013, in another hospital demonstrated well-marginated mass-like high-intensity opacity at the basilar segment of the right lower lung lobe, in a size of about 51 mm × 44 mm, with lobulation and spikes. There were also patchy high-intensity opacity at the anterior and lateral basilar segment of the right lower lung lobe and no thickening of the vascular and bronchial bundles at both lungs. Lymph nodes were demonstrated to be enlarged at the right hilum and subcarina, and the bronchi at the right lower lung lobe narrowed due to compression. Nodular low-intensity opacity was demonstrated at the right side of the 12th thoracic vertebra with slight marginal sclerosis.

11.4.2.4 Initial Diagnosis

The initial diagnosis was opacity at the right lower lung lobe, which was suspected to be neoplasm or tuberculosis and lung infection.

11.4.3 Diagnosis and Treatment

After admission, the patient was given biapenem for infection and symptomatic support against cough and expectoration. Laboratory tests showed rheumatoid factors negative, antistreptolysin O negative, and D-dimer 0.1 mg/L (normal range 0–0.3 mg/L). The sputum culture for fungi showed negative, for Gram-negative bacteria negative, and for Gram-positive bacteria negative. The assay for antibody of

Treponema pallidum showed negative, for antibody of HIV negative, for antibody of *Mycoplasma pneumoniae* IgM negative, and for antibody of *Legionella pneumophila* IgM negative. The blood sugar level was within normal limits. To further define the diagnosis, chest CT scan was performed on September 11, 2013. It demonstrated poorly defined mass opacity of soft tissue intensity at the right lower lung lobe, which showed heterogeneous enhancement after administration of contrast medium. Flakes of ground-glass opacity and cords opacity were also demonstrated (Fig. 11.14). The lobular septa were thickened at the right lower lung lobe, and lymphadenectasis was demonstrated at the right hilum and seventh mediastinal area. The inferior thoracic spine was demonstrated with confined low-intensity opacity. The condition was suspected to be tuberculosis, lung carcinoma with lymphatic metastasis, inflammation at the right middle and lower lung lobes, and lateral bone destruction of the interior thoracic spine.

The patient was a young woman with recurrent cough, expectoration, and accompanying fever for 6 months. Anti-infection therapy and antituberculosis therapy were administered, but the condition improved and deteriorated. In combination with the chest radiology, the diagnosis was suspected to be pulmonary abscess, but lung carcinoma and tuberculosis cannot be excluded. To further define the diagnosis, CT-guided puncture of the right lung was performed on September 11, 2013, for biopsy. Microscopy demonstrated large quantities of hyphae and spores and the hyphae twined into mass. The surrounding tissues were demonstrated with infiltration of inflammatory cells. The hyphae were arranged in filamentous or radiating form, with even thickness. The bilateral hyphae walls were parallel, with septa. Some hyphae showed branching with 45° angle, and the spores were scattering (Fig. 11.15). By PAS staining, the external membrane of hyphae was stained red (Fig. 11.15). The pathological diagnosis was fungal infection, and the condition was morphologically consistent to pulmonary aspergillosis.

The final diagnosis was pulmonary aspergillus infection.

11.4.4 Discussion

Pulmonary aspergillosis is a clinically rare lung infection. However, along with widespread applications of antibiotics, hormone, and anticarcinogen and the increasingly improved diagnostic technology, its incidence and detecting rate have been increasing [17]. Pulmonary aspergillosis shows a high incidence in populations with compromised immunity. And it also occurs in populations with competent immunity but basic lung diseases such as bronchiectasis and pulmonary tuberculosis. In this case, the patient was immunocompetent and suffered from no basic lung disease, which is extremely rare. The case indicated that pulmonary aspergillosis may also occur in populations with competent immunity and no basic lung disease [18].

The clinical symptoms of IPA include persistent fever, cough, chest pain, and possible hemoptysis. CT scan demonstrates early IPA as halo sign, namely, consolidation with surrounding ground-glass opacity. And CT demonstrations of IPA mainly include singular or multiple nodules, segmental or subsegmental consolidation, diffuse ground-glass opacity, and small cavity opacity [19–21].

In this case, CT scan demonstrated mass opacity of soft tissue intensity with inner patchy low-intensity area. Enhanced scan demonstrated obvious marginal enhancement and irregular central non-enhancement that was considered as necrosis. The condition should be radiologically differentiated from peripheral lung carcinoma, pulmonary tuberculosis including primary syndrome or secondary pulmonary tuberculosis, and pulmonary abscess. The diagnosis and treatment course that the patient experienced was also the course of their differentiation. During the 6-month illness course, the patient had been diagnosed with pulmonary tuberculosis and then received antituberculosis therapy for more than 3 months but with poor therapeutic efficacy. Reexamination of CT scan indicated possible pulmonary abscess, and the patient then received anti-infection therapy. Reexamination of CT scan demonstrated absorption of lesions, but the condition improved and deteriorated. The patient then was hospitalized in a hospital of PLA, and reexamination of CT scan there indicated space-occupying lesion at the right lower lung. The diagnosis was considered to be peripheral lung carcinoma. Since then, the illness course lasted for almost 6 months. In our hospital, puncture of the right lung for biopsy defined the diagnosis as pulmonary aspergillosis. Radiologically, the case can be differentiated from saprophytic aspergilloma and allergic bronchopulmonary aspergillosis. By CT scan, saprophytic aspergilloma is demonstrated as round or round-like dense opacity in lung cavity or cavum, crescent-shaped or ring-shaped translucent opacity between the cavity walls, and the round-like dense opacity. In the cases with sufficiently large cavity or cavum, the round-like dense opacity is movable along with body postures [18–20]. And by CT scan, allergic bronchopulmonary aspergillosis is demonstrated as recurrent multiple migratory intrapulmonary infiltrations, central bronchiectasis, and formation of mucous clog in the dilated bronchus [19, 20]. In this case, radiology demonstrated mass-like consolidation and central patchy necrosis. In combination with the case history for 6 months and puncture with following biopsy, the diagnosis was finally defined as subacute invasive pulmonary aspergillosis.

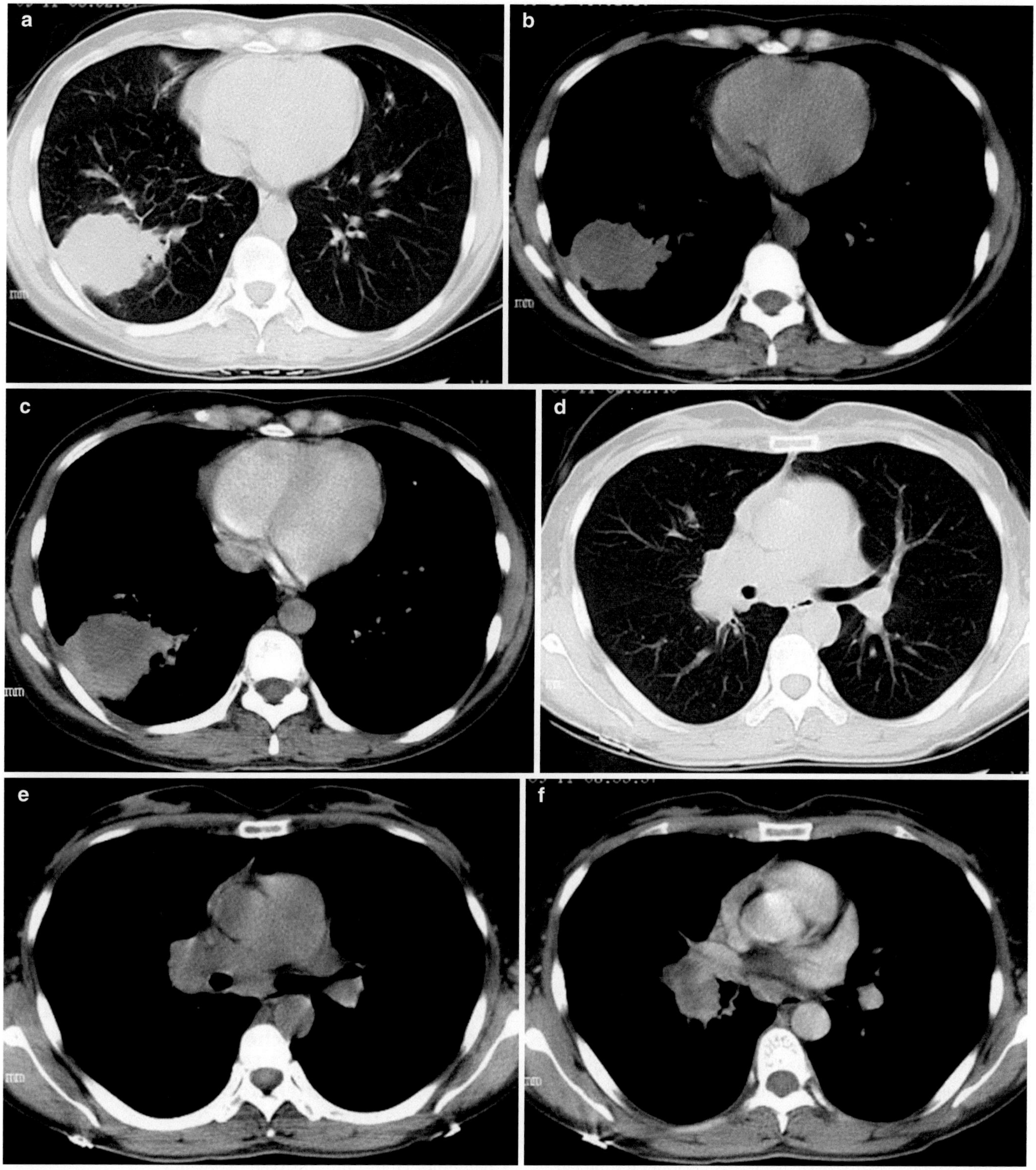

Fig. 11.14 (**a**–**f**) Chest CT scan. (**a**) The lung window demonstrates mass opacity of soft tissue intensity at the basilar segment of the right lower lung lobe with superficial lobulation, in a size of about 51 mm × 44 mm, adjacent pleural thickening, and flakes of ground-glass opacity at the right middle lung lobe near cardiac border. (**b**) The mediastinum window demonstrates mass opacity of soft tissue heterogeneous intensity, with slightly lower central intensity. By plain scanning, the CT value is around 22 Hu. The lateral mass opacity is locally connected with the lateral pleura. (**c**) CT scan with administration of contrast medium demonstrates obviously enhanced margin of the mass opacity, with irregular non-enhanced area at the center. (**d**, **e**) Lymphadenectasis is demonstrated at the R10 area and seventh area. (**f**) Enhanced CT scan demonstrates obvious enhancement of the enlarged lymph nodes

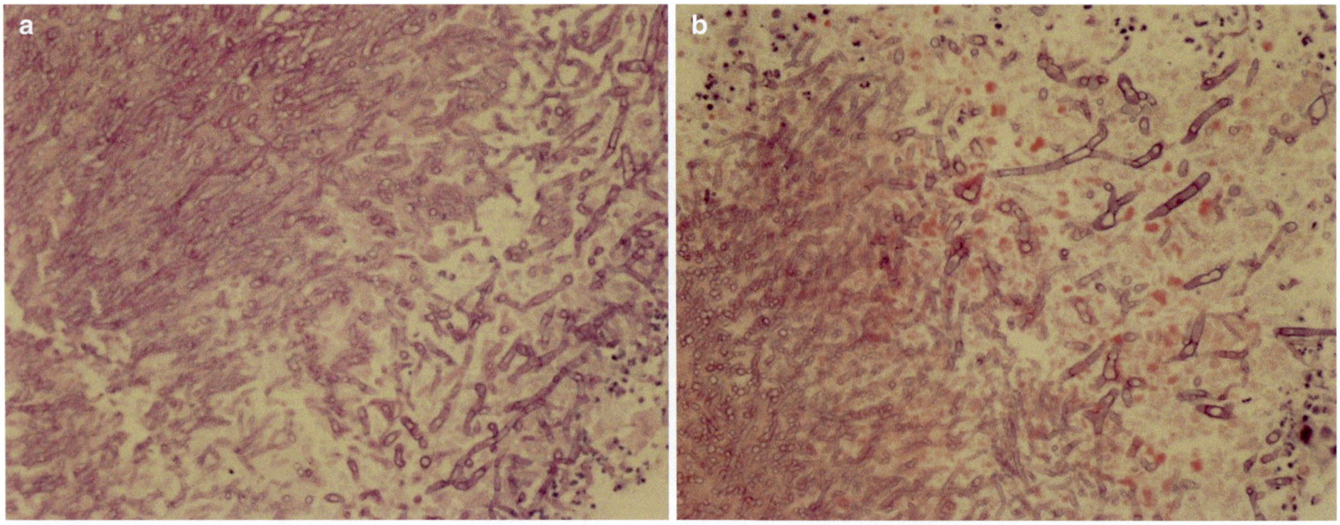

Fig. 11.15 (**a**, **b**) Pathology of the lung tissue. (**a**) Large quantities of hyphae and spores are demonstrated, and the hyphae, with septa and branch of 45°, twine into mass (H&E staining). (**b**) Large quantities of hyphae and spores are demonstrated, and the hyphae, with septa and branch of 45°, twine into mass. The external membrane of hyphae is stained red (PAS staining)

11.4.5 Comments

In this case, the condition was misdiagnosed as pulmonary tuberculosis, pulmonary abscess, and lung carcinoma, and the treatment was then delayed for up to 6 months. The diagnosis was finally defined as IPA by pathology. Based on its illness course, the condition can be categorized into chronic necrotizing pulmonary aspergillosis or semi-invasive pulmonary aspergillosis. The following two points should be noted by the clinicians.

1. The patient was a young woman, with no basic disease and structural lung disease. It was indicated that pulmonary aspergillosis may also occur in healthy people. The clinicians should inquire the history of occupational disease carefully because people working in some special occupation are at high risk of inhaling a large quantity of aspergillus that induces infection. Aspergillus grows and reproduces rapidly in damp rotted straws or rotted tree leaves. Therefore, large quantities of aspergillus exist in barns, cattle pens, and stables, which may induce primary pulmonary aspergillosis. In this case, the condition can be categorized into primary pulmonary aspergillosis.
2. In this case, CT scan demonstrated mass opacity at the lung, which was firstly suspected as peripheral lung carcinoma. But the clinical symptoms are mainly infection. The secondly suspected diseases included pneumonia, pulmonary abscess, and pulmonary tuberculosis. But both anti-infection and antituberculosis therapies showed poor therapeutic efficacy, and the condition improved and deteriorated. When the patient was hospitalized in our hospital, the disease had prolonged for 6 months. The diagnosis was finally defined by puncture of the lung with following biopsy. In this case, the diagnosis and treatment that the patient experienced indicated that for the cases that the clinical symptoms and radiology fail to be cross verified, especially when the therapeutic efficacy is poor, the thinking way for diagnosis should be changed and further investigations should be ordered. In this case, the clinical symptoms indicated infection. However, radiology, anti-infection therapy, and antituberculosis therapy did not support the diagnosis of infection. The diagnostic and therapeutic plan should be changed then. The patients with lung carcinoma also experience symptoms of fever, cough, and expectoration. If the diagnosis cannot be defined within 6 months, the optimal opportunity for treatment may be missed. In this case, pulmonary aspergillosis can be hardly considered in the differential diagnosis. But due to poor therapeutic efficacy of the anti-infection and antituberculosis therapies, further investigations are necessary to define the diagnosis.

11.5 Case 5: Joint Ache of the Four Limbs for More Than 1 Month as Well as Cough and Accompanying Fever for 3 Days

Chengying Hong, Junmin Wen, Xueyan Liu, Shi-Ping Wu, Pu-Xuan Lu, and Guan-Xun Cheng

11.5.1 Presenting Complaint

Joint ache of the four limbs for more than 1 month as well as cough and accompanying fever for 3 days.

11.5.2 Brief Case History

A 39-year-old woman was admitted to our hospital on October 21, 2012, due to presenting complaints of joint ache of the four limbs for more than 1 month as well as cough and accompanying fever for 3 days.

One month ago, the patient experienced joint ache of the four limbs with no known causes. But she experienced no joint swelling and restricted movements, no fever, and skin rash. Half a month ago, she began to experience fatigue of the four limbs that disabled her movement, and she then remained completely bedridden. Three days ago, she began to show cough, expectoration of yellowish white mucous sputum in a large quantity, and accompanying fever but no aversion to cold or chill. The highest body temperature was up to 38.7 °C, and she presented in the outpatient department of our hospital. And her blood pressure was 70/40 mmHg. The condition was considered to be infectious shock and she was hospitalized. After admission, the patient received anti-infection therapy with medication of piperacillin sodium and tazobactam sodium, supplementation of blood volume, nutritional support, and symptomatic support. But the fever persisted with the highest body temperature of 39 °C and unstable blood pressure. Intravenous infusion of dopamine was continued. On October 26, her partial pressure of oxygen decreased, and her SPO_2 was around 70% with face mask for high-flow oxygen inhalation. Tracheal incubation for mechanical ventilation was given, and the patient was transferred to general ICU for further treatment.

11.5.2.1 Past Medical History

She denied history of special diseases and reported a history of obvious hair loss.

11.5.2.2 Physical Examination

Physical examination when she was transferred to ICU showed a body temperature of 37.5 °C, a pulse rate of 140/min, respiration rate of 20/min, blood pressure 103/74 mmHg, SPO_2 95%, and FIO_2 50%. Peroral tracheal incubation for mechanical ventilation was given, and a large quantity of mucous thick sputum was aspirated from the airway. She was typically developed with average nourishment and anemic appearance. The patient was conscious with sparse hair on her head. The ventral surface of toes showed scattering dark reddish macula that was more obvious on the left foot and faded when pressed. The superficial lymph nodes were unpalpable with no enlargement. The respiration sounds of both lungs were coarse with moist rales and wheezing rale. The heartbeat was rhythmic, 140/min with no pathological murmur. The abdomen was soft, with no tenderness and rebound pain. Bowel sounds were positive. The meningeal irritation sign was negative. No pathological reflexes were induced.

11.5.2.3 Auxiliary Investigation

Laboratory Test

Routine blood test showed WBC 16.44 × 10^9/L, platelet 98.0 × 10^9/L, and hemoglobin concentration 72 × 10^9 g/L.

Blood chemistry showed GOT 214 U/L, ALT 59 U/L, and serum albumin 21.8 g/L. The kidney function test showed PCT 4.46 ng/ml on October 21, 8.23 ng/ml on October 24, and 27.55 ng/ml on October 26. C-reactive protein (CRP) was 35.4 mg/L. ESR was 78 mm/h.

Pathogenic investigations showed blood 1-3-β-D glucan 188.5 pg/ml on October 22. The blood antibody for *Mycobacterium tuberculosis* was negative. The blood IgM antibody for *Mycoplasma pneumoniae* was negative.

Blood immunological assay for rheumatism showed nuclear homogeneous type 1:100 positive, cytoplasmic granular type 1:100 positive, anti-double-stranded DNA antibodies positive, anti-PR3 antibody, anti-MPO antibody, and anti-GBM-IgG antibody negative.

The sputum culture on October 24 showed no growth of bacteria.

Radiology

Chest X-rays are shown on Figs. 11.16 and 11.17.

Chest CT scans are shown in Fig. 11.18.

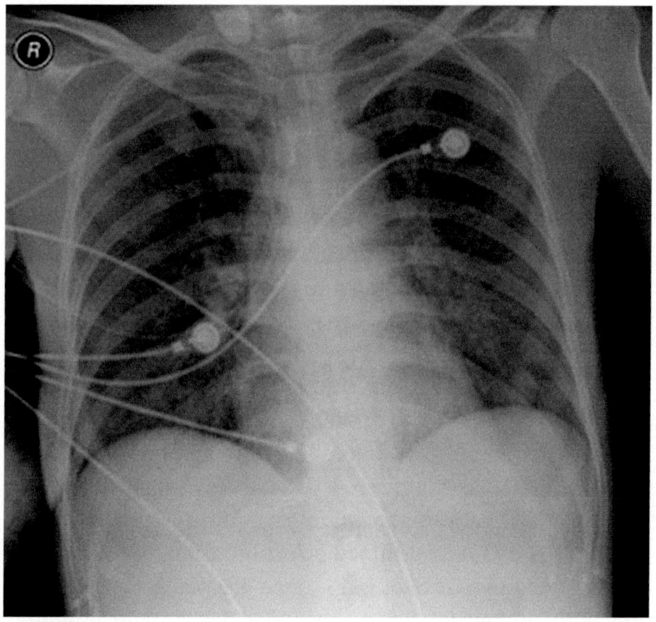

Fig. 11.16 Chest X-ray. Chest X-ray demonstrates increased and thickened lung markings in both lungs that are poorly defined. The left lung hilum is demonstrated to be ill defined, and the right lung hilum is demonstrated to be not enlarged. The mediastinum is demonstrated to be not widened. The bilateral diaphragmatic surfaces are demonstrated to be smooth, with sharp costophrenic angle. The condition was considered to be multiple infections at both lungs

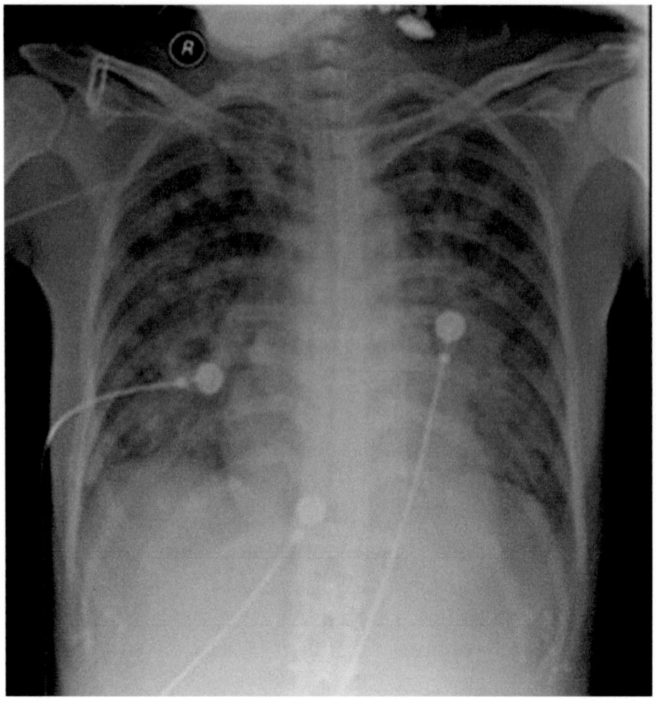

Fig. 11.17 Chest X-ray. Chest X-ray demonstrates decreased transparency of both lungs as well as thickened and deranged lung markings that are poorly defined. Both lungs are demonstrated with multiple poorly defined patchy exudations. And the heart opacity is enlarged

11.5.2.4 Initial Diagnosis

The initial diagnosis was systemic lupus erythematosus (SLE), lung infection, and respiratory failure of type I.

11.5.3 Diagnosis and Treatment

After admission, the patient experienced persistent fever, low blood pressure, dyspnea, and aspiration of bloody mucous sputum in a large quantity. Based on chest X-ray and chest CT scan, SLE was considered, and lupus pneumonia could not be excluded. Methylprednisolone, cytoxan, and large dose of intravenous immunoglobulin were given as pulse therapy. But due to obviously increased levels of blood PCT and peripheral WBC, complication of pulmonary bacterial infection was considered. Due to obviously increased level of blood 1-3-β-D glucan, the condition is more likely to be bacterial and fungal mixed infection. Imipenem was then administered at a dose of 0.5 g once every 6 h, in combination with fluconazol 0.6 g, once per day as anti-infection therapy. Meanwhile, pathogenic investigations were ordered, including blood bacterial and fungal cultures, sputum bacterial and fungal cultures, as well as BALF bacterial and fungal cultures. Re-examination on 27 October 2012 showed that bilateral pulmonary infection, bilateral lower pulmonary insufficiency, bilateral pleural effusion and pericardial effusion were all more advanced, which compared with the CT film on 24 October 2012 (Fig. 11.19).

By the abovementioned therapy, the airway bleeding volume decreased, and the patient began to experience expectoration of yellowish purulent sputum. To further define the lung condition, bedside fibrobronchoscopy was performed on October 29. Under the bronchoscope, there were mucosa congestion and erosion at the lower trachea, with adherence of purulent moss. Mucous biopsy and brushing test were performed at the opening of dorsal segment at the right lower lung lobe with purulent moss. In combination with radiological and bronchoscopic findings, aspergillus infection of lungs was suspected. Fluconazol was then withdrawn on October 29, and voriconazole was administered via intravenous infusion of 6 mg/kg every 12 h at the first day, followed by 4 mg/kg every 12 h.

On October 30, reexamination of blood 1-3-β-D glucan showed 222.1 pg/ml. On November 2, biopsy of bronchial mucosa indicated aspergillus infection (Fig. 11.20). On November 3, the bronchoscopic sputum culture showed growth of *Aspergillus fumigatus*.

The sputum cultures on November 1 and November 14, 2012, demonstrated Acinetobacter baumannii. The drug sensitivity test indicated that it was resistant to antibacterial drugs except cefoperazone/sulbactam and ampicillin/sulbactam mediator. On November 1, 2012, cefoperazone/sulbactam was added in a dose of 3.0 q8h. The blood cultures on November 4 and November 8 indicated growth of Acinetobacter baumanii that was resistant to all antibacterial drugs including tigecycline. On November 11, the BALF culture indicated growth of Acinetobacter baumanii and the drug sensitivity test showed the same results as the sputum culture.

Based on results of pathogenic investigations and drug sensitivity test, medications of imipenem, cefoperazone/sulbactam, and voriconazole were continued. The body temperature decreased and the autonomous respiration improved. On November 10, 2012, the respirator was withdrawn. And on November 11, tracheal incubation was withdrawn, and the medication to increase the blood pressure was discontinued.

Reexamination of chest CT on November 19, 2012, demonstrated decreased pleural effusion, complete atelectasis and consolidation of the right lower lung lobe, and decreased exudation and consolidation at the left lower lung lobe. The other parts of the lungs were demonstrated with multiple cavities which progressed compared to previous CT scan and nodule in large cavity. The condition was suspected to be complication of fungal infection (Fig. 11.21).

The final diagnosis was systemic lupus erythematosus (SLE), acute invasive pulmonary aspergillosis, baumanii infection of lungs, sepsis, and multiple organ dysfunction syndrome.

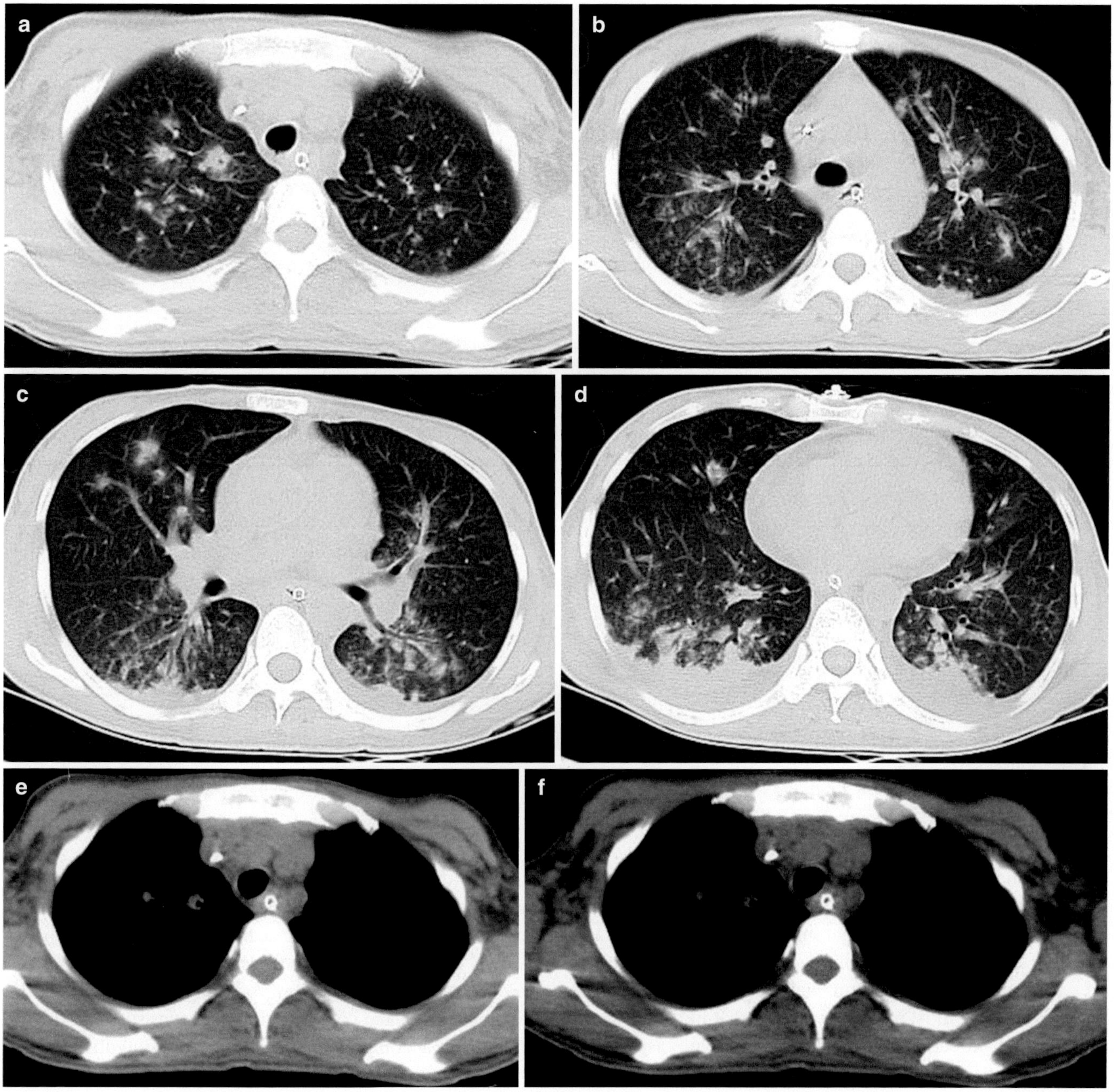

Fig. 11.18 (**a**–**f**) Chest CT scan. Both lungs are demonstrated with nodular and flakes of opacity in different sizes that are predominantly located at the middle and lower lung fields. There are also atelectasis of both lower lungs, bilateral pleural effusion, and multiple small lymph nodes at the mediastinum and bilateral axilla. Pericardial effusion is demonstrated in a small quantity

11.5.4 Discussion

Pulmonary aspergillosis is clinically classified into noninvasive pulmonary aspergillosis and invasive pulmonary aspergillosis. Noninvasive pulmonary aspergillosis includes aspergilloma and allergic bronchopulmonary aspergillosis. The condition of IPA is dangerous with rapid progression, and it commonly occurs in critically ill patients with compromised immunity. In patients with neutropenia, aspergillus infection of the lungs tends to induce pulmonary abscess or formation of granuloma. The use of glucocorticoid is the most common risk factor of invasive pulmonary aspergillosis in critically ill patients with no neutropenia. In such condition, aspergillus infection of the lungs commonly does not involve vascular wall, with comparatively chronic progression. The clinical manifestations and radiological demonstrations are atypical, which renders its early diagnosis challenging [22]. Autopsy of the death case in ICU has been

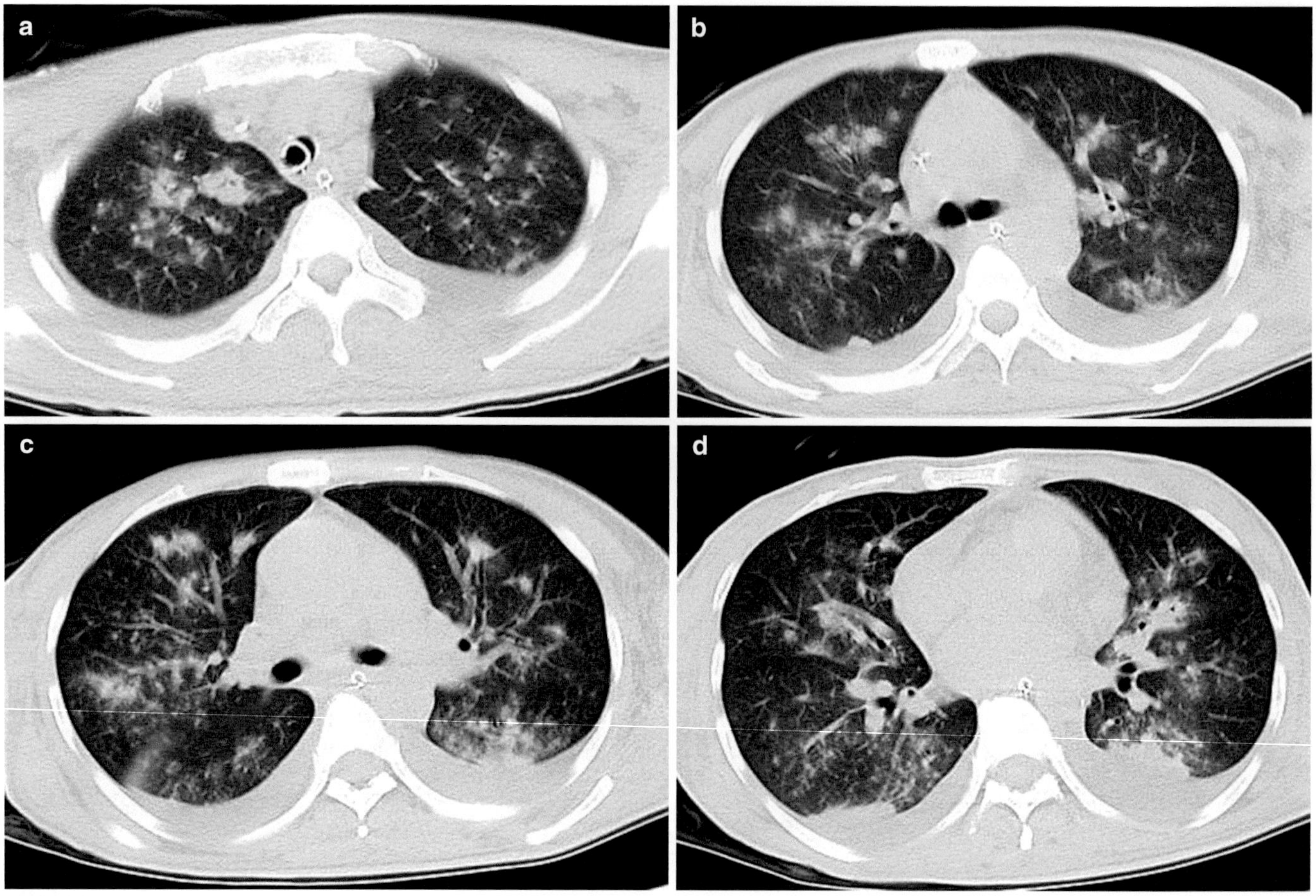

Fig. 11.19 (**a–d**) Chest CT scan. (**a–d**) Both upper, middle, and lower lungs are demonstrated with poorly defined patchy high-intensity opacity and bilateral pleural effusion

reported that IPA is the most commonly miss diagnosed infection in ICU [23]. In patients with SLE, the incidence of complicating pulmonary fungal infections has been increasing due to the application of glucocorticoid, immunosuppressant, and wide-spectrum antibiotics, among which aspergillus is the most important fungus that induces pulmonary fungal infections [24]. The pathogenic aspergillus includes *Aspergillus fumigatus* and *Aspergillus flavus*. *Aspergillus fumigatus* is the more common pathogen that induces aspergillus infection of the lungs [25]. In this case, the pathogen of pulmonary aspergillus infection was *Aspergillus fumigatus*.

The early clinical manifestations of SLE complicated by IPA are non-specific, and the condition progresses rapidly. It can be hardly differentiated from lupus pulmonary vasculitis or SLE complicated by pulmonary bacterial infections. Therefore, the critically or seriously ill patients admitted to critical care department should receive assessment of fungal infections, especially IPA. The radiological demonstration of IPA include (1) early subpleural nodular consolidation with increased intensity that shows halo sign several days later. About 10–15 days later, the consolidation of the lungs is subject to liquefaction and necrosis to show cavity shadow or crescent sign [4]. (2) The CT scan demonstrations of airway invasion include minor airway lesion, consolidation of tissues surrounding the airway, bronchiectasis or bronchial wall thickening, and consolidation of tissues surrounding the airway with accompanying cavity. And the diagnosis should be based on at least one of these demonstrations. (3) Mixed invasion is demonstrated with both (1) and (2) by CT scan. (4) Undefined type of invasion is demonstrated with none of above signs by CT scan [26]. IPA secondary to non-hematological disease is commonly demonstrated as signs of bronchial pneumonia with invasion of ground-glass opacity and consolidation along airway [27]. It should be noted that CT demonstrations of the lungs dynamically change in the cases of pulmonary aspergillosis and dynamic observation is clinically significant.

CT scan or HRCT of the lungs is valuable in the diagnosis of invasive fungal infections of the lungs. But early diagnosis of IPA based only on CT demonstrations is confined. CT scan, in combination with serum antigen detection including

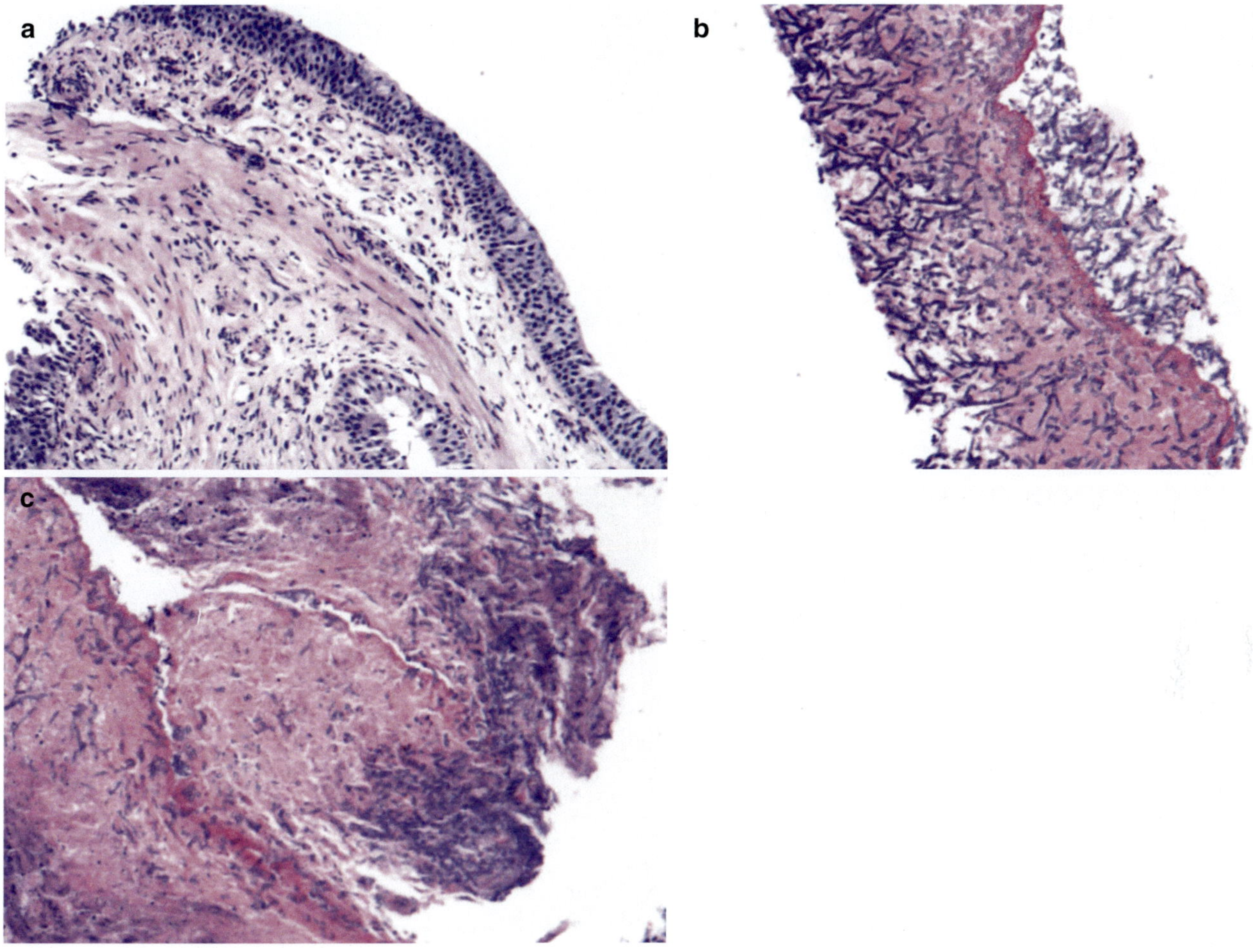

Fig. 11.20 (**a**–**c**) Pathology of the lung tissue. Biopsy at the dorsal segment at the right lower lung lobe demonstrates fungal mass, which is morphologically consistent to aspergillus (H&E staining)

blood 1-3-β-D glucan, serum GM test, and BALF GM test, is valuable in the early diagnosis of IPA. Xu et al. [27] have reported that in the diagnosis of IPA, the sensitivity of CT characteristic signs is 30%, while the sensitivity of combined CT characteristic signs with GM test is equivalent to simple GM test, being 47.5% and 50.0%, respectively. However, the specificity of combined CT characteristic signs with GM test is significantly higher than that of the simple GM test, being 100% and 84.2%, respectively. Therefore, for suspected cases of IPA with no agranulocytosis, combination of GM test with CT scan has certain sensitivity and favorable specificity. Du et al. [28] have reported that with GM value of 10 as positive threshold value, both specificity and predicted positive value of BALF GM test and serum GM test can reach 100%. However, both sensitivity and predicted negative value of BALF GM test (66.7% and 90.1%, respectively) are significantly higher than those of serum GM test (28.6% and 81.0%, respectively). When patients with SLE show symptoms and signs of lung infection as well as radiological demonstrations of new infiltration lesions, blood G test, blood GM test, and BALF GM test should be performed for early diagnosis. In such a way, the success rate of emergency rescue can be improved in the critically and seriously ill patients.

In this case, the patient suffered from a basic disease of SLE, and the patient had compromised immunity. Especially at the stage of active lupus and immunosuppression, patients with SLE are high-risk population of IPA. Patients with SLE and aggravating respiratory tract infection, if early radiological changes are atypical but blood 1-3-β-D glucan obviously increases, should be considered with invasive pulmonary fungal infection. In this case, the successful emergency rescue indicated that fibrobronchoscopic sputum culture and fibrobronchoscopic biopsy should be performed. In these ways, microbiological and histopathological evidence can be provided to define the diagnosis of IPA. Based on the results of investigations, the treatment plan should be changed accordingly. Only in such a way, the mortality rate of IPA can be reduced. But in this case, the symptoms were greatly improved by 4 weeks treatment, but radiology still

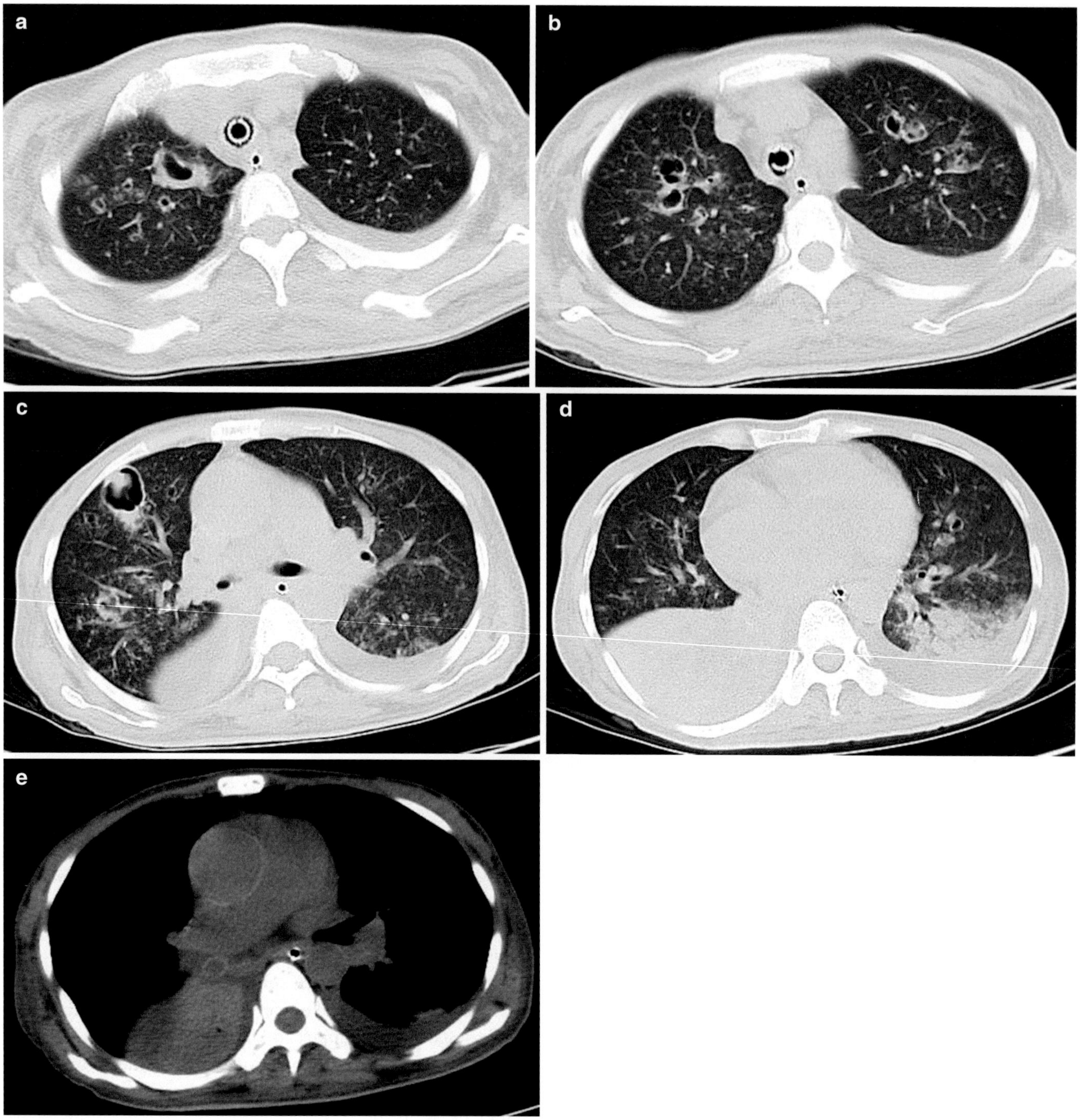

Fig. 11.21 (**a**–**e**) Chest CT scan. (**a**–**d**) The lung window demonstrates multiple newly emerging cavity opacities at both lungs that are in different sizes. Some large cavities are demonstrated with nodular opacity. There is also atelectasis of the right lower lung lobe that progresses compared to the previous CT scan. (**e**) The mediastinum window demonstrates atelectasis of the right lower lung and pleural effusion at the left lower thorax

demonstrated progression of the lesions, indicating patients with IPA and compromised immunity need prolonged therapeutic course. In clinical practice, medication should be sufficiently administered to avoid recurrence of lesions. In addition, IPA tends to involve vascular vessels to cause major hemorrhage and even threaten the life. In this case, CT scan indicated radiological signs of vascular invasion, and dynamic reexamination of chest CT scan should be ordered for close monitor of the lesions. If necessary, surgical operation can be performed for active intervention.

11.5.5 Comments

In this case, the diagnosis is definitive, and the patient suffered from a basic disease of SLE and complicating pulmonary bacterial infection and aspergillus infection (acute invasive pulmonary aspergillosis). In this case, 1 month prior to her admission, the patient experienced the onset of symptoms, including joint ache of the four limbs, fatigue of the four limbs, and difficulty moving. Three days prior to her admission, the patient began to experience symptoms of cough, fever, and even shock. After admission, large doses of hormone and other immunosuppressants were administered due to the diagnosis of lupus pneumonia. The questions are "Does complicating pulmonary fungal infection occur before or after her admission?" and "How to differentiate lupus pneumonia and fungal lung infection?"

SLE is an autoimmune disease commonly occurring in young women. Immunologically, it manifests as decreased T lymphocytes, dysfunctional T-cell inhibition, and excessive proliferation of B cells. About 30% of patients with SLE show accompanying *hyperglobulinemia*. The serum IgG level increases during active stage of the disease, while complements C3, C4, and CH50 decrease during the active stage of the disease, which is associated with consumption of complements during formation of immune complexes. Therefore, the immunologic changes of SLE are generally immune disorder of organism instead of immune deficiency. SLE complicated by infection, especially fungal infection, is rare. In this case, the pulmonary changes on admission are possibly lupus pneumonia.

SLE tends to be complicated by infection mostly due to the application of steroid hormone and immunosuppressant, especially large dose of steroid hormone for pulse therapy at the reduced remission stage. The immunity of patients is deeply suppressed and the patients are susceptible to infections. In this case, the patient received methylprednisolone and cyclophosphamide as the pulse therapy due to the diagnosis of active SLE and possible lupus pneumonia. Reexamination of lung CT scan on October 27 demonstrated progression of lesions at both lungs, which indicated complicating infection. If the symptoms improved and radiology demonstrated improved condition but fever and pulmonary symptoms recurred and aggravated with radiological signs of progression in patients receiving large doses of steroid hormone and immunosuppressant, infection, especially fungal infection, should be suspected.

If CT scan of the lungs demonstrates early subpleural nodular consolidation opacity of high intensity, surrounding halo sign several days later and liquefaction and necrosis of consolidation and emergence of cavity opacity or crescent sign 10–15 days later, a diagnosis of pulmonary aspergillus infection can be made. Based on the atypical radiological demonstrations of the lungs, pulmonary aspergillus infection can be hardly differentiated from the primary disease such as lupus pneumonia. The key point is that the clinicians should know more about pulmonary aspergillus infection, and pathogenic and pathologic investigations should be ordered as early as possible. 1-3-β-D glucan test, serum GM test, and BALF GM test are extremely important for the early diagnosis of IPA. If possible, these investigations should be ordered. In this case, the successful emergency rescue is based on timely fibrobronchoscopic sputum culture and fibrobronchoscopic biopsy, which provide microbiologic and pathologic evidence for the diagnosis of IPA.

11.6 Case 6: Fever and Expectoration of Yellowish Sputum for 1 Month

Wei Gao, Guan-Xun Cheng, Dandan Chen, Xueyan Liu, Chengying Hong, and Xuemei Han

11.6.1 Presenting Complaint

Fever and expectoration of yellowish sputum for 1 month.

11.6.2 Brief Case History

A 30-year-old man, farmer, was admitted to our hospital on September 13, 2013, due to presenting complaints of fever and expectoration of yellowish sputum for 1 month. One month ago, the patient began to experience fever with no known causes, and the highest body temperature was 41 °C. The associate symptoms include cough, expectoration of yellowish sputum with a small quantity of blood streak, chest distress, breathlessness, and incapability of violent sports. In another hospital, chest X-ray demonstrated pneumonia of the right lower lung. Chest plain CT scan demonstrated possible pulmonary abscess of the right lung. Intravenous infusion of medication was given (specifically unknown), and the condition was not improved. For further diagnosis and treatment, he presented in the outpatient department of our hospital and was admitted due to mass in the right lower lung.

11.6.2.1 Past Medical History

He was definitively diagnosed with diabetes on September 6, 2013, and was receiving insulin therapy. And he denied medical histories of hepatitis and tuberculosis. He also denied habitual smoking and drinking.

11.6.2.2 Physical Examination

Physical examination showed a body temperature of 36.0 °C, pulse rate 95/min, respiration rate 18/min, and blood pressure 118/74 mmHg. The patient was typically developed, with good nourishment and natural expression. His spiritual state was good and he is well cooperated with the physical examination. The systemic superficial lymph nodes were unpalpable with no enlargement. The thorax showed no abnormality. The sternum showed no tenderness. The respiration movements and intercostal space were normal. The vocal fremitus of the right lung increased. By percussion, the right lung showed partial flatness. The respiration sound of the left lung was clear with a small quantity of moist rales. The respiration sound of the right lung was weak, with a large quantity of moist rales. The precordial area showed no protrusion. The border of cardiac dullness was normal, with heartbeat of 95/min, rhythm. By auscultation, the valvular areas showed no pathological murmur. The abdomen was soft, with no tenderness. The liver and spleen were subcostally unpalpable. Both lower limbs showed no edema.

11.6.2.3 Auxiliary Investigation

Laboratory Test

ESR was 70 mm/h and CRP 10.9 mg/L on September 13, 2013.

Radiology

Chest X-ray on August 28, 2013, in another hospital demonstrated pneumonia of the right lower lung.

Chest plain CT scan on September 7, 2013, in another hospital demonstrated pulmonary abscess of the right lung.

11.6.2.4 Initial Diagnosis

The initial diagnosis was space-occupying lesion of the right lung, which was suspected to be fungal infection or neoplasm, and type II diabetes.

11.6.3 Diagnosis and Treatment

After admission, blood sugar level was closely monitored, and subcutaneous injection of insulin was given for active control of blood sugar. Routine blood test on September 14, 2013, showed no abnormality. The neoplasm biomarkers were Cyfra 21-1 1.55 ng/ml, NSE 15.41 ng/ml, and CEA 2.02 μg/L. Repeated sputum smears showed no growth of bacteria and acid fast bacilli. The sputum culture for fungi and identification on September 16, 2013, showed no growth of *Monilia*. Chest X-ray on September 13, 2013, demonstrated thick wall cavity at the dorsal right middle lung field, poorly defined flakes of high-intensity opacity at its inferior margin, as well as thickened, increased, and deformed lung markings of the right lower lung (Fig. 11.22).

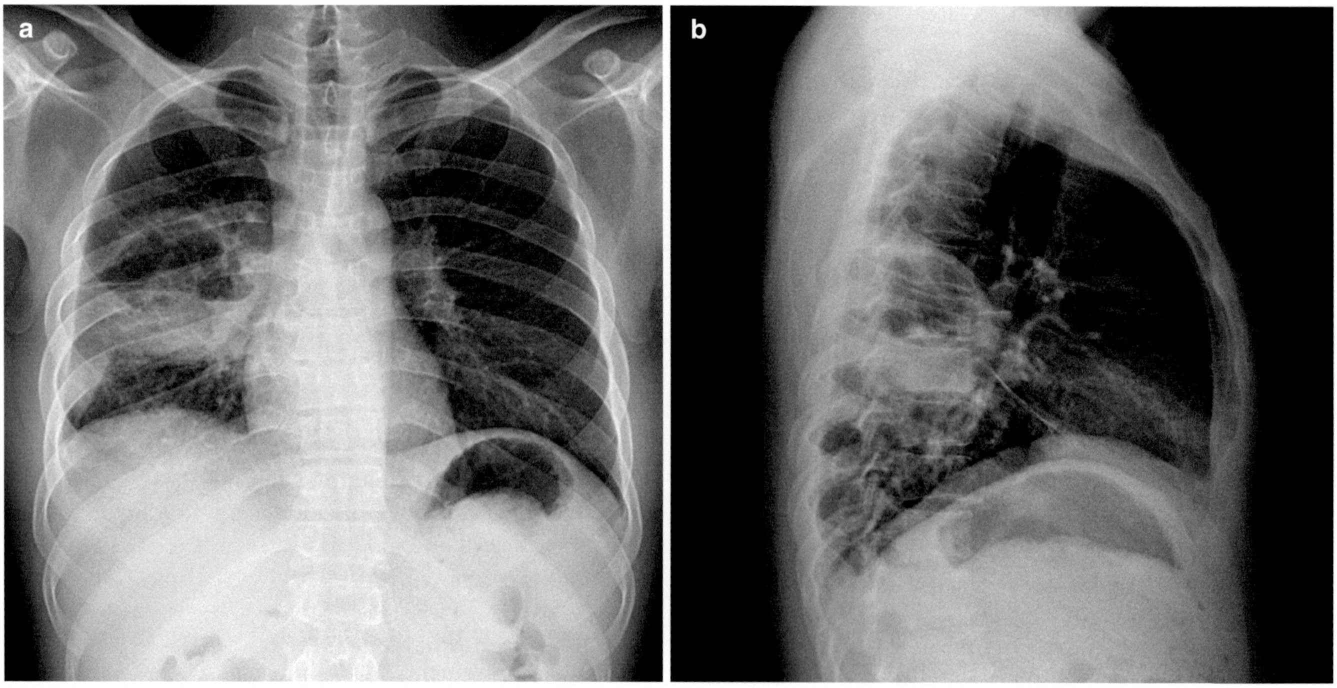

Fig. 11.22 (**a**, **b**) Chest X-ray. The dorsal part of the right middle lung field is demonstrated with thick wall cavity and poorly defined flakes of high-intensity opacity at its inferior margin. In combination with the lateral chest X-ray, the lesion is located at the dorsal segment of the right lower lung lobe

Chest CT scan on September 18, 2013, demonstrated mass-like high-intensity opacity at the dorsal segment of the right lower lung lobe in size of about 0.7 cm × 0.6 cm, with inner air crescent sign. The inner wall of the mass-like high-intensity opacity was smooth, with filiform opacity inside. The mass-like high-intensity opacity was poorly defined, and adjacent lung markings were blurry, presented as small flake of ground-glass opacity. Some lung tissues were demonstrated with consolidation, with air bronchogram inside. The adjacent pleura was thickened. By enhanced scanning, the cystic wall of the lesion showed moderate enhancement, and the inner necrotic area showed no enhancement. The basilar segment of the right lower lung lobe was demonstrated with multiple poorly defined spots and strips of high-intensity opacity, which were more obvious in the posterior basilar segment of the right lower lung lobe. The right lung hilum was demonstrated with several calcified lymph nodes. And the tracheal bifurcation was demonstrated with enlarged lymph node opacity with a transverse diameter of about 2.9 cm. At the dorsal part of bilateral thorax, a small quantity of arch-shaped liquid intensity opacity was demonstrated (Fig. 11.23).

The diagnosis was made based on the radiological findings. The cavity at the dorsal segment of the right lower lung lobe and the multiple patchy opacities at the basilar segment of the right lower lung lobe were considered to be pulmonary abscess. And the soft tissue intensity opacity at the right lung hilum was possibly lung carcinoma.

Due to his medical history of diabetes, fungal infection was not excluded. And voriconazole was given at a dose of 20 ml, once per day, as antifungal therapy. Fibrobronchoscopic brushing test showed aspergillus. In combination with chest CT demonstrations of pulmonary abscess, the diagnosis was suspected to be aspergillus infection complicated by pulmonary abscess. Due to the poor therapeutic efficacy and risk of major hemoptysis of palliative therapy, surgical operation was recommended. At day 12 after admission, thoracoscopic wedge removal of the right lower and upper lung was performed. Postoperative pathology demonstrated fungal pneumonia of the right lower lung, which was morphologically consistent to aspergillus infection, with accompanying chronic purulent inflammation and formation of cavity (Fig. 11.24).

The diagnosis on admission was chronic necrotizing pulmonary aspergillosis and type II diabetes.

After the operation, the patient showed no surgical complications, and the incision was favorably healed. The patient recovered and was discharged.

11.6.4 Discussion

Invasive pulmonary aspergillosis commonly occurs in populations with suppressed immunity, such as patients with diabetes, connective tissue disorder, alcoholism, malnutrition, elderly, chronic granuloma, or receiving glucocorticoid. Chronic necrotizing pulmonary aspergillosis (CNPA) is also known as subacute invasive aspergillosis (SAIA). During its early stage, it presents as inflammatory nodule, formation of granuloma, and accompanying halo sign, with secondary cavity in the consolidation area that gradually enlarges. The disease commonly progresses slowly in months or shows acute onset within weeks. In this case, the patient suffered from diabetes, and the onset of symptoms lasted for more than 1 month. The clinical symptoms include fever, cough, expectoration, hemoptysis, and breathlessness. Laboratory tests showed elevated levels of inflammatory indices. By chest CT scan, lesions of infection and accompanying formation of cavity were demonstrated. Fibrobronchoscopic brushing demonstrated aspergillus. And postoperative pathology defined the diagnosis of aspergillus infection. Clinically, the condition was consistent to the diagnostic key points of CNPA [29].

The clinical symptoms of CNPA resemble to those of active pulmonary tuberculosis, atypical mycobacteriosis, and pulmonary histoplasmosis. Its definitive diagnosis is based on histopathologic examination or tissue culture. Pathologically, it is characterized by infiltration of aspergillus hyphae in lung tissue, accompanying bleeding, tissue necrosis, formation of microabscess, and infiltration of inflammatory cells. By CT scan, it is typically demonstrated as the most common consolidation with formation of cavity at the upper lung lobe as well as filiform, cotton wool-like, and spongy lesions in the cavity. Emergence of new consolidations, honeycomb-like lesion, and pleural effusion around the cavity indicates progression of the disease. For patients with chronic lung disease and compromised immunity, emergence of small flake of ground-glass opacity and small nodule at the upper lung lobe with surrounding halo sign should be considered as early lesions of CNPA [30]. In this case, the patient showed a nodular high-intensity opacity and patchy ground-glass opacity at the dorsal segment of the right lower lung lobe and air crescent sign in the nodule, which were consistent to the diagnostic key points of CNPA by chest CT scan.

Clinically, CNPA should be differentiated from pulmonary aspergilloma. The key points for differentiation include the following: (1) Histopathological examination is the golden standard for diagnosis. In the cases of CNPA, aspergillus may infiltrate the lung tissue to induce tissue bleeding and necrosis, formation of microabscess, and infiltration of inflammatory cells. However, aspergilloma only grows in cavity or cystic lumen. (2) The common symptoms of CNPA include cough, expectoration, and hemoptysis. In most cases of CNPA, the condition is complicated by systemic toxic symptoms such as low-grade fever, weight loss, night sweat, and fatigue. However, the common symptoms of aspergilloma include hemoptysis, cough, and expectoration.

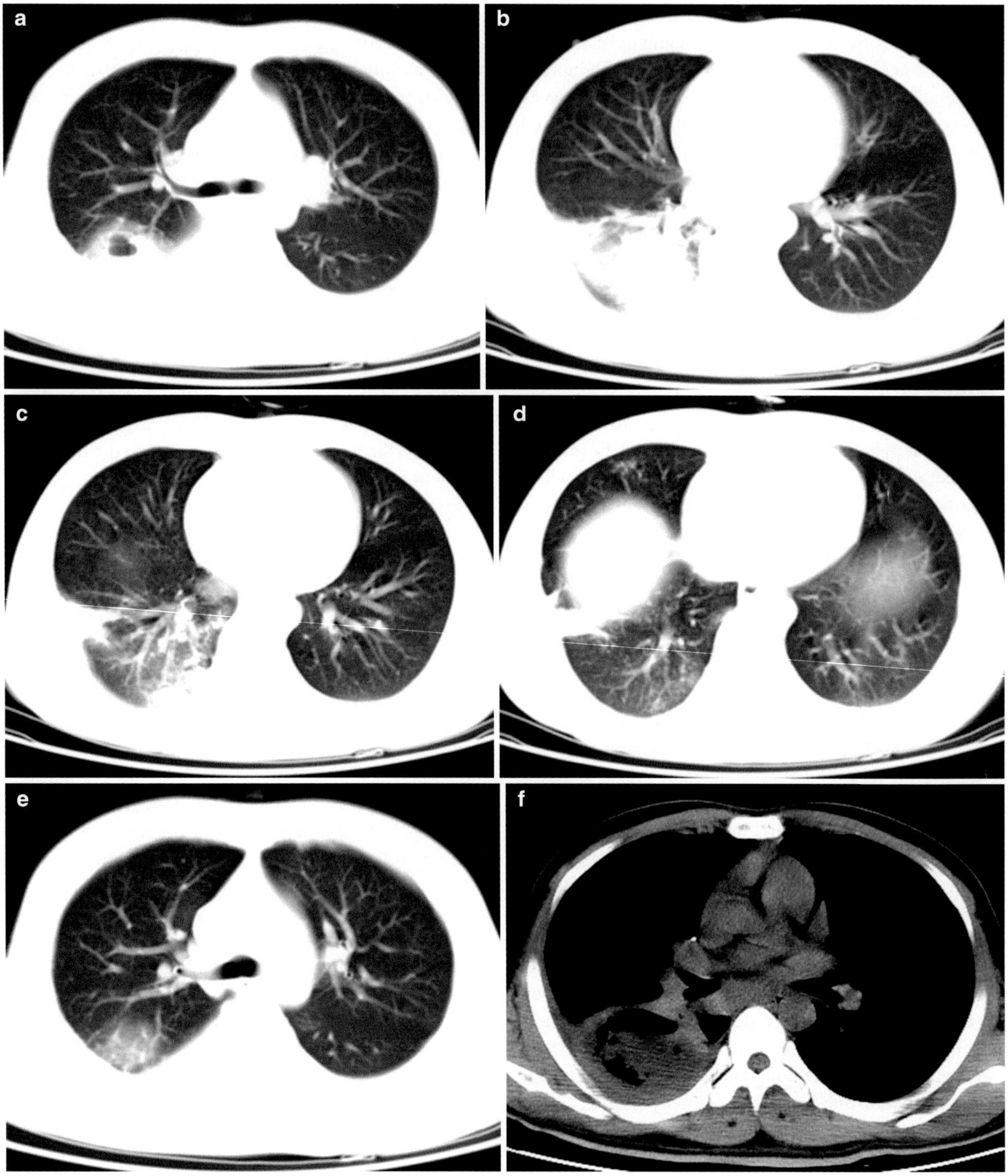

Fig. 11.23 (**a**–**i**) Chest CT scan. (**a**) The lung marking adjacent to lesion at the dorsal segment of the right lower lung lobe is blurry, presented as small flake of ground-glass opacity. (**b**) The dorsal segment of the right lower lung lobe is demonstrated with a mass-like high-intensity opacity in size of about 0.7 cm × 0.6 cm, with air crescent sign inside. (**c**) The surrounding lung tissues of the high-intensity lesion at the dorsal segment of the right lower lung lobe are demonstrated with consolidation opacity, with air bronchogram. (**d**, **e**) The basilar segment of the right lower lung lobe is demonstrated with multiple poorly defined spots and strips of high-intensity opacity, which are more obvious at the posterior basilar segment of the right lower lung lobe. (**f**, **g**) The mediastinum window demonstrates mass-like high-intensity opacity at the dorsal segment of the right lower lung lobe, with smooth inner wall and filiform opacity inside. The lesion has poorly defined margin and some lung tissues show consolidation opacity. The adjacent pleura is thickened. (**h**) The right lung hilum is demonstrated with several calcified lymph nodes. And the tracheal bifurcation is demonstrated with an enlarged lymph node opacity with a transverse diameter of about 2.9 cm. (**i**) Enhanced mediastinum window demonstrates high-intensity opacity at the dorsal segment of the right lower lung lobe, moderate enhancement of the cystic wall, and no enhancement of the inner necrosis

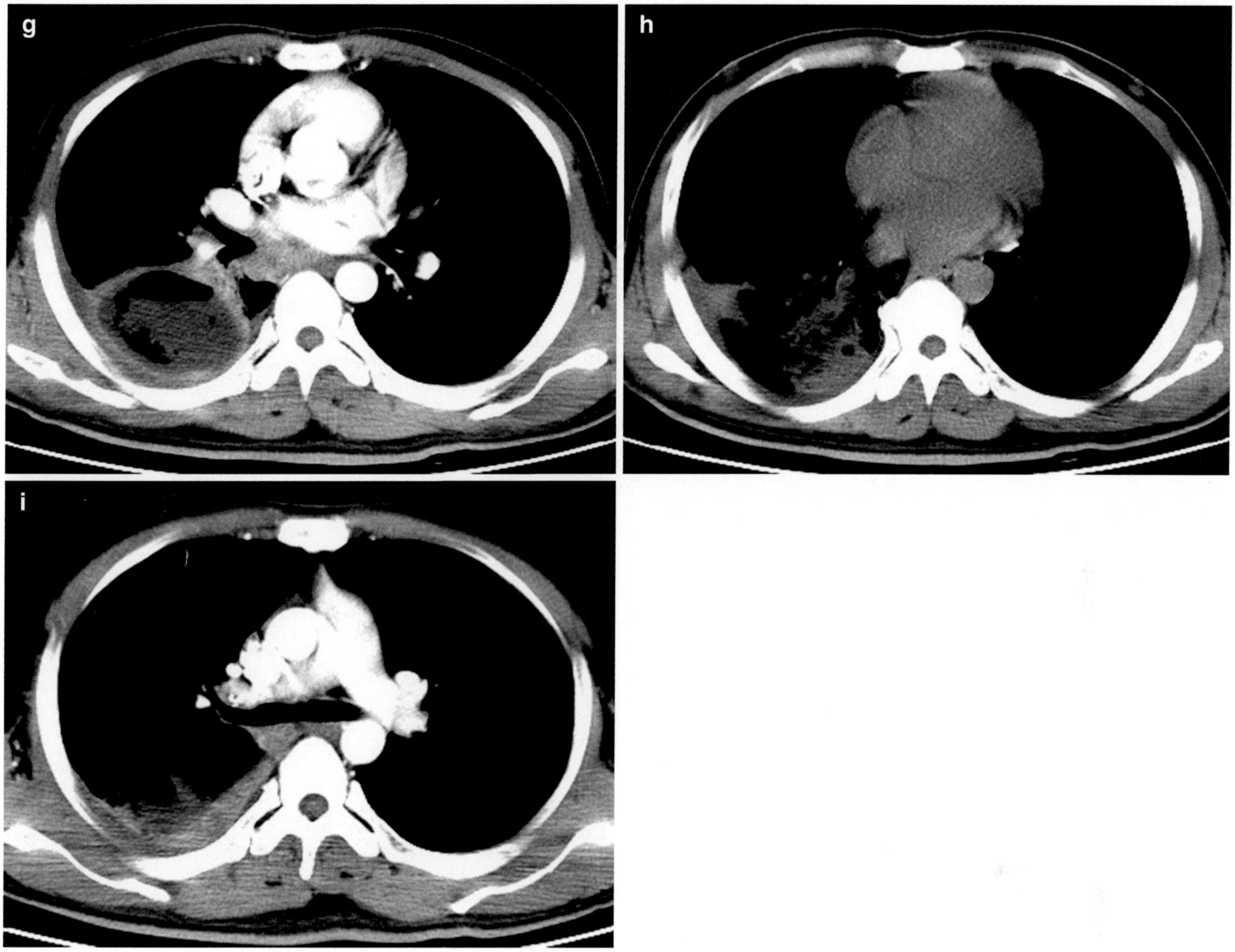

Fig. 11.23 (continued)

(3) Radiological demonstration of air crescent sign indicates both CNPA and pulmonary aspergilloma [31]. However, the cavity in the cases of CNPA is commonly thick wall cavity with irregular wall and surrounding infiltration opacity. In the cases of pulmonary aspergilloma, the cavity wall is comparatively thin, with regular wall and rare surrounding infiltration opacity. Along with the progression of the disease, pulmonary aspergilloma hardly changes. But in the cases of CNPA, the cavity may enlarge with pulmonary fibrosis that finally progresses into chronic fibrous cavitary pulmonary aspergillosis. Therefore, dynamic observation by radiology is necessary. Other common radiological demonstrations of CNPA and pulmonary aspergilloma include nodular or mass-like opacity. The nodular or mass-like opacity in the cases of CNPA commonly has a large area that possibly develops into lobar or segmental consolidation, with accompanying air bronchogram. The nodular or mass-like opacity in the cases of pulmonary aspergilloma has a small area, rarely with air bronchogram. However, the condition in some cases of pulmonary aspergilloma may develop into CNPA when the immunity of patients is compromised. (4) Acute inflammatory markers such as C-reactive protein and blood viscosity facilitate the differentiation of CNPA and pulmonary aspergilloma. These indicators increase in patients with CNPA [32].

CNPA also needs to be differentiated from tuberculosis. The two diseases share some commonalities in CT scan demonstrations, including common location at the upper lung lobes, formation of cavity, and fibrosis. Therefore, their differentiation is challenging. The following key points facilitate the differentiation: (1) In the cases of old pulmonary tuberculosis with accompanying chronic necrotizing pulmonary aspergillosis, lung consolidation occurs based on primary lesions of tuberculosis, with emergence of huge cavity in about 2 weeks. In the cases of tuberculosis, tuberculoma firstly forms with following formation of cavity in several weeks or months. The size of cavity is associated with the size of tuberculoma. In addition, the

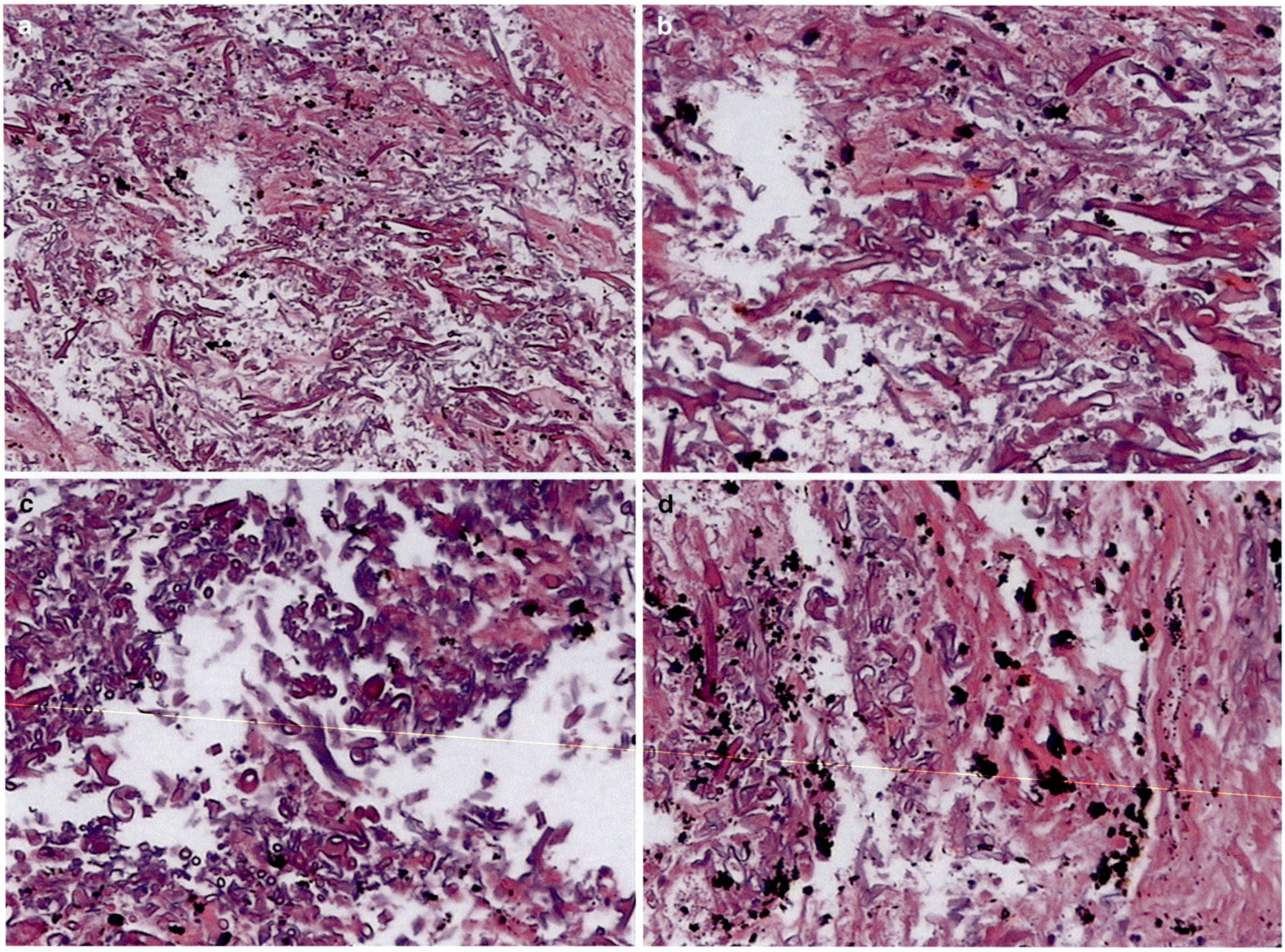

Fig. 11.24 (**a**–**d**) Pathology of lung tissue. H&E staining demonstrates hyphae with septa and branching in 45° angle

lesions of caseous pneumonia in the cases of tuberculosis are mainly insect erosive small cavity. (2) In the cases of CNPA, the cavity has thick and irregular wall with unsmooth inner and outer walls. Filiform opacity is attached to the inner wall and in the cavity. In the cases of tuberculosis, the cavity may be thick wall cavity, but no filiform opacity is attached to the inner wall and in the cavity. (3) In the cases of tuberculosis, satellite lesions are common, while the lesions of CNPA are surrounded by consolidation and fibrosis. Therefore, the cases with formation of huge cavity at upper lung lobe within a short period of time, filiform opacity in the cavity, and no satellite lesions around the cavity are commonly diagnosed with CNPA. Differential diagnosis can be made in combination with case history and radiological changes [33].

The therapies for treatment of CNPA include medication, surgical removal, and interventional therapy.

1. Medication: Patients with CNPA need systemic antifungal therapy with prolonged therapeutic course or even lifelong antifungal therapy. To prevent progression and relapse of the disease, collaborative medications of two from polyenes, triazoles, and echinocandins should be administered if necessary.
2. Surgical removal: The indications of surgical removal include large cavity or formation of abscess, poor therapeutic efficacy by medication with accompanying major hemoptysis, or nodular opacity at the lung that is incapable of differentiating from neoplasm. Surgical removal is only indicated to patients with reserved pulmonary function. And antifungal medication should be administered along with surgery.
3. Interventional therapy: The cavity filling therapy is injection of mixed antifungal medication and gel into cavity via fibrobronchoscope or CT-guided percutaneous puncture into the cavity to create an oxygen-free environment in the cavity. For patients with major hemoptysis but contraindicated to surgery, bronchial artery embolization can be chosen. In such a way, 75–90% of the patients show immediate hemostasis. However, the long-term

recurrence rate is high, and follow-ups for at least 3 years are recommended. Due to vascular invasion of aspergillus, it is believed that the recurrence rate of CNPA is higher [34].

11.6.5 Comments

Subacute invasive aspergillosis (SAIA) is also known as semi-invasive pulmonary aspergillosis. It commonly occurs in patients with slightly compromised immunity or extremely weak condition, such as patients with diabetes, malnutrition, alcoholism, elderly, COPD, connective tissue disorder, *Mycobacterium tuberculosis* infection of the lungs, and HIV infection as well as receiving long-term medication of hormones, other immunosuppressant, and radiotherapy. Concerning diabetes as a risk factor of pulmonary aspergillosis, the clinical guidelines show national or regional variance. Diabetes has not been listed as a risk factor of pulmonary aspergillosis in the 2007 consensus on diagnosis and treatment of pulmonary mycosis in China and the latest 2016 clinical guideline for diagnosis and treatment of aspergillosis by the IDSA. However, diabetes has been listed as the first high risk factor in the 2015 clinical guideline for diagnosis and treatment of chronic pulmonary aspergillosis jointly issued by the ESCMID and ERS.

Patients with diabetes show immune disorder. The high level of blood sugar suppresses phagocytosis of the neutrophil granulocytes, which compromised the immunity against infections. The high blood sugar environment also promotes growth and reproduction of fungi. In recent years, more cases of diabetes complicated by invasive pulmonary aspergillosis have been reported. According to released data, the incidence rate of invasive pulmonary aspergillosis in patients with diabetes is 3–4 times as high as that in healthy population. In this case, the patient was a young man who had just been diagnosed with diabetes before his admission to our hospital. His family history of diabetes remained unknown. During the treatment for pulmonary aspergillosis, the level of blood sugar was closely monitored, and a nearly normal level of blood sugar was maintained.

A detailed inquiry of his recent housing and daily life was made for possible exposure to environment with a large quantity of aspergillus spores or inhalation of a large quantity of aspergillus spores from crops and/or soil. Due to the onset at a young age, HIV screening should also be considered.

For diagnosis of aspergillosis, the sputum culture has a low positive rate. But BALF investigation or brushing facilitates detecting the pathogen.

In this case, the radiological demonstrations included consolidation, cavity, and abscess. No risk factor of surgical operation was found except diabetes. The patient showed favorable cardiopulmonary functions. By surgical removal, long-term cure was achieved, hemoptysis and local expansion of lesions were avoided, and the survival rate was improved.

11.7 Case 7: Fever, Cough, and Sputum with Blood Streak for 1 Month

Mengjie Feng, Yuemei Lu, Minjie Yang, Wei-Dong Song, Jiezhu Ding, and Hui Yin

11.7.1 Presenting Complaints

Fever, cough, and sputum with blood streak for 1 month.

11.7.2 Brief Case History

A 56-year-old man was admitted to our hospital due to complaints of fever, cough, and sputum with blood streak for 1 month. One month ago, the patient began to experience fever (body temperature unknown), cough, expectoration of yellowish purulent sputum, and sputum with blood streak. Half a month ago, the patient received chest X-ray in another hospital, demonstrating large flake of high-intensity opacity at the left upper lung, which was considered to be pulmonary tuberculosis of the left upper lung. Levofloxacin was administered for treatment but the symptoms were not improved. Reexamination of chest X-ray demonstrated obviously increased lesions at the left upper lung. Chest CT scan demonstrated bronchiectasis and infection at the left upper lung. Cefoperazone/sulbactam in combination with amikacin and imipenem/cilastatin and piperacillin/sulbactam in combination with levofloxacin were consecutively administered as anti-infection therapy and symptomatic support. But the patient still experienced cough and fever. Reexamination of chest CT scan on December 6, 2014, demonstrated enlarged area with lesions and bilateral pleural effusion of small quantities. For further diagnosis and treatment, the patient was admitted to our hospital. Since the onset of symptoms, the patient showed poor appetite and sleep. The bowel movements were normal, with no obvious weight loss.

11.7.2.1 Past Medical History

He reported a past medical history of hypertension and left nephrectomy due to atrophy of the left kidney.

11.7.2.2 Physical Examination

Physical examination showed a body temperature of 37.2 °C, pulse rate 97/min, respiration rate 20/min, and blood pressure 106/64 mmHg. The respiration sounds of both lungs were coarse. By auscultation, the left lung showed moist rales, and the right lung showed no obvious dry and/or moist rales. The heartbeat rate was 97/min, rhythm. The valvular areas showed no pathological murmur by auscultation. The abdomen was soft, with no tenderness and rebound pain. Both lower limbs showed no edema.

11.7.2.3 Auxiliary Investigation

Laboratory Test

Routine blood test showed WBC 12.1×10^9/L and N 80.9%. Routine urine test showed occult blood (+++), WBC (±), urobilinogen (±), and protein (±). Blood gas analysis showed pH 7.491, PCO_2 30.2 mmHg, PO_2 55.2 mmHg, and FIO_2 21%. Hs-CRP 161.97 mg/L. The liver function test showed ALB 28.1 g/L. The glycosyl antigen 125 was 46.09 U/ml. The procalcitonin PCT was 0.21 ng/ml. ESR was 113 mm/h. Antibody against *Mycobacterium tuberculosis* was positive. Total cholesterol was 2.86 mmol/L. The high-density lipoprotein HDL was 0.67 mmol/L. The blood electrolytes, myocardial enzyme, kidney function test, AFP, carcinoembryonic antigen, glycosyl antigen 19-9, Cyfra 21-1, neuro-specific enolase, antibody against *Mycoplasma pneumoniae*, fungal 1-3-β-D glucan, antibody against AIDS, antibody against syphilis, series of vasculitis, ANA series, and antibody spectrum against ENA were within normal limits. The Widal's reaction and Weil-Felix reaction were negative. The antibody against tuberculosis was negative. The sputum smear for acid fast bacillus was negative. The sputum cultures showed growth of *Micrococcus catarrhalis* and alpha streptococcus. The sputum smear showed pairs of Gram-negative cocci, strains of Gram-positive cocci, and occasional Gram-negative small *Bartonella* bacteria but no yeasts. Non-repeated sputum culture of qualified sputum specimen showed *Aspergillus fumigatus*.

Radiology

Color Doppler ultrasound of the abdomen demonstrated slight hepatic adipose infiltration, multiple hepatic cysts, multiple right kidney stones, no left kidney, and slightly enlarged prostate gland. Color Doppler ultrasound of the heart demonstrated aortic sclerosis, aneurysmal dilatation of ascending aorta, dysfunctional left ventricular diastole, well functional left ventricular systole, and no obvious ventricular wall motion abnormality at resting.

11.7.2.4 Initial Diagnosis

The initial diagnoses were bronchiectasis and infection, type I respiratory failure, and respiratory alkalosis.

11.7.3 Diagnosis and Treatment

After admission, the patient received enhanced chest CT scan on November 15, 2014, which demonstrated mass and flake of consolidation at the left upper lung lobe, with air crescent sign inside. The diagnosis was considered to be possible fungal infection. Both lungs were demonstrated with segmental slight bronchiectasis with accompanying infection. And bilateral pleural effusion in small quantities was also demonstrated (Fig. 11.25). By bronchoscopy, mucosa congestion and swelling were demonstrated at the segments of right upper lung lobe as well as bronchial opening of the left lower lung lobe. The bronchial opening of the right middle lung lobe was subject to protrusion of local mucosa. The pathology of bronchial mucosa at the left upper lung lobe demonstrated epithelial squamous metaplasia that was well differentiated, hyperplastic inflammatory granulation tissue under the epithelium, no changes of tuberculosis, and acid-fast staining negative. Fibrobronchoscopic harvest of sputum for smear and the sputum smear showed no acid fast bacillus.

Based on chest CT scans, the diagnosis was made to be aspergillus infection of the lungs. Voriconazole was then administered for anti-infection treatment. The symptoms of cough and expectoration were improved, hemoptysis was cured, and the body temperature returned to normal. The patient was discharged due to stable condition.

The diagnosis on discharge was invasive pulmonary aspergillosis, bronchiectasis, and type I respiratory failure.

After discharge, voriconazole in combination with acetylcysteine was continued, with regular follow-ups. The symptoms of cough and expectoration were obviously improved. Reexamination of chest CT scan on January 15, 2015, demonstrated slightly improved lesion at the left lung and absorption of bilateral pleural effusion (Fig. 11.26).

On April 20, 2015, the patient presented in our hospital complaining aggravating cough and expectoration during the recent 1 month. He coughed up dark yellow purulent sputum. Reexamination of chest CT scan demonstrated slightly enlarged space-occupying lesion at the apex of left lung. He was admitted again and received bronchoscopy on April 30, 2015. Pathology of bronchoscopic brushing is shown in Fig. 11.27. And pathology of fibrobronchoscopic lung tissue is shown in Fig. 11.28.

Pathology of fibrobronchoscopic lung tissue demonstrates hyperplasia of fibrous tissue as well as infiltrations of many lymphocytes, neutrophil granulocytes, and histocytes in the interstitium. The changes are demonstrated as chronic inflammation. By IHC, CD68 histocytes show positive and CK epithelium positive. By histochemistry, methenamine silver is negative (H&E staining).

To further define the diagnosis, percutaneous puncture of the lung for biopsy was performed on May 5, 2015, and the

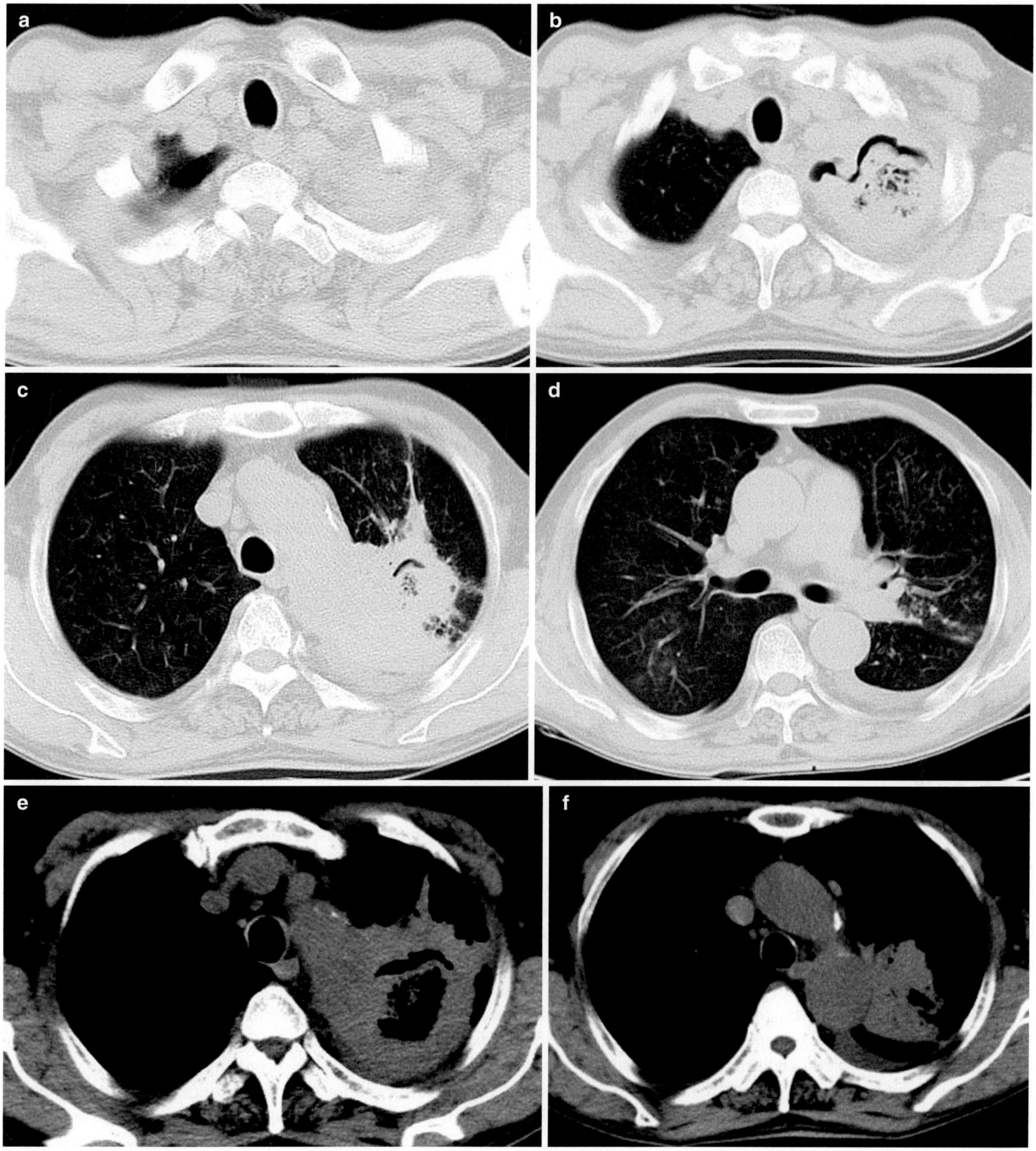

Fig. 11.25 (**a**–**h**) Plain and enhanced chest CT scan. (**a**–**d**) The lung window demonstrates mass and flake of consolidation at the left upper lung lobe, with air crescent sign inside. The consolidation is surrounded by acinar nodular opacity. Bilateral pleural effusion of small quantities is demonstrated. (**e**, **f**) The left upper lung field is demonstrated with huge thick wall cavity opacity whose surrounding tissues connect with mediastinum and lateral pleura. (**g**, **h**) Enhanced scanning demonstrates heterogeneous enhancement of the thick wall and no obvious enhancement of the inner low-intensity lesion

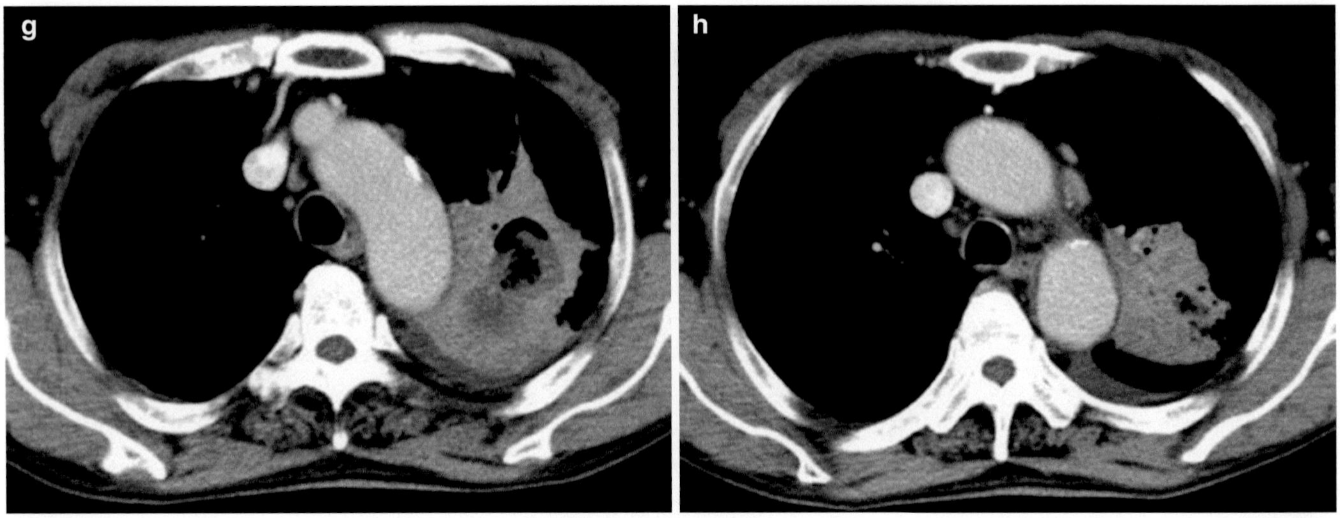

Fig. 11.25 (continued)

pathology is shown in Fig. 11.29. Bacterial and fungal cultures of tissues harvested by percutaneous puncture of the lung indicated growth of *Actinomyces dentocariosus* and measles like bacilli which were sensitive to penicillin and minocycline.

The lung tissue is demonstrated with hyperplastic fibrous tissue. Local lesions show inflammatory infiltration. The interstitium shows infiltrations of many neutrophil granulocytes and lymphocytes. The lesions are presented as chronic inflammation (H&E staining).

After admission, oral intake of voriconazole was continued. In addition, penicillin and minocycline were administered for *Actinomyces dentocariosus* and measles like bacilli. But the patient still experienced cough, expectoration of greenish purulent sputum, poor appetite, and general fatigue. Reexamination of chest CT scan on May 20, 2015, demonstrated thick wall cavity at the apical segment of the left upper lung lobe and accompanying surrounding infiltrative consolidation, which were consistent to aspergillus infection of lung (Fig. 11.30).

Due to unobvious improvement of the symptoms by medication of voriconazole, thoracoscopic removal of the left upper lung, cautery of pleural adhesion, and intercostal nerve block were performed on May 20, 2015, under general anesthesia. On June 4, 2015, when the patient was brushing his teeth after getting up, he suddenly experienced squeezing chest pain that persisted for about 40 min, with accompanying chest distress, breathlessness, and dyspnea. Bedside electrocardiography demonstrated elevated ST-T of V1-6 lead by 0.2–0.5 mV and complete right bundle branch block. The diagnosis was acute coronary syndrome, and anticoagulation, blood pressure rise, blood volume supplement, and symptomatic support were immediately administered. At 9:10, the patient was suddenly unconscious. The cardiac monitoring showed ventricular fibrillation. The emergency rescuing was ineffective and death occurred.

11.7.4 Discussion

In recent years, due to increase of patients with compromised immunity, the incidence of aspergillus infection has been increasing. Research study showed that the cases of aspergillus infection account for more than 50% of fungal infection and 90% cases of aspergillus infection show pulmonary infection, which is known as pulmonary aspergillosis [35]. Pulmonary aspergillosis can be classified into three types: (1) invasive pulmonary aspergillosis which can be further classified into three subtypes of invasive pulmonary aspergillosis, invasive tracheal and bronchial aspergillosis, and chronic necrotizing pulmonary aspergillosis; (2) chronic and saprophytic aspergillosis, which can be further divided into aspergilloma and chronic cavitary pulmonary aspergillosis (CCPA); and (3) allergic bronchopulmonary aspergillosis. CCPA occurs commonly in patients with basic disease. Without timely diagnosis and appropriate antifungal treatment, the 5-year mortality rate is up to 80%. Specialist in the respiratory department should know about the diagnosis and treatment of CCPA to improve the survival rate and quality of life of the patients [36].

Currently in China, based on host factors, clinical characteristics, microbiology, and histopathology, the diagnosis of

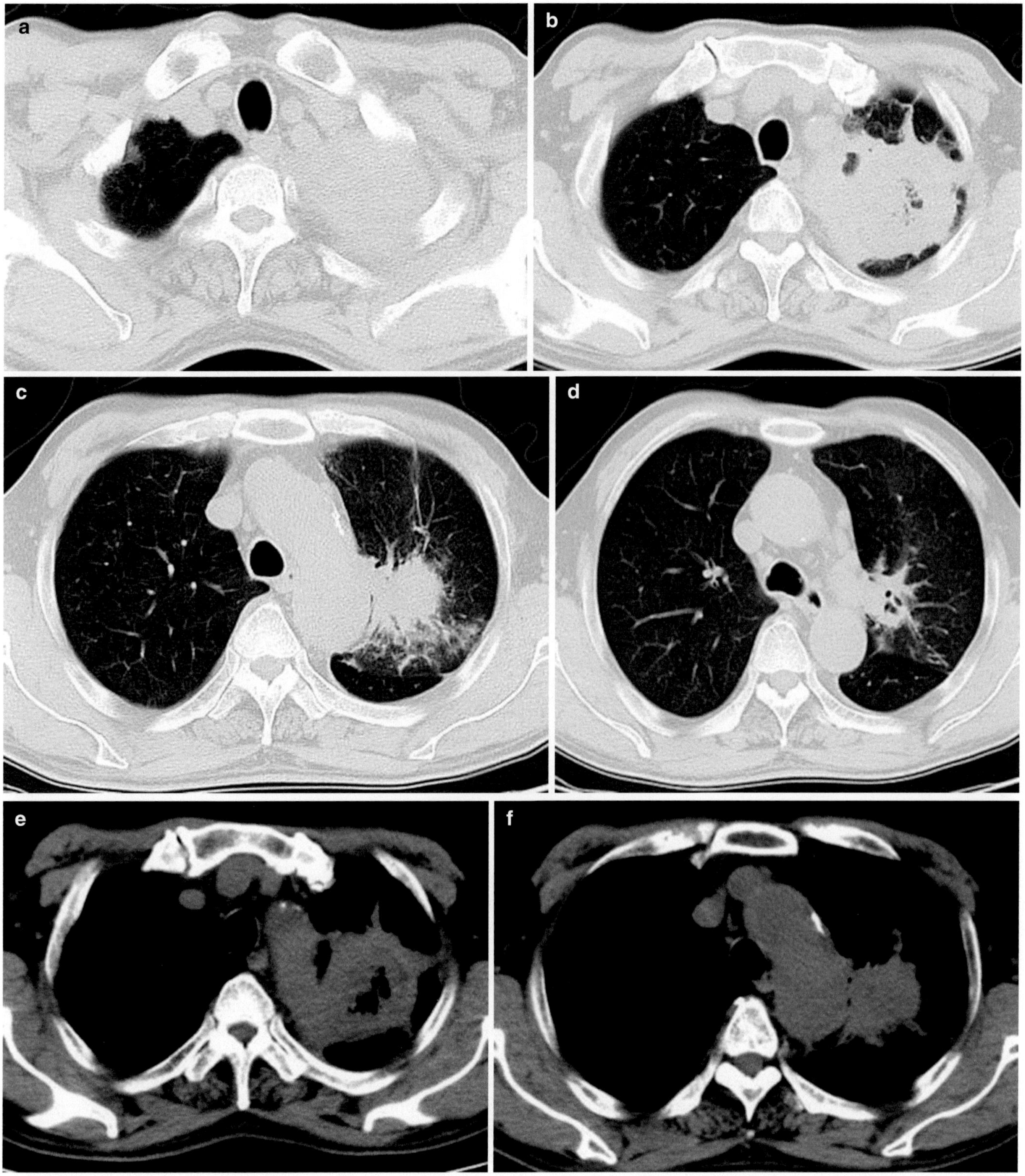

Fig. 11.26 (**a**–**f**) Reexamination of chest CT scan. (**a**–**d**) The lung window demonstrates shrinkage of mass and flake of consolidation at the left upper lung lobe and no cavity opacity. (**e**, **f**) The mediastinum window demonstrates thick wall cavity opacity at the left upper lung lobe that shrinks compared to previous CT scans

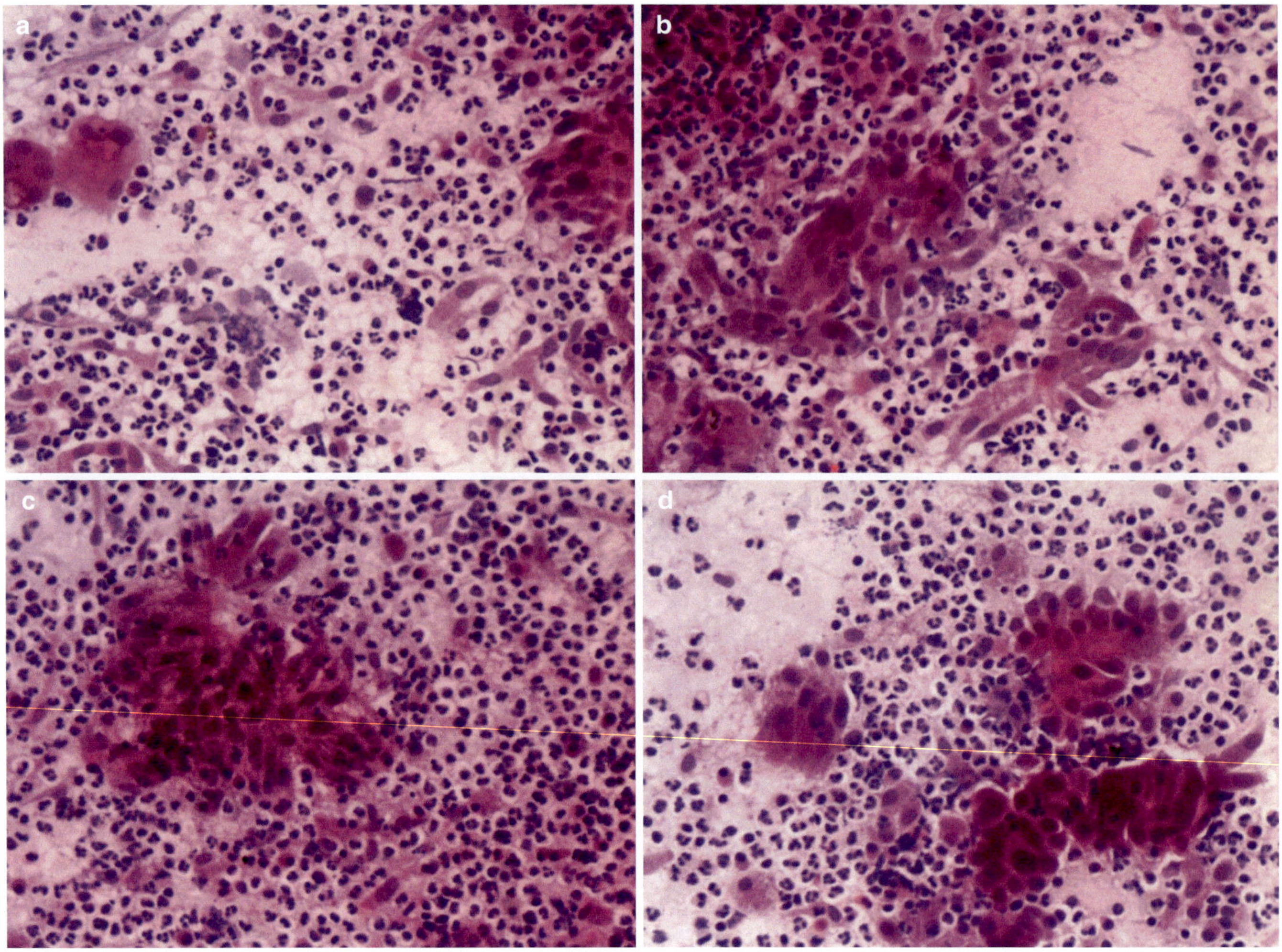

Fig. 11.27 (**a**–**d**) Microscopy following bronchoscopic brushing. (**a**–**d**) The smear demonstrates ciliated columnar epithelial cells, beaker cells, alveolar phagocytes, a large quantity of neutrophil leukocytes, lymphocytes, and polykaryocytes (H&E staining)

pulmonary aspergillosis is classified into suspected diagnosis, clinical diagnosis, and definitive diagnosis [37]. In this case, it lasted for more than 5 months from the onset of symptoms to pathological diagnosis, which was also a course from clinical diagnosis to definitive diagnosis. Meanwhile, it was also a course of development from acute invasive pulmonary aspergillosis to chronic cavitary pulmonary aspergillosis. In November 2014, the initial onset of symptoms occurred, with manifestations of fever, cough, and expectoration of sputum with blood streak. Chest CT scan demonstrated mass and flake of consolidation at the left upper lung lobe, with air crescent sign inside. Based on these findings, the clinical diagnosis was made as acute invasive pulmonary aspergillosis. After medication of voriconazole, the body temperature of the patient gradually returned to normal, with decreased cough and expectoration and disappearance of hemoptysis. Dynamic reexamination of chest CT scan demonstrated shrinkage of the lesions at the lungs. However, after medication of voriconazole for 3 months, the condition aggravated. Chest CT scan demonstrated enlarged lesions at the lungs. Fibrobronchoscopy and percutaneous puncture of the lung failed to define the diagnosis. Thoracoscopic wedge removal of lung lesions and following pathology confirmed the diagnosis of aspergillus infection.

Voriconazole is an antifungal medication of triazoles, and its antifungal spectrum include *Candida*, *Cryptococcus*, *Aspergillus*, *Fusarium*, and other pathogenic fungi. It is indicated to patients with serious fungal infection and immunosuppression, such as patients with invasive pulmonary aspergillosis. In this case, voriconazole was administered for 3 months, but the condition of the patient improved and aggravated, which may be associated with the following reasons: (1) The patient continued smoking and drinking in large quantities and the risk of lung infection persisted. (2) The percutaneous puncture of the lung and following investigation when he was admitted to our hospital for second time showed growth of *Actinomyces dentocariosus* and measles like bacilli, indicating CCPA complicated by

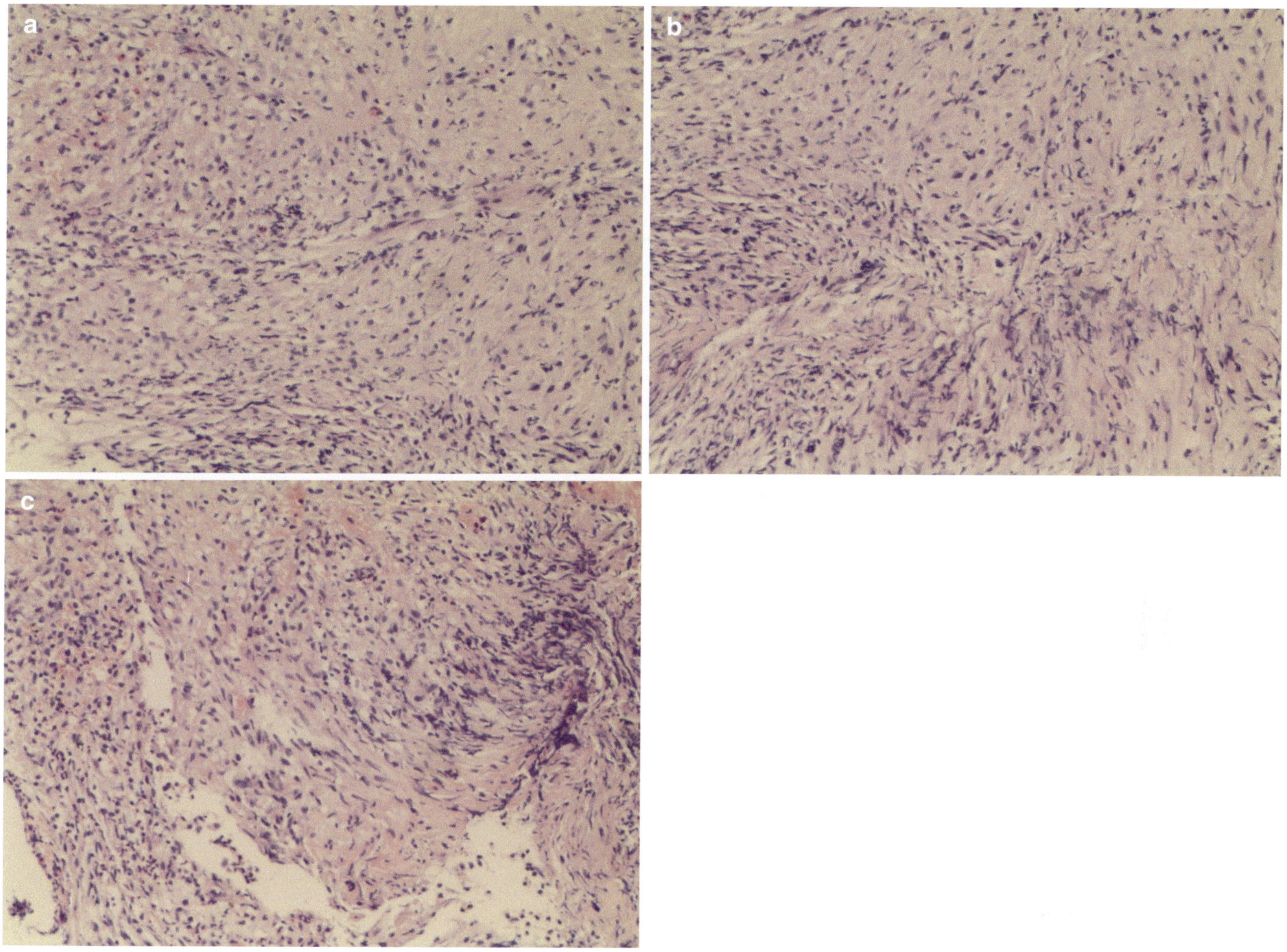

Fig. 11.28 (**a**–**c**) Pathology of fibrobronchoscopic lung tissue

infections of *Actinomyces dentocariosus* and measles like bacilli. Infection of *Actinomyces dentocariosus* is a special infection, which is a progressive purulent granulomatous subacute to chronic infection. It is characterized by local dissemination, purulent or granulomatous inflammation, multiple abscesses, and sinus fistula. And the first choice medication for it is penicillin. *Tetracycline* and erythromycin antibiotics can be administered as alternatives for patients allergic to penicillin [38]. (3) The patient may be resistant to voriconazole. In the cases of CPA, the antifungal medications commonly come slowly into effects. In most patients, the medication is effective at the sixth month, during which the patients with aggravating conditions may experience therapeutic failure by the primary therapy [39]. Resistance to azoles is an important reason for failed long-term antifungal therapy. Molecular biological investigation of drug-resistant mutation in respiratory specimens may provide guidance for therapeutic decision-making [40]. In addition, research study showed that interferon-mediated impaired immune response plays an important role in pathogenesis of chronic pulmonary aspergillosis. The patients may suffer from IFN-γ defect [41].

Surgery is a therapy for CCPA. However, the risk of death and incidence of postoperative complications are high due to the poor general condition of the patients. In this case, the patients sustained concurrent *Aspergillus fumigatus* infection and actinomycotic infection, and the symptoms progressively aggravated after medications. Radiology demonstrated enlarged cavity at the lung, and the patient was at high risk of major hemoptysis. Based on these considerations, surgical removal of the left upper lung lobe was performed. Due to postoperative complication of acute myocardial infarction and ineffective emergency rescuing, death occurred. Therefore, preoperative assessment should be carefully performed, especially the cardiopulmonary functions, to effectively decrease the mortality rate [42].

Based on the experience of diagnosis and treatment in this case, we summarized the following key points: (1) For the cases with highly suspected clinical diagnosis of aspergillus infection and exclusion of lung carcinoma, pulmonary

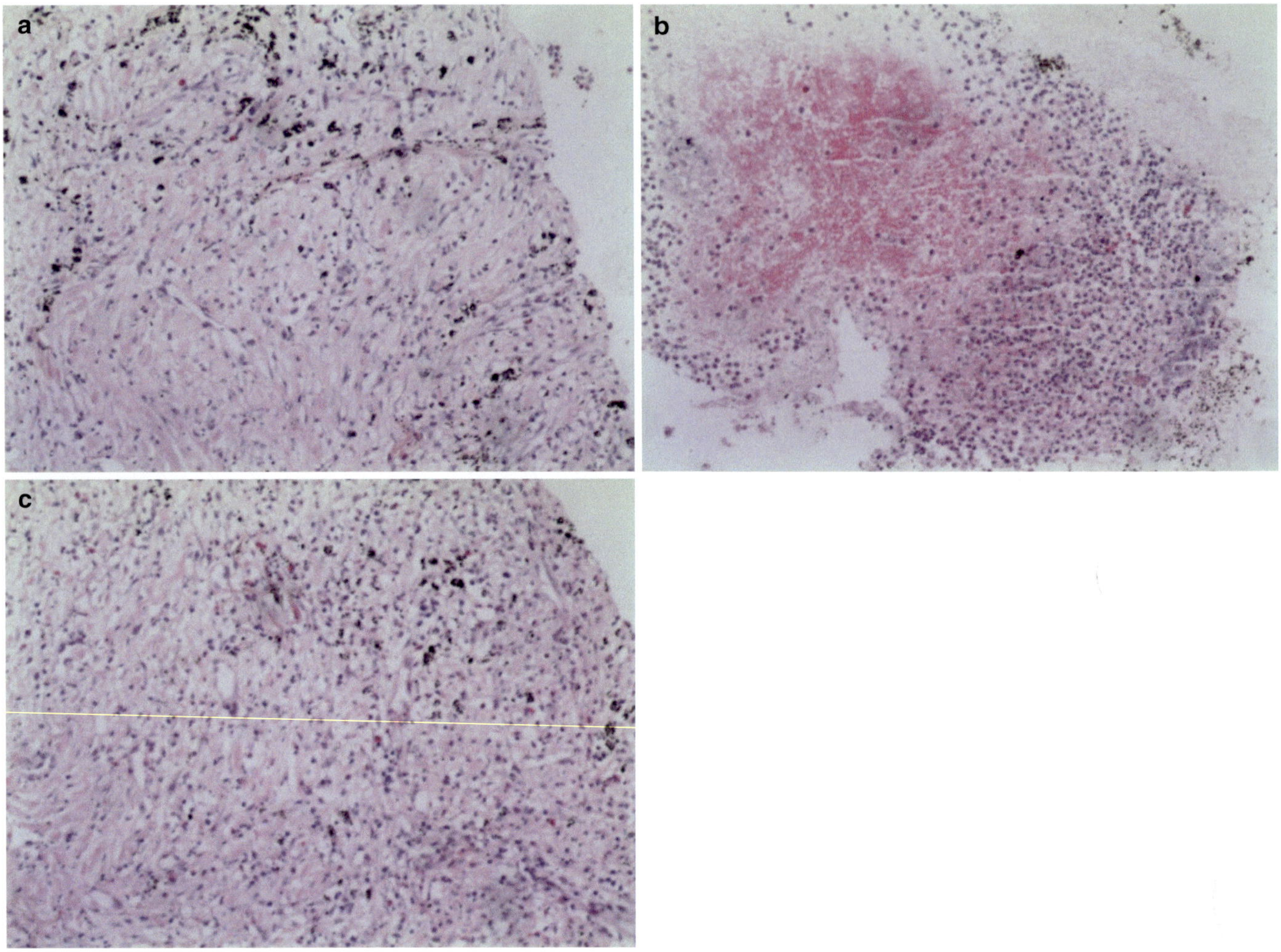

Fig. 11.29 (**a**–**c**) Pathology of lung tissue

tuberculosis, and bacterial infection of the lung, antifungal medication should be administered as early as possible. (2) Lung infection in patients with compromised immunity may be infection of multiple microorganisms. Qualified sputum specimens, BALF specimens, and lung tissue specimens via percutaneous puncture of the lung should be repeatedly harvested for culture to define its etiology. (3) Voriconazole or itraconazole is a favorable choice of medication for patients with pulmonary aspergillus infection and compromised immunity. However, if the condition aggravates after improvement, resistance to medication should be suspected. Echinocandins or amphotericin B can be administered as alternative. In addition, recent study has demonstrated that local cavity infusion of medication is indicated to patients showing no effects or side effects to general antifungal medication [43]. (4) The cardiopulmonary function plays a vitally important role in surgery for patients with CCPA. Preoperative assessment of cardiopulmonary function should be carefully performed.

11.7.5 Comments

For initial treatment of invasive pulmonary aspergillosis, oral intake of voriconazole can be chosen. For the patients with serious conditions, intravenous infusion of voriconazole is recommended, and oral intake of voriconazole or itraconazole can be started as sequential therapy after the condition is improved. If the initial therapy is ineffective, rescue therapy of caspofungin or micafungin, liposome amphotericin B, posaconazole, or itraconazole can be administered based on definitive diagnosis. However, for patients with IPA but therapeutic failure by itraconazole, voriconazole is not recommended as rescue therapy. In the initial treatment, combined medications are not recommended as routine therapy. But combined medications are recommended for the patients with intolerance to standard therapy, multidrug-resistant bacterial infection, or extensive infection. In addition, when rescue therapy is administered, new antifungal medication can be added on the current therapy.

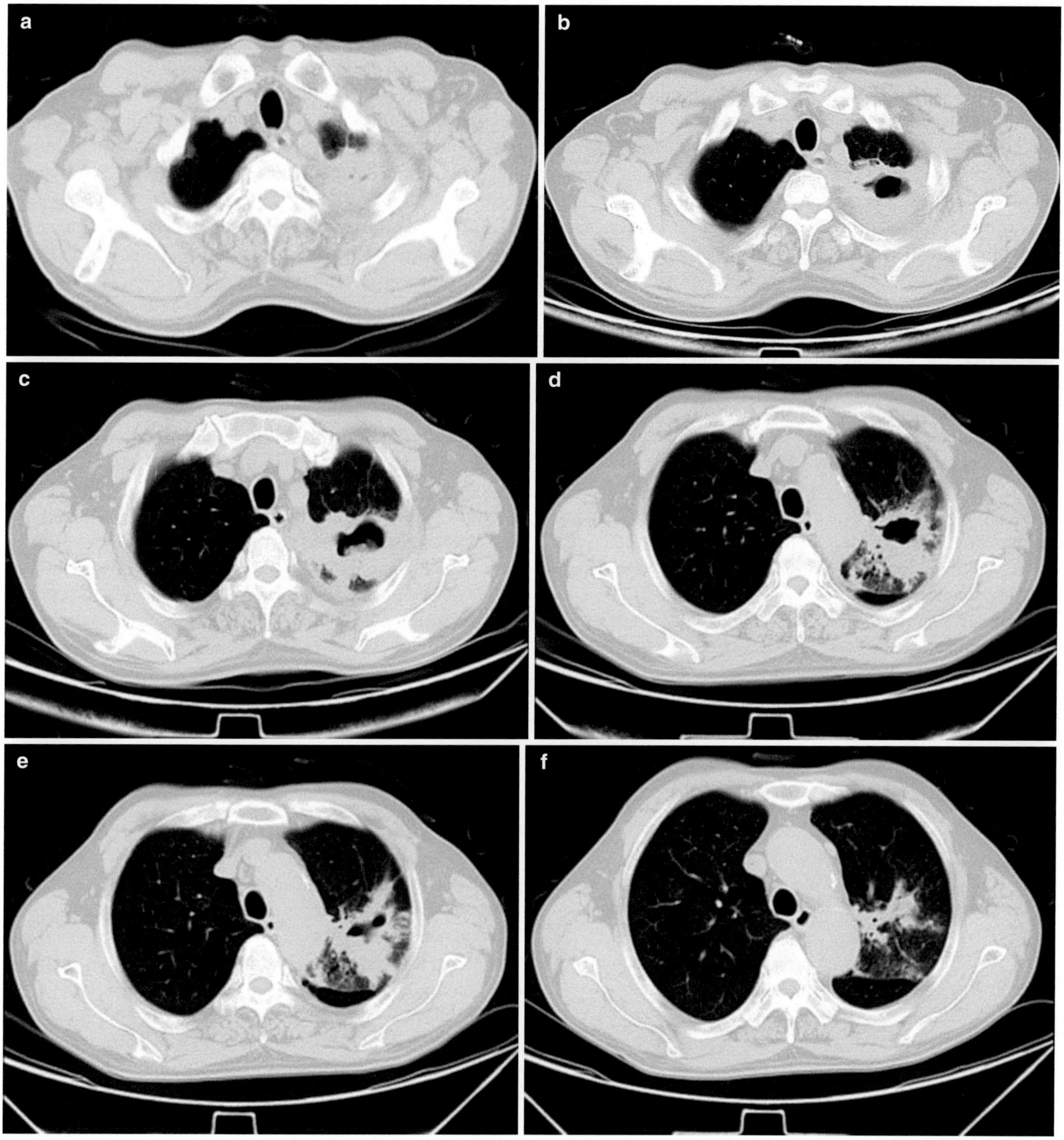

Fig. 11.30 (**a**–**f**) Chest CT scan. (**a**–**f**) The lung window demonstrates thick wall cavity opacity at the apical segment of the left upper lung lobe with surrounding infiltrative lesions. Compared to chest CT scan on January 15, 2015, the lesions are shown to be slightly absorbed

In this case, the patient was immediately administered voriconazole after the diagnosis of invasive pulmonary aspergillosis. The symptoms and radiologic demonstrations were ever improved, indicating favorable therapeutic efficacy. But 5 months after treatment, the lesions of the lung enlarged, indicating poor therapeutic efficacy, which may be associated with host factors. Although he experienced no agranulocytosis and definitive immunosuppression, his concurrent actinomycotic infection as well as smoking and drinking in large quantities may negatively affect the therapeutic efficacy. In this case, the condition gradually developed from acute invasive pulmonary aspergillosis into CCPA.

Combined surgery and medication can be administered to patients with CCPA. However, compared to pulmonary aspergilloma, the incidence of postoperative complications obviously increases. Therefore, sufficient systemic assessment should be performed before the surgery.

During recent years, some new therapies provide more choice for patients with chronic pulmonary aspergillosis but contraindications to surgery or showing unfavorable therapeutic efficacy to routine medications. For instance, some scholars have attempted infusion of antifungal medications into cavity via bronchoscope. Some other scholars have attempted infusion of amphotericin B into cavity via CT-guided percutaneous intubation. Both have achieved favorable therapeutic efficacy. Meanwhile, the development of interventional therapy provides new therapies for patients with chronic pulmonary aspergillosis. For instance, patients with major hemoptysis can choose bronchial artery embolization. Along with the development of bronchoscopic intervention, elimination of aspergilloma under bronchoscope is possible. Some scholars have shown that aspergilloma can be observed, clamped, irrigated, and treated by amphotericin B under bronchoscope by technologies of X-ray localization, microwave, and electric coagulation. In addition to the simultaneous oral intake of antifungal medication, aspergilloma in cavity is successfully eliminated.

11.8 Case 8: Fever and Cough for 5 Days

Zhengqiang He, Fei Shi, Shusong Peng, Jian Yang, Rong Huang, and Shi-Ping Wu

11.8.1 Presenting Complaint

Fever and cough for 5 days.

11.8.2 Brief Case History

A 21-year-old man was admitted to our hospital on September 4, 2005, due to complaints of fever and cough for 5 days. Five days ago, the patient began to experience irregular fever with no known causes, and the highest body temperature was 39 °C. He also experienced cough and expectoration of yellowish purulent sputum in a small quantity. He then consulted in another hospital and was administered anti-infection therapy of cephalosporins. But the therapeutic efficacy was unfavorable and the symptoms aggravated. The patient began to experience even breathlessness and hoarseness. Since the onset of symptoms, he experienced no hemoptysis, chest pain, and night sweat. His bowel movements were normal and he experienced no obvious weight loss.

11.8.2.1 Past Medical History

One year ago, he had received circumcision and suffered from postoperative complication of infection. He then was cured after anti-infection therapy for more than 1 month. He had worked in a factory of electric welding rod for 3 years.

11.8.2.2 Physical Examination

Physical examination showed a body temperature of 36.7 °C, respiration rate 20/min, pulse rate 82/min, and blood pressure 104/72 mmHg. He was well conscious, with emaciation. Soybean-sized lymph node was palpable under the right mandible, movable and well defined, with tenderness with slightly pressed and smooth surface. The posterior wall of the pharynx was congested. The tonsils showed swelling of degree I. Both lungs showed coarse respiration sounds, with scattering moist rales and inspiratory dry rales. The heart rate was 82/min, rhythm. The valvular areas showed no pathological murmur by auscultation. The abdomen was soft with no tenderness. The liver and spleen were subcostally unpalpable.

11.8.2.3 Auxiliary Investigation

Laboratory Test

Routine blood test showed WBC 5.9 × 109/L, neutrophil granulocytes 50.8%, and eosinophile granulocytes 0.1%. ESR was 35 mm/h. The liver function and kidney function tests showed no abnormality. The bone marrow examination showed reactive myelogram. The analysis of lymphocyte immunophenotype showed no abnormality, with CD3+ 73.8%, CD4+ 24.4%, CD8+ 48.9%, CD19+ 13.2%, CD16+ 56 10.2%, and CD4/CD8 0.5%. HIV antibody was negative. PPD was negative. Repeated sputum test for acid fast bacilli showed negative. Repeated blood culture showed negative.

Radiology

Chest X-ray on September 5, 2005, demonstrated poorly defined patchy opacity along lung markings in medial and middle parts of bilateral middle and lower lung fields. The diagnosis was suspected to be infection of the lungs (Fig. 11.31).

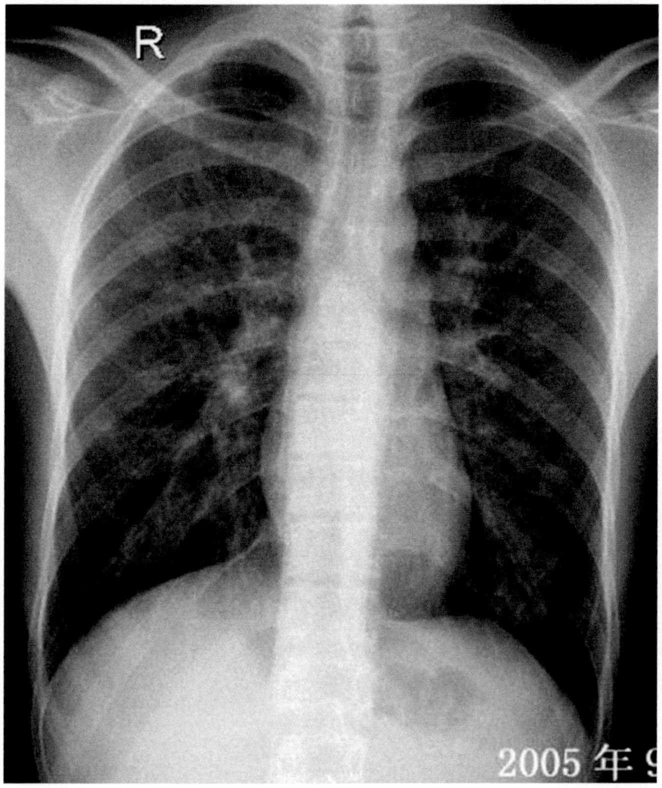

Fig. 11.31 Chest X-ray. Chest X-ray demonstrates poorly defined patchy opacity along lung markings in medial and middle parts of bilateral middle and lower lung fields

Chest CT scan on September 6, 2005, demonstrated multiple patchy opacities in both lungs that were distributed along lung markings (Fig. 11.32).

11.8.2.4 Initial Diagnosis

The initial diagnosis was infection of the lungs.

11.8.3 Diagnosis and Treatment

After admission, ciprofloxacin and azithromycin dispersible tablets were administered for anti-infection therapy, but the condition was not improved. Isoniazid, rifampin, and pyrazinamide were then continued for diagnostic therapy for tuberculosis. But the condition aggravated, with higher body temperature and increased quantity of sputum.

Due to aggravation of his condition, infection of special pathogen was not excluded. On September 7, 2005, electronic bronchoscopy was performed, which demonstrated multiple ulcerations and accompanying necrosis at the bilateral vocal cords, trachea, and bilateral bronchi (Fig. 11.33). Biopsy of bronchial mucosa demonstrated multifocal necrosis of bronchial mucosa and a large quantity of fungi in necrotic substances, which was considered to be aspergillus (Fig. 11.34). The diagnosis of primary invasive pulmonary aspergillosis was then made, and antifungal medication of itraconazole was administered.

After medication of itraconazole, the condition was still not improved. Chest X-ray on September 11 demonstrated aggravating infection of the lungs (Fig. 11.35). On September 12, his breathlessness aggravated, with poor spiritual state and an SPO_2 of 89%. Inhalation of oxygen was then administered and symptomatic support was reinforced. On September 15, the symptoms further aggravated. Chest X-ray on September 21 demonstrated further aggravation of the lesions at the lungs (Fig. 11.36). The sputum culture following bronchoscopy demonstrated growth of *Aspergillus fumigatus*. The drug sensitivity test with meat soup demonstrated resistance to fluconazol, suspected resistance to itraconazole, and sensitivity to 5-flurocytosine and amphotericin B. Itraconazole was then withdrawn and voriconazole was administered. The symptoms were then improved, with decreased body temperature and decreased quantity of whitish sputum. His spiritual state, voice hoarseness, and breathlessness were greatly improved.

The final diagnosis was invasive pulmonary aspergillosis.

On September 28, the patient was discharged and oral intake of voriconazole was continued. But the patient withdrew the medication 3 days later by himself. Reexamination of chest X-ray on October 11, 2005, demonstrated obvious absorption of inflammatory lesions of both lungs. Reexamination of bronchoscopy on October 19, 2005, demonstrated disappearance of ulcerations and necrosis in the airway and two polyps at local tracheal mucosa. On December 8, 2005, there were no symptoms presented. Reexamination of chest CT demonstrated obvious absorption of inflammatory exudation at both lungs compared to chest CT scan on September 6, 2005 (Fig. 11.37). Reexamination of bronchoscopy on December 12, 2005, demonstrated no abnormalities in the airway (Fig. 11.38).

11.8.4 Discussion

Aspergillus exists extensively in the natural world and is a parasitic fungus of the human upper respiratory tract. The common pathogenic aspergillus includes *Aspergillus fumigatus*, *Aspergillus flavus*, and *Aspergillus niger*. And human can be infected by aspergillus via two ways. The first is primary infection caused by inhalation of aspergillus-contaminated air, soil, and water. The second is opportunistic

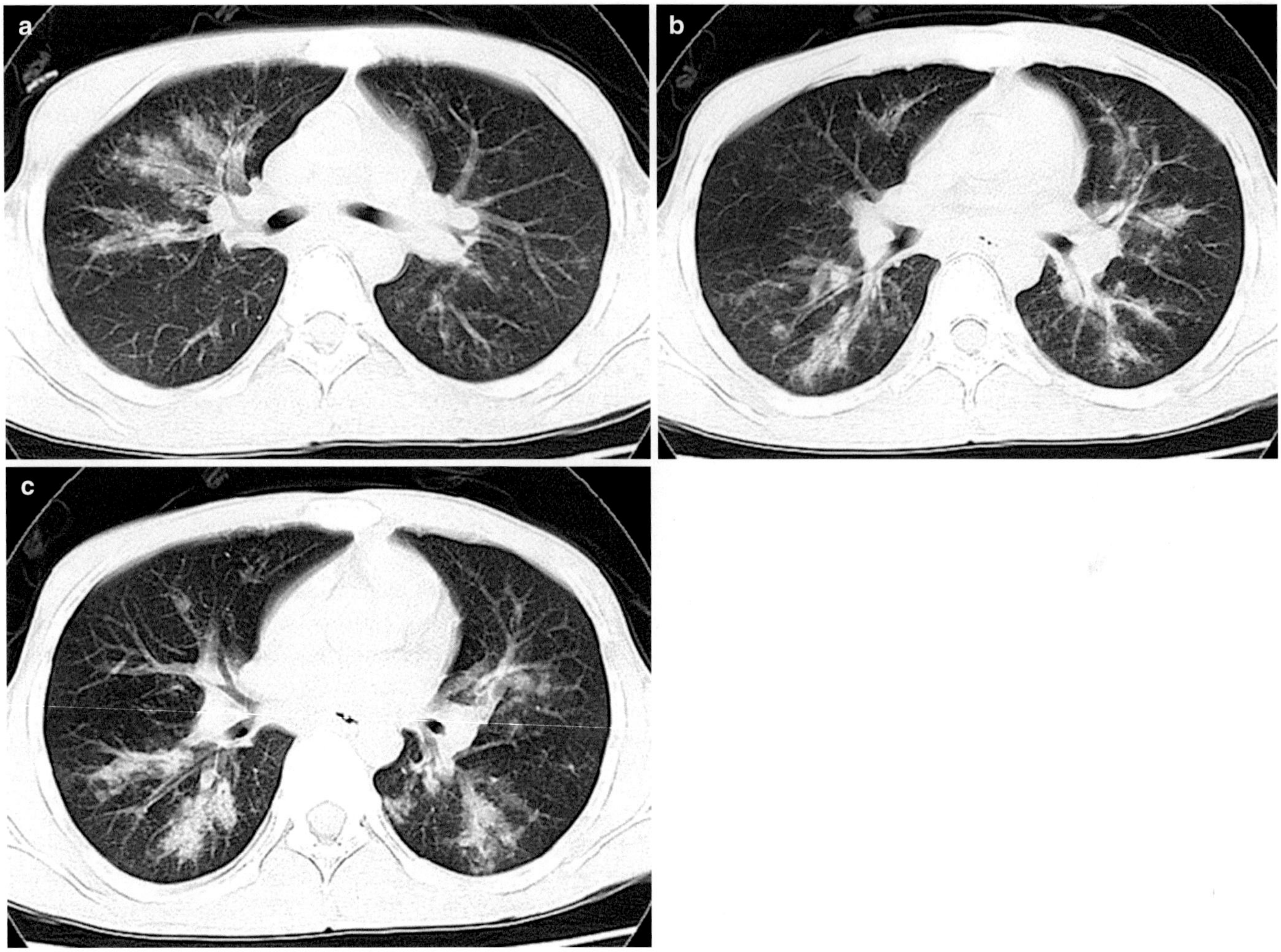

Fig. 11.32 (**a**–**c**) Chest CT scan. (**a**) CT scan demonstrates multiple patchy opacities and acinar nodular opacity at the right lung. (**b**) CT scan demonstrates multiple patchy opacities at both lungs that are more obvious at the right lingual lobe and dorsal segment of bilateral lower lung lobes. (**c**) CT scan demonstrates multiple patchy and nodular opacities at both lungs that are more obvious at the left lingual lobe and dorsal segment of bilateral lower lung lobes

infection of aspergillus due to compromised immunity of human body induced by long-term use of immunosuppressant or glucocorticoid. Clinically, pulmonary aspergillosis can be classified into pulmonary aspergilloma, allergic bronchopulmonary aspergillosis (ABPA), and invasive pulmonary aspergillosis (IPA) [40]. Along with the use of immunosuppressant, glucocorticoid, and large dose of antibiotic, the incidence of IPA has been increasing, and its mortality rate is higher than other types of pulmonary aspergillosis. In recent years, cases of primary pulmonary aspergillosis in immunocompetent individuals have been also increasingly reported [44]. In this case, the patient was immunocompetent with no systemic disorders and no history of using immunity-related medications. He worked in a factory of electric welding rod for several years, which had a poorly hygienic working environment. However, he showed no definitive inhalation of aspergillus-contaminated substances, and the case was clinically rare.

The clinical manifestations of IPA are diverse, which are non-specific and mainly associated with biological properties of aspergillus and immune responses of its host. Histopathological changes of the lungs in the cases of aspergillosis include vascular infiltration and airway invasion. But in cases with hyperreactive or hyporeactive host immune responses, the histopathological changes of the lungs include destructed organ or excessive inflammatory reaction. The interaction of aspergillus with host is demonstrated in clinical signs and symptoms of IPA [45]. In this case, the patient showed obvious airway invasion with invasive destructions of the vocal cords, trachea, as well as major and minor bronchi. The respiratory symptoms include cough, obvious breathlessness, and even respiratory failure, with

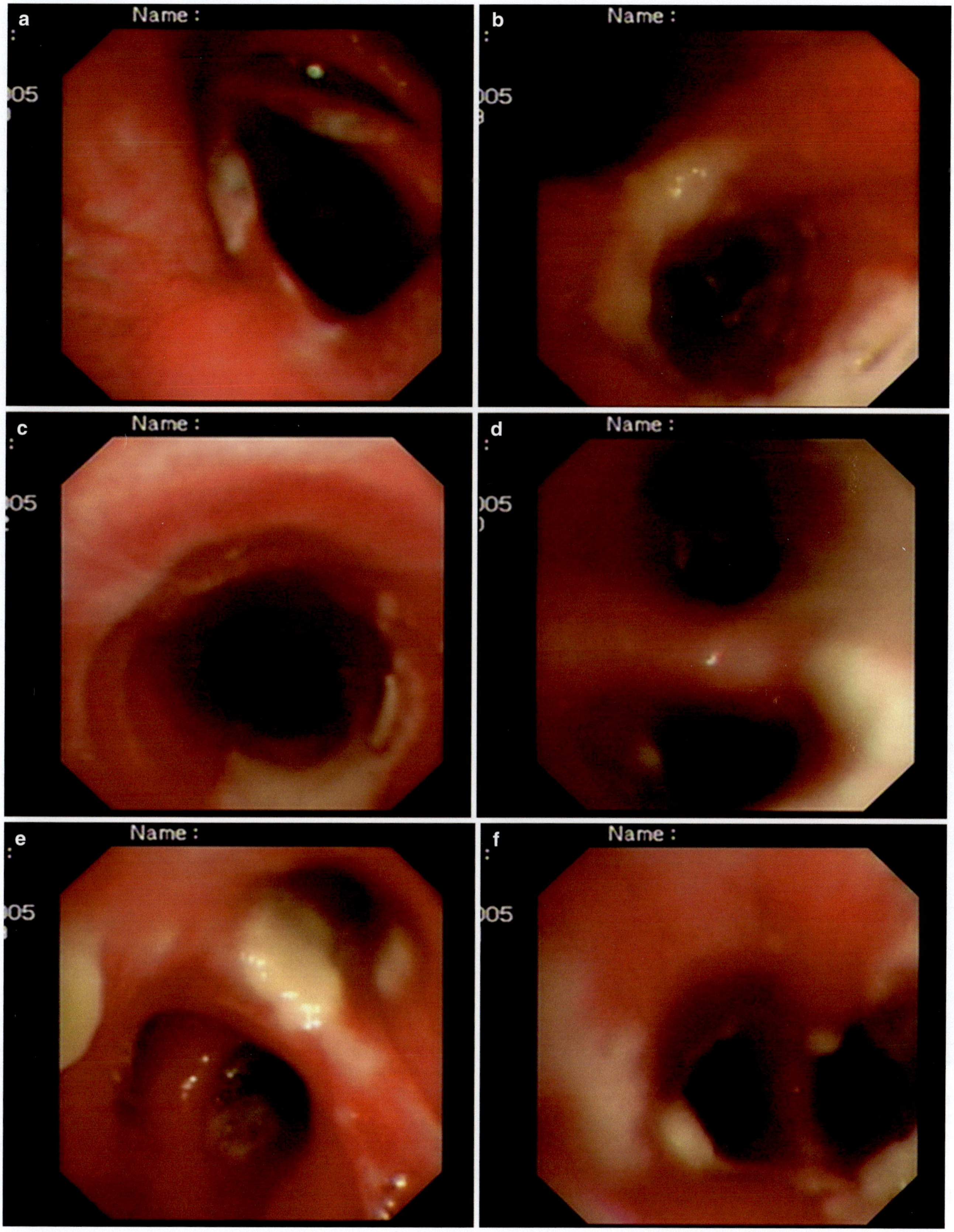

Fig. 11.33 (a–f) Bronchoscopy. Bronchoscopy demonstrates multiple ulcerations that are coated by necrotic substances at the bilateral vocal cords, tracheal mucosa, and bilateral bronchial mucosa

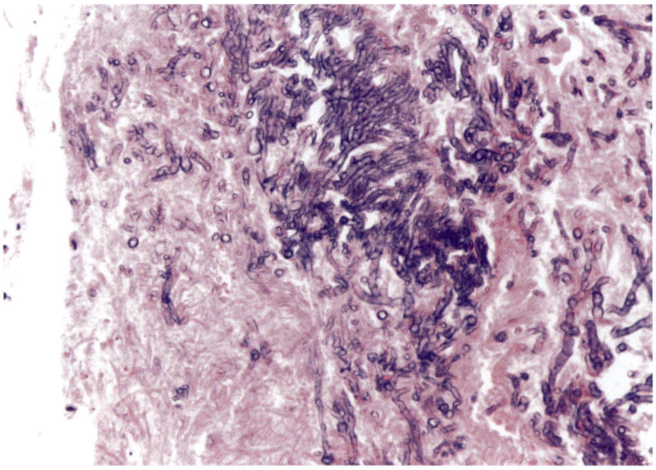

Fig. 11.34 Pathology of lung tissue. Pathology of lung tissue demonstrates multifocal necrosis of bronchial mucosa and a large quantity of fungi in the necrotic substances, which was considered to be aspergillus infection (H&E staining)

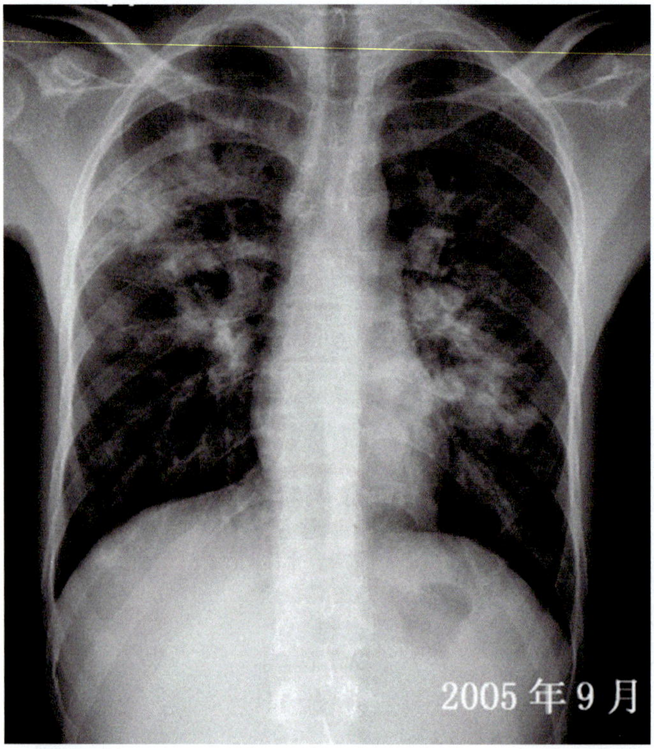

Fig. 11.35 Chest X-ray. Chest X-ray demonstrates obviously increased patchy exudations at both lungs, with progression compared to the chest X-ray on September 5, 2005

rapid progression. In addition, the systemic inflammatory responses were obvious, with recurrent high fever and persistently increasing inflammatory indices. The chest X-ray demonstration of IPA is also non-specific and commonly

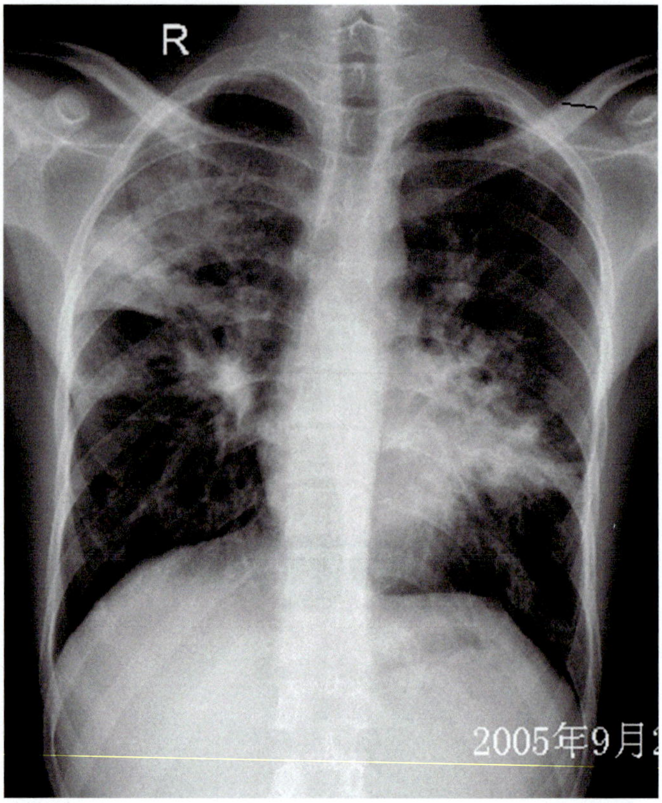

Fig. 11.36 Chest X-ray. Chest X-ray demonstrates increased patchy exudations at both lungs, with further progression compared to the chest X-ray on September 11

includes patchy opacity, nodular opacity, and cavity. During its early stage, chest X-ray demonstrates even no abnormality. Typical chest CT demonstrations include halo sign at its early stage and air crescent sign 3 weeks after onset. However, the halo sign and air crescent sign are clinically uncommon. A study by Xu et al. [46] have shown that the common early CT demonstrations in 64 cases of IPA are ground-glass opacity or consolidation opacity, which accounts for 56.9%. In addition, halo sign is demonstrated in 32.3% of IPA cases, and nonmalignant blood disease is demonstrated in 12.9% of IPA cases. And IPA patients with nonmalignant blood disease tend to show invasion of airway, which accounts for 67.8%. In this case, the chest X-ray and chest CT scan of the patient demonstrated patchy opacity along lung markings, which were non-specific. His bronchoscopy demonstrated serious involvement of the airway, which resembled to the bronchoscopic findings of bronchial tuberculosis. Their differentiation depends on histopathology and microbiological culture.

The main therapy for IPA is antifungal therapy. Itraconazole is one of the oral intake antifungal triazoles that has therapeutic efficacy for aspergillosis. However, in this case, itraconazole was ineffective and the drug sensitivity

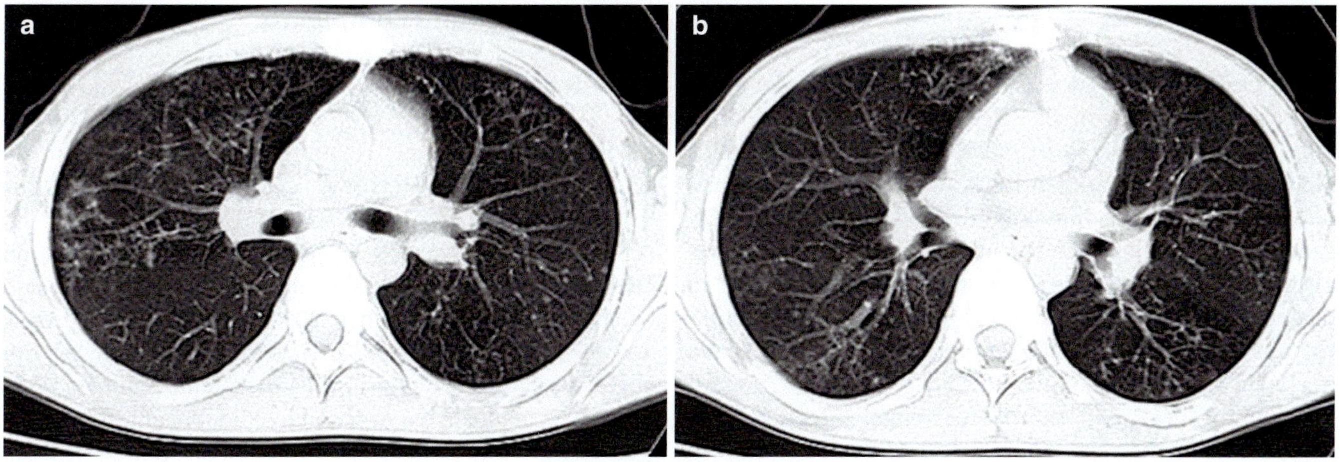

Fig. 11.37 (**a**, **b**) Chest CT scan. Chest CT scan demonstrates scattering spots of opacity in both lungs, with absorption of lesions and improvement compared to chest CT scan on September 6, 2005

Fig. 11.38 (**a**–**d**) Bronchoscopy demonstrates no abnormality in the airway

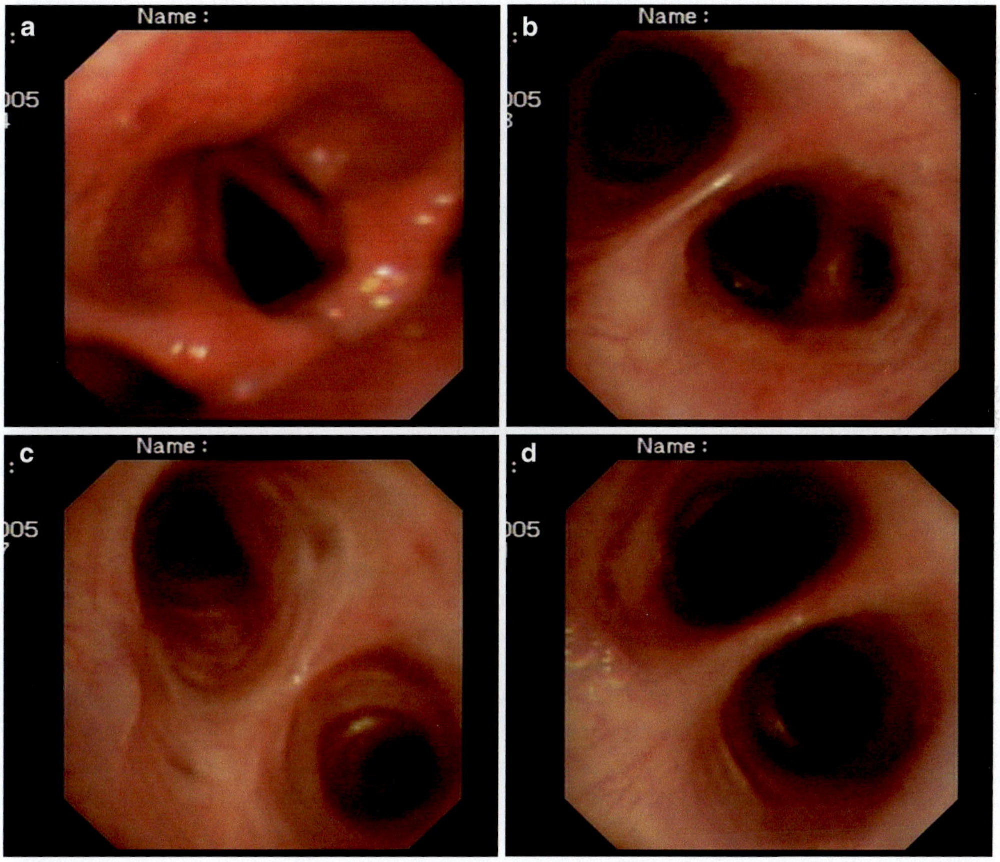

test showed resistance. Amphotericin B has favorable therapeutic efficacy but with serious side effects. Concerning the therapeutic efficacy and safety of medication, voriconazole is optimal. In this case, the condition of the patient obviously improved after intravenous infusion of voriconazole. But the patient discontinued the medication by himself due to presence of side effects. The therapeutic course of antifungal medication was short in this case, lasting for less than 3 weeks. Follow-ups showed no relapse of the symptoms, which may be related to competent immunity of the patient.

11.8.5 Comments

In this case, the patient was a young man, with no definitive medical history of basic diseases. The symptoms included only fever and cough. Chest radiology demonstrated multiple patchy opacities at both lungs, which distributed along lung markings. After admission, common antibacterial medications were administered for infection. But the symptoms of the patient aggravated. The therapy was then changed to diagnostic therapy for tuberculosis. Based on the early clinical manifestations and laboratory test, the diagnosis and treatment were reasonable.

Recently, the cases of invasive fungal infection have been increasingly reported. The clinicians have known more about the disease based on their clinical experience. Most cases of primary invasive aspergillosis are community-acquired infection, and the patients may not show risk factors and basic disease of fungal infection. During its early stage, the clinical manifestations and radiological demonstrations are not special. Chest radiology may demonstrate patchy opacity, nodular opacity, or cavity. Typical chest CT scan demonstrations of invasive aspergillosis may include halo sign and air crescent sign. Based on the clinical guideline for invasive mycosis, the diagnosis of invasive mycosis is classified into definitive diagnosis, clinical diagnosis, and suspected diagnosis. In this case, the condition was definitively diagnosed as invasive aspergillosis based on histopathological evidence. Biopsy of bronchial mucosa demonstrated necrosis of bronchial mucosa and a large quantity of fungi inside, which was considered to be aspergillus infection.

The diagnostic evidence for invasive aspergillosis also includes GM test positive and/or G test positive as well as CT scan demonstrations of pulmonary aspergillosis. In this case, no laboratory evidence was obtained but bronchoscopy was timely performed. The diagnosis was defined based on histopathology. The diagnostic experience merits attention.

The shortest therapeutic course of invasive aspergillosis is 6–12 weeks. And the antifungal medication can be withdrawn based on absorption of lesions by radiology, elimination of aspergillus, and regained immunity. In this case, the patient had no immunosuppression, and the condition was still in its early stage. In addition to the timely diagnosis and treatment, the therapeutic course should be based on the therapeutic responses of the patient.

11.9 Case 9: Fever, Cough and Breathlessness for More Than 20 Days

Zhengqiang He, Chengying Hong, Di Wu, Jian Yang, Di Wu, and Minjie Yang

11.9.1 Presenting Complaints

Fever, cough, and breathlessness for more than 20 days.

11.9.2 Brief Case History

A 40-year-old woman was admitted to our hospital on October 15, 2009, due to complaints of fever, cough, and breathlessness for more than 20 days. More than 20 days ago, the patient began to experience irregular high fever with no known causes, with the highest body temperature of up to 39.3 °C, accompanying aversion to cold, breathlessness that was aggravating, cough, expectoration of yellowish thick sputum with difficulty coughing up, chest pain, and vomiting during severe coughs. Chest X-ray in another hospital demonstrated infection of bilateral lower lungs. The blood culture on October 3, 2009, demonstrated growth of *Pseudomonas aeruginosa*. The sputum culture on October 7, 2009, showed growth of *Pseudomonas aeruginosa*. The diagnosis in this hospital was pneumonia of the bilateral lower lungs, bronchial asthma, and pyemia. Cefamandole, cefoperazone/tazobactam, and levofloxacin were consecutively administered for infection, but the condition was not improved. For further diagnosis and treatment, the patient was transferred into our hospital. Since the onset of symptoms, the patient was in a poor spiritual state, with poor appetite. Her bowel movements were normal, with a weight loss of 3 kg.

11.9.2.1 Past Medical History

She reported attack of asthma 1 year ago but did not present to hospital for diagnosis and treatment. Eight months ago, she received hemorrhoidectomy.

11.9.2.2 Physical Examination

Physical examination showed body temperature of 36.9 °C, blood pressure 93/71 mmHg, respiration rate 21/min, and pulse rate 104/min. The superficial lymph nodes were unpalpable with no enlargement. The trachea was at the midline. The respiration sounds of both lungs were coarse. And by auscultation, both lungs showed moist rales and wheezing sounds. The heartbeat was 104/min, with rhythm. The valvular areas showed no pathological murmur by auscultation. The abdomen was soft, with no tenderness and rebound pain. The liver and spleen were subcostally unpalpable.

11.9.2.3 Auxiliary Investigation

Routine blood test showed WBC 11.4 × 10^9/L, neutrophil granulocytes 92.4%, lymphocytes 4.4%, eosinophile granulocytes 0.1%, and D-dimer 2044.51 ng/ml. CRP was 123.8 mg/L and ESR was 113.0 mm/h. The blood gas analysis showed pH 7.46, PCO_2 35 mmHg, PO_2 61 mmHg, and

FIO_2 29%. The antibody against *Mycoplasma pneumoniae* was 1:320 positive. The blood IgE was 166.0 IU/ml, IgG 16.2 g/L, and complement C3 1.77 g/L, all within normal limits. The 1-3-β-D glucan was 157 pg/ml. The liver function test, kidney function test, and thyroid function test showed no abnormalities. PPD skin test was negative. Repeated sputum tests for acid fast bacilli showed negative.

11.9.2.4 Initial Diagnosis

The initial diagnosis was infection of the lungs and bronchial asthma.

11.9.3 Diagnosis and Treatment

After admission, tests and investigations were ordered. The lung function test showed FEV1 53% and FEV1/FVC 60%, which was suspected as moderate obstructive ventilation dysfunction. Color Doppler ultrasound of the heart demonstrated no abnormality. Ceftazidime and moxifloxacin were administered for infection and symptoms, but the condition was not improved. Anterior-posterior chest X-ray on October 15, 2009, demonstrated multiple patchy exudation opacities, which were more obvious at the left upper lung and bilateral lower lung fields (Fig. 11.39).

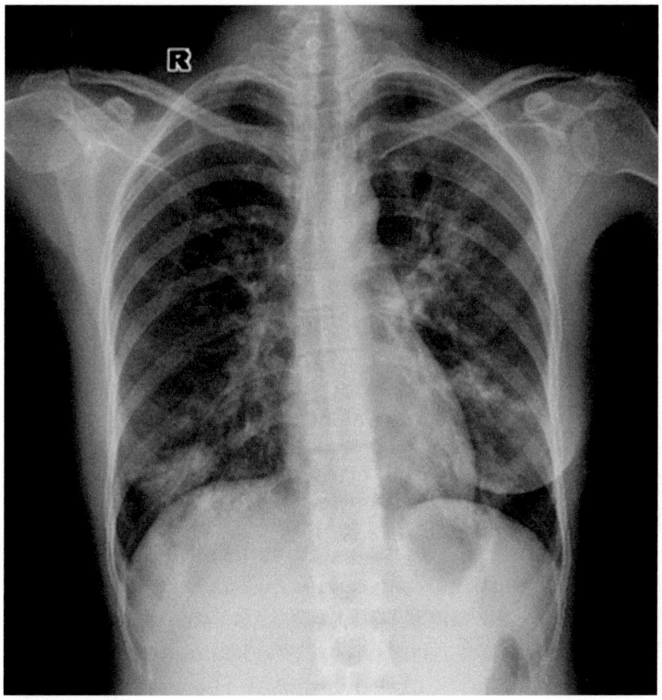

Fig. 11.39 Anterior-posterior chest X-ray. Anterior-posterior chest X-ray demonstrates multiple patchy exudation opacities at both lungs, which are more obvious at the left upper lung and bilateral lower lung fields

To further define the diagnosis, bronchoscopy was performed on October 16, 2009, demonstrating congestion of tracheal mucosa and bilateral bronchial mucosa and multiple erosion with coating of yellowish white necrotic substances (Fig. 11.40). Biopsy of bronchial mucosa demonstrated a large quantity of fungi, necrosis, and inflammatory exudates, and the fungi were morphologically consistent to aspergillus (Fig. 11.41). Fibrobronchoscopy and following sputum culture demonstrated growth of *Aspergillus fumigatus*. Injection of voriconazole was administered and standard therapy for bronchial asthma was given. The condition was gradually improved, with relieved asthma and obviously relieved cough.

Reexamination of CT scan on October 26, 2009, demonstrated multiple spots, patchy, and cord-like opacity with high intensity, which were more obvious at the left upper lung and bilateral lower lungs (Fig. 11.42).

The final diagnosis was invasive pulmonary aspergillosis and asthma.

After discharge on October 30, oral intake of voriconazole was administered, with follow-ups. Reexamination of CT scan on November 16, 2009, demonstrated absorption of lesions, compared to CT scan on October 26, 2009 (Fig. 11.43). Reexamination of CT scan on March 1, 2010, demonstrated the absorption of lesions and less old lesions in bilateral lower lungs, compared to previous CT scans (Fig. 11.44). Reexamination of bronchoscopy on September 19, 2010, demonstrated disappearance of previous bronchial erosions and necrosis. In addition, there were scar-like changes at the mucosa of b subsegmental opening of anterior basilar segment at the right lower lung lobe and b subsegmental opening of the inferior lingual segment at the left upper lung lobe (Fig. 11.45).

11.9.4 Discussion

Pulmonary aspergillosis is a common fungal infection of the lungs. Based on its clinical manifestations, it can be classified into aspergilloma, allergic bronchopulmonary aspergillosis (ABPA), and invasive pulmonary aspergillosis (IPA). IPA is a necrotic inflammation induced by invasion of aspergillus into the trachea and bronchi via airway (rarely along with blood flow), which commonly occurs in patients with compromised immunity. It has been reported that IPA also occurs in immunocompetent individual when he/she inhales a large quantity of aspergillus. In recent years, reports of primary pulmonary aspergillosis in immunocompetent individuals have been increasing [47]. In this case, radiology and bronchoscopy demonstrated involvement of trachea, bronchi, and lung parenchyma. Pathology of mucosa harvested by bronchoscopy demonstrated growth of a large quantity of aspergillus, inflammatory necrosis, and destructed bronchi.

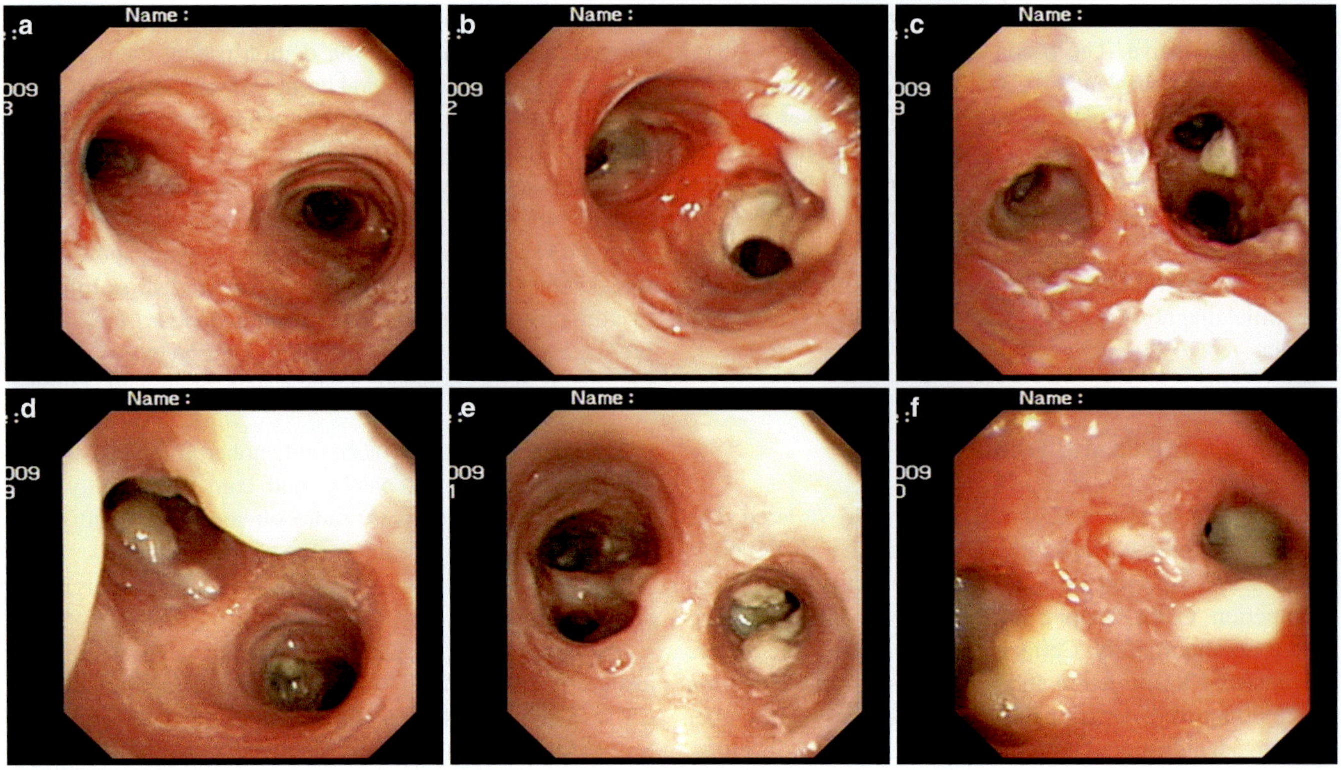

Fig. 11.40 (**a–f**) Bronchoscopy. Bronchoscopy demonstrates multiple mucosal erosions and their coating by yellowish white necrotic substances at the inferior trachea and bilateral bronchi

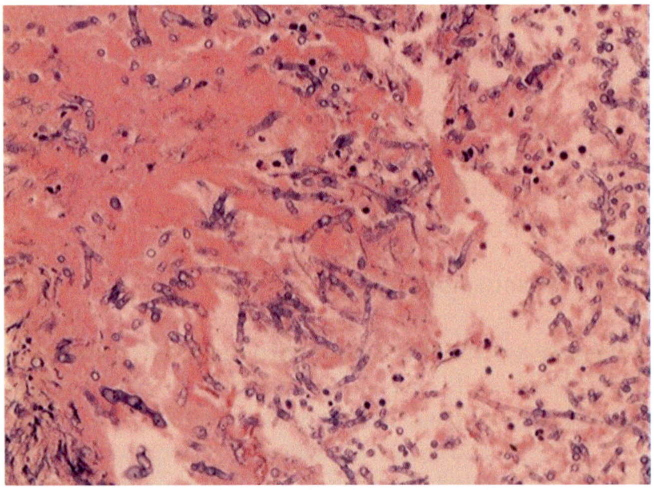

Fig. 11.41 Pathology of lung tissue. Pathology of lung tissue demonstrates a large quantity of fungi, necrosis, and inflammatory exudates at the bronchial mucosa. And the fungi are morphologically consistent to aspergillus (H&E staining)

Based on these findings, the diagnosis of IPA can be defined. The clinical manifestations of IPA are diverse. In this case, the patient experienced asthma-like symptoms as well as infiltrations of the trachea, bronchi, and lungs, which may be misdiagnosed as ABPA. The diagnostic criteria of ABPA mainly include (1) recurrent episodes of asthma, (2) increased eosinophile granulocytes in peripheral blood, (3) skin test for aspergillus antigen immediately positive, (4) serum antibody against *Aspergillus fumigatus* precipitation positive, (5) increased serum IgE, (6) serum antibody against aspergillus-specific IgG and IgE positive, (7) a history of migratory infiltration opacity at the lungs, and (8) central bronchiectasis. The secondary diagnostic criteria of ABPA include the sputum culture for aspergillus positive, expectoration of brownish sputum bolt, and delayed positive in skin test. The diagnosis can be defined based on any six items in the above eight [48]. In this case, the skin test and aspergillus-specific antibody test were not performed because the hospital was not well equipped for these tests. But the eosinophile granulocytes in peripheral blood and IgE were normal, and CT scan demonstrated immobile infiltration with no central bronchiectasis. Based on the diagnostic criteria, ABPA can be excluded.

In this case, the patient had had a history of asthma-like condition 1 year ago, with obvious wheezing symptom during her hospitalization. Wheezing sound was auscultated in both lungs. By lung function test, moderate obstructive ventilation dysfunction was demonstrated. The blood gas analysis confirmed existence of respiratory failure. The diagnosis on discharge was asthma complicated by IPA. Asthma is chronic inflammation of the airway, with local immune dysfunction of the airway. Research study has demonstrated that

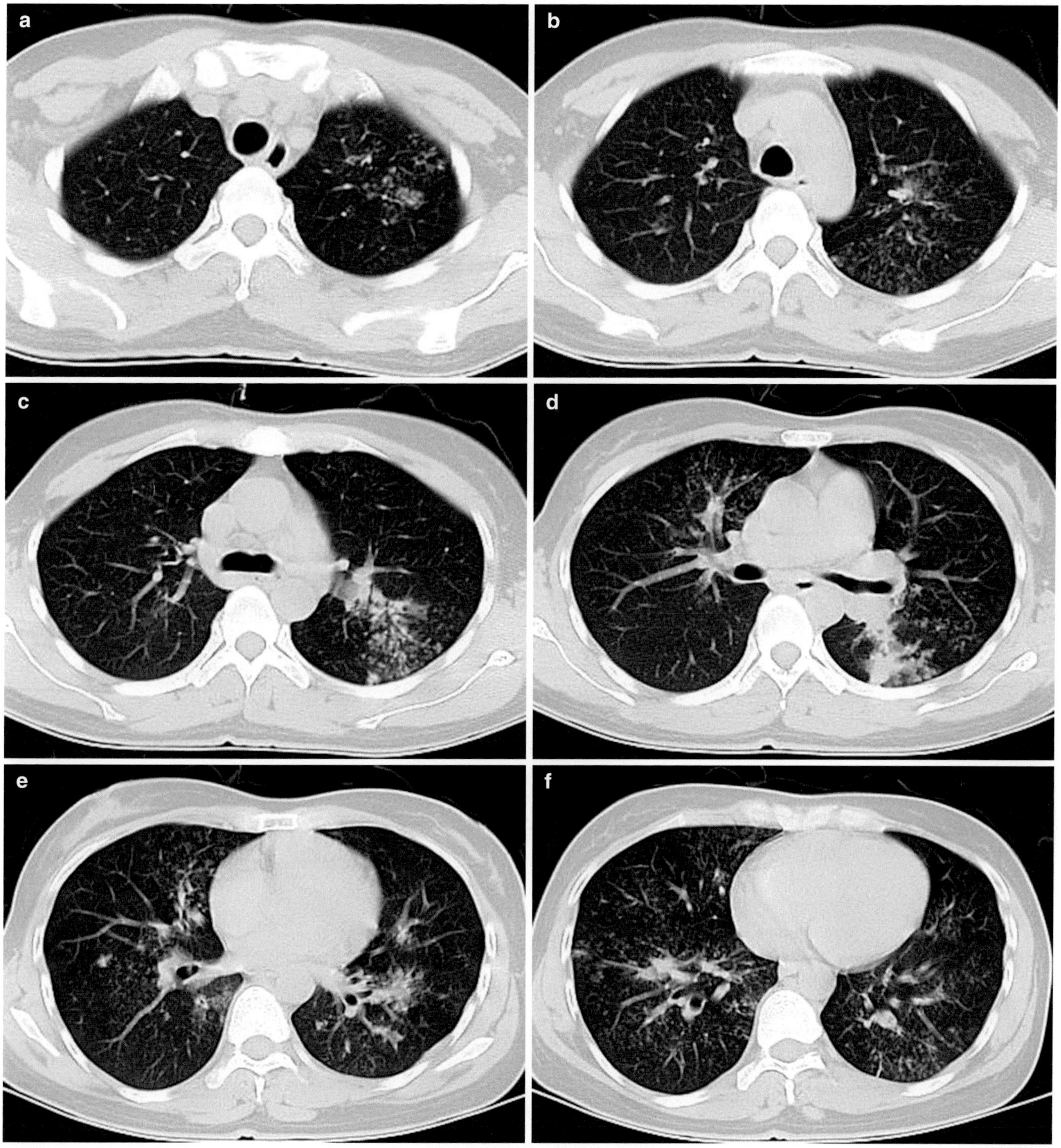

Fig. 11.42 (**a**–**f**) Chest CT scan. (**a**–**f**) The lung window demonstrates multiple spots, patchy, and cord-like opacity with high intensity at both lungs, which are more obvious at the left upper lung and the bilateral lower lungs

fungi can be isolated from the sputum in 54% of patients with asthma. The allergenicity of fungi may induce persistent respiratory symptoms in patients with asthma, which may also be related to pulmonary dysfunction [49]. Across the world, over 6.5 million of patients with serious asthma show fungal allergenicity [50], and thus asthma tends to be complicated by fungal infection. But in this case, the diagnosis of asthma needs to be confirmed. Although the patient experienced asthma-like episode 1 year before her admission to our hospital, she received no standard diagnosis and

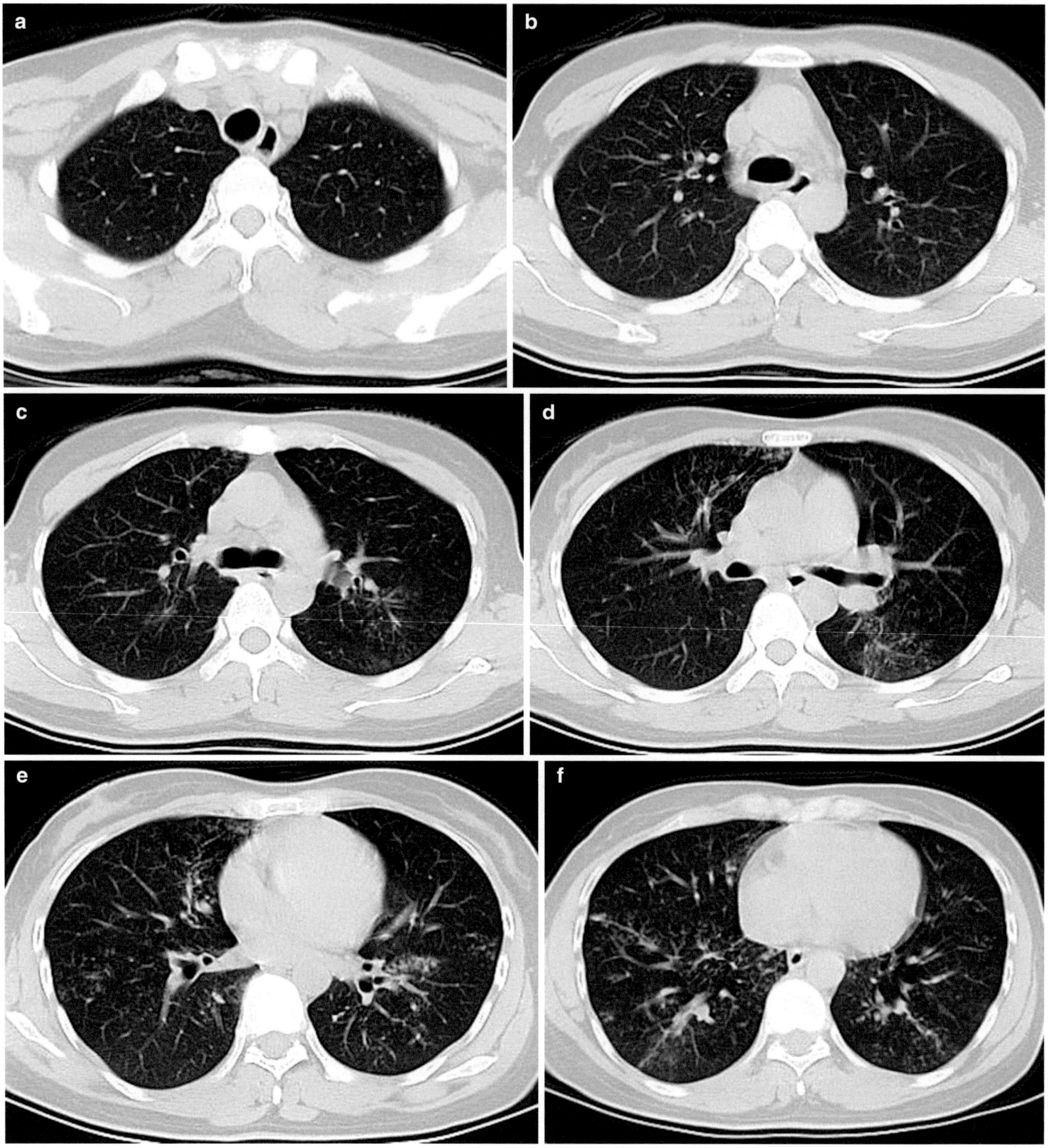

Fig. 11.43 (**a**–**f**) Chest CT scan. (**a**–**f**) The lung window demonstrates multiple spots of opacity at both lungs, with obvious absorption of lesions compared to CT scan on October 26, 2009

treatment. Furthermore, involvement of bronchus by IPA induces inflammatory edema and thick jelly-like secretions in a large quantity at the airway, which obstruct the airway to show pulmonary obstructive ventilation dysfunction. Therefore, the existence of asthma still needs long-term follow-ups. After standard antifungal medication, the pulmonary and bronchial provocation test can be performed to further confirm the diagnosis of asthma.

The treatment for IPA is mainly antifungal therapy. The treatment for ABPA is intended to protect the structure and

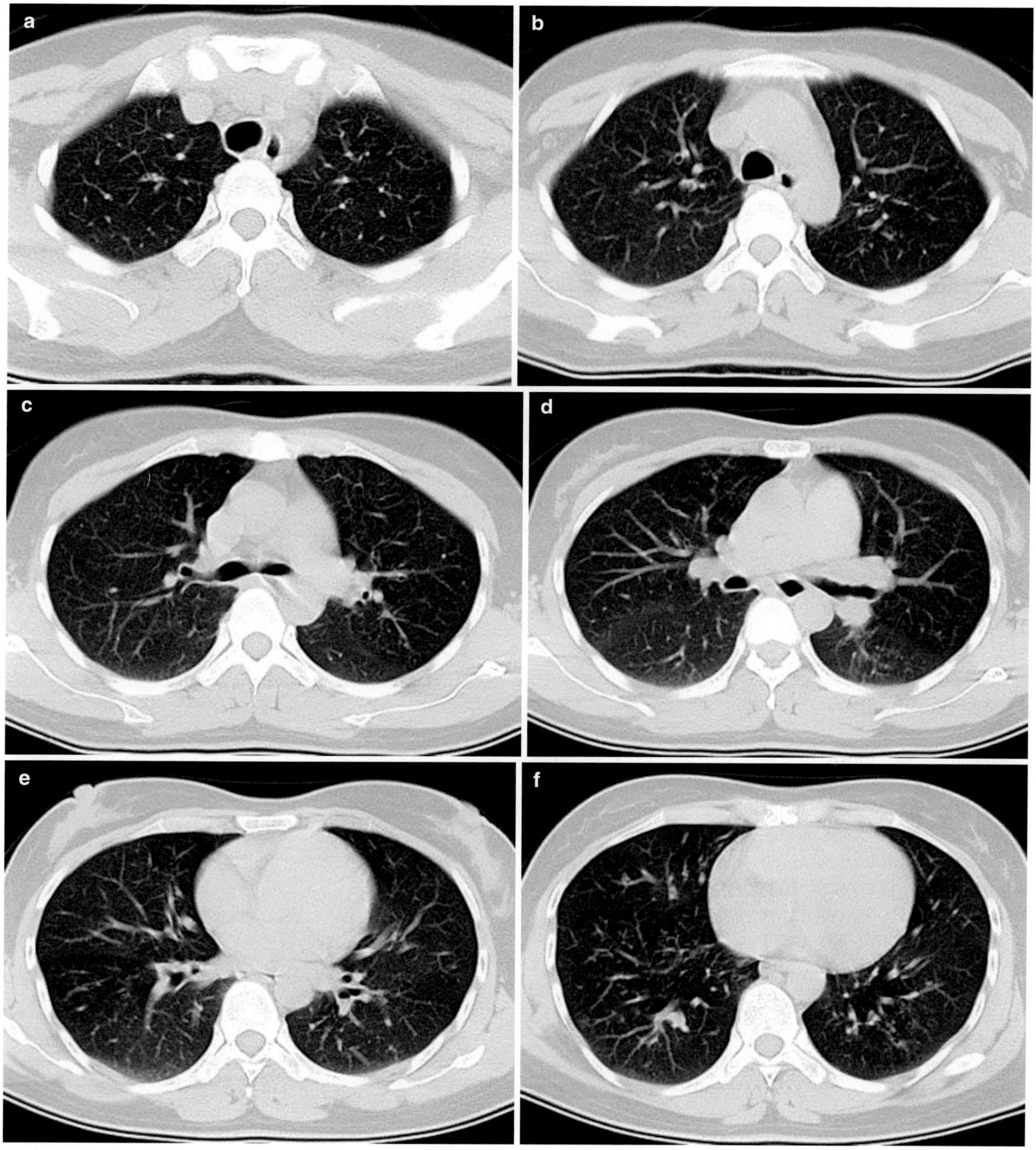

Fig. 11.44 (**a**–**f**) Chest CT scan. (**a**–**f**) The lung window demonstrates absorption of lesions at both lungs, with obvious absorption of lesions compared to CT scan on November 16, 2009

function of the airway and lung tissue, which is commonly administration of glucocorticoid instead of antifungal medication. In addition to standard treatment for asthma, antifungal therapy facilitates to control fungal infection, provides symptomatic support for asthma, stabilizes the lung functions, decreases the systemic inhalation of corticosteroid, and improves serum inflammatory indices [51]. In this case, the diagnosis of asthma cannot be defined and cannot be

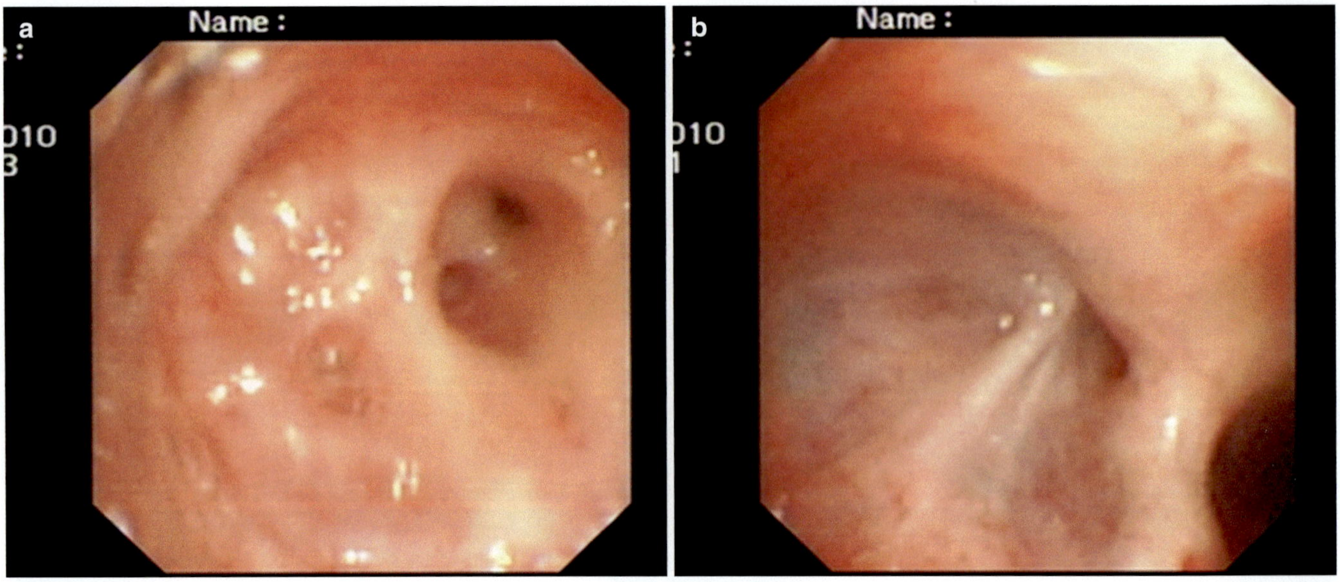

Fig. 11.45 (**a**, **b**) Bronchoscopy. (**a**) Anterior basilar segment of the right lower lung lobe. (**b**) The subsegmental opening and the lingual segment of the left lower lung lobe. (**c**) Scar-like changes at the mucosa of subsegmental bronchi

excluded. The condition of the patient was critical during its early stage, with respiratory failure. The medication of voriconazole and standard treatment for asthma are appropriate, with favorable therapeutic efficacy.

11.9.5 Comments

Pulmonary aspergillosis is commonly secondary to other respiratory diseases, such as pulmonary tuberculosis and pulmonary sarcoidosis. Without active treatment, the mortality rate in 5 years is high. Therefore, the clinicians should get systemic knowledge about pulmonary aspergillosis for its early diagnosis and appropriate treatment. Only in such a way, its mortality rate can be decreased.

In this case, the patient was admitted to the hospital due to complaints of fever, cough, and breathlessness for more than 20 days. Chest CT scan demonstrated multiple spots, patchy, and cord-like high-intensity opacity at both lungs. Clinically, the diagnosis tends to be bacterial pneumonia. But anti-infection therapy showed unfavorable therapeutic efficacy, and 1-3-β-D glucan was positive (157 pg/ml), indicating fungal infection. The diagnosis was finally defined based on bronchoscopy and following biopsy of bronchial mucosa.

A recent study has shown that over 80 species of fungi can induce allergic respiratory disease and are obviously related to the severity of asthma. *Aspergillus* is the most common fungi, and *Aspergillus fumigatus* is the independent risk factor of serious asthma. In this case, the patient had a history of asthma, which should be differentiated from ABPA. The laboratory findings for the diagnosis of ABPA include skin test for aspergillus antigen immediately positive, serum aspergillus precipitin positive, and serum antibody against aspergillus-specific IgE positive. For patients with bronchial asthma, especially patients with serious asthma or intractable asthma, when antiasthmatic therapy shows unfavorable therapeutic efficacy, aspergillus infection should be suspected. Smear and culture for fungi, serum GM test and/or G test, and antibody against aspergillus test should be performed.

References

1. Xu S, Dong X, Bahetnisa, et al. Initial CT scanning in patients with invasive pulmonary aspergillosis. Chin J Intensive Care Emerg Med. 2013;25(4):229–32.
2. Liu Z, Wang Y, Wu Y, et al. Effect of diabetes complicated by lung infection on immunity and its risk factors. Chin J Diabetes. 2003;11(02):67–8.
3. Xiao Z, Liao J, Diao X, et al. Effects of diabetes complicated by lung infection on immunity and prevention of infection. Chin J Endocrinol Metab. 2000;16(05):19–22.
4. Park SY, Lim C, Lee S, et al. Computed tomography findings in invasive pulmonary aspergillosis in non-neutropenic transplant recipients and neutropenic patients, and their prognostic value. J Infect. 2011;63(6):447–56.
5. Walsh TJ, Petraitis V, Petraitiene R, et al. Diagnostic imaging of experimental invasive pulmonary aspergillosis. Med Mycol. 2009;47(s1):S138–45.
6. Greene R. The radiological spectrum of pulmonary aspergillosis. Med Mycol. 2005;43(s1):147–54.
7. Shi Y. Re-recognition about the diagnosis and treatment of invasive lung mycosis. Chin J Tuberc Respir. 2011;34(2):83–5.
8. Long J, Zhang Y. Clinical analysis of lung fungal infection during 2008–2012. Chin J Hosp Infect. 2013;24(13):3240–342.
9. Deeren DH. The importance of previous CT scans in the diagnosis of invasive pulmonary aspergillosis. Ther Adv Hematol. 2011;2(2):121–2.

10. Walsh TJ, Anassie EJ, Denning DW, et al. Treatment of aspergillosis: clinical practice guidelines of the Infectious Diseases Society of America. Clin Infect Dis. 2008;46(3):327–60.
11. Wu N, Huang Y, Li Q, et al. Isolated invasive aspergillus tracheobronchitis: a clinical study of 19 cases. Clin Microbiol Infect. 2010;16(6):689–95.
12. Qu WX, Feng XW, Li Z. Successful treatment of larynx-tracheobronchial-pulmonary aspergillosis in an immunocompetent host: a case report. Genet Mol Res. 2014;13(4):9308–14.
13. Fernandez-Ruiz M, Silva JT, San-Juan R, et al. Aspergillus tracheobronchitis: report of 8 cases and review of the literature. Medicine (Baltimore). 2012;91(5):261–73.
14. Zou M, Tang L, Zhao S, et al. Systematic review and meta-analysis of detecting Galactomannan in bronchoalveolar lavage fluid for diagnosing invasive aspergillosis. PLoS One. 2012;7(8):e43347.
15. Ramos A, Segovia J, Gomez-Buen M, et al. Pseudomembranous aspergillus tracheobronchitis in a heart transplant recipient. Transpl Infect Dis. 2010;12(1):60–3.
16. Li Y, Chen C, Ye M, et al. Bronchoscopic and chest CT scan demonstrations of invasive airway aspergillosis in immunocompetent patients. Chin J Tuberc Respir. 2009;32(6):439–43.
17. Zhuo S, Luo B. Diagnosis and treatment of pulmonary aspergillosis. Chin J Mod Med. 1998;8(7):31–2.
18. Alexey A, Navatha K, Anthony GS. Aspergillus-related lung disease. Respir Med CME. 2008;1(3):205–15.
19. Chabi ML, Goracci A, Roche N, et al. Pulmonary aspergillosis. Diagn Interv Imaging. 2015;96(5):435–42.
20. Fernando FG, Bruno H, Luiz CS, et al. High-resolution computed tomographic findings of Aspergillus infection in lung transplant patients. Eur J Radiol. 2014;83:79–83.
21. Curbelo J, Galván JM, Aspa J. Up-dates on aspergillus, pneumocystis and other opportunistic pulmonary mycoses. Arch Bronconeumol. 2015;51(12):647–53.
22. Kosmidis C, Denning DW. The clinical spectrum of pulmonary aspergillosis. Postgrad Med J. 2015;91:403–10.
23. Winters B, Custer J, Galvagno SM Jr, et al. Diagnostic errors in the intensive Care Unit: a systematic review of autopsy studies. BMJ Qual Saf. 2012;21:804–902.
24. Zhang L, Jiang Y, Zeng X. Connective tissue disorders complicated by invasive pulmonary aspergillosis: a clinical analysis of 20 cases. Beijing Med. 2010;32(3):194–6.
25. The Editorial Committee of Chinese Journal of Internal Medicine. The diagnostic criteria and treatment principles of invasive fungal infection of lungs. Chin J Intern Med. 2006;45(8):697–700.
26. Xu S, Dong X. Initial CT scan demonstrations of invasive pulmonary aspergillosis. Chin J Crit Care Emerg Med. 2013;25(4):229–32.
27. Xu P, Zhou J, Zhou H, et al. Combined serum antigen investigation with lung CT scan for the diagnosis of invasive pulmonary aspergillosis. J Zhejiang Univ (Ed Med). 2012;41(3):332–7.
28. Du J, Gao W, Feng Q, et al. Value of bronchoalveolar lavage fluid GM test in the early diagnosis of invasive pulmonary aspergillosis. J Pract Med. 2013;29(10):1677–9.
29. Denning DW, Cadranel J, Beigelman-Aubry C, et al. Chronic pulmonary aspergillosis: rationale and clinical guidelines for diagnosis and management. Eur Respir J. 2016;47(1):45–68.
30. Zheng Y, Zhou J. Chronic necrotizing pulmonary aspergillosis. Int J Respir. 2006;26(04):293–5.
31. Yella LK, Krishnan P, Gillego V. The air crescent sign: a clue to the etiology of chronic necrotizing pneumonia. Chest. 2005;127(1):395–7.
32. Zheng Y, Ding W, Zhou J. Chronic necrotizing pulmonary aspergillosis and pulmonary aspergilloma: a clinical pathological comparison. Chin J Infect Dis. 2008;26(5):305–8.
33. Bao Q, Li M, Xu M, et al. CT scan demonstrations of chronic necrotizing pulmonary aspergillosis. J Med Rev. 2011;17(12):1902–3.
34. Zheng Y, Wang X, Ding W, et al. Diagnosis and treatment of chronic necrotizing pulmonary aspergillosis. Chin J Tuberc Respir. 2006;29(2):92–5.
35. Pagano L, Caira M, Candoni A, et al. The epidemiology of fungal infections in patients with hematologic malignancies: the SE-IFEM-200 study. Haematologica. 2006;91(8):1068–75.
36. Denning DW, Cadranel J, Beigelman-Aubry C, et al. Chronic pulmonary aspergillosis: rationale and clinical guidelines for diagnosis and management. Eur Soc Clin Microbiol Infect Dis Eur Respir Soc. 2016;47(1):45–68.
37. The Editorial Committee of Chinese Journal of Internal Medicine. The diagnostic criteria and treatment principles of invasive pulmonary fungal infection (draft). Chin J Intern Med. 2006;45:697–9.
38. Li X, Li X, Liao W. Research development on actinophytosis. Chin J Mycol. 2006;3(3):189–92.
39. Felton TW, Baxter C, Moore CB, et al. Efficacy and safety of posaconazole for chronic pulmonary aspergillosis. Clin Infect Dis. 2010;51:1383–91.
40. Kosmidis C, Denning DW. The clinical spectrum of pulmonary aspergillosis. Thorax. 2015;70(3):270–7.
41. Döffinger R, Harris C, Lear S, et al. Impaired Th1 and Th17 immunity in chronic pulmonary aspergillosis. In: NHS England National Commission Group Chronic Pulmonary Aspergillosis national service, The National Aspergillosis Centre Annual Report 2013–2014. London: NHS England; 2014.. Available from: http://www.uhsm.nhs.uk/nac/news/Documents/NAC%20annual%20report%202013-4%20web.pdf.
42. Farid S, Mohamed S, Devbhandari M, et al. Results of surgery for chronic pulmonary aspergillosis, optimal antifungal therapy and proposed high risk factors for recurrence – a National Centre's experience. J Cardiothorac Surg. 2013;8(1):1–9.
43. Kravitz JN, Berry MW, Schabel SI, et al. A modern series of percutaneous intracavitary instillation of amphotericin B for the treatment of severe hemoptysis from pulmonary aspergilloma. Chest. 2013;143:1414–21.
44. Zhang R, Wang S, Lu H, et al. Misdiagnosis of invasive pulmonary aspergillosis: a clinical analysis of 26 immunocompetent patients. Int J Clin Exp Med. 2014;7(12):5075–82.
45. Warris A. The biology of pulmonary aspergillus infections. J Infect. 2014;69(Suppl 1):S36–41.
46. Xu SC, Dong XN, Baihetinisha T, et al. The initial CT findings in patients suffering from invasive pulmonary aspergillosis. Chin J Crit Care Emerg Med. 2013;25(4):229–32.
47. Agarwal R, Aggarwal AN, Garg M, et al. Cut-off values of serum IgE (total and A. fumigatus-specific) and eosinophil count in differentiating allergic bronchopulmonary aspergillosis from asthma. Mycoses. 2014;57(11):659–63.
48. Pashley CH. Fungal culture and sensitisation in asthma, cystic fibrosis and chronic obstructive pulmonary disorder: what does it tell us? Mycopathologia. 2014;178(5–6):457–63.
49. Agarwal R. Severe asthma with fungal sensitization. Curr Allergy Asthma Rep. 2011;11(5):403–13.
50. Denning DW, Pashley C, Hartl D, et al. Fungal allergy in asthma-state of the art and research needs. Clin Transl Allergy. 2014;4:14.
51. Parulekar AD, Diamant Z, Hanania NA. Antifungals in severe asthma. Curr Opin Pulm Med. 2015;21(1):48–54.

12 Pulmonary Aspergillosis with Presenting Symptom of Hemoptysis

Shi-Ping Wu and Ling-Wei Wang

Hemoptysis is one of the most common respiratory symptoms. The main cause of hemoptysis had been previously believed to be pulmonary tuberculosis, bronchiectasis, and lung carcinoma. During recent years, due to improved technology and increasing knowledge of the clinicians about pulmonary aspergillosis, hemoptysis has been increasingly reported to be caused by pulmonary aspergillosis. Actually, hemoptysis is the most common symptom of pulmonary aspergillosis, with an incidence rate of up to 80% and an incidence rate of life-threatening major hemoptysis of about 30%. Pulmonary aspergilloses that most commonly induce hemoptysis include pulmonary aspergilloma and chronic cavitary pulmonary aspergillosis, followed by invasive pulmonary aspergillosis. Strictly speaking, aspergilloma is a radiological diagnosis, which is characterized by nodular or spherical opacity with moderate intensity in irregular cavity with unsmooth inner wall. Singular aspergilloma (SA) can be categorized into chronic pulmonary aspergillosis, referring to parasitic singular aspergillosis with slight or no clinical symptoms and no dynamic radiological changes during at least 3 months observation.

Both chronic cavitary pulmonary aspergillosis and singular aspergilloma are most commonly secondary to bronchiectasis and old pulmonary tuberculosis. In literature reports, hemoptysis with clinical significance presents in 50% of patients with aspergilloma, which is commonly self-limited and intermittent. Therefore, it tends to be neglected in clinical practice. Hemoptysis is commonly attributed to primary disease of the patients instead of possible occurrence of secondary pulmonary aspergilloma. The volume of blood coughed up by patients with aspergilloma ranges from blood streak in sputum to a fatally large quantity. And the other symptoms include cough, expectoration, and rarely occurring weight loss and fever, which are non-specific. In the cases of the cavity in the lungs being larger than 2 cm in diameter, the risk of aspergilloma is 15–20%. In about 42% of patients with aspergilloma, the lesion is located at the right upper lung. Persistent existence of intrapulmonary cavity after antituberculosis therapy is the structural basis for occurrence of pulmonary aspergilloma. The blood that is coughed up in the patients with aspergilloma is mostly from the bronchial artery and sometimes from the pulmonary artery. In addition to primary disease, hemoptysis may be also associated with friction of the movable aspergilloma with vascular vessels in the cavity wall or endotoxin and pro-

The corresponding author of section 12.1 is Na Li,
Email: lanying5204@sina.com.
The corresponding author of section 12.2 is Wenhui Tang,
Email: 13902444613@163.com.
The corresponding author of section 12.3 is Jingjing Li,
Email: 54891948@qq.com.
The corresponding author of section 12.4 is Yulin He,
Email: 33heyulin@163.com.
The corresponding author of section 12.5 is Di Wu,
Email: wudi315817@163.com.
The corresponding author of section 12.6 is Di Wu,
Email: wudi315817@163.com.
The corresponding author of section 12.7 is Fei Shi,
Email: shifei2003@126.com.
The corresponding author of section 12.8 is Wendi Huang,
Email: vickdi@163.com.
The corresponding author of section 12.9 is Ping Xu,
Email: Xuping750621@163.com.
The corresponding author of section 12.10 is Yazhou Cai,
Email: 562870847@qq.com.
The corresponding author of section 12.11 is Hongtao Chen,
Email: 843139770@qq.com.
The corresponding author of section 12.12 is Guoxin Huang,
Email: szhuanggx@hotmail.com.
The corresponding author of section 12.13 is Yuemei Lu,
Email: szhuanggx@hotmail.com.
The corresponding author of section 12.14 is Ying-Yun Fu,
Email: yingyunf2013@163.com.
The corresponding author of section 12.15 is Dong-Na Su,
Email: sudona@qq.com.
The corresponding author of section 12.16 is Guoxin Huang,
Email: szhuanggx@hotmail.com.
The corresponding author of section 12.17 is Dong-Na Su,
Email: sudona@qq.com.

S.-P. Wu (✉) · L.-W. Wang
Second Clinical Medical College of Jinan University,
Shenzhen, Guangdong, China

C. Qiu et al. (eds.), *Pulmonary Aspergillosis*, https://doi.org/10.1007/978-981-13-3435-1_12

tease produced by aspergillus. Moreover, abundant vascular network due to inflammatory stimulation around aspergilloma and even angioma, along with mechanical stimulation of respiratory movement, can also induce vascular rupture.

In the cases of invasive pulmonary aspergillosis, especially in the cases of acute invasive pulmonary aspergillosis, hemoptysis is also common. Compared to chronic pulmonary aspergillosis, the systemic and respiratory symptoms of invasive pulmonary aspergillosis are more obvious, commonly accompanied by acute onset of high fever, cough, expectoration of purulent sputum, and hemoptysis of blood streak in sputum instead of major hemoptysis. The cause of these symptoms is necrotic pneumonia. Being different from hemoptysis induced by aspergilloma, the pathological changes of hemoptysis in the cases of invasive pulmonary aspergillosis include infiltrative inflammation, tissue necrosis and suppuration, formation of multiple small abscesses, and even small focal infarction.

In this section, a total of 17 cases of pulmonary aspergillosis with presenting symptom of hemoptysis are analyzed and discussed. The presenting symptom of hemoptysis shows no significant gender variance. Concerning the typing, hemoptysis commonly presents in the cases of singular aspergilloma and chronic cavitary pulmonary aspergillosis. In these 17 cases, only 1 case was diagnosed with acute invasive bronchopulmonary aspergillosis, indicating rare occurrence of hemoptysis in the cases of acute invasive bronchopulmonary aspergillosis. Their illness course ranged from 1 month to 20 years, and the most common basic disease is old pulmonary tuberculosis. Before the diagnosis was finally defined, the condition had been misdiagnosed as pulmonary tuberculosis, lung carcinoma, and bronchiectasis. In laboratory test, the WBC count was commonly not high, and the ESR was not high or slightly high. The sputum culture for fungi showed low positive rate, which is considered to be related to noncommunication of aspergilloma with bronchus. G test also showed low positive rate, which is consistent to the noninvasiveness of aspergilloma. Because some hospitals were not well equipped for GM test, the data of GM test was absent. According to literature reports, the sensitivity of serum GM test may be higher in patients with aspergilloma and presenting symptom of hemoptysis (38%) than in patients with aspergilloma but no presenting symptom of hemoptysis. It was speculated to be related to release of GM into blood after invasion of aspergillus into blood vessels. Radiologically, pulmonary aspergillosis with presenting symptom of hemoptysis should be differentiated from lung carcinoma, pulmonary tuberculoma, or cavitary pulmonary tuberculosis. High-resolution CT scan can more favorably demonstrate cavity wall and aspergilloma in the cavity than routine CT scan. But actually, the definitive diagnosis was commonly made based on surgery and postoperative pathology.

Generally speaking, the key points for pulmonary aspergillosis with presenting symptom of hemoptysis are as the following:

1. Hemoptysis is the most common clinical symptom of chronic cavitary pulmonary aspergillosis and simplex aspergilloma, which should be differentiated from old pulmonary tuberculosis with presenting symptom of hemoptysis. In the cases of old pulmonary tuberculosis with repeated sputum culture for bacteria negative, DNA of *Mycobacterium tuberculosis* negative, radiological sign of characteristic air crescent sign, and spherical substance in cavity, pulmonary aspergillosis should be considered. Laboratory tests provide limited diagnostic value. For patients with good general condition, surgery is recommended for radical treatment and pathological diagnosis.
2. Hemoptysis in the cases of IPA commonly presents as accompanying symptom, and the symptoms of fever, cough, and expectoration of purulent sputum may be typical. Serum GM test shows high sensitivity (75%) to pulmonary aspergillosis in patients with or receiving persistent agranulocytosis and allogeneic hematopoietic stem cell transplantation. And BALF GM test shows high diagnostic value in patients with pulmonary aspergillosis and non-agranulocytosis, with a sensitivity of above 90%.

Patients' consents have been obtained for images or other clinical information relating to the cases to be published.

12.1 Case 1: Cough and Expectoration of Sputum with Blood Streak for 1 Month

Na Li, Songming Zhuo, Wenhui Tang, Jin Xu, Dong-Na Su, Chen Qiu, and Guan-Xun Cheng

12.1.1 Presenting Symptom

Cough and expectoration of sputum with blood streak for 1 month.

12.1.2 Brief Medical History

A 71-year-old woman was admitted to our hospital on January 7, 2015, due to presenting complaints of cough and expectoration of bloody sputum. One month ago, the patient began to experience cough and expectoration of sputum with blood streak with no known causes. She experienced no fever, fatigue, night sweat, chest distress, breathlessness, and chest pain. On December 14, 2014, she received chest X-ray in a local hospital, demonstrating peripheral lung carcinoma at the posterior segment of the right lower lung lobe that needed to be differentiated from pulmonary tuberculosis. On December 15, 2014, enhanced chest CT scan in another hospital demonstrated lesion at the posterior segment of the right lower lung lobe, which was considered to be tuberculosis, which needed to be differentiated from peripheral lung carcinoma. Hemocoagulase was administered for 2 days for hemostasis, but with poor therapeutic efficacy. On December 19, 2014, puncture of the lung for biopsy demonstrated pulmonary aspergillosis. For further diagnosis and treatment, the patient was admitted to our hospital. Since the onset of symptoms, the patient showed no weight loss, with quite good appetite. Her urinations and bowel movements were normal.

12.1.2.1 Physical Examination

Physical examination showed a body temperature of 36.5 °C, pulse rate 66/min, respiration rate 21/min, and blood pressure 137/71 mmHg. The SPO_2 was 99%. She was well conscious, with smooth respirations. She answered to the questions and well cooperated in physical examination. The sclera and systemic skin showed no yellowish stain, with no bleeding spot. The superficial lymph nodes were not enlarged. The respiration sounds of both lungs were clear, with no dry and/or moist rales. The heart, liver, and spleen as well as the abdomen showed no abnormalities. Both lower limbs showed no edema.

12.1.2.2 Auxiliary Investigation

Laboratory Test

On December 16, 2014, the test for biomarkers of neoplasm showed that the CEA, CA153, CA19-9, CA724, NSE, and CYFRA21-1 were within normal limits. PCT was 0.05 ng/ml within normal limits. On December 17, 2014, the immunologic assay for tuberculosis showed that the three items were within normal limits. The DNA of *Mycobacterium tuberculosis* was normal. The sputum culture for *Mycobacterium tuberculosis* showed negative. On December 19, 2014, the routine blood test showed that the indices were within normal limits.

Radiology

On December 19, 2014, CT scan of the lungs (Fig. 12.1) demonstrated mass-like opacity with soft tissue intensity at the right lower lung lobe in a size of about 20 mm × 22 mm. Its margin was lobulated, with spikes and spinous processes in different lengths. There was pleural adhesion adjacent to the mass. The right middle lung lobe and subpleural part of the right lower lung lobe were demonstrated with multiple small nodular opacity of soft tissue intensity. Both lungs were demonstrated with local light flakes of high intensity opacity. The mediastinum was demonstrated with no obviously enlarged lymph nodes. The space between superior vena cava and trachea was demonstrated with opacity of liquid intensity in size of about 14 mm × 17 mm and a CT value of about 12 Hu. Based on the demonstrations, the diagnosis was made to be space-occupying lesion at the right lower lung lobe that was possibly peripheral lung carcinoma, less inflammation of the left upper lung lobe, less chronic inflammation of both lungs, and bilateral pleural effusion of small quantities.

On December 19, 2014, CT-guided lung puncture for biopsy demonstrated fungal hyphae and spores in the specimen, indistinct branching and septa of the hyphae, hyperplasia of alveolar epithelium of the adjacent lung tissue, interstitial fibrosis, and infiltration of lymphocytes with carbon dust deposition. By special staining, methenamine silver staining showed positive and gram staining negative. Histologically, the changes were consistent to pulmonary aspergillosis (Fig. 12.2).

12.1.2.3 Initial Diagnosis

The initial diagnosis was pulmonary aspergillus infection.

12.1.3 Diagnosis and Treatment

After admission, the investigations were performed. The G test on January 9, 2015, showed under 50.0 pg/ml, negative. The sputum investigation on January 9, 2015, demonstrated fungal hyphae. Voriconazole was administered after her admission in a dose of intravenous dripping of 200 mg every 12 h for antifungal therapy. Reexamination of CT scan on January 21, 2015 (Fig. 12.3), demonstrated absorption of consolidation opacity at the right lower lung lobe and absorption of multiple nodules at the right middle lung lobe and subpleural part in the right lower lung lobe. The patient required transfer to the hospital of higher grade for surgery, but she finally gave up surgical operation.

The diagnosis on discharge was aspergillus infection at the right lower lung lobe.

After discharge, her condition was stable. The telephone follow-up on January 8, 2016, demonstrated that the patient was capable of managing daily life and working, with no hemoptysis and other symptoms. But she was unwilling to pay clinic visit.

12.1.4 Discussion

In this case, the patient presented due to cough and expectoration of bloody sputum. Chest CT scan demonstrated mass-like opacity of soft tissue intensity at the right lower lung.

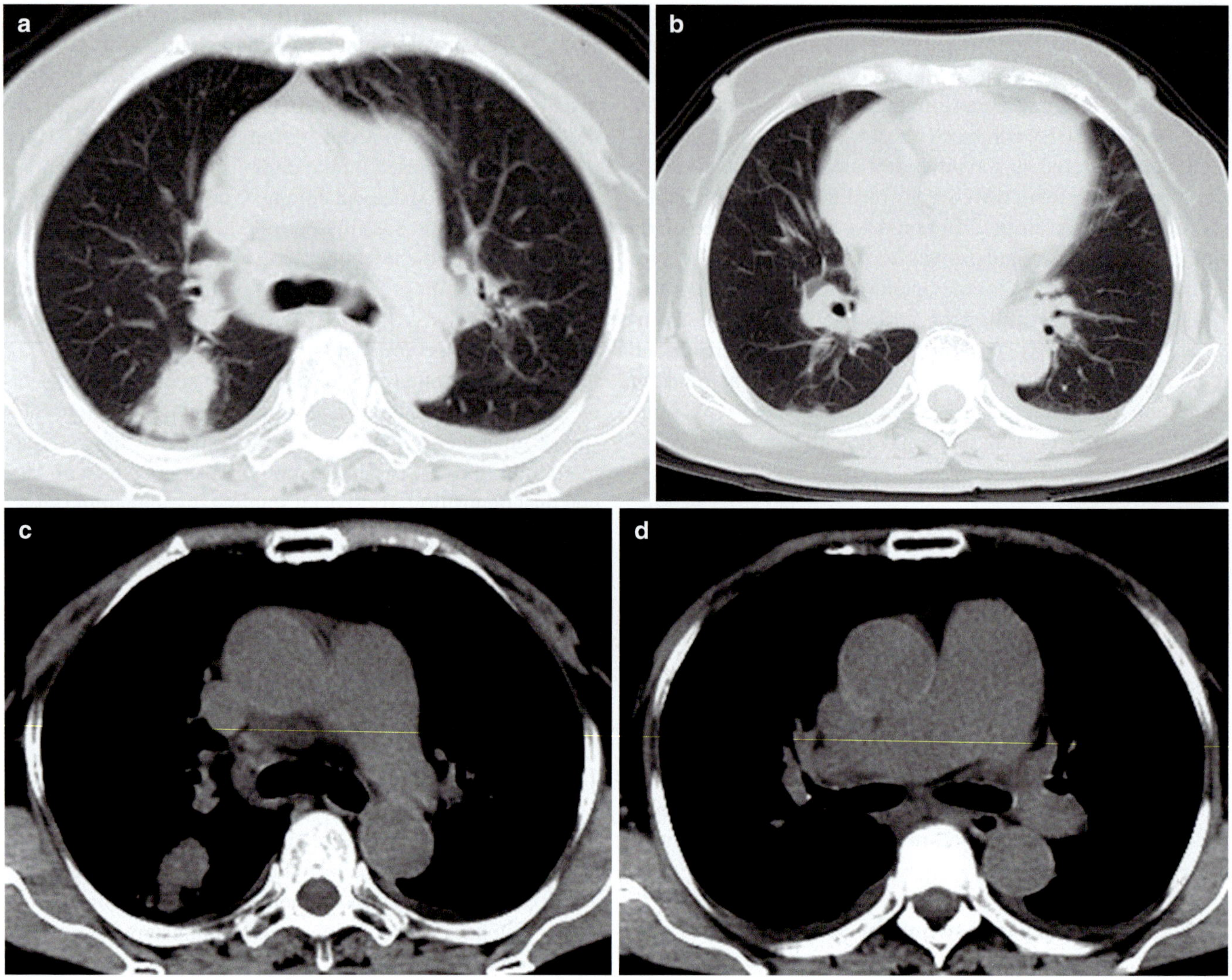

Fig. 12.1 (**a**–**d**) Chest CT scan. (**a**) A mass-like dense opacity was demonstrated at the right lower lung, which was connected with the posterior pleura. (**b**) The pleura at the right lower lung lobe is demonstrated with multiple small nodular opacity. (**c**) The mediastinum window demonstrates irregular nodular opacity with quite homogeneous soft tissue intensity at the right lower lung. (**d**) The bilateral pleura are demonstrated with thickening

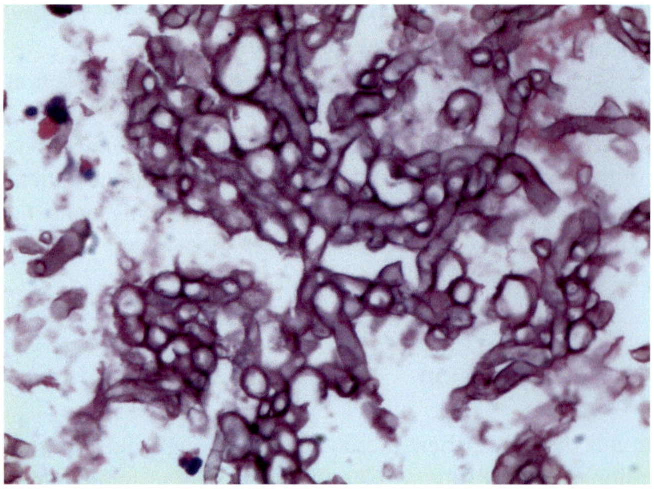

Fig. 12.2 Lung tissue culture for aspergillus. There were observable hyphae and spores (H&E staining)

By puncture of the lung for biopsy, the pathological diagnosis was made to be aspergillus infection. And the diagnosis was finally defined.

Radiologically, the patient was demonstrated with mass-like opacity with soft tissue intensity at the right lower lung that was lobulated with spikes and spinous processes but no crescent sign. The condition should be firstly differentiated from lung carcinoma. For patients with lung lesions and clinically recurrent hemoptysis but unfavorable therapeutic efficacy by medications, the condition should be suspected to be pulmonary aspergillosis. Radiology, especially CT scan, has important diagnostic value [1]. In this case, voriconazole was administered, showing favorable therapeutic efficacy, and hemoptysis did not occur after withdrawal of medication for 1 year. Lung carcinoma was less likely. However, literature reports show possible concurrence of pulmonary aspergillosis and lung carcinoma [2]. Therefore, lung carcinoma

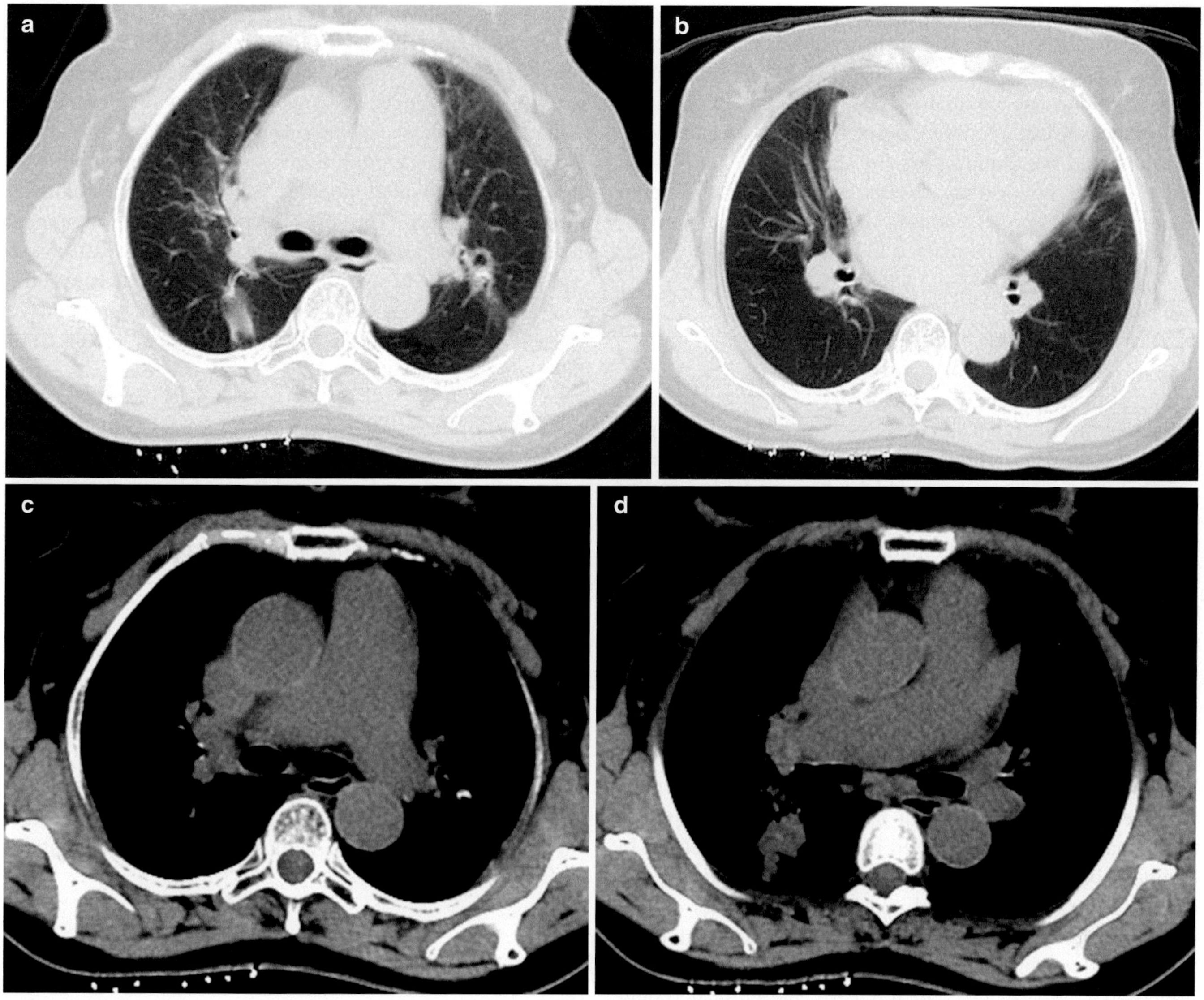

Fig. 12.3 (**a**–**d**) Chest CT scan. (**a**, **b**) The lung window demonstrates shrinkage of the consolidation opacity at the right lower lung lobe and shrinkage of multiple small nodules at the right middle lung lobe and subpleural part in the right lower lung lobe. (**c**, **d**) The mediastinum window demonstrates irregular nodular opacity with heterogeneous intensity, with slight absorption compared to previous chest CT scan

may be misdiagnosed. Formation of cavity due to infarction of lung tissue induced by aspergillus infection should be differentiated from cavity induced by tuberculosis and lung carcinoma. The space formed by liquefaction of tuberculoma is commonly located at side of lung hilum, while the space induced by aspergillus infection is commonly located superior to the cavity. And the cavity induced by lung carcinoma is commonly eccentric, which is far away from the side of lung hilum with unsmooth inner wall. This is the key point for their radiological differentiation.

In this case, the G test showed negative, and sputum investigation for fungus showed positive, with finding of fungal hyphae, which indicated possible G test negative due to focal parasitic aspergillosis. In this case, the finding of fungal hyphae in sputum specimen should not be the basis for definitive diagnosis. Contamination of specimens should be excluded. According to literature reports, the positive rate of sputum culture for pulmonary aspergillosis is only 10–30%. The sensitivity of fibrobronchoscopic biopsy or BALF biopsy is about 40–70%. Currently, surgery is recommended for patients with chronic parasitic pulmonary aspergillosis to remove primary lung lesion and parasitic aspergillosis and prevent bleeding [3]. For the patients with chronic parasitic pulmonary aspergillosis, surgery has favorable therapeutic efficacy and prognosis. Antifungal medication after elimination of the lesion can reinforce the therapeutic efficacy. Currently, no definitive guideline for therapeutic course of medication has been internationally issued. Voriconazole or itraconazole can be administered for 6–12 weeks based on the condition of the patients as well as radiological demonstrations [4]. According to literature reports, for the patients with primary pulmonary lesion or other conditions that may cause recurrence or dissemination of aspergillosis due to extensive lesion and rupture of cavity during the surgical operation, prophylactic antifungal medication should be administered for above 8 weeks. For the patients with no primary disease and complete surgical removal of the isolated lesion, antifungal medication for 4 weeks should be administered [5].

12.1.5 Comments

In this case, the patient was an elderly woman, with presenting symptoms of cough and expectoration of bloody sputum for 1 month. Radiology demonstrated space-occupying lesion at the right lower lung, which was a mass-like opacity with soft tissue intensity. Radiologically, the lesion is likely to be lung carcinoma, with marginal lobulation, spikes, and spinous processes in different lengths and adjacent pleural adhesion. In addition, there were multiple small nodular opacities of soft tissue intensity at the right middle lung lobe and subpleural part in the right lower lung. In the cases of lung carcinoma, the lesion is obviously enhanced by enhanced radiology. However, in this case, the lesion showed no enhancement by enhanced radiology, which did not support the diagnosis of lung carcinoma. In this case, the nodules were surrounded by light halo sign, which supported hemorrhagic infarction induced by aspergillus infection. In combination to case history, pathology, and radiological demonstrations of subpleural nodules in a diameter of less than 3 cm, accompanying halo sign, local necrosis and liquefaction, and tendency of cavity formation, aspergillus infection should be suspected. In this case, the clinical typing should be aspergillus nodule of chronic pulmonary aspergillosis. Aspergillus nodule is a rare type of chronic pulmonary aspergillosis. Resembling to tuberculoma, lung carcinoma, lung metastasis, *Cryptococcus* nodule, coccidioidomycosis, and other diseases caused by rare pathogen, the diagnosis can only be defined based on histopathology. In this case, the diagnosis was defined based on puncture of the lung for biopsy.

In this case, one medication of voriconazole was administered for antifungal treatment, which showed favorable therapeutic efficacy. The patient experienced shrinkage of aspergillus nodule and no recurrence of hemoptysis. Close follow-ups should be performed after treatment to observe the absorption of the lesions induced by aspergillus. Due to poor compliance of the patient, routine follow-ups were not performed. Here, we emphasize the importance of follow-ups after antifungal treatment. It is recommended that follow-up should be performed every 3–6 months after commencement of antifungal treatment, followed by reduced frequency of follow-ups. Reexamination of radiology is necessary when any change occurs clinically. Within less than 3 months after antifungal treatment, radiology demonstrates no significant change. The signs of improving chronic pulmonary aspergillosis include decreased pleural thickening, decreased substances in the cavity, more smooth inner wall of the cavity, smaller nodule, and smaller consolidation around the cavity. The signs indicating failed treatment include enlarged cavity, emergence of new cavity, fusion of cavity, formation of aspergilloma, and enlarged consolidation around the cavity. The longitudinal progression of lesions can be assessed via volume quantification with computer software package.

12.2 Case 2: Recurrent Cough, Expectoration and Breathlessness for 5 Years, Which Aggravated with Accompanying Hemoptysis for 8 Months

Wenhui Tang, Na Li, Songming Zhuo, Jin Xu, Dong-Na Su, Xueyan Liu, and Xuemei Han

12.2.1 Presenting Symptom

Recurrent cough, expectoration, and breathlessness for 5 years, which aggravated with accompanying hemoptysis for 8 months.

12.2.2 Brief Case History

A 66-year-old man, a retired worker from Jiangxi province, was admitted to our hospital for the second time on May 24, 2014, due to complaints of recurrent cough, expectoration, and breathlessness for more than 5 years with aggravation and accompanying hemoptysis for 8 months. Five years ago, the patient began to experience cough, expectoration of yellowish white sputum, and breathlessness. In February 2014, he was admitted to a local hospital in Ji'an of Jiangxi province due to aggravation of cough and expectoration of bloody sputum. The diagnosis was aggravating stage of chronic obstructive pulmonary disease and pneumonia. Cefuroxime and moxifloxacin were consecutively administered for infection, hemostasis, breathlessness, and other symptoms. But the symptoms of cough and expectoration were not improved. On March 4, 2014, bronchoscopy was performed in our hospital, with a diagnosis of pulmonary aspergillosis. And voriconazole was administered with favorable therapeutic efficacy, and the patient was discharged. After discharge, oral medication of voriconazole and mucosolvin were continued, and he still experienced cough and expectoration of bloody sputum.

12.2.2.1 Past Medical History

He denied histories of hypertension and diabetes. And he reported a medical history of pulmonary tuberculosis 10 years ago (specifically unknown).

12.2.2.2 Physical Examination

Physical examination showed a body temperature of 36.8 °C, pulse rate 86/min, respiration rate 20/min, and blood pressure 125/70 mmHg. The oxygen saturation of blood was 98% (with no inhalation of additional oxygen). The patient showed barrel chest, with stable respirations. The bilateral thoracic wall showed no mass. There were no subcutaneous edema and widened intercostal space. The respiration movements were rhythmic and bilaterally symmetric. By palpation, the vocal fremitus were weakened. By percussion, both lungs showed hyperresonant note. By auscultation, the breathing sounds of both lungs were weakened, with no dry and/or moist rales.

12.2.2.3 Auxiliary Investigation

Laboratory Test

Routine blood test showed WBC 4.08 × 109/L, neutrophil granulocytes 57.0%, eosinophile granulocytes ratio 2.0%, hemoglobin 98 g/L, and platelets 380 × 109/L. The ESR was 135 mm/h. And the antigen test for aspergillus was 0.467 μg/L, antigen test for candida 0.063 μg/L, and antigen test for cryptococcus less than 0.5 μg/L. The sputum smear and culture for common bacteria, *Mycobacterium tuberculosis*, and fungi were negative. G test for fungus was 86.3 pg/ml, and the GM test showed negative.

Radiology

Chest plain and enhanced CT scan on March 5, 2014 (Fig. 12.4), demonstrated many tracted and dilated bronchi with thickened bronchial wall in both lungs and a thick wall cavity in size of about 55 mm × 50 mm with unsmooth inner wall and a small quantity of liquid intensity opacity inside. Enhanced CT scan demonstrated enhancement of the cavity wall. Both lungs were demonstrated with multiple thin wall cavities in different sizes and the largest one in size of about 44 mm × 29 mm. The transparency of both lungs increased, and the lung markings of both lungs were thickened and deranged. High signal shadows of multiple cords, stripes, spots and nodules were seen in both lungs. And patchy consolidation was demonstrated at the posteroapical segment of the right upper lung lobe, medial segment of the right middle lung lobe, and dorsal segment and posterolateral basilar segment of the right lower lung lobe. In the patchy opacity, there were multiple honeycomb-like opacity, spots of calcification opacity, and air bronchogram. The trachea and bronchi were not obstructed, and the lung hilum opacity was not enlarged. The mediastinal lymph nodes were not enlarged, and no sign of pleural effusion was demonstrated. The heart opacity showed

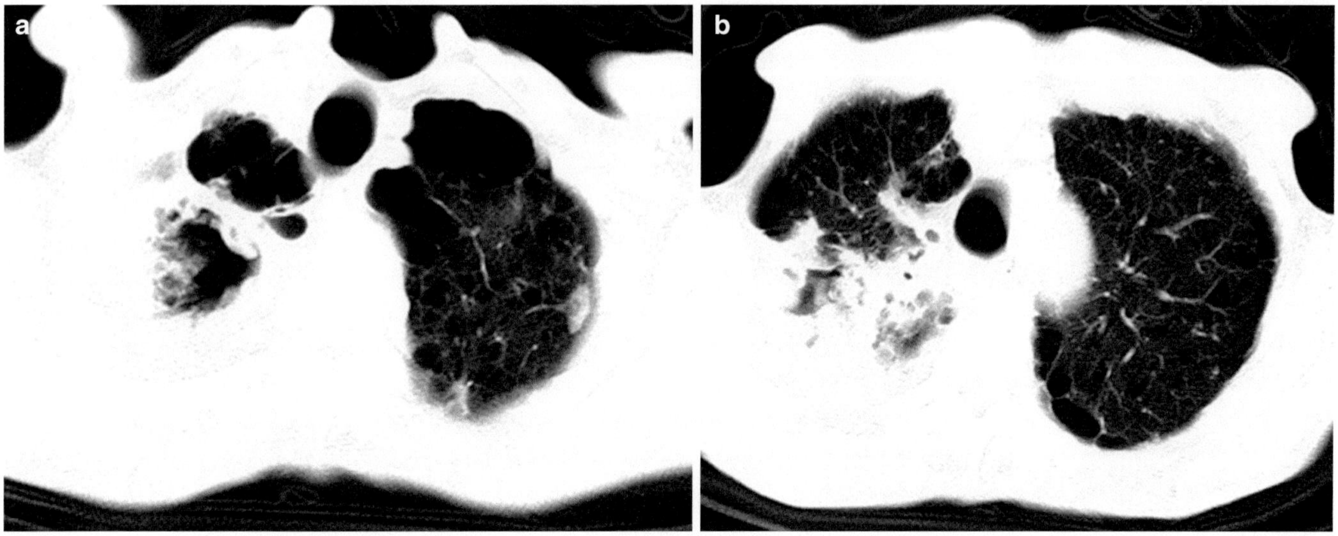

Fig. 12.4 (**a**–**h**) Chest CT scan. (**a**–**c**) The lung window demonstrates a thick wall cavity at the right upper lung in size of about 55 mm × 50 mm with unsmooth inner wall and a small quantity of liquid intensity opacity inside. (**d**, **e**) Patchy consolidation opacity is demonstrated at the medial segment of the right middle lung lobe and dorsal segment and posterolateral basilar segment of the right lower lung lobe. There are multiple honeycomb-like opacities, spots of calcification opacity, and air bronchogram in the patchy consolidation opacity. (**f**, **g**) The mediastinum window demonstrates huge thick wall cavity opacity at the right upper lung lobe. And its surrounding tissue is connected with pleura. (**h**) Enhanced CT scan demonstrates spots of vascular opacity and slight enhancement of the cavity wall

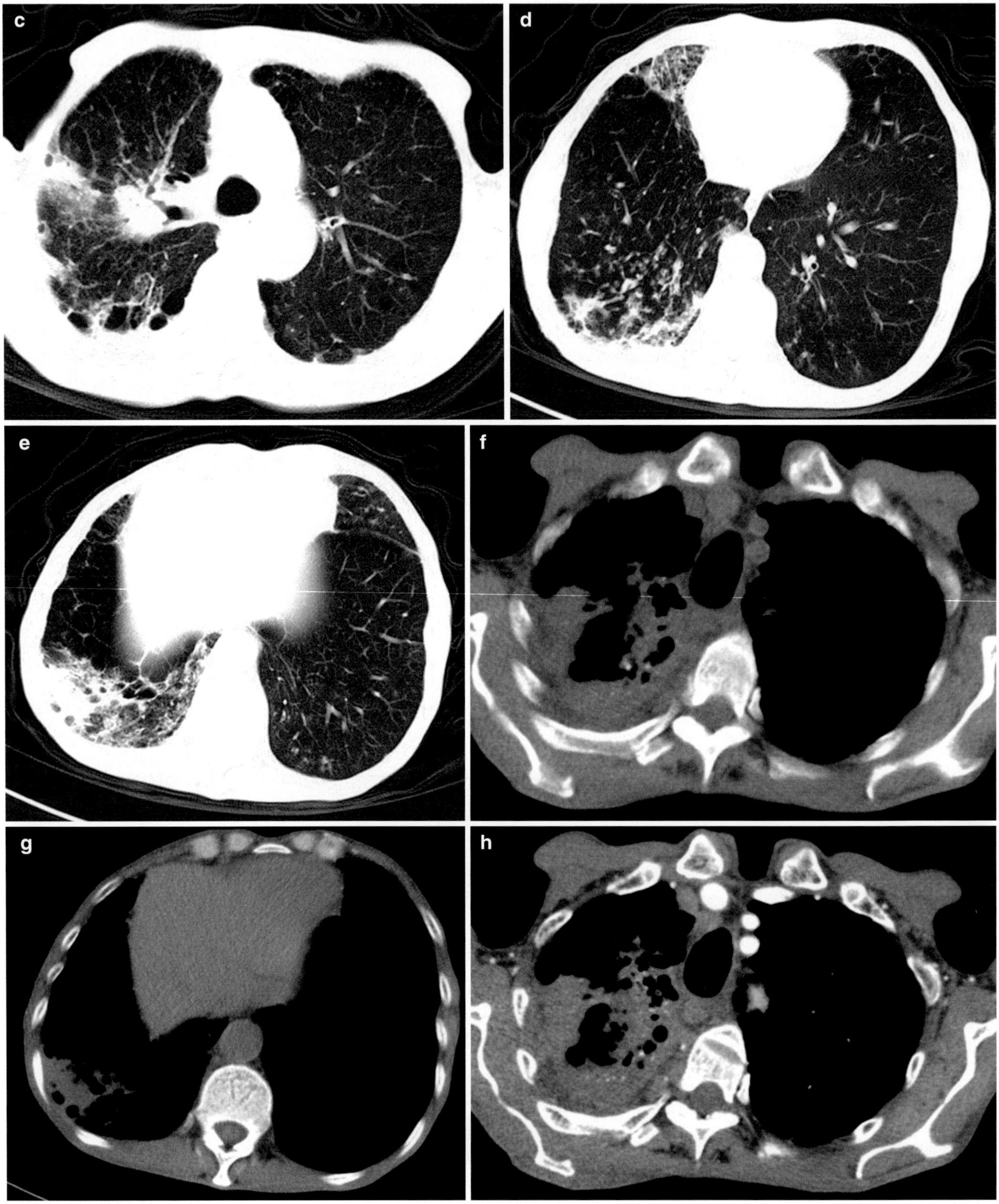

Fig. 12.4 (continued)

no abnormality. The bilateral pleura were thickened. The radiological diagnosis was chronic fibro-cavitary tuberculosis of the right upper lung with complicating fungal infection not excluded, secondary tractive bronchiectasis of both lungs, chronic bronchitis and emphysema, multiple bullae at both lungs, and multiple opacities at bilateral lower lungs which needed differentiation between disseminating lesions of tuberculosis and inflammation. Reexamination after treatment was recommended.

Pathology

Bronchoscopic biopsy of the lateral basilar segment of the right lower lung lobe was performed on March 7, 2014 (Fig. 12.5).

The pathology demonstrated pathological changes of the lateral basilar segment of the right lower lung lobe, which was consistent to pulmonary aspergillosis (Fig. 12.6).

12.2.2.4 Initial Diagnosis

The initial diagnoses were chronic fibro-cavitary pulmonary tuberculosis, complicating formation of aspergilloma in the cavity, secondary tractive bronchiectasis of both lungs, and aggravating stage of chronic obstructive pulmonary disease.

12.2.3 Diagnosis and Treatment

After admission, piperacillin/tazobactam was administered for infection. Etamsylate, aminomethylbenzoic acid, and vitamin C were administered for hemostasis. Injection and tablets of voriconazole were consecutively administered for a total of 84 days for fungal infection. The cough was improved occasionally with hemoptysis. Chest plain and enhanced CT scan on May 26, 2014 (Fig. 12.7), Transparency increased with multiple cords, stripes, spots and nodules in

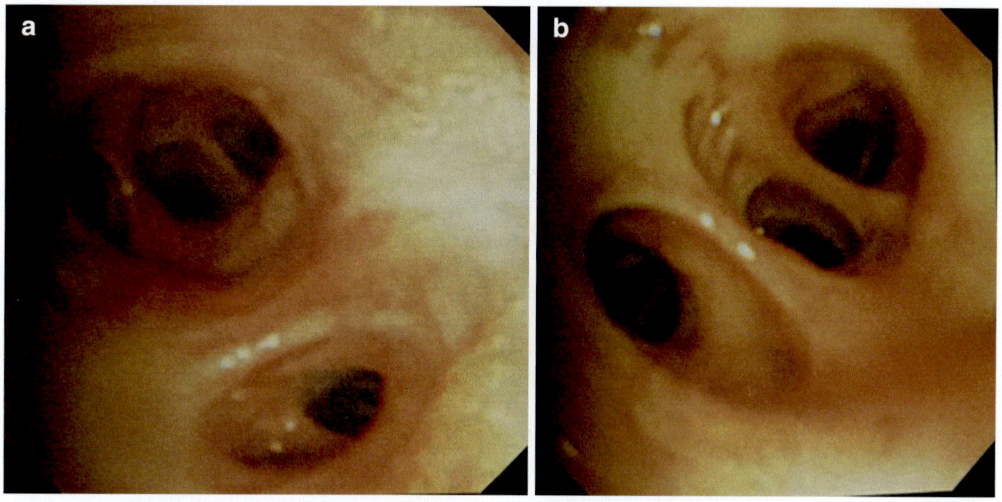

Fig. 12.5 (a, b) Fibrobronchoscopy. Fibrobronchoscopy demonstrates smooth tracheal and bronchial mucosa, with unobstructed lumen and no neoplasm in the lumen. Biopsy of the lateral basilar segment of the right lower lung lobe was performed via fibrobronchoscopy

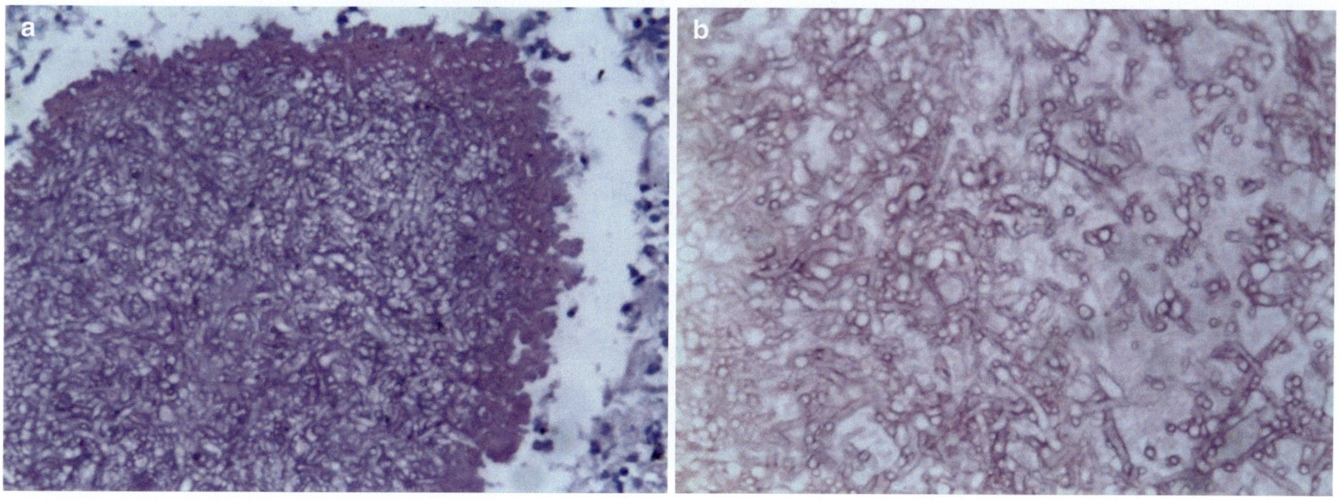

Fig. 12.6 (a–d) Pathology of the lung tissue. The lateral basilar segment of the right lower lung lobe is demonstrated with granulation of lung tissue. There are a small quantity of organic lesions and well-marginated class-A epithelial lesions in the alveolar cavity. Hyphae and spores are demonstrated at the center, with even thickness of the hyphae and sharp angle branching of the hyphae (H&E staining). By special stainings, acid fast staining shows negative, methenamine silver staining positive, AB staining negative, and PAS staining positive

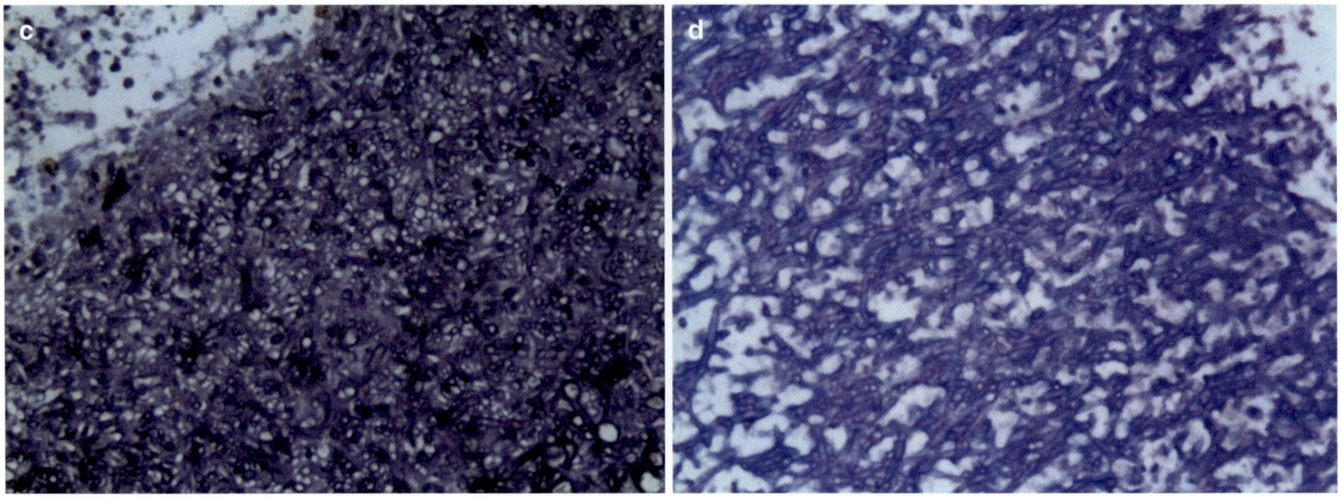

Fig. 12.6 (continued)

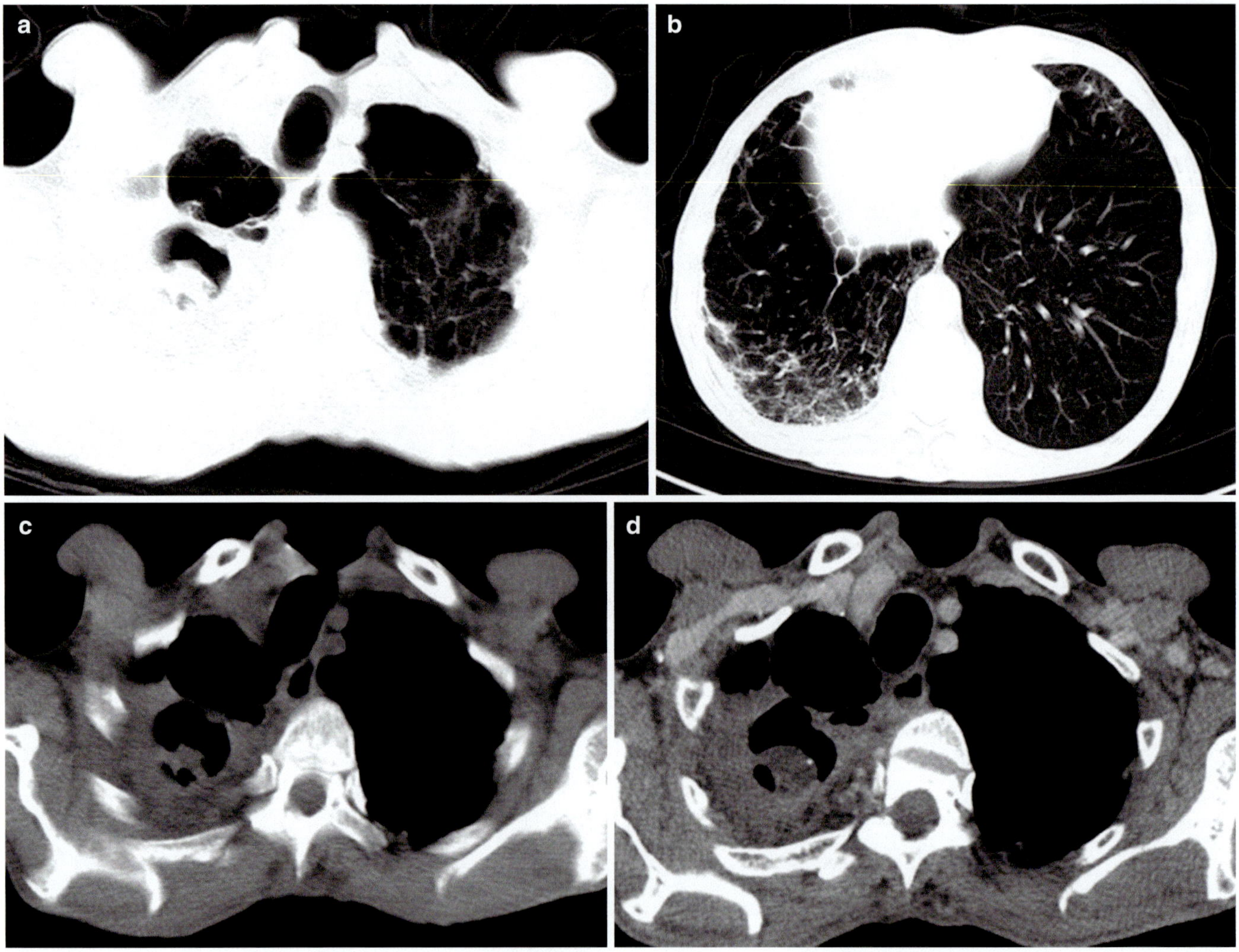

Fig. 12.7 (**a–d**) Chest CT scan. (**a**, **b**) The posteroapical segment of the right upper lung lobe is demonstrated with cavity opacity. And the medial segment of the right middle lung lobe and dorsal segment of the right lower lung lobe are demonstrated with grid-like cords opacity. The interlobular septa are obviously thickened. (**c**) The mediastinum window demonstrates a thick wall cavity at the right upper lung in size of about 55 mm × 56 mm, which is slightly enlarged compared to previous CT scan demonstration. (**d**) Enhanced CT scan demonstrates slight enhancement of the thick wall

both lungs. with multiple cords, spots, and nodular high intensity opacities. The patchy consolidation opacities at the posteroapical segment of the right upper lung lobe, medial segment of the right middle lung lobe, and dorsal segment of right lower lung lobe were almost the same as previously demonstrated. The patchy consolidation opacities at the posterior lateral segment of the right lower lung lobe decreased compared to the previous CT scan demonstrations, with multiple honeycomb-like opacities, spots of calcifications, and air bronchogram inside. Both lungs were demonstrated with many tracted and dilated bronchi, with thickened bronchial wall. A thick wall cavity was demonstrated at the right upper lung and lateral segment of the right middle lung lobe, separately. The larger cavity was located at the right upper lung in size of about 55 mm × 56mm, which was slightly enlarged compared to the previous scan demonstration, with unsmooth inner wall and air crescent sign and nodular opacity inside. The nodular opacity was in size of about 22 mm × 20 mm, with no enhancement by enhanced CT scan. Both lungs were also demonstrated with multiple thin wall cavities in different sizes, the largest in size of about 44 mm × 29 mm, which was almost the same as previously demonstrated. The trachea and bronchi were not obstructed. And lung hilum opacity was not enlarged. The mediastinal lymph nodes were not enlarged. No sign of pleural effusion was demonstrated. And the heart opacity showed no abnormality. The bilateral pleura were thickened. The radiological diagnoses include (a and b) Cavity shadows were seen in the posterior segment of the right upper pulmonary apex, reticulated stripes were seen in the medial and dorsal segments of the right middle lobe, and the interlobular septum was markedly thickened; (c) mediastinal window: A thick-walled cavity was seen in the right upper lung, about 55 mm × 56 mm in size, slightly larger than the previous one; (d) Slight enhancement of thick wall was seen on enhanced CT.

The final diagnoses were (1) chronic fibro-cavitary pulmonary tuberculosis with complicating aspergilloma in the cavity, (2) secondary tractive bronchiectasis of both lungs, and (3) acute aggravating stage of chronic obstructive pulmonary disease.

After discharge, the condition of the patient was stable, and no hemoptysis occurred during follow-ups.

12.2.4 Discussion

Pulmonary aspergillosis is a group of acute or chronic lung diseases induced by aspergillus infection. Aspergillus is a conditional pathogen, which commonly infects human when the immunity is inhibited or impaired. Pulmonary aspergillosis is commonly secondary to basic lung disease, such as bronchial cyst, bronchiectasis, pneumonia, and pulmonary abscess. Primary aspergillus infection is rare. In some serious cases, aspergillus may cause death due to systemic dissemination along with blood flow. Clinically, pulmonary aspergillosis can be classified into invasive pulmonary aspergillosis, aspergilloma, and allergic bronchopulmonary aspergillosis.

Based on its pathomechanism, aspergilloma can be classified into:

1. Parasitic cavitary aspergilloma, which is secondary growth of aspergillus in cavity within lung. The hyphae, spores, mucous cellulose, and inflammatory cells form aspergilloma, which is a common type of pulmonary aspergillosis. It is commonly secondary in the cavity induced by pulmonary tuberculosis, pulmonary abscess, bronchiectasis, and bullae.
2. Primary aspergilloma, which is caused by reproduction and growth of aspergillus in the cavity induced by infarction and necrosis of lung tissue after aspergillus infection.

There is also another type of formation of cavity in the cases of aspergilloma. The lesion is initially irregular poorly defined infiltration of local lung tissue. The infiltration gradually progresses into well marginated round in shape to form cavity. This type is extremely rare. In this case, the condition can be categorized into parasitic cavitary aspergilloma, which was secondary to chronic fibro-cavitary pulmonary tuberculosis. Currently, it has been confirmed that obstructed drainage promotes growth of aspergillus in the cavity. The patients commonly have history of long-term medication of antibiotic, medication for tuberculosis, chemotherapy, or medication of hormone.

The clinical manifestations of pulmonary aspergilloma are non-specific. It commonly presents as the primary disease, and it, therefore, tends to be misdiagnosed as pulmonary tuberculosis, bronchiectasis, and lung carcinoma. The common symptoms of pulmonary aspergilloma include hemoptysis, cough, chest pain, and fever. Hemoptysis is especially common in clinical practice. The causes of hemoptysis include:

1. The surrounding tissue of pulmonary aspergilloma is subject to inflammatory stimulation to form abundant vascular network or even angioma. Along with mechanical stimulation from respiration movements, vascular rupture is induced.
2. The endotoxin and protease produced by aspergillus induce necrosis and lysis of the tissue.
3. The primary disease induces bleeding.

The diagnosis of pulmonary aspergilloma is challenging with high rate of misdiagnosis. The diagnosis is commonly defined based on postoperative pathology. Because the antifungal medication can hardly reach the curative concentration in the cavity, the therapeutic efficacy of medication is poor. Several scholars from China [6] have recommended surgical operation as the first choice for treatment, with favorable therapeutic efficacy.

To reverse immune-suppressive state such as neutropenia is a necessary condition in treatment of aspergillosis. Due to existence of immunosuppression in most patients with fungal infection, maximally decreased use of immunosuppressant is the first consideration in infection control, and immunoenhancers should be administered. Long therapeutic course is needed for treatment of pulmonary aspergilloma, with favorable therapeutic efficacy and prognosis. Due to higher rate of survival and favorable therapeutic efficacy, voriconazole is currently the first choice medication for pulmonary aspergilloma [7]. Amphotericin B is a conventional medication for aspergillosis but has been rarely applied in clinical practice due to its obvious side effects. Caspofungin shows favorable safety and therapeutic efficacy. When amphotericin B and its liposome as well as voriconazole fail to treat aspergillosis or the patient is intolerant to amphotericin B, caspofungin is the first choice as remedial therapy. The patients with pulmonary aspergilloma who receive surgical operation of the lesions do not need postoperative antifungal medication [8].

In this case, the patient initially received treatment for pneumonia. But consecutive medications of cefuroxime, moxifloxacin, and piperacillin-tazobactam showed no therapeutic efficacy for infection, and the condition showed progression. After the diagnosis was defined, injection and tablets of voriconazole were administered for 84 days for fungal infection. The condition was then stabled, and the patient showed no hemoptysis during follow-ups.

12.2.5 Comments

In this case, the patient suffered from aspergilloma in cavity based on chronic fibro-cavitary pulmonary tuberculosis. Pulmonary tuberculosis tends to be complicated by aspergillus infection, and the reasons are as the following:

1. The bronchial mucosal epithelium is impaired, which weakens the cleanup effect, and the fungi in oropharynx tend to move downward to invade the lung tissue.
2. Long-term use of broad-spectrum antibiotics, antituberculosis drugs and hormones induces respiratory tract flora imbalance, decreasing of T lymphocyte number and function, suppression of immune response in vivo, and spread of pathogenic bacteria such as Aspergillus to the respiratory system.
3. Exudation, hyperplasia, caseous necrosis, cavity, and other lung lesions induced by pulmonary tuberculosis facilitate the growth and reproduction of fungi. The aspergillus spores are inhaled into the respiratory tract and stay in cavity induced by pulmonary tuberculosis. Due to deficient immunologic active substances in the cavity and favorable humidity and temperature in the cavity, aspergillus tends to grow in the cavity and reproduce in a large quantity. Their mixture with fibrin, hemorrhagic, and necrotic substances in the cavity, mucosal epithelia, and mucus forms aspergilloma.

In the 2015 Clinical Guideline for the Diagnosis and Treatment of Chronic Pulmonary Aspergillosis jointly issued by ERS and ESCMID, surgical removal is recommended for singular aspergilloma. If surgical removal is incomplete, anti-aspergillus medication should be administered. For the cases of multiple aspergilloma or nodules, antifungal medication and regular follow-ups are recommended. In this case, the patient showed multiple cavities. Figure 12.7 demonstrated slightly enlarged thick wall cavity at the right upper lung compared to previously demonstrated and new irregular small cavity opacity at the lateral segment of the right middle lung. The clinical typing of chronic cavitary pulmonary aspergillosis is appropriate. In the medical history of the patient, a history of pulmonary tuberculosis 10 years ago was reported, and the appropriateness of antituberculosis therapy was unknown. During treatment of aspergillosis, activeness of primary pulmonary tuberculosis should be assessed for necessity of simultaneous antituberculosis therapy.

12.3 Case 3: Recurrent Cough and Hemoptysis for 20 Years, Which Onset Again for 1 Day

Jingjing Li, Jian Zheng, Hui Wang, Chang'e Jin, Xiongfei Sun, and Mengjie Li

12.3.1 Presenting Symptoms

Recurrent cough and hemoptysis for 20 years, which onset again for 1 day.

12.3.2 Brief Case History

A 50-year-old man was admitted to our hospital on June 19, 2014, due to presenting complaints of recurrent cough and hemoptysis for 20 years, which onset again for 1 day. Twenty years ago, the patient began to experience cough and hemoptysis, and he presented in a local hospital for diagnosis and treatment. The diagnosis there was pulmonary tuberculosis. Antituberculosis medication of 3HRZES/9HRE was administered. The patient was cured, and the medication was discontinued. But since then, the patient still experienced recurrent cough, expectoration of whitish mucous sputum in a small quantity, and recurrent sputum with blood streak. The symptomatic medication was administered for hemostasis, but antituberculosis therapy was not administered. One day before his admission to our hospital, he experienced aggravating cough and several times hemoptysis. Since the onset of the symptoms, the patient experienced no fever, aversion to cold, chill, flush after noon, night sweat, chest pain, and breathlessness. His spiritual state and appetite were quite good. The urinations and bowel movements were normal. The body weight showed no obvious change.

12.3.2.1 Physical Examination

Physical examination showed a body temperature of 37.4 °C, pulse rate 108/min, respiration rate 21/min, and blood pressure 118/69 mmHg. He was well conscious but poorly nourished. The superficial lymph nodes were unpalpable with no enlargement. The respiration sound of both lungs was weakened. By auscultation, the left upper lung showed slight and moderate moist rales and dry wheezing. The liver and spleen were unpalpable. The bowel sound was normal.

12.3.2.2 Auxiliary Investigation

Laboratory Test

The WBC count was 7.56 × 109/L, neutrophil granulocytes 71.4%, lymphocytes 21%, hemoglobin concentration 142 g/L, and platelet 158 × 109/L. The C-reactive protein quantification by immunoturbidimetry was 33.72 mg/L. The liver function test, kidney function test, electrolytes, CEA, CA19-9, and the two-item biomarkers for neoplasm in respiratory tract were within normal limits. The four-item blood coagulation was within normal limits. Repeated sputum investigation for acid fasting bacilli for three times showed negative. The sputum smears for bacteria and fungi showed negative. The sputum culture for fungi showed growth of yeast-like fungi.

Radiology

Chest CT scan on June 19, 2014 (Fig. 12.8), demonstrated a large cavity opacity at the left upper lung, with crescent sign and a nodular opacity with uniform intensity in the cavity. And the chest X-ray was demonstrated in Fig. 12.9.

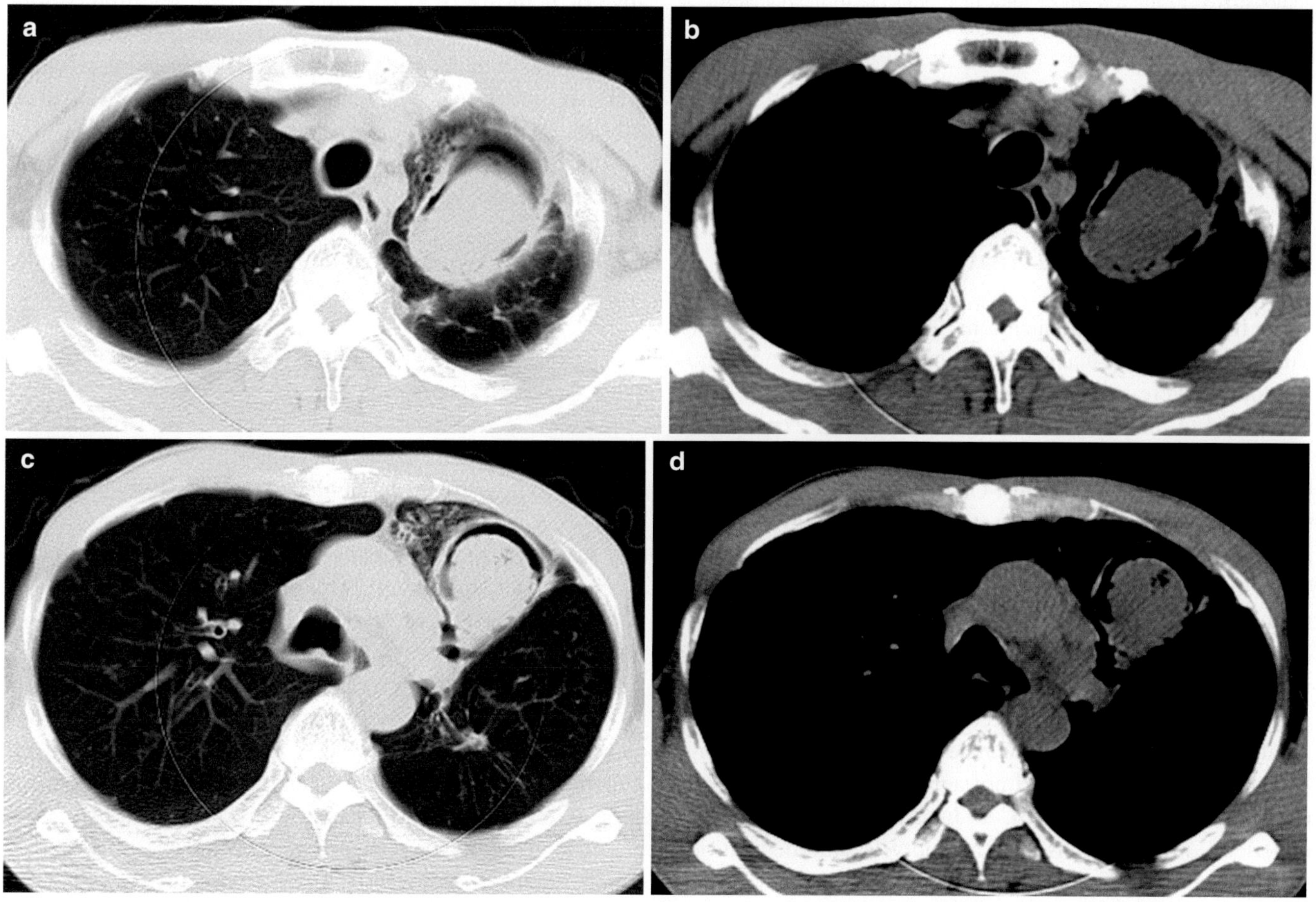

Fig. 12.8 (**a**–**d**) Chest CT scan. (**a**) The lung window demonstrates large cavity opacity at the left upper lung, with crescent sign and nodular opacity with uniform intensity in the cavity. (**b**) The mediastinum window demonstrates crescent sign around the nodular opacity at the left upper lung lobe, with uniform intensity. (**c**) The lung window demonstrates scattering strips of opacity in the cavity opacity at the right upper lung lobe. (**d**) The mediastinum window demonstrates small necrotic translucent area in the nodular opacity at the left upper lung lobe

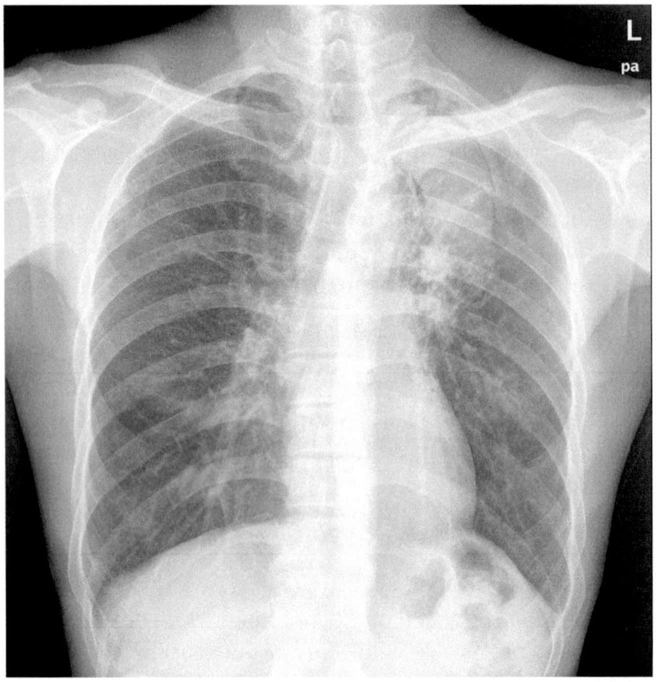

Fig. 12.9 Chest CT scan. Large flakes of high intensity opacity are demonstrated at the left upper lung field adjacent to heart margin. A sign resembling to crescent sign is demonstrated

12.3.2.3 Initial Diagnosis

The initial diagnosis was pulmonary aspergilloma of the left upper lung and bronchiectasis complicated by hemoptysis.

12.3.3 Diagnosis and Treatment

After his admission, medications for hemostasis including Yunnan white medicinal powder, tranexamic acid, and hemocoagulase were administered. Cefuroxime sodium was administered for infection. But the patient still experienced intermittent hemoptysis of fresh red blood in a small quantity. To exclude malignancies, CEA, CA19-9, and biomarkers for neoplasm in the respiratory tract were investigated, and the results were within normal limits. The four-item blood coagulation was within normal limits. Immunologic three-item for tuberculosis was within normal limits. Repeated sputum investigations for acid fasting bacilli for three times as well as sputum smears for bacteria and fungi showed negative. For timely control of hemoptysis, bronchial artery embolization was recommended for the patient, but his family members did not agree to receive the procedure. During June 23, 2014, to June 30, 2014, the patient experienced repeated onsets of hemoptysis, and medications showed unfavorable therapeutic efficacy. The patient was then transferred to the surgery department. On July 2, 2014, thoracoscopy-assisted surgical removal of the left upper lung lobe was performed under general anesthesia. During the operation, extensive adhesion of left thorax was observed, which was more serious at the left upper lung lobe, with multiple cellulosic adhesions and dense adhesion of lung apex. The left upper lung lobe was in size of about 20 cm × 10 cm × 10 cm, with reddish color and poor elasticity. Within the left upper lung lobe, there was a mass in size of 15 cm × 6 cm × 6 cm, which was oval in shape with moderate density. The left lower lung lobe was in generally good color, density, and elasticity. And the oblique fissure was poorly developed. By pathology (Fig. 12.10), the lung tissue was demonstrated with multiple dilated bronchi, with shedding of most coating mucosal epithelium. In the dilated bronchial lumen, fungal hyphae and spores were observed. The bronchial mucosa and its surrounding tissues were congested, with proliferation of fibrous tissue and infiltrations of lymphocytes and plasmocytes. No tubercles and caseous necrosis were observed. By special stains, methenamine silver staining showed positive and acid fast staining negative. The pathological diagnosis was bronchiectasis of the left upper lung lobe and fungal infection, which was considered to be aspergillus infection.

After the operation, medication of voriconazole and therapy for hemostasis were administered. In addition, symptomatic supports were given. Reexamination of chest X-ray (Fig. 12.11) demonstrated favorable recovery of the left lung after the operation. The patient was cured and discharged on July 26, 2014.

The final diagnosis was bronchiectasis complicated by hemoptysis and pulmonary aspergilloma at the left upper lung.

After discharge, the condition of the patient was stable. And follow-ups showed no recurrence of hemoptysis.

12.3.4 Discussion

In this case, the patient showed recurrent hemoptysis. Chest CT scan demonstrated bronchiectasis of the left upper lung lobe, with dense mass opacity and crescent sign. A clinical diagnosis of bronchiectasis complicated by pulmonary aspergilloma can be made. The pathology of specimen harvested by surgical removal of the left upper lung further confirmed the diagnosis.

Pulmonary aspergilloma is a type of pulmonary aspergillosis, which is commonly secondary to bronchial cyst, bronchiectasis, pulmonary abscess, and tuberculous cavity. Aspergilloma is composed of large quantities of fungal hyphae, inflammatory cells, fibrin, mucus, and tissue debris [9]. The patients may experience symptoms of irritating cough, recurrent hemoptysis, and even lift-threatening major hemoptysis. In this case, the clinical symptoms of the patient were in consistence with the common symptoms of pulmonary aspergilloma. In this case, the patient experienced a

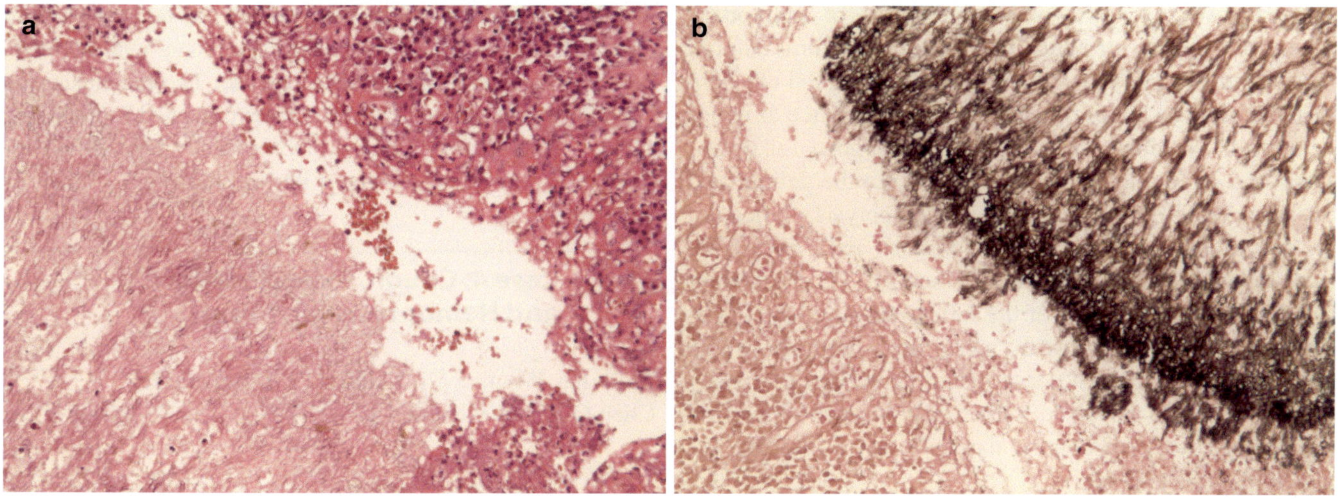

Fig. 12.10 (**a**, **b**) Pathology of the lung tissue. (**a**) H&E staining. (**b**) PASM staining. The lung tissue is demonstrated with multiple dilated bronchi, with shedding of coating mucosal epithelium. In the dilated lumen, there are hyphae and spores of aspergillus. The bronchial mucosa and its surrounding tissue are congested with proliferation of fibrous tissue and infiltrations of lymphocytes and plasmocytes. No tubercles and caseous necrosis are observed. By special stains, methenamine silver staining shows positive and acid fast staining negative

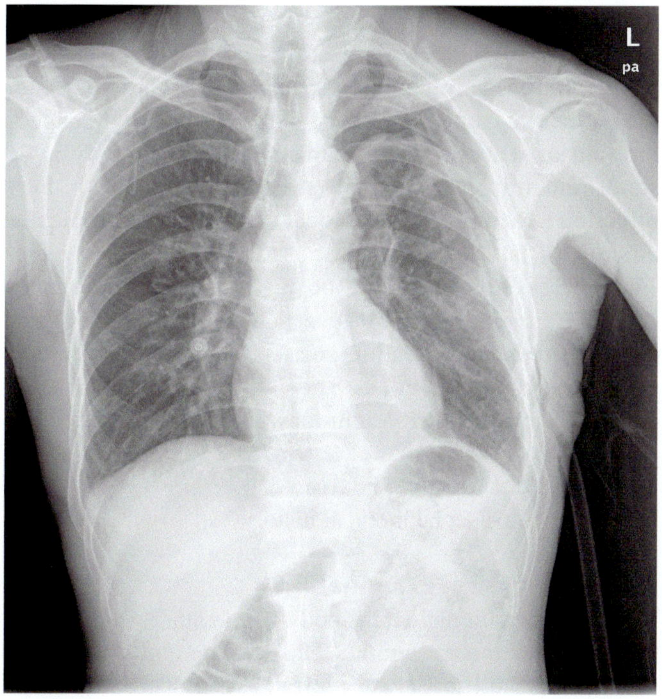

Fig. 12.11 Chest DR. After surgical removal of aspergilloma at the left upper lung field, the lesions disappear, with observable drainage tube at the left thoracic wall

comparatively long history of illness, with recurrence hemoptysis that was incurable by medications. Due to noncommunication of aspergilloma with bronchi, the sputum was in a small quantity, and aspergillus can hardly be detected in the sputum. The clinical manifestations of pulmonary aspergilloma depend on two factors: underlying lung disease and immunity of the patient. Pulmonary aspergilloma commonly occurs in immunocompromised patients with pulmonary tuberculosis or other diseases with lung cavity. The patients with pulmonary aspergillosis account for certain percentage in patients with pulmonary tuberculosis [10]. In this case, pathology demonstrated no tubercles and caseous necrosis, indicating cured pulmonary tuberculosis [11]. It can be hardly identified that aspergillus infection occurred before tuberculosis was cured or secondary aspergillus infection due to bronchiectasis after tuberculosis was cured. Pulmonary aspergilloma can be favorably demonstrated by radiology, and CT scan showed characteristic [12] signs of sphere-in-sphere sign:

1. Round or round-like dense opacity in lung cavity or space.
2. Crescent sign or ring-shaped translucent area between lung cavity or space and its content; when the cavity is large enough, movable inner content is observable along with body posture change.
3. The size of pulmonary aspergilloma may be constant with calcification.

The combination of radiology with culture for fungi facilitates the diagnosis, while the diagnosis can be defined by pathology. For patients with pulmonary aspergilloma and hemoptysis, surgical operation is the treatment of first choice. By research studies [13, 14], the indications of surgery include clinically defined cases or highly suspected cases of pulmonary aspergilloma. Because the antifungal medication can hardly penetrate into the lesion, the clinically defined cases or highly suspected cases of pulmonary aspergilloma with or with no clinical symptoms should receive surgery as early as possible. Early surgical can help to avoid progression of the disease and occurrence of major hemoptysis. In this case, symptomatic supports for hemostasis and infection were administered, but the patient still experienced long-term intermittent hemoptysis, indicating uncontrollable hemoptysis by mediations and unfavorable therapeutic efficacy of palliative therapy. Thoracoscopy-assisted surgical removal of the left upper lung lobe under general anesthesia was then performed, with favorable therapeutic efficacy. The case history indicated that early diagnosis should be made with timely surgical operation for patients with pulmonary aspergilloma to improve the patients' quality of life.

12.3.5 Comments

This is a case of bronchiectasis complicated by aspergillus infection, and the patient was successfully treated. Based on the case analysis, the thinking ability for the diagnosis and treatment of chronic lung disease should be improved. In this case, the patient had characteristic chest radiological changes, such as air crescent sign. The diagnosis was finally defined by pathology, and the clinical typing was pulmonary aspergilloma.

The cases of pulmonary aspergilloma account for about 10–15% of the cases with chronic cavitary lung disease. The basic diseases that induce formation of lung cavity are commonly cavitary pulmonary tuberculosis and bronchiectasis in China. In this case, the patient had a history of bronchiectasis. Such structural lung disease is the basis of pulmonary aspergilloma.

Hemoptysis is one of the common clinical symptoms whose causes include pulmonary tuberculosis, bronchiectasis, and lung carcinoma. Hemoptysis is also a common symptom of pulmonary aspergilloma, which tends to be neglected. In this case, the patient had a history of recurrent hemoptysis of sputum with blood streak for more than 20 years. Only symptomatic support for hemostasis but no radiologic examination delayed the diagnosis and detection of pulmonary aspergillus infection.

In this case, the lesion was located in the left upper lung lobe, which is also common location of pulmonary tuberculosis. Therefore, the diagnosis of pulmonary tuberculosis more than 20 years ago was correct. Pathology demonstrated no tubercles and caseous necrosis, indicating cured tuberculosis. Bronchiectasis secondary to tuberculosis further induces aspergillus infection.

According to the latest clinical guideline, the patients at low risks of surgery can be permanently cured by surgery. In addition, hemoptysis and local cavity enlargement can be avoided. In such a way, the survival rate can be improved. In this case, the patient was a middle-aged man, with no obvious breathlessness and no basic disease. The diagnosis was singular aspergilloma. All of the facts indicated low risks of surgery. And surgery, instead of bronchial artery embolization, should be the treatment of first choice.

12.4 Case 4: Cough, Expectoration and Hemoptysis for 1 Year

Yulin He, Wanling Qi, Xiaofen Li, Dong-Na Su, Chen Qiu, and Mengjie Li

12.4.1 Presenting Symptom

Cough, expectoration, and hemoptysis for 1 year.

12.4.2 Brief Case History

A 69-year-old man was admitted to our hospital on January 9, 2015, due to presenting complaints of cough, expectoration, and hemoptysis for 1 year. One year ago, the patient began to experience paroxysmal cough, expectoration of whitish sputum, and recurrent hemoptysis of small quantity with blood streak. He received anti-infection therapy in a local hospital (specifically unknown), but the therapeutic efficacy was unfavorable. Then he presented in our hospital. During the illness course, he experienced no fever, chest pain, night sweat, chest distress, and breathlessness. His spiritual state and appetite were quite good. The bowel movements were normal. There was no weight loss.

12.4.2.1 Past Medical History

He reported no special medical history.

12.4.2.2 Physical Examination

By physical examination, his body temperature was 36.4 °C, pulse rate 84/min, respiration rate 18/min, and blood pressure 128/72 mmHg. He was typically developed, with moderate nourishment. The patient was well conscious. The oral mucosa showed no cheese-like white spots. The pharynx was not congested, and the bilateral tonsils were not enlarged. The thorax was bilaterally symmetric with no deformity. By auscultation, the respiration sounds of both lungs were clear, with no dry and/or moist rales. The precordial area showed no protrusion, and the vocal fremitus was unpalpable. The heart was not enlarged, with a heartbeat rate of 84/min, rhythmic. The heart sounds were normal, and the valvular areas showed no pathological murmur by auscultation.

The abdomen was soft, with no tenderness and rebound pain. The liver and spleen were subcostally unpalpable. The liver and kidney areas were not sensitive to percussion. The shifting dullness was negative. The bowel sounds were 5/min. The joints of four limbs were not deformed, with no redness and swelling. There was no clubbing finger. The nervous system showed no abnormalities.

12.4.2.3 Auxiliary Investigation

Routine blood test and blood biochemistry showed WBC4.38 × 109/L, RBC3.57 × 1012/L, HB112g/L, PLT190 × 109/L, and ESR24mm/h. The liver function test showed ALT13U/L and AST20U/L. The kidney function test showed Cr63.5 μmol/L (the normal range 43–115 μmmol/L). And the procalcitonin (PCT) was 0.66 ng/ml.

12.4.2.4 Initial Diagnosis

The initial diagnosis was hemoptysis possibly due to pulmonary tuberculosis or bronchiectasis.

12.4.3 Diagnosis and Treatment

After admission, tests and investigations were performed for diagnosis. On January 10, 2015, the sputum specimen showed acid fast staining negative. To further define the cause of hemoptysis, chest CT scan was performed on January 10, 2015. It demonstrated a cystoids translucent opacity at the apical segment of the right upper lung lobe, with a spherical parasitism inside in size of about 2.7 cm × 2.5 cm. Linear translucent air opacity was around the spherical parasitism. By enhanced scanning, the spherical parasitism in the cyst showed no enhancement, with necrotic change of low intensity. The adjacent lung field was shown with ill-defined ground-glass opacity. The diagnosis was suspected to be cystoid bronchiectasis of the apical segment of the right upper lung lobe complicated by aspergilloma and alveolar blood at the apical segment of the right upper lung lobe (Fig. 12.12).

After completing the relevant examinations, the right upper lobectomy was performed after multidisciplinary consultation considered that it had surgical indications. Surgical removal of the right upper lung lobe was performed then. By intraoperative exploration, the right thoracic adhesion was observed in a small quantity, and the lesion was located at the apical segment in a size of about 3.5 cm × 2.5 cm. The lesion was tenacious and was wedge removed, which was sent intraoperatively for freezing. During the operation, gel-like substance was observed in the cyst. Under thoracoscope, the bronchi were dilated to be cystoid, with large quantities aspergillus hyphae and spores inside. Some bronchi showed no epithelium but large quantities of granulation tissue, neutrophile granulocytes, lymphocytes, and plasmocytes (Fig. 12.13). Surgical removal of the right upper lung lobe was performed based on a diagnosis of benign lesion. The pathological diagnosis was cystoid bronchiectasis at the apex of the right lung complicated by aspergilloma and inflammation of the right upper lung.

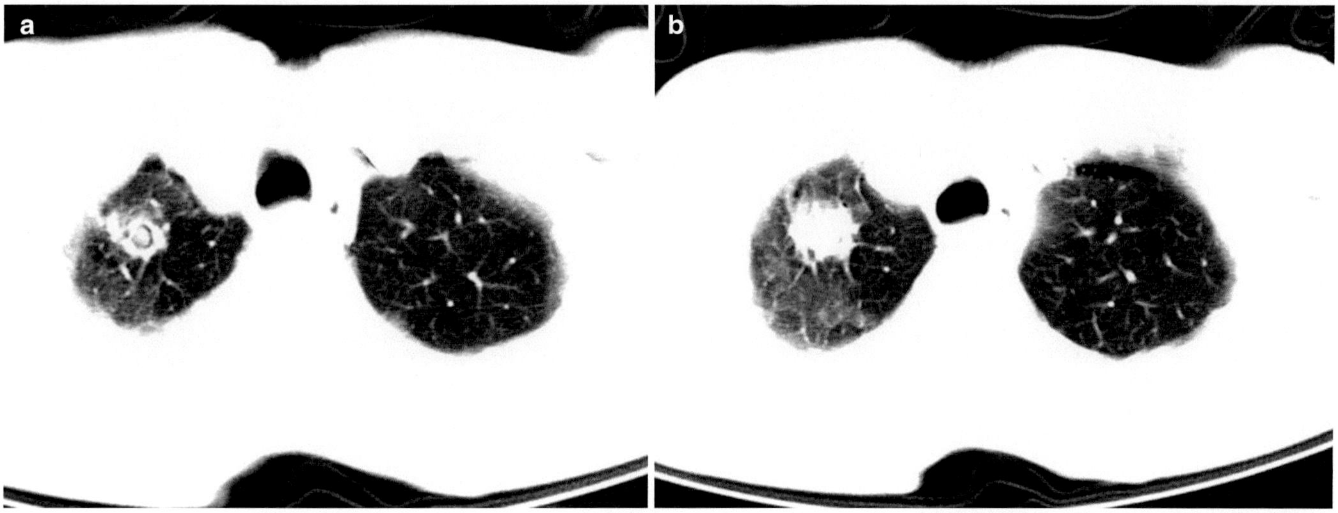

Fig. 12.12 (**a–h**) Chest CT scan. (**a**, **b**) The lung window at the thoracoclavicular joint level demonstrates cavity opacity with a spherical content inside at the apical segment of the right upper lung lobe. On the margin of the spherical content, there is a linear translucent air opacity. The adjacent lung field is demonstrated with ground-glass opacity. (**c**, **d**) The mediastinum window by plain scan of the thoracoclavicular joint level demonstrates anopacity with slightly lower soft tissue intensity at the apical segment of the right upper lung lobe and a surrounding linear translucent air opacity. (**e–h**) The mediastinum window of the arterial and venous phases by enhanced scanning at the thoracoclavicular joint level demonstrates no enhancement of the spherical content in the cavity at the apical segment of the right upper lung lobe

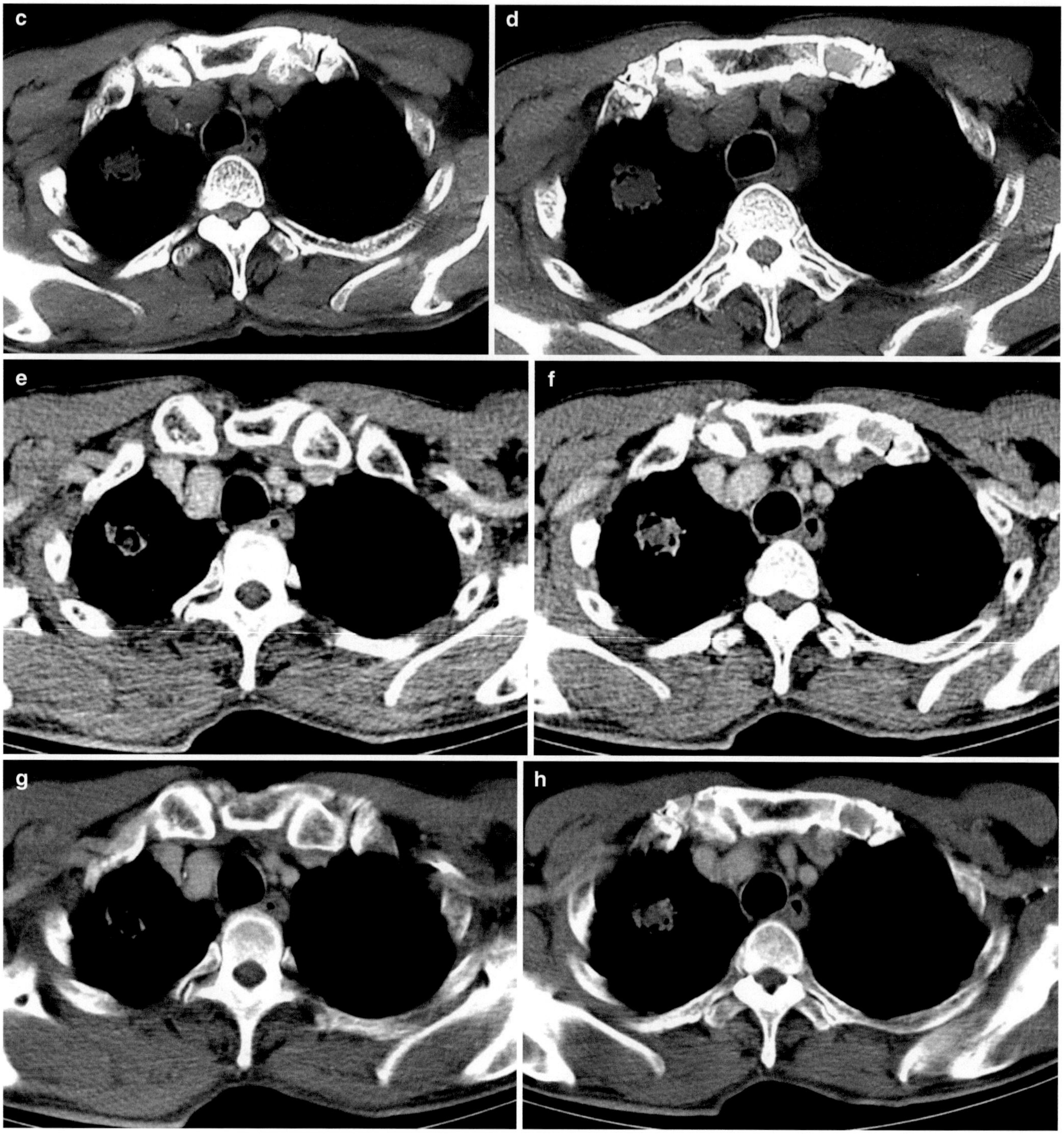

Fig. 12.12 (continued)

The final diagnosis was cystoid bronchiectasis at the apex of the right lung complicated by simplex aspergilloma and inflammation of the right upper lung.

After discharge, the condition of the patient was stable. He showed no recurrence of hemoptysis during follow-ups.

12.4.4 Discussion

Pulmonary aspergilloma is a special type of pulmonary aspergillosis, which commonly occurs based on primary lung disease. Cavitary pulmonary tuberculosis and bronchiectasis are the most common basic diseases based on which

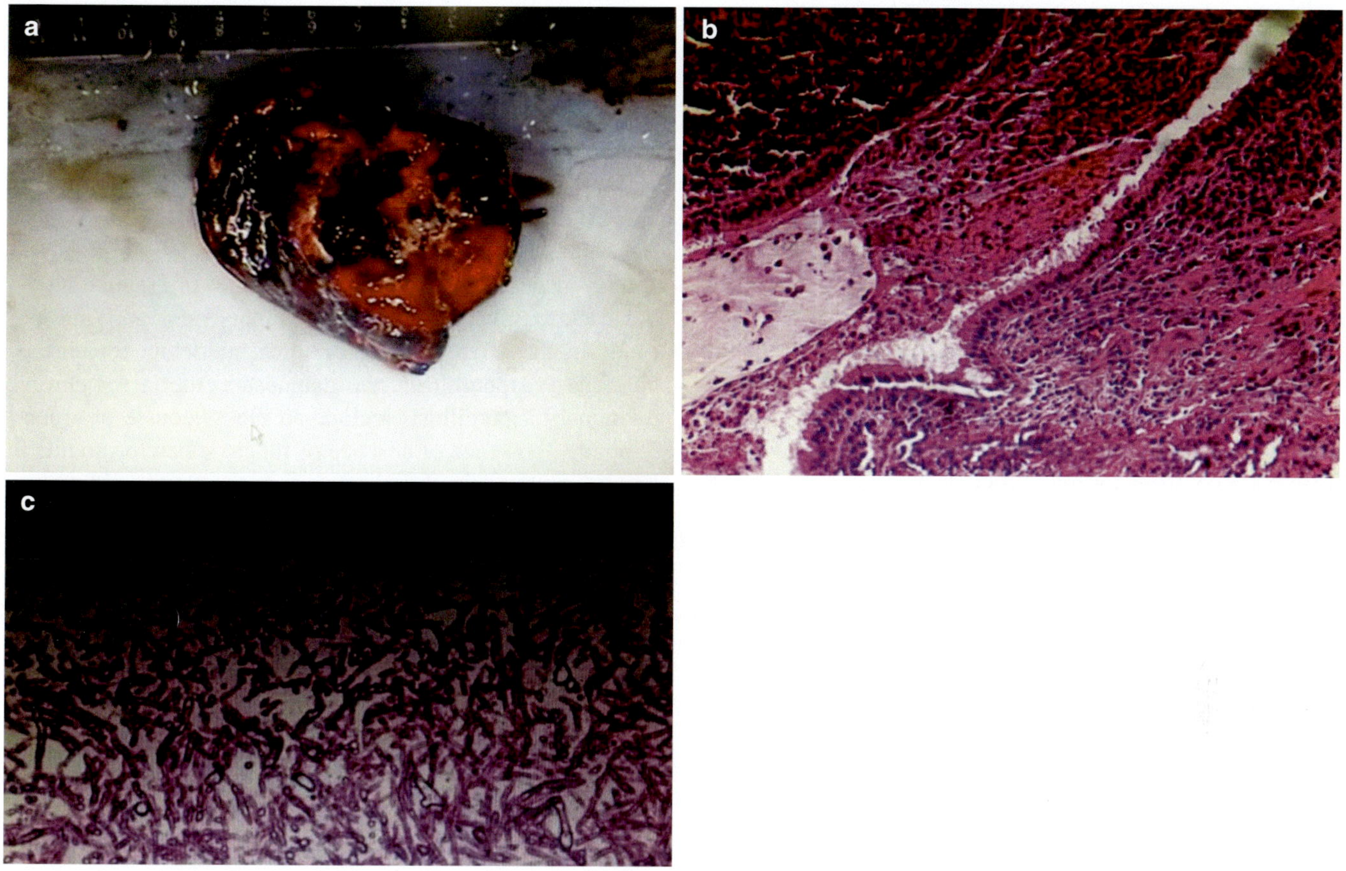

Fig. 12.13 (**a**–**c**) Pathology of the lung tissue. (**a**) The gross specimen for pathology. (**b**) By H&E staining, the bronchi are dilated to be cystoid, with large quantities of aspergillus hyphae and spores inside. (**c**) By H&E staining, some bronchi are demonstrated with no epithelium but large quantities of granulation tissue, neutrophile granulocytes, lymphocytes, and plasmocytes

aspergilloma occurs [15]. Most patients with aspergilloma showed no obvious systemic symptoms, and hemoptysis is the most common clinical symptom. The blood that is coughed up comes mostly from rupture and bleeding of the bronchial artery, which is commonly self-limited and intermittent. In addition to primary disease, the cause of hemoptysis is possibly also related to friction of movable aspergilloma with vascular vessels at the cavity wall or histolysis induced by aspergillus produced endotoxin and protease [16].

Chest CT scan has great diagnostic value for pulmonary aspergilloma. According to reports by Zeng et al. [17], the signs of aspergilloma by chest CT scan include air crescent sign, air ring sign, air-in-sphere sign, and rolling-ball sign. Due to noninvasiveness of aspergilloma to the cavity wall, its volume is commonly smaller than the cavity. Due to gravity, aspergilloma is commonly located at the bottom of the cavity, with formation of crescent-shaped air containing space between the sphere and the superior wall of the cavity, namely, the air crescent sign. If the sphere is completely separated from the cavity wall, the sphere is surrounded by a ring-shaped space, namely, the air ring sign. The sphere is movable in a certain degree that location change of the sphere can be observed along with change of body posture. By scanning after body posture changes, the sphere can be observed to be located at the near-ground position, which is known as the rolling-ball sign. The air-in-sphere sign is possibly caused by loose mixture of aspergillus hyphae with fiber, mucus, cell debris, and protein during the early and middle stage of hyphae development. Some residue air remains in the mixture, which is radiologically demonstrated as sponge-like or honeycomb-like air opacity of aspergilloma nodule. Aspergilloma is mainly composed of aspergillus hyphae, fibrin, cell debris, and mucus, which is commonly spherical or spongy in size of about 3.0–4.0 cm. Due to no blood supply to aspergilloma, enhanced scanning demonstrates no enhancement [18]. In this case, aspergilloma parasitized in the cystoid bronchiectasis, which almost fully filled in the cyst, with typical radiological demonstrations. Although CT scan has high diagnostic value for pulmonary aspergilloma, the rate of missed diagnosis is high. Due to common noncommunication of aspergilloma with bronchi, the sputum detection shows a low positive rate. Due to existence of aspergillus in upper respiratory tract of healthy human, findings of aspergillus in sputum cannot define the diagnosis. The findings of aspergillus hyphae by pathology can define the diagnosis. In this case, the diagnosis was defined based on postoperative pathology.

Radiologically, aspergilloma should be differentiated from peripheral lung carcinoma. Peripheral lung carcinoma is commonly demonstrated as lobulated parenchymal singular nodule in lung, with fine short spikes, pleural indentation sign, and vacuole. By enhanced scanning, moderate enhancement can be demonstrated. However, in the cases of pulmonary aspergilloma, radiology demonstrates spherical substance in cyst or cavity, which shows no enhancement by enhanced scanning. In addition, aspergilloma should also be differentiated from cystoid bronchiectasis complicated by bacterial infection. The clinical symptoms of cystoid bronchiectasis include fever and expectoration of purulent and foul-smelling sputum. By CT scanning, the bronchial wall is obviously thickened, with emergence of broadly large gas liquid level in the cyst. In the cases with multiple lesions, typical honeycomb-like changes can be demonstrated. Aspergilloma should be also differentiated from pulmonary sclerotic angioma. If a middle-aged woman shows singular nodule or mass with intact and well-defined margin as well as air crescent sign, which can be enhanced by enhanced scanning, pulmonary sclerotic angioma should be considered.

Because medications can hardly penetrate into the lung cavity to eliminate aspergillus and great toxicity of antifungal medications, systemic antifungal therapy shows unfavorable therapeutic efficacy for pulmonary aspergilloma [19]. For patients with major hemoptysis, emergency bronchial artery embolization can be performed to save life. Currently, surgical operation is still the main treatment for pulmonary aspergillosis [20]. Surgical removal of confined lesion is the main way for the treatment of pulmonary aspergilloma. Surgical removal of lung lobe and wedge or partial removal of the lesion are the main surgical procedures. In the cases with thoracic wall involved, surgical removal of the thoracic wall should be performed. Application of thoracoscopy or thoracoscopy-assisted noninvasive surgery shows advantages of small incision, rapid recovery from surgery, and less bleeding due to easy intraoperative hemostasis [21]. For patients with many concurrent diseases or pulmonary dysfunctions, surgery is contraindicated. For such patients, percutaneous injection of antifungal medication into cavity can be attempted, but the success rate is low. In this case, the patient received surgical removal of the right upper lung lobe and wedge removal of the lesion. After the operation, a closed thoracic drainage tube was placed at the seventh intercostal auxiliary midline to prevent the occurrence of postoperative complications. During follow-ups, no symptoms relapsed, which confirmed that the treatment was successful.

12.4.5 Comments

In this case, the patient was an elderly man, with a chronic illness course of up to 1 year. His respiratory symptoms were typical, including cough, expectoration, and hemoptysis of sputum with blood streak. Pathology demonstrated dilated bronchi into cyst, with large quantities of aspergillus hyphae and spores inside. And the epithelium of some bronchi was absent. Instead, there were large quantities of granulation tissue, neutrophile granulocytes, lymphocytes, and plasmocytes. In the 2015 European clinical guideline for chronic pulmonary aspergillosis, the diagnostic criteria for chronic pulmonary aspergillosis include an illness course of at least 3 months, presence or absence of fungal sphere or nodule in one or more cavity by chest radiology, direct evidence of aspergillus infection by microscopy, culture for biopsy or immune response of aspergillus strain, and exclusion of other conditions. Currently, chronic pulmonary aspergillosis can be classified into aspergillus nodule, singular aspergilloma, chronic cavitary pulmonary aspergillosis, and chronic fibrotic pulmonary aspergillosis. In this case, the illness course exceeded 3 months, and there was formation of granuloma in the lesion, which indicated chronic aspergillosis. Aspergillus infection was confined within dilated bronchi. By radiology, there was necrotic translucent area in the spherical nodule, which was clinically typed as singular aspergilloma.

In the latest 2016 clinical guideline for aspergillosis issued by IDSA, asymptomatic patients with singular aspergilloma and no progression of cavity in the past 6–24 months need only clinical observation. But for symptomatic patients, especially with serious hemoptysis, surgical removal of the lesion should be performed if with no contraindications to surgery. Perioperative or postoperative antifungal medication is not routinely required. But for patients with moderate risk of intraoperative rupture of aspergilloma, voriconazole or echinocandin is recommended to prevent aspergillar empyema. In this case, the patient experienced obvious symptoms. Surgical removal of the lesion should be the therapy of first choice. Antifungal medication should be administered when the nodule was not completely removed.

12.5 Case 5: Recurrent Hemoptysis for More Than 2 Years and Onset Again for 3 Months

Di Wu, Hongtao Jin, Fuqiang Zhu, Shi-Ping Wu, Minjie Yang, and Chang'e Jin

12.5.1 Presenting Symptom

Recurrent hemoptysis for more than 2 years and onset again for 3 months.

12.5.2 Brief Case History

A 57-year-old woman was admitted to our hospital on May 24, 2013, due to complaints of recurrent hemoptysis for more than 2 years and onset again for 3 months. More than 2 years ago, the patient began to experience recurrent hemoptysis once each day to several times each week. The blood volume was also variant, ranging from blood streak to tens milliliters. She experienced no symptoms of fever, chest pain, breathlessness, night sweat, and emaciation. One year ago, she was diagnosed with bronchiectasis in a local hospital. Medications were administered (specifically unknown), and her condition was slightly improved. So she paid less attention to it. Three months before her admission this time, she presented recurrent hemoptysis of fresh red blood or with dark red blood clot. The blood that she coughed up was in a small quantity, with intermittent yellowish sputum. And she experienced no symptoms of fever and breathlessness. The traditional Chinese medicine was administered with unfavorable therapeutic efficacy. In recent days, hemoptysis was more frequent, and the blood volume increased. For further diagnosis and treatment, she was admitted to our hospital. Since the onset of the symptoms, her spiritual state, appetite, and sleep were unfavorable. The urinations and bowel movements were normal. She experienced no obvious weight loss.

12.5.2.1 Past Medical History

In the year of 2007, she was diagnosed with nasopharyngeal tuberculosis and was cured after 2 years standard antituberculosis therapy. She reported histories of chronic nasosinusitis and chronic pharyngitis. And she denied histories of hypertension and diabetes. There were no histories of surgery, trauma, and blood transfusion. The history of vaccination was unknown.

12.5.2.2 Physical Examination

Physical examination showed a body temperature of 36.2 °C, respiration rate of 20/min, pulse rate 89/min, blood pressure 132/78 mmHg, and SPO_2 98%. She was well conscious. The skin mucosa showed no abnormality. The systemic superficial lymph nodes were not enlarged. The respirations were quite smooth. The respiration sounds of both lungs were coarse, with no obvious dry and/or moist rales. The heart rate was 89/min, rhythmic. The valvular areas showed no pathological murmur. The abdomen was soft, with no tenderness and rebound pain. The liver and spleen were not enlarged. And both lower limbs showed no edema.

12.5.2.3 Initial Diagnosis

The initial diagnosis was bronchiectasis complicated by hemoptysis.

12.5.3 Diagnosis and Treatment

After admission, therapies for infection and hemostasis were firstly administered. Laboratory tests showed indices of routine blood test within normal limits. Blood coagulation and ESR were within normal limits. The procalcitonin (PCT) and D-Dimer were within normal limits. The blood electrolytes, blood sugar, liver function, kidney function, and BUA were normal. The blood antibody against *Mycobacterium tuberculosis* was negative. The antibody against mycoplasma pneumonia IgM was negative. The sputum smear and culture for bacteria were negative. Nasopharynx and chest CT scan on May 25, 2013, demonstrated left deviation of the nasal septum, mucosal thickening of bilateral inferior concha, several nodular opacities, and a cavity near hilum of the left lower lung lobe (Fig. 12.14).

To further define the diagnosis, fibrobronchoscopy was performed on May 28, 2013, which demonstrated tracheal and bronchial inflammation. Bronchoscopic brushing for smear showed no acid fast bacilli. The culture of sputum harvested by fibrobronchoscopy showed negative. The clinical diagnosis was suspected to be secondary pulmonary tuberculosis or pulmonary aspergillosis. Due to undefined reason of hemoptysis, differentiation of pulmonary tuberculosis and pulmonary aspergilloma was clinically considered. The patient was transferred to the thoracic surgery department on May 31, 2013, for surgical operation. Since June 3, 2013, voriconazole was administered. Reexamination of chest CT scan on June 15, 2013, demonstrated several nodular opacities and cavity near the hilum of the left lower lung lobe, which were slightly smaller but similar small strip of calcification at the left lower lung lobe compared to previous chest CT scan (Fig. 12.15).

Based on the changes of chest CT scan before and after the treatment, the diagnosis was more likely to be pulmonary aspergillosis. On June 18, 2013, thoracoscopic removal of the dorsal segment of the left lower lung lobe and cautery of intercostal nerve block and pleural adhesion were performed under general anesthesia. Intraoperative exploration showed adhesion of the left lung with the thoracic wall, grayish lung surface at the dorsal segment of the left lower lung. Removal of the dorsal segment of the left lower lung was performed, and the specimen was sent for pathology and bacteriology.

Pathology of the dorsal segment of the left lower lung demonstrated grayish lung tissue in size of about 5.5 cm × 4 cm × 1.5 cm, with slight bronchiectasis and grayish red brittle shedding substances inside, no nodule or mass, and observable anastomosis nail. Under a microscope, there were ciliated columnar epithelium-coated bronchial mucosa, well-differentiated cells, and infiltrations of many lymphocytes, plasmocytes, and less polykaryocytes around the bronchi, with calcium deposition. The bronchial lumen was shown with fungal mass. The hyphae were in even thickness

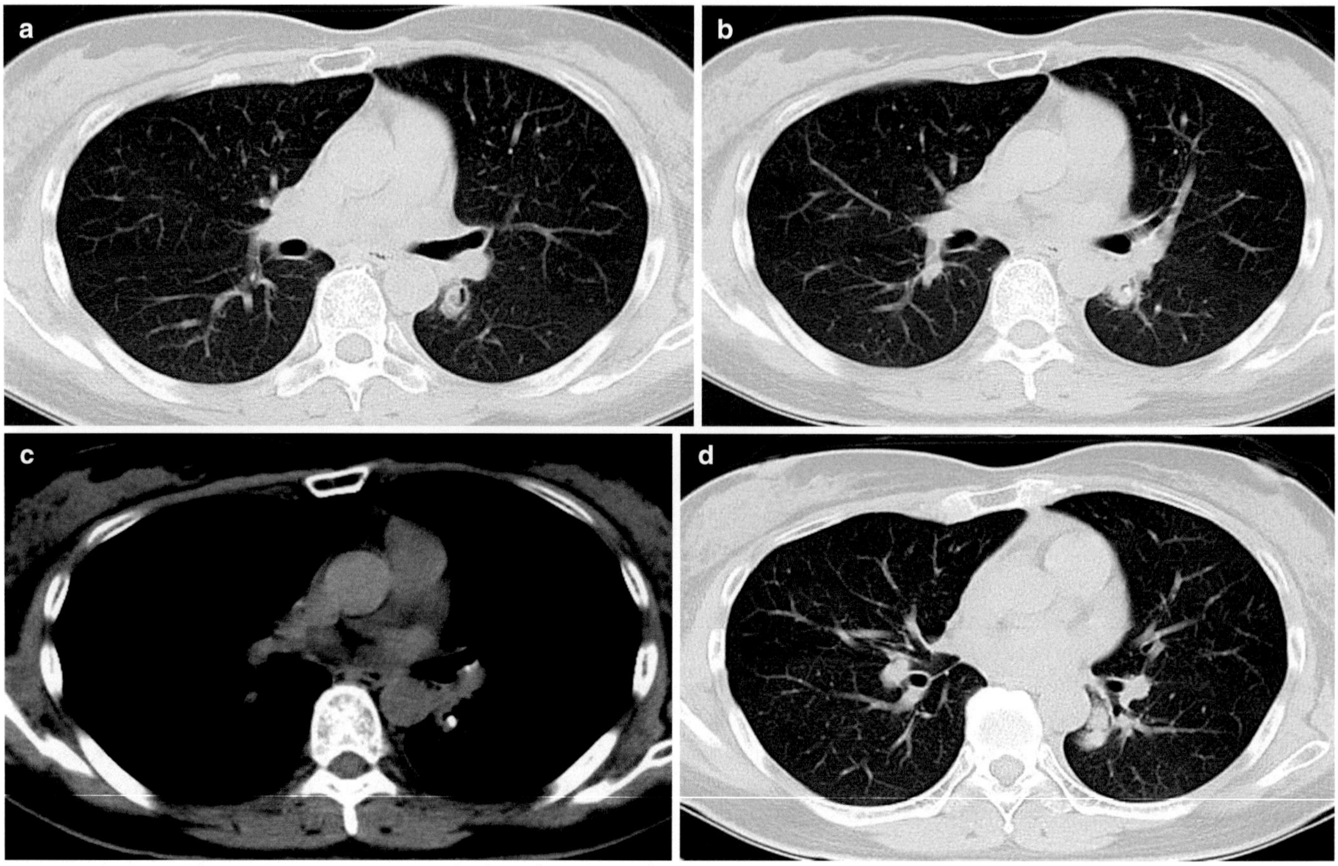

Fig. 12.14 (**a**–**d**) Chest CT scan. (**a**) The lung window demonstrates small cavity opacity near aorta at the dorsal segment of the left lower lung lobe, with small nodular opacity inside. (**b**) The nodule at the left lower lung lobe is shown to be anteromedially connected with the hilar vascular vessels. (**c**) The mediastinum window demonstrates calcification of cavity wall at the left lower lung lobe. (**d**) The posterolateral part of the nodule at the left lower lung lobe is irregular

and oriented arrangement, with branching in about 45° angle and many transverse septa. There were small round spores. By special stains, the PAS staining was positive and the methenamine silver staining positive. The pathological diagnosis was fungal disease of the lung, which was likely to be aspergillus infection (Fig. 12.16).

After the operation, oral intake of voriconazole was administered for fungal infection. And the patient was discharged on July 2, 2013.

The final diagnosis was chronic cavitary pulmonary aspergillosis.

After discharge, the condition of the patient was stable and showed no hemoptysis during follow-ups.

12.5.4 Discussion

Hemoptysis is a common acute and serious respiratory symptom. The diseases that cause hemoptysis include pulmonary tuberculosis, bronchiectasis, lung carcinoma, and lung infection [22]. In this case, the patient presented recurrent hemoptysis. She had a medical history of nasopharyngeal tuberculosis but was cured after 2 years of standard antituberculosis treatment. And her condition was diagnosed as bronchiectasis in a local hospital. The initial diagnosis was then made to be bronchiectasis complicated by hemoptysis. However, chest CT scan during her hospitalization demonstrated formation of cavity at the left lung with calcified cavity wall but no signs of bronchiectasis, which did not support the diagnosis of bronchiectasis complicated by hemoptysis. Cavity is a common radiological sign of pulmonary diseases, such as pulmonary tuberculosis, fungal infection, lung carcinoma, and other benign or malignant pulmonary diseases. Cavity is the most commonly induced by pulmonary tuberculosis. By epidemiological study, cavity is shown in about 40% patients with pulmonary tuberculosis among adults. In this case, the patient had a post medical history of nasopharyngeal tuberculosis and present conditions of hemoptysis, formation of cavity in the lung, and calcification of cavity wall. Based on these findings, secondary tuberculosis was suspected. Several research studies [23, 24] have demonstrated that secondary fungal infection may occur

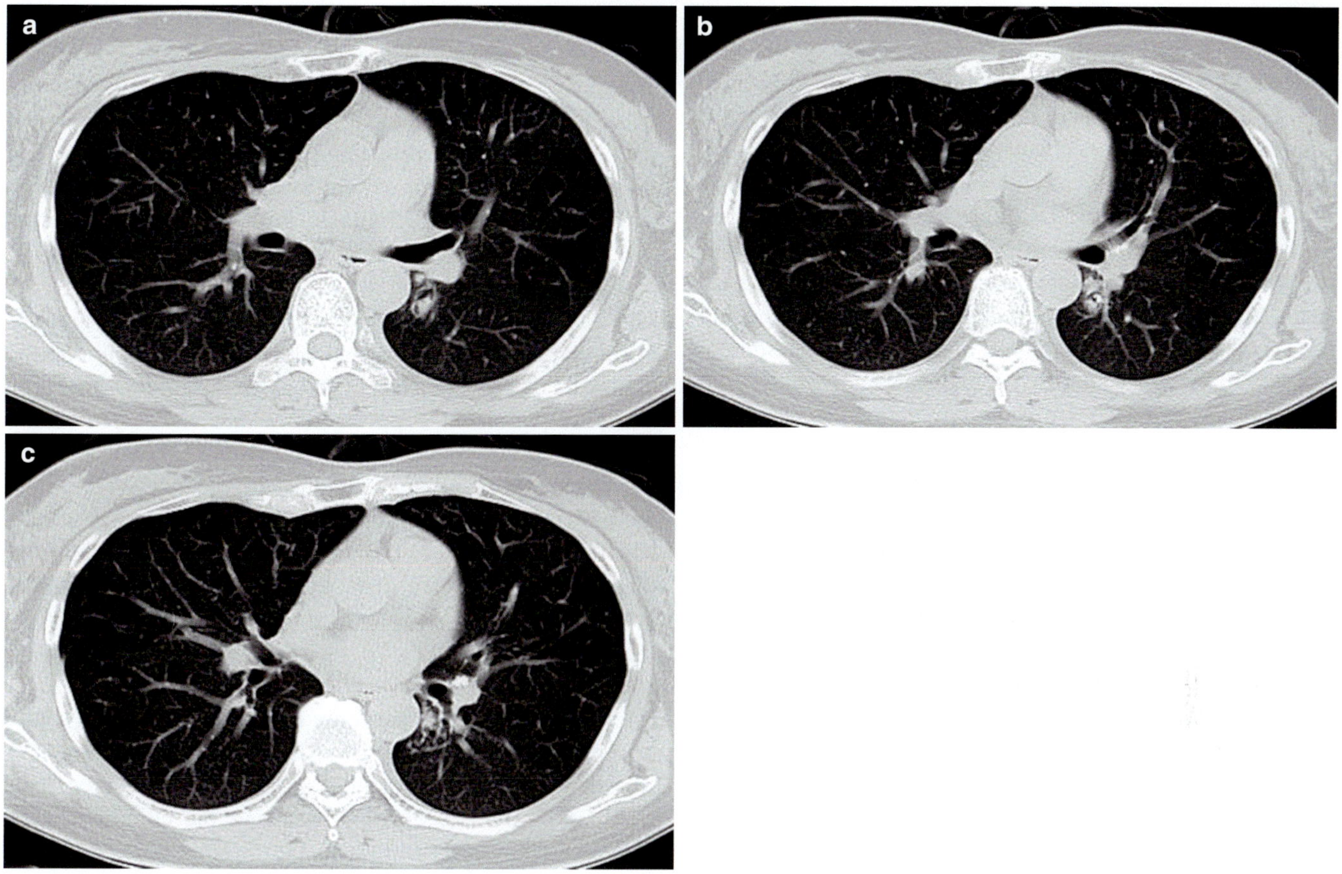

Fig. 12.15 (**a**–**c**) Chest CT scan. (**a**) Slight shrinkage of the cavity at the left lower lung lobe. (**b**) Better defined nodules at the left lower lung lobe. (**c**) Absorption of the surrounding lesions of the nodules at the left lower lung

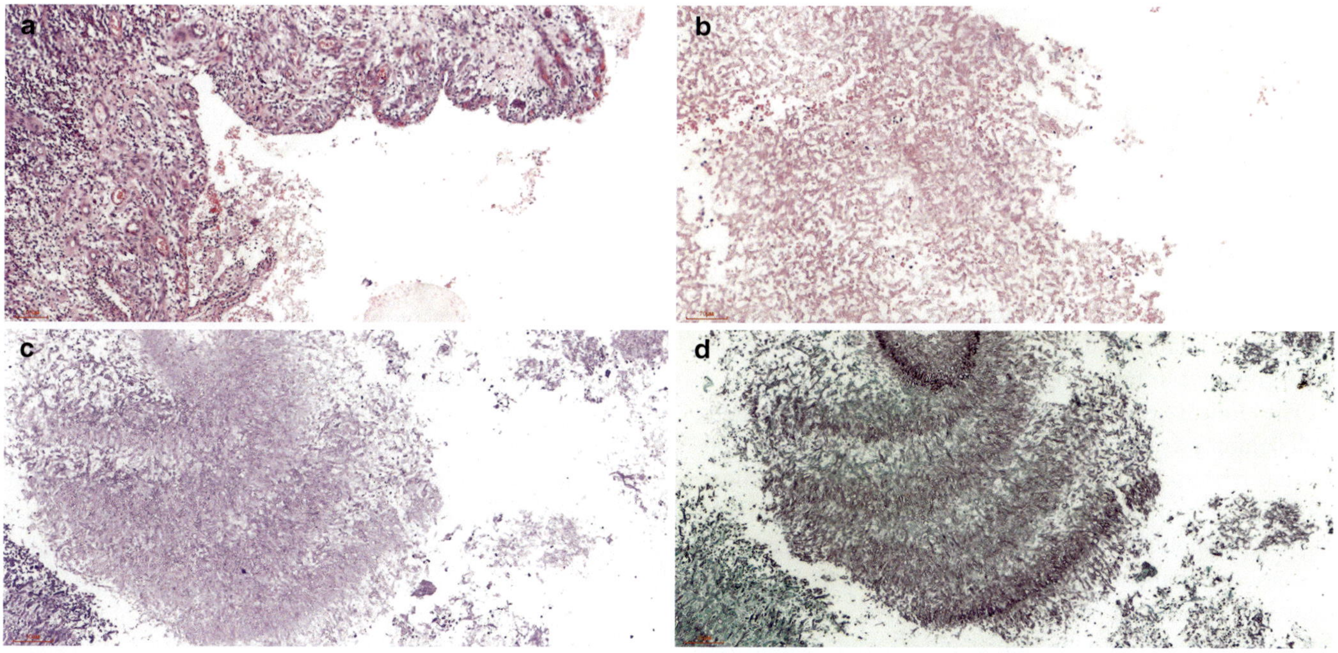

Fig. 12.16 (**a**–**d**) Pathology of the lung tissue. (**a**) H&E staining demonstrates infiltration of many inflammatory cells around the bronchi. (**b**) H&E staining demonstrates fungal hyphae in the cyst lumen. (**c**) PAS staining. (**d**) PASM staining

based on tuberculosis, especially aspergillus infection. Therefore, bronchoscopy was performed to demonstrate presence of active tuberculosis and to exclude fungal infection. In this case, radiology demonstrated nodule and cavity, with no typical polymorphous change of tuberculosis. In addition, repeated sputum smears and cultures showed no evidence of tuberculosis. Therefore, the diagnosis was more likely to be aspergillus infection. Voriconazole was then administered. Reexamination of chest CT after 12 days treatment showed absorption of the lesions and improved condition of the patient. The diagnosis of pulmonary aspergillosis was initially confirmed. The patient was then treated by surgery, and the postoperative pathology defined the diagnosis of aspergillus infection.

Pulmonary aspergillosis is a lung disease caused by aspergillus infection, which is commonly secondary to chronic bronchitis, bronchiectasis, pulmonary tuberculosis, pulmonary abscess, advanced lung carcinoma, and patients with immunosuppression. In recent years, the incidence of pulmonary aspergillosis has been increasing [25]. Aspergillus exists extensively in soils, foods, and indoor environment. The common pathogenic aspergillus that induces invasive pulmonary aspergillosis is *Aspergillus fumigatus*. The typical clinical manifestations of invasive pulmonary aspergillosis include fever, cough, dyspnea, chest distress, and hemoptysis [26]. The radiological demonstrations of pulmonary aspergillosis are diverse, including patchy opacity, nodular opacity, mass opacity, and cavity. And the typical radiological signs include halo sign and air crescent sign. However, halo sign is commonly demonstrated at days 5–7 after onset, and the crescent sign is commonly demonstrated at days 10–15 after onset. If the period of time is missed, the typical radiological signs can hardly be demonstrated. Therefore, their diagnostic value is limited. Clinically, the diagnosis of pulmonary aspergillosis is based on combination of the clinical manifestations, laboratory findings (including culture and serology), and radiology. But the diagnosis can only be defined based on histopathological evidence. In this case, pathology demonstrated hyphae with branching in 45° angle. In combination to the results of immunohistochemistry, the diagnosis of pulmonary aspergillosis can be defined.

The clinical experience of this case indicated that patients with hemoptysis and cavity but negative findings in repeated sputum smears for acid fast bacilli, especially the patients showing unfavorable therapeutic response to antituberculosis therapy, should be suspected with aspergillus infection. In this case, the patient experienced recurrent hemoptysis and showed formation of cavity in the lung. The condition may probably develop into life-threatening major hemoptysis. Therefore, active surgical operation should be performed along with medication.

12.5.5 Comments

The key point of this case is actually differential diagnosis of hemoptysis. Hemoptysis is a common acute and serious clinical symptom in departments of respiration, emergency, and tuberculosis. The common diseases that induce hemoptysis include pulmonary tuberculosis, bronchiectasis, lung infection, pulmonary abscess, and lung carcinoma.

For patients with hemoptysis, chest X-ray and chest CT scan should be performed. The chest X-ray demonstrations of round bronchus opacity and double track sign support the diagnosis of bronchiectasis. The chest X-ray demonstration of gas liquid level supports the diagnosis of pulmonary abscess. The demonstration of mass-like opacity supports the diagnosis of malignant neoplasm in the lung. In this case, the patient received no chest X-ray and CT scan in a local hospital 1 year before her admission to our hospital. The diagnosis of bronchiectasis and corresponding treatment actually delayed accurate diagnosis and appropriate treatment.

After admission to our hospital on May 25, 2013, chest CT scan demonstrated several nodular opacities and a cavity near hilum of the left lower lung lobe. Based on the chest CT scan demonstrations, the radiologist should suspect the diagnosis of pulmonary aspergillosis, and the communication between radiologists and physicians is important. However, chest X-ray demonstrations are non-specific, and the diagnosis should be based on its combination with case history, sign, and other investigations. The characteristic CT signs such as halo sign and air crescent sign can indicate the diagnosis of pulmonary aspergillosis. However, these characteristic CT signs can also be demonstrated in other pathogen infections, such as *Pseudomonas aeruginosa* infection and nocardia infection. Therefore, these signs demonstrated by CT scan are not evidence for definitive diagnosis of pulmonary aspergillosis.

In the clinical guideline issued by IDSA, aspergilloma is classified into singular aspergilloma and chronic cavitary pulmonary aspergillosis (CCPA). Singular aspergilloma is demonstrated with thin wall cavity rarely with surrounding lesions of lung parenchyma. CCPA is characterized by multiple thick wall cavities, with or with no aspergilloma inside and common surrounding lesions of lung parenchyma. In this case, the CT scan demonstrations should be categorized into CCPA.

In this case, voriconazole was administered for fungal infection before surgical operation. Reexamination of chest CT scan demonstrated slight shrinkage of several nodules and cavity near hilum of the left lower lung lobe, indicating favorable therapeutic response. In consideration of recurrent hemoptysis and formation of cavity that probably develop into life-threatening major hemoptysis, surgery was indicated. Hemoptysis is a serious complication of pulmonary aspergillosis. In the clinical guideline for diagnosis and treatment of aspergillosis issued by IDSA, surgical removal of lesions of aspergillosis facilitates to define the diagnosis, and radical elimination of local infection is possible.

In this case, the patient received voriconazole before surgery. Medication during perioperative period has not reached agreement. There was research study experimenting cavernostomy and myoplasty to treat complex aspergilloma, with medication of itraconazole during 2 weeks before the operation and 3 months after the operation, which showed effectiveness. However, there was also research study indicating no improvement of the condition after postoperative medication. Further studies are needed to elucidate the effectiveness of medication before or after the surgery.

12.6 Case 6: Cough and Expectoration for More Than 1 Year and Hemoptysis for 8 Days

Di Wu, Zhengqiang He, Guoxin Huang, Shi-Ping Wu, Hongtao Chen, and Jingshan Gong

12.6.1 Presenting Symptom

Cough and expectoration for more than 1 year and hemoptysis for 8 days.

12.6.2 Brief Case History

A 39-year-old woman was admitted to our hospital on March 16, 2012, due to complaints of cough and expectoration for more than 1 year and hemoptysis for 8 days. During the past 1 year, the patient experienced recurrent cough and expectoration of white foamy sputum. But there were no fever, breathlessness, chest pain, hemoptysis, night sweat, and emaciation. She had received anti-infection therapy for several times in another hospital (specifically unknown), but the condition improved and aggravated. Eight days ago, the cough aggravated, and she coughed up sputum with blood streak. And she experienced no fever, breathlessness, chest pain, and night sweat. CT scan on March 10, 2012, in another hospital demonstrated type III pulmonary tuberculosis of both lungs with accompanying bronchiectasis. For further diagnosis and treatment, she was transferred to our hospital. Since the onset of symptoms, her spiritual state and appetite were average. The urinations and bowel movements were normal, and she experienced no weight loss.

12.6.2.1 Past Medical History

She reported a medical history of pulmonary tuberculosis 20 years ago and received standard antituberculosis therapy for 1 year.

12.6.2.2 Physical Examination

Physical examination showed a body temperature of 36 °C, pulse rate 108/min, respiration rate 20/min, and blood pressure 100/78 mmHg. She was typically developed with average nourishment. She was well conscious, with active position, and well cooperative with physical examination. The systemic superficial lymph nodes were unpalpable and not enlarged. The thorax was bilaterally symmetric. By percussion, both lungs showed clear sounds. And both lungs showed coarse respiration sounds, with no dry and/or moist rales and no pleural rubs. The heartbeat was 108/min, with rhythm. The valvular areas showed no pathological murmur. The abdomen was soft, with no tenderness. The liver and spleen were subcostally unpalpable.

12.6.2.3 Auxiliary Investigation

Chest CT scan in another hospital on March 19, 2012, demonstrated type III pulmonary tuberculosis of both lungs with accompanying bronchiectasis.

12.6.2.4 Initial Diagnosis

The initial diagnosis was left upper lung infection and hemoptysis and old pulmonary tuberculosis of the left upper lung.

12.6.3 Diagnosis and Treatment

After admission, the tests and investigations were performed. The routine blood test showed WBC 6.8 × 109/L and neutrophile granulocytes 61.8%. The ESR was 26 mm/h. The liver function test, the kidney function test, electrolytes, and blood coagulation were normal. The blood gas analysis showed pH 7.43, PCO_2 36.8 mmHg, and PO_2 82.4 mmHg. The sputum culture was negative. The sputum test for acid fast bacilli was negative. Chest CT scan on March 18, 2012, demonstrated multiple cords, strips, and flakes of soft tissue lesions at bilateral upper lungs and dorsal segment of the left lower lung, suspected formation of cavity at the left upper lung, and multiple calcifications of both lungs. The mediastinum was demonstrated with no enlarged lymph nodes. And there was no pleural effusion. The diagnosis was considered to be tuberculosis of bilateral upper lungs with suspected formation of cavity at the left lung and scattering multiple old lesions in the other parts of the lungs (Fig. 12.17).

After admission, in combination with case history, physical examination, and auxiliary investigation, pulmonary tuberculosis was suspected. Surgical removal of the left

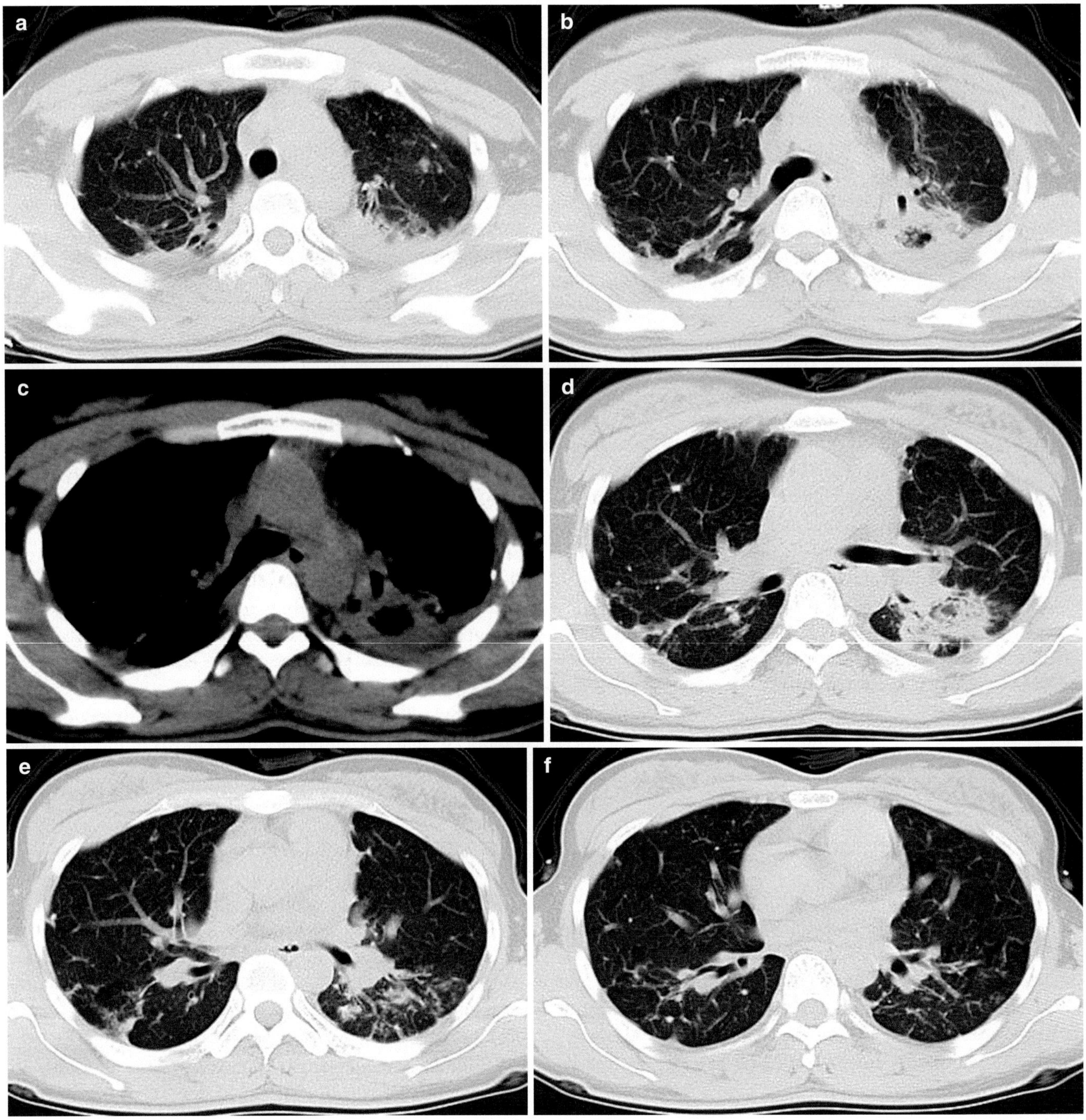

Fig. 12.17 (**a**–**f**) Chest CT scan. (**a**) The posteroapical segment of the bilateral upper lungs is demonstrated with less cords opacity, with bilateral pleural effusion in small quantities. (**b**) The right upper lung is demonstrated with cords opacity and flakes of opacity. The lung window at the carina level demonstrates large flake of consolidation opacity and flake of ground-glass opacity at the left upper lung. In the consolidation opacity, there is irregular cavity opacity. (**c**) The mediastinum window at the carina level demonstrates thick wall cavity at the left upper lung, with nodular opacity inside. There is left pleural effusion in a small quantity. (**d**) The left upper lung is demonstrated with mass-like soft tissue opacity with heterogeneous intensity, with honeycomb-like change. (**e**) The dorsal segment of bilateral lower lungs is demonstrated with cords and patchy opacity. (**f**) The bilateral lower lungs are demonstrated with spots and cords like opacity, which is adhered with local pleura

upper lung and dorsal segment of left lower lung lobe was performed on March 21, 2012, under general anesthesia. The postoperative pathology demonstrated grayish lung tissue in a size of about 13 cm × 6 cm × 4 cm. The bronchial mucosa was smooth, and a grayish white nodule was observed on the section, which was in a size of about 4 cm × 2 cm × 2 cm with formation of cavity inside. There were caseous necrotic substances in the cavity. Under a microscope, there were formation of local cyst in lung tissue and hyperplasia of fibrous tissue at the cystic wall with many accompanying necrosis. Around the necrosis, there was infiltration of many inflammatory cells and formation of granuloma. In the cyst, fungal hyphae were observed, with even thickness, branching in about 45° angle, and oriented arrangement. Small round spores were observed. By special staining, PAS staining showed positive and methenamine silver staining positive. The pathological diagnosis was mycosis at the left upper lung and the dorsal segment of the left lower lung, which was morphologically consistent to aspergillosis (Fig. 12.18).

The final diagnosis was chronic cavitary pulmonary aspergillosis at the left lung and old pulmonary tuberculosis at the right upper lung.

After discharge, the condition of the patient was stable. Repeated reexaminations of chest CT scan demonstrated only postoperative changes.

12.6.4 Discussion

Aspergillus widely distributes in soil, foods, and indoor environment. The common pathogenic aspergillus includes *Aspergillus fumigatus*, *Aspergillus flavus*, and *Aspergillus niger*. Bronchopulmonary aspergillosis is commonly caused by inhalation of aspergillus spores, which is the most commonly *Aspergillus fumigatus* [27]. Pulmonary aspergillosis is commonly secondary to chronic bronchitis, bronchiectasis, pulmonary tuberculosis, pulmonary abscess, advanced stage of serious lung disease, and patients with immunosuppression. In recent years, the incidence of pulmonary aspergillosis has been increasing [25]. An epidemiological survey conducted in China has demonstrated that the top four basic diseases that tend to be complicated by pulmonary mycosis include neoplasm (including solid tumor and malignant hematonosis), COPD, pulmonary tuberculosis, and diabetes [28, 29]. Research study has shown that 50% of aspergillus infection come from intensive care unit (ICU), and IPA accounts for 50%. The onset of IPA depends on the toxicity of aspergillus, quantity of inhaled aspergillus, immunity of the host, and presence of basic disease. Once onset, the condition progresses rapidly with high mortality rate [30].

In this case, the patient was a young woman, with chronic illness course. She had a past medical history of pulmonary

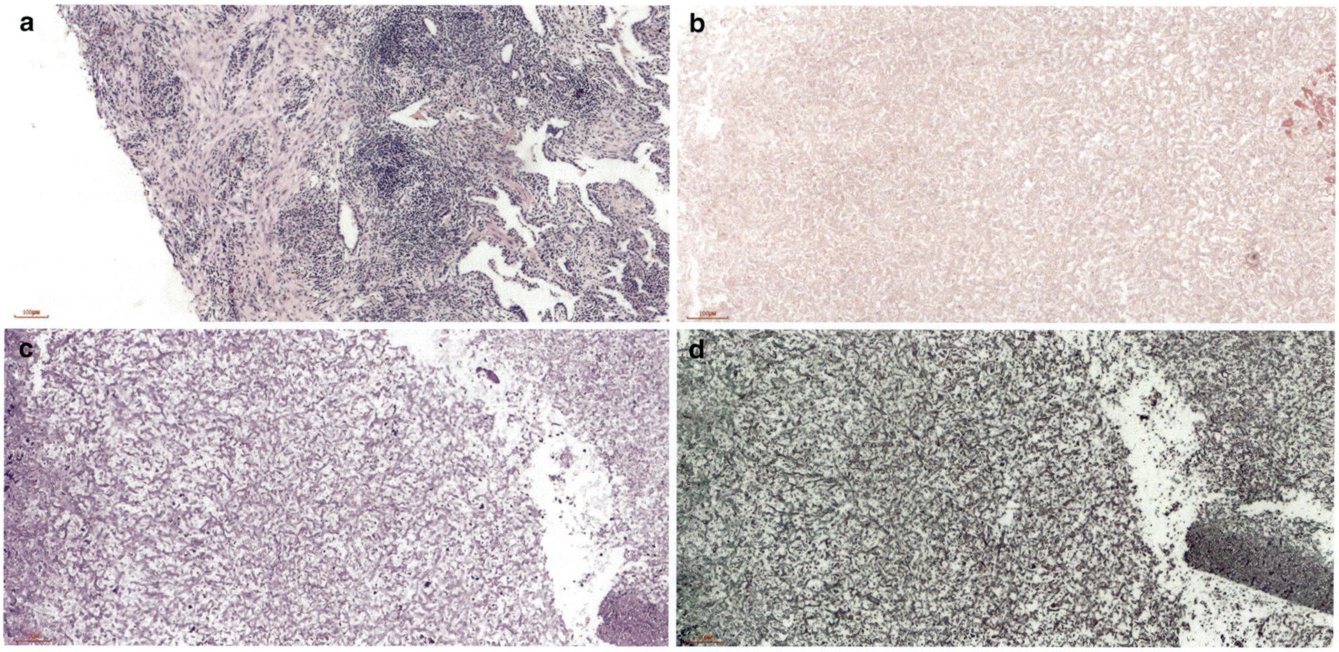

Fig. 12.18 (**a–d**) Pathology of lung tissue. (**a**) H&E staining demonstrates infiltration of many inflammatory cells around the cyst. (**b**) H&E staining demonstrates aspergillus hyphae in the cyst. (**c**) PAS staining. (**d**) PASM staining

tuberculosis. CT scan demonstrated lesion at the dorsal segment of the left lower lung lobe, which is a common location of tuberculosis. In addition, there were multiple cord opacity, flakes of exudation, multiple small calcifications at both lungs, and formation of cavity. Therefore, the diagnosis was suspected to be pulmonary tuberculosis based on finding by CT scan. However, the patient experienced no flush after noons, night sweat, fatigue, weight loss, and other symptoms of tuberculosis poisoning. ESR showed unobvious increase. CT scan demonstrated no obvious calcification of the cavity, no liquid level, lobulation, spikes, and other typical signs of tuberculosis. Further sputum smear and culture showed no *Mycobacterium tuberculosis*. To further define the diagnosis, fibrobronchoscopy was performed for biopsy of lung tissue. Due to the formation of cavity in the lung, percutaneous puncture was at a high risk. And the patient was young with favorable pulmonary functions. Due to her possible tolerance to surgical operation, surgical operation was performed to remove the lesions.

Lung CT scan or high-resolution CT scan is a convenient and rapid way for early diagnosis of IPA. The radiological demonstrations of pulmonary aspergillosis are diverse. The most common radiological demonstrations include ground-glass opacity, consolidation, and nodule. The typical demonstrations include early subpleural nodule or consolidation, surrounding halo sign in several days, liquefaction and necrosis of consolidation in 10–15 days, cavity or crescent sign, and enhancement of cavity wall by enhanced CT scan. However, the typical radiological demonstrations are not common. Especially in patients with nongranulocytic deficiency, the common radiology demonstrations include nodule, consolidation, and cavity. Pulmonary aspergillosis can hardly be differentiated from pulmonary tuberculosis during its early stage. The accurate differentiation in experienced radiologists is only 61–78% [31]. Therefore, if CT scan demonstrates singular or multiple nodules with formation of cavity, halo sign around nodule, and air crescent sign, IPA should be highly suspected. Timely pathogenic histopathological investigations should be performed. In this case, the patient showed formation of cavity with caseous necrotic substances inside. But under a microscope, fungal hyphae with branching of about 45° angle were observed. In addition to PAS staining positive and methenamine silver staining positive, the diagnosis can be defined as pulmonary aspergillosis.

Medications of voriconazole and other triazoles, amphotericin B, and echinomycin can be administered for pulmonary aspergillosis. For patients with surgical removal of lung lobe or whole lung, follow-ups of 3–6 months should be performed for inflammatory biomarkers, aspergillus antigen, and precipitin. Since then, regular follow-ups every 6 months should be performed in the following 3 years for early detection of recurrent lesion.

12.6.5 Comments

In this case, the patient showed clinical manifestations of cough, expectoration, and hemoptysis, which were non-specific. Chest CT scan on March 18, 2012, demonstrated multiple cords, strips, and flakes of soft tissue lesions at bilateral upper lungs and the dorsal segment of left lower lung, suspected formation of cavity at the left upper lung, and multiple calcifications of both lungs. Based on CT scan, a diagnosis of pulmonary tuberculosis was reasonable. However, postoperative pathology demonstrated formation of cyst in local lung tissue and hyperplasia of fibrous tissue in the cystic wall with many accompanying necrosis. Around the necrosis, there were infiltration of many inflammatory cells, formation of granuloma, and fungal hyphae in the cyst. The pathological diagnosis was pulmonary aspergillosis, and the diagnosis was then defined.

In this case, pulmonary aspergillosis possibly complicated the basic disease of pulmonary tuberculosis. Pulmonary tuberculosis complicated by pulmonary aspergillosis is not uncommon. Because pulmonary tuberculosis is a chronic consumptive disease, the patients are commonly poorly nourished, with compromised immunity. Due to tuberculosis, the lung tissue and bronchial tissue are subject to structural changes that the patients are vulnerable to fungal infection. In December 2011, a briefing issued by WHO indicated that lung cavity occurs in about one third of patients with pulmonary tuberculosis, which makes them vulnerable to aspergillus infection. In recent years, aspergillus, as a conditional pathogenic fungus, causes increasing incidence of aspergilloma in cavity induced by tuberculosis. About 25–30% patients with cavity induced by pulmonary tuberculosis show aspergilloma due to invasion of aspergillus. The cavity induced by pulmonary tuberculosis has a poor blood supply. In addition to bleeding of destructed lung tissue, the destructions facilitate growth and reproduction of aspergillus in the cavity. In this case, the patient had received multiple anti-infection therapies in another hospital due to long-term cough and expectoration, which may promote occurrence of fungal infection.

Concurrence of pulmonary tuberculosis and pulmonary aspergillosis showed atypical clinical manifestations, non-specific radiological demonstrations. Therefore, the clinical diagnosis is challenging. The onset of pulmonary aspergillus is insidious, with common symptoms of chronic cough, expectoration, and hemoptysis, which are similar to those of pulmonary tuberculosis. Due to the non-specific symptoms, the condition tends to be misdiagnosed as progression of pulmonary tuberculosis. In this case, the patient received chest CT scan on March 10, 2012, in another hospital, demonstrating type III pulmonary tuberculosis of bilateral upper lungs and accompanying bronchiectasis. Another chest CT scan on March 18 demonstrated pulmonary tuberculosis of bilateral upper lungs. Repeated chest CT scans demonstrated pulmonary tuberculosis, indicating the difficulty in differentiating the two diseases.

If chest CT scan demonstrates spherical lesion in cavity, a diagnosis of complicating pulmonary aspergillosis is not challenging. Changeable crescent-shaped translucent sign along with body postures is typical CT sign of aspergilloma. For patients with atypical signs by lung CT scan, the differential diagnosis of cavity induced by pulmonary tuberculosis from pulmonary aspergillosis is challenging. Repeated sputum investigations for aspergillus or fibrobronchoscopy facilitate the diagnosis. Postoperative pathology defines the diagnosis. In this case, the diagnosis was defined based on postoperative pathology.

Based on this case, we know that pulmonary tuberculosis complicated by aspergillus infection is not uncommon. For the patients with no improved condition by active anti-tuberculosis therapy or recurrent hemoptysis with no known reasons and radiological demonstration of formation of cavity, if aspergilloma cannot be excluded, pathogenic or pathological investigations should be ordered to define the diagnosis.

12.7 Case 7: Paroxysmal Cough and Hemoptysis for 3 Months

Fei Shi, Yuemei Lu, Zhiqiang Cheng, Shi-Ping Wu, Ruming Xie, and Xuemei Han

12.7.1 Presenting Symptom

Paroxysmal cough and hemoptysis for 3 months.

12.7.2 Brief Case History

A 27-year-old woman, a clerk, was admitted to our hospital on April 15, 2013, due to complaints of paroxysmal cough and hemoptysis for 3 months. Three months ago, the patient began to experience paroxysmal cough and expectoration of yellowish white mucous sputum with dark red blood streak with no known reasons. She experienced no chest pain, breathlessness, fever, night sweat, and emaciation. In another hospital, chest CT scan was performed, indicating mass at the left upper lung. For further diagnosis and treatment, she was admitted to the thoracic surgery department in our hospital. Since the onset of the symptoms, her spiritual state was quite good, but the appetite was slightly poor. During recent 3 months, she experienced no obvious weight loss.

12.7.2.1 Past Medical History

Two years ago, she was diagnosed with pulmonary tuberculosis at both lungs in another hospital and received antituberculosis therapy (specifically unknown). And she denied histories of hypertension and diabetes. She smoked for more than 3 years, 10 cigarettes per day.

12.7.2.2 Physical Examination

Physical examination showed body temperature of 36.3 °C, pulse rate of 78/min, respiration rate 20/min, and blood pressure 105/71 mmHg. The patient was typically developed and averagely nourished. She was well conscious, with average spiritual state and active position. She was well cooperated with the physical examination. The skin showed no yellowish stain. The systemic superficial lymph nodes were not enlarged. The sclera showed no yellowish stain. The oral lips showed no cyanosis. The neck was soft, with no distended jugular vein. By percussion, both lungs showed clear sounds. By auscultation, both lungs showed coarse respiration sounds, with less moist rales at the left upper lung and no dry rales. The precordial area showed no protuberance, and the heart was not enlarged, with rhythmic heartbeat of 78/min. The valvular areas showed no pathological murmur. The abdomen was soft, with no tenderness and rebound pain. The liver and spleen were subcostally unpalpable. The liver and kidney were not sensitive to percussion. And both lower limbs showed no edema.

12.7.2.3 Auxiliary Investigation

Laboratory blood test showed WBC 5.0 × 109/L, N% 33.7%, L% 53.8%, and HB 101 g/L. HSCRP was less than 5 mg/L. ESR was 43.00 mm/h, and 1,3-ß-D glucan was 234.0 pg/ml.

Microbiology of the sputum, including sputum culture for common bacteria, fungi, and *Mycobacterium tuberculosis*, showed negative.

12.7.2.4 Initial Diagnosis

The initial diagnosis was space-occupying lesion at the left upper lung, which was suspected to be aspergilloma or lung carcinoma and old pulmonary tuberculosis at both lungs.

12.7.3 Diagnosis and Treatment

After admission, the investigations were performed. The liver and kidney function tests showed negative. The blood coagulation was normal. Inhalation of oxygen, voriconazole, and levofloxacin were administered, and the symptoms of cough and hemoptysis were slightly improved. To define the reason of hemoptysis, enhanced chest CT scan was performed on April 17, 2013, which indicated space-occupying lesion at the apex of left lung, which was consistent to pulmonary

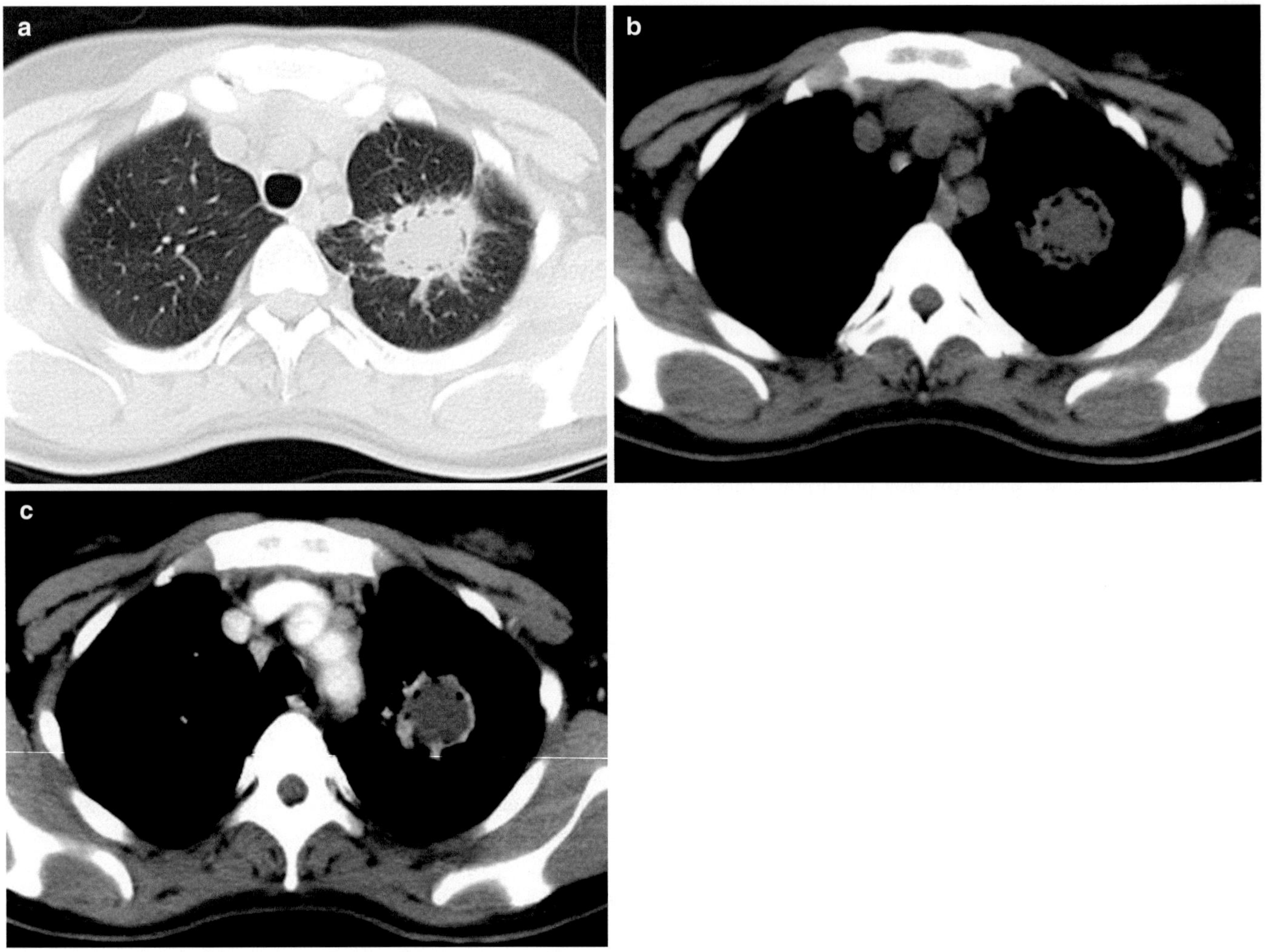

Fig. 12.19 (**a**–**c**) Chest CT scan. (**a**) The left upper lung is demonstrated with mass-like opacity with heterogeneous intensity and unsmooth margin. (**b**) The mediastinum window demonstrates cavity opacity at the left upper lung, which is similar to crescent sign, and central nodular opacity with homogeneous intensity. (**c**) Enhanced chest CT scan demonstrates ring-shaped enhancement of the mass opacity at the left upper lung

aspergilloma, old pulmonary tuberculosis at the apex of right lung, and scattering infection lesions at both lungs (Fig. 12.19).

Due to suspected diagnosis of pulmonary aspergilloma and the symptoms of recurrent cough and hemoptysis, surgical removal of the left upper lung, cautery of pleural adhesion, and intercostal nerve block were performed on April 21, 2013, under thoracoscope. The postoperative pathology demonstrated chronic inflammation of the mucosa of the dilated bronchi with accompanying epithelial hyperplasia, aspergillus hyphae in the lumen with even thickness, many branching in about 45° angle, septa, and oriented arrangement. There were also small round spores. By special staining, PAS staining showed positive and methenamine silver staining positive. The pathological diagnosis was aspergillosis at the left upper lung (Fig. 12.20).

After the operation, the patients showed favorable recovery, and she was discharged on April 27, 2013. The condition was stable after discharge, and no cough, expectoration, and hemoptysis relapsed during follow-ups.

The final diagnosis was pulmonary aspergilloma at the left upper lung and old pulmonary tuberculosis at both lungs.

12.7.4 Discussion

Due to compromised cellular immunity and long-term use of antituberculosis medication, patients with pulmonary tuberculosis are also susceptible population to complications of conditional fungal infection, especially aspergillus infection [32]. In recent years, more and more clinical evidence support occurrence of aspergillus infection secondary to old pulmonary

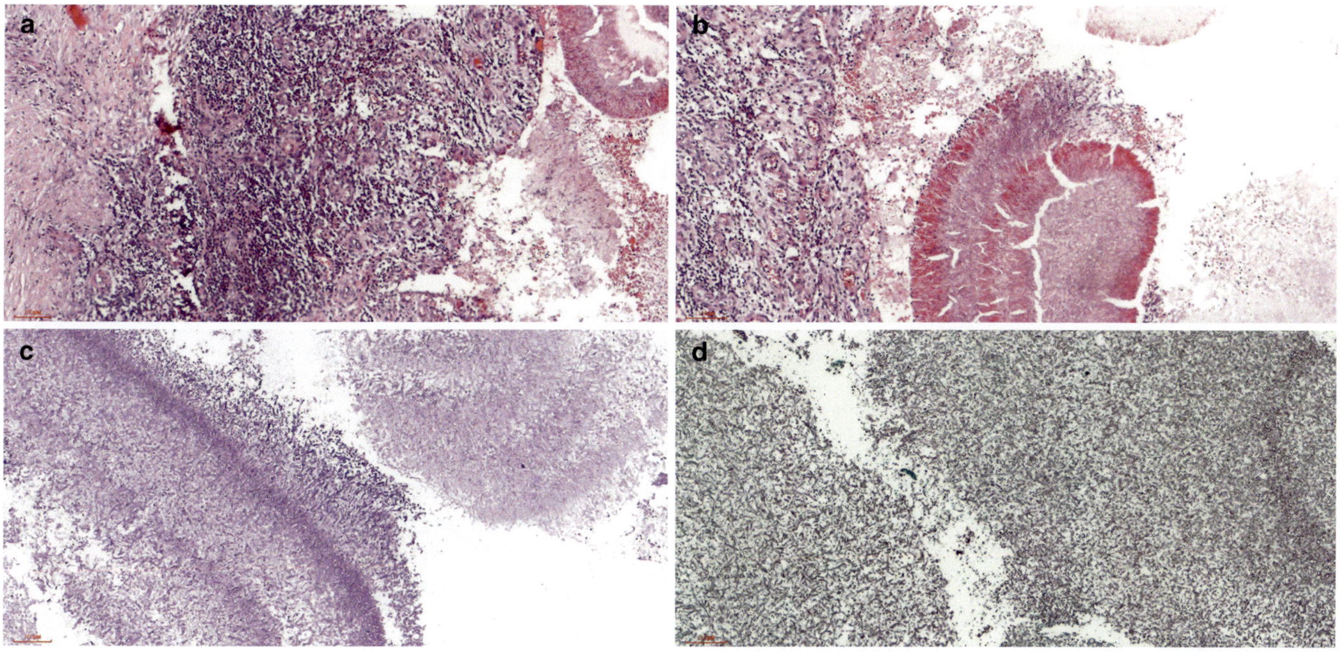

Fig. 12.20 (**a**–**d**) Pathology of lung tissue. (**a**) H&E staining demonstrates infiltration of inflammatory cells at the bronchial mucosa. (**b**) H&E staining demonstrates aspergillus hyphae in the tracheal lumen. (**c**) PAS staining. (**d**) PASM staining

tuberculosis. Old pulmonary tuberculosis complicated by aspergillus infection presents as some respiratory symptoms, which are non-specific. Therefore, its early diagnosis is challenging. And it tends to be misdiagnosed as relapse of pulmonary tuberculosis or neoplasm and thus appropriate treatment is delayed, with high mortality rate. A research study by Kim et al. [32] has demonstrated that CT scan demonstrations of pulmonary aspergillosis are almost identical to those of pulmonary tuberculosis and their differentiation can be hardly made. Therefore, to summarize the clinical features and key points of diagnosis and treatment of old pulmonary tuberculosis complicated by aspergillus infection facilitates improving its diagnosis and decreasing its mortality rate.

In this case, the initial symptoms were chronic cough and expectoration of bloody sputum. Chest CT scan in another hospital demonstrated mass at the left upper lung. In combination to her medical history of pulmonary tuberculosis, it tends to be misdiagnosed as relapse of pulmonary tuberculosis. However, the patient had normal body temperature, with no obvious flush after noons, night sweat, and other symptoms of tuberculosis poisoning. There was no typical lesion of pulmonary tuberculosis. All these findings did not support the diagnosis of pulmonary tuberculosis.

Because the antifungal medication can hardly permeate into the lesion of pulmonary aspergilloma and pulmonary aspergilloma can hardly discharged via obstructed or narrowed draining bronchus, simple administration of antifungal medication shows unfavorable therapeutic efficacy. Surgical removal has been the only way to radically treat pulmonary aspergilloma [33]. The surgical approaches include cavity closure, surgical removal of the lung lobe, and surgical removal of the whole lung. The choice of surgical approach depends on the condition of the patients. For patients with peripheral localized lesion of the lung, surgical removal of lung lobe or segment can be performed. For patients of elderly with cardiopulmonary dysfunction and lung cavity who are intolerant to surgical removal of lung lobe, simplex cavity closure can be performed. After the operation, antifungal medication of voriconazole should be administered based on the severity of infection. In addition, standard follow-ups for 6–24 months should be performed to observe possible relapse of the symptoms.

In this case, the key points are summarized as the following:

1. Patients with old pulmonary tuberculosis are immunocompetent. But local structural change of lung induced by tuberculosis may be the important reason of aspergillus infection.
2. For patients with old pulmonary tuberculosis and intrapulmonary nodular lesion but no symptoms of tuberculosis poisoning, complication of pulmonary aspergillus infection should be suspected. Bronchoscopy- or CT-guided lung puncture should be performed for biopsy to define the diagnosis.
3. CT scan is an important technique in the diagnosis of pulmonary aspergillus infection. But because nodular opacity

can also be demonstrated in patients with pulmonary tuberculosis, its diagnostic value is limited [33].

4. Surgical removal is the radical therapy for pulmonary aspergilloma. Therefore, for patients with pulmonary tuberculosis complicated by pulmonary aspergilloma, active surgical operation should be performed if indicated no matter the condition is slight or serious. After the operation, antifungal medication of voriconazole should be administered, and follow-ups should be reinforced to avoid its relapse.

12.7.5 Comments

In this case, the diagnosis and treatment are not complex. After admission, chest CT scan was performed, and the diagnosis was suspected to be pulmonary aspergilloma, indicating possible diagnosis of pulmonary aspergilloma by chest X-ray or chest CT scan. Lung X-ray or lung CT scan demonstrates pulmonary aspergilloma as round dense opacity in lung cavity, with translucent halo opacity at its margin. If the cavity is large, pedicle of the spherical lesion can be observed to be connected with cavity wall. Resembling to pendulum, the spherical opacity is movable along with change of body posture. If the cavity is small with spherical lesions that filled most of the cavity, the halo opacity is possibly small, demonstrated as a narrow and long crescent-shaped translucent area. Typical X-ray sign has high diagnostic value in the diagnosis of pulmonary aspergilloma. Experienced radiologists can suspect the diagnosis of pulmonary aspergilloma based only on X-ray demonstrations, and their suspect can remind the clinicians of further investigations to define the diagnosis.

In some cases, chest X-ray demonstrations are not typical, especially in the cases of pulmonary aspergilloma secondary to tuberculosis cavity. Its diagnosis may be challenging. The chest X-ray demonstrates pulmonary aspergilloma secondary to tuberculosis cavity as irregular cavity with unsmooth inner wall and nodular or spherical opacity in large flakes of lesion. Some scholars have reported that high-resolution CT is more favorable than conventional CT in demonstrating cavity wall of tuberculosis and aspergilloma in the cavity. Especially when aspergilloma is large and almost fully fill in the cavity, high-resolution CT scan facilitates detecting arch-shaped translucent space between aspergilloma and inner wall of cavity. And the arch-shaped translucent space plays a critical role in early diagnosis of pulmonary aspergilloma. Although pulmonary aspergilloma has characteristic radiological sign, clinically it should be differentiated from other mass-like lesions such as tuberculoma, hamartoma, lung carcinoma, and pulmonary abscess.

In this case, the disease was cured by surgical operation, which was undoubtedly successful. However, the best therapy for pulmonary aspergilloma has not reached consensus. Conventional prophylactic surgical operation remains controversial both domestically and internationally. Generally speaking, asymptomatic patients with aspergilloma need regular observation instead of special treatment. However, some scholars believe that all patients with pulmonary aspergilloma, if have no contraindications, should receive surgical operation due to the risk of hemoptysis. Some other scholars believe that surgery is indicated to patients with serious hemoptysis. In this case, the patient did experience symptom of hemoptysis, and the surgery is necessary.

12.8 Case 8: Recurrent Cough and Expectoration of Sputum with Blood Streak for More Than 1 Year

Wendi Huang, Wei-Dong Song, Hui Yin, Huaisheng Chen, Minjie Yang, and Xuemei Han

12.8.1 Presenting Symptom

Recurrent cough and expectoration of sputum with blood streak for more than 1 year.

12.8.2 Brief Case History

A 58-year-old woman was admitted to our hospital on January 20, 2015, due to complaints of recurrent cough and expectoration of sputum with blood streak for more than 1 year. One year ago, the patient began to experience cough and occasional expectoration of sputum with blood streak with no known reasons. She experienced no symptoms of fever, night sweat, chest distress, breathlessness, and chest pain. She had been treated in a local hospital (specifically unknown), and the symptoms were improved and aggravated. One week ago, she received chest CT scan in another hospital, demonstrating space-occupying lesion at the right upper lung. And she presented in our hospital for diagnosis and treatment. Since the onset of symptoms, her spiritual state, appetite, and sleep were generally good. The urinations and bowel movements were normal. And she experienced no obvious weight loss.

12.8.2.1 Past Medical History

She reported a medical history of diabetes for more than 4 years and was receiving insulin therapy. And the subjective blood sugar control was quite good.

12.8.2.2 Physical Examination

Physical examination showed a body temperature of 36.4 °C, pulse rate 78/min, respiration rate 18/min, and blood pressure 134/82 mmHg. She was typically developed, well-nourished, and conscious. The systemic superficial lymph nodes were unpalpable and were not enlarged. The thorax was not deformed. The respiration sounds of both lungs were clear, with no dry and/or moist rales. The heart and abdomen showed no abnormality. Both lower limbs showed no edema. There was no clubbing finger. The nervous system showed no abnormality.

12.8.2.3 Auxiliary Investigation

Chest CT scan on January 13, 2015, demonstrated space-occupying lesion at the right upper lung.

12.8.2.4 Initial Diagnosis

A space-occupying lesion at the right upper lung whose reason was to be detected and type II diabetes.

12.8.3 Diagnosis and Treatment

After admission, the blood test, urine test, and feces test showed no abnormality. The ALT was 50 U/L and albumin 33.4 g/L. The urea nitrogen was 8.49 mmol/L and creatinine 78 μmol/L (normal range: 45–84 μmol/L). The fasting blood glucose was 5.41 mmol/L. The sputum culture and sputum smear for fungi and acid fast bacilli showed no abnormality. Chest CT scan on January 22, 2015, is shown in Fig. 12.21.

After admission, anti-infection therapy and atomization were administered, but the symptoms were not improved. She still experienced intermittent hemoptysis. By multidisciplinary meeting with specialist from the thoracic surgery department, it was believed that surgery is indicated to the patient. Surgical removal of the right upper lung lobe was performed on January 23, 2015, under thoracoscope and general anesthesia. The postoperative pathology indicated a lung tissue in size of about 14 cm × 8 cm × 5 cm with a cyst

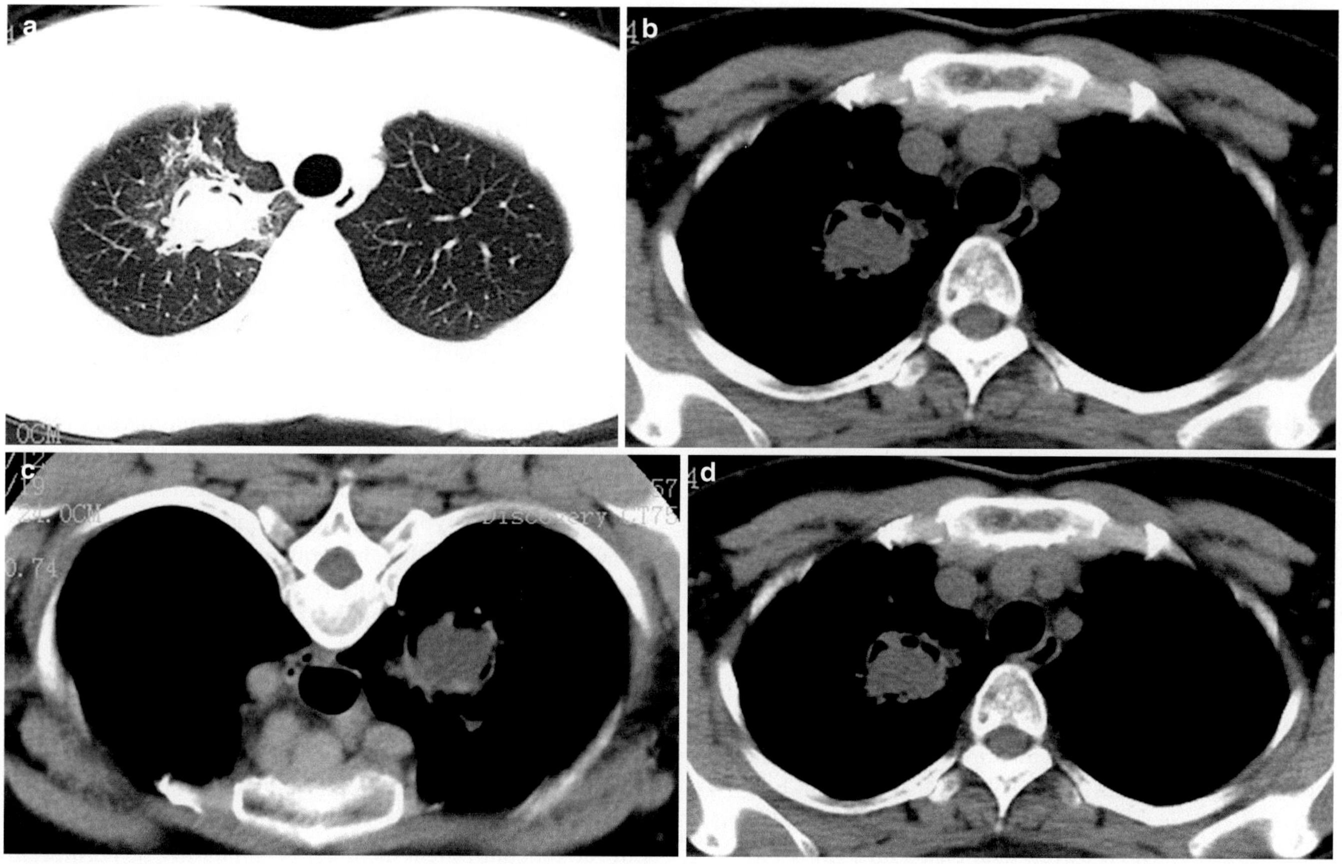

Fig. 12.21 (**a–d**) Chest CT scan. (**a**) The lung window at the sternoclavicular joint level demonstrates a round-like cavity opacity at the apical segment of right upper lung lobe, with smooth inner wall and mass-like slightly high intensity opacity inside, and crescent sign. The lesion was in size of about 3.4 cm × 2.5 cm, with heterogeneous intensity and a CT value of about 23 Hu. Around the lesion, there are strips, flakes, and cotton wool-like opacity with increased intensity. (**b**) The mediastinum window at the sternoclavicular joint level demonstrates cavity opacity at the apical segment of right upper lung lobe, with mass-like opacity inside, and crescent sign. The lesion has heterogeneous intensity, with a CT value of about 23 Hu. (**c**, **d**) The sternoclavicular joint level demonstrates movable mass-like opacity in the cavity when the patient is in prone position

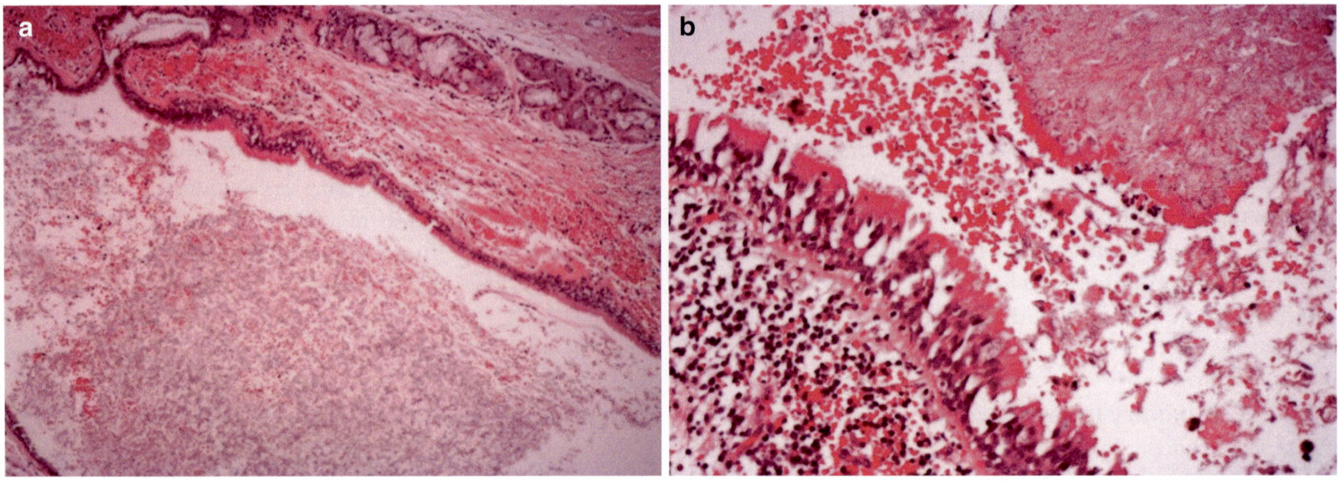

Fig. 12.22 (**a**, **b**) Pathology of lung tissue. The bronchus is demonstrated with a large quantity of fungal masses, which is morphologically consistent to aspergillus (H&E staining)

in size of 1.5 cm × 2 cm on its section, with bean dregs like substance inside. Under a microscope, there were large quantity of fungal masses in the bronchus, which was morphologically consistent to aspergillus (Fig. 12.22).

The final diagnosis was pulmonary aspergilloma of the right lung and type II diabetes.

After the surgical operation, voriconazole and symptomatic support were administered for fungal infection. After treatment, the symptoms of cough and hemoptysis were improved. The patient experienced no chest distress, chest pain, and fever. The postoperative recovery was favorable, and the patient was discharged.

12.8.4 Discussion

In recent years, along with widespread use of broad-spectrum antibiotic, glucocorticoid, and immunosuppressant, the incidence of pulmonary aspergillosis has been increasing. It is generally believed that pulmonary aspergillosis has a high incidence in immunocompromised populations. Aspergillus infection occurs due to compromised immunity of the patients when they suffer from underlying systemic diseases such as blood system diseases, malignancies, and desmosis [34]. Diabetes is also a risk factor of pulmonary aspergillosis. Diabetes has not been listed as the host risk factor of pulmonary fungal infection in the clinical guideline of China [35]. However, data based on 11,881 cases of invasive fungal infection from more than 1000 medical institutions of America indicated the patients with COPD have the highest incidence of invasive fungal infection (22.2%), followed by diabetes (21.7%) [36]. In this case, the patient had an underlying basic disease of type II diabetes and symptoms of recurrent cough and hemoptysis of sputum with blood streak. The diagnosis was then defined to be pulmonary aspergillosis. Therefore, patients with diabetes and chest CT scan demonstrations of space-occupying lesion in the lung with accompanying cavity should be suspected with pulmonary abscess, tuberculosis, malignancies, and fungal infection.

Patients with pulmonary aspergilloma generally have no obvious systemic symptoms. Clinically, hemoptysis is the most common. According to literature report, the incidence of hemoptysis with clinical significance is up to 50.3% [37]. The volume of blood ranges from a small quantity to fatally large quantity. And the other symptoms include cough and expectoration as well as rare symptoms of weight loss and fever. Generally speaking, the symptoms are non-specific. Clinically, it should be differentiated from pulmonary tuberculosis, bronchiectasis, and lung carcinoma. Chest CT scan has great significance in the clinical diagnosis of pulmonary aspergilloma. The typical chest CT demonstrations include lung cavity or spherical high intensity opacity in the cavity or crescent-shaped low intensity opacity. And movable spherical opacity in the cavity along with body postures is unique CT scan demonstration of aspergilloma [38]. In this case, the chest CT scan demonstrations were consistent to the characteristic demonstrations of pulmonary aspergilloma (Fig. 12.21). Therefore, the clinical diagnosis can be made. But the patient experienced recurrent cough and hemoptysis, and further treatment was necessary. It has been generally believed that antifungal medication can hardly be permeated into the cavity. For the patients with hemoptysis and generally favorable condition, surgical operation is the first choice for treatment to prevent fatal major hemoptysis [39]. Other approaches for hemoptysis include medication for hemostasis and interventional bronchial artery embolization. However, medication shows unfavorable therapeutic efficacy for hemoptysis. And hemoptysis tends to relapse after bronchial artery embolization. In this case, surgical operation was performed after palliative therapy showed unfavorable therapeutic efficacy. Some scholars have indicated that postoperative antifungal medication should be administered for 4–8 weeks to reduce the risk of postoperative relapse. In this case, the patient received antifungal medication of voriconazole, and the recovery was favorable. The symptoms of cough and hemoptysis were improved.

12.8.5 Comments

The patient was a middle-aged woman, with a past medical history of diabetes. She was admitted to the hospital due to complaints of recurrent cough and hemoptysis of sputum with blood streak for more than 1 year. After her admission, chest CT scan demonstrated typical characteristic changes of pulmonary aspergillosis, which was cavity opacity at the apical segment of right upper lung lobe, with mass opacity inside, and crescent sign. Based on these findings, pulmonary aspergillus infection was suspected. In this case, the patient failed to provide previous CT scan images in another hospital before her admission. The reason of missed diagnosis in that hospital remained unknown. Actually, her condition was misdiagnosed for a long period of time. In this case, the patient had a past medical history of diabetes, which may be a susceptible factor of invasive fungal infection. But the presence of other susceptible factors needed further inquiries about her housing, peripheral blood WBC count, and lymphocyte count as well as immunosuppression. These data were not analyzed in the case study. Radiological changes are the important basis for the diagnosis of pulmonary aspergillosis. In this case, chest CT scan after her admission demonstrated characteristic changes of pulmonary aspergillosis, including cavity opacity at the apical segment of right upper lung lobe, with mass opacity inside, and crescent sign. Before admission to the hospital, she presented to another hospital, and chest CT scan was performed. The clinicians in another hospital obviously neglected these typical radiological changes.

Based on clinical guideline, surgical operation was indicated to the patient, and indications include signs of pulmonary aspergilloma and recurrent hemoptysis. For patients with singular pulmonary aspergilloma, clinical observation can be performed after complete removal of the lesion. And antifungal medication is not necessary. So far, there has no evidence supporting therapeutic efficacy of medication of triazoles after surgical removal of singular aspergilloma. After surgical removal of singular aspergilloma, if no leakage of fungal substances during the operation, auxiliary antifungal medication is not necessary. If the surgical operation is complex with possible leakage of fungal substances, antifungal medication can be administered several weeks before the operation. However, for those with uncertainty about complete removal of the lesion, antifungal medication is recommended to prevent relapse. In this case, the successful treatment depended on the sufficient knowledge about pulmonary aspergilloma, careful differentiation of radiological demonstrations, and appropriate management.

12.9 Case 9: Recurrent Cough and Hemoptysis for 1 Year and Aggravation for 20 Days

Ping Xu, Wei-Dong Song, Guan-Xun Cheng, Xuemei Han, Ying-Yun Fu, and Chang'e Jin

12.9.1 Presenting Symptom

Recurrent cough and hemoptysis for 1 year and aggravation for 20 days.

12.9.2 Brief Case History

A 63-year-old woman, an environmental sanitation worker, was admitted to our hospital due to complaints of recurrent cough and hemoptysis for 1 year and aggravation for 20 days. One year ago, the patient began to experience cough, expectoration of a small quantity whitish mucous sputum, and hemoptysis of sputum with blood streak in a small quantity. Hemoptysis was improved after medication of cefaclor by herself, but she experienced recurrent hemoptysis, which was not treated. Twenty days ago, hemoptysis aggravated in a volume of about 30–50 ml/d, with accompanying fever and the highest body temperature of 38.1 °C. She experienced no dyspnea and chest pain. She ever presented in a local hospital, and the chest CT scan there demonstrated enlarged left hilum and opacity adjacent to the left lung hilum. She then received medication for treatment (specifically unknown), but the symptoms were not improved. And she presented in our hospital and was admitted due to chest CT scan demonstration of mass opacity inferior to the hilum of left upper lung. Since the onset of the symptoms, her spiritual state and appetite were poor, with a weight loss of about 3 kg.

12.9.2.1 Past Medical History

She had a past medical history of percutaneous vertebroplasty of T12 for compression fracture of lumbar vertebra in November 2012. And she denied histories of hepatitis, tuberculosis, and diabetes.

12.9.2.2 Personal History

She denied histories of smoking and alcoholism. And she worked as an environmental sanitation worker.

12.9.2.3 Physical Examination

Physical examination showed a body temperature of 36.2 °C, pulse rate 95/min, respiration rate 20/min, and blood pressure 141/72 mmHg. The respiration was stable and smooth. The superficial lymph nodes were not enlarged. The trachea was at the midline, and the thorax was bilaterally symmetric with no deformity. The bilateral vocal fremitus was bilaterally symmetric. By percussion, both lungs showed clear sounds. And by auscultation, both lungs showed coarse respiration sounds, with no dry and/or moist rales. The heartbeat was 95/min, rhythmic, with no pathological murmur. The abdomen was soft, with no tenderness and rebound pain. The liver and spleen were subcostally unpalpable. And both lower limbs showed no edema.

12.9.2.4 Initial Diagnosis

The space-occupying lesion at the hilum of left lung possibly due to lung carcinoma, pulmonary tuberculosis, or pulmonary inflammatory pseudoneoplasm.

12.9.3 Diagnosis and Treatment

After admission, the WBC count was 3.20 × 109/L and the neutrophile granulocytes 66.9%. The liver function test showed no abnormality, with urea nitrogen 2.19 mmol/L and creatinine 68.4 μmol/L. The hs-CRP was 14.32 mg/L and ESR 40 mm/h. The antibodies against tuberculosis, mycoplasma pneumonia, chlamydia, and legionella were negative. The antistreptolysin O and rheumatoid factors were negative. The ENA autoantibody series and ANA were within normal limits. The blood culture showed no growth of pathogenic bacteria. G test and GM test showed negative. Repeated sputum smears showed no acid fast bacilli and fungi. And the sputum culture showed no growth of bacteria. PPD skin test was positive.

Chest CT scan on May 4, 2013, demonstrated bronchostenosis at the lingual segment of left upper lung lobe, with accompanying formation of mass in a size of about 36 mm × 25 mm. The lung tissue distal to the mass was demonstrated with small flake of blurry opacity (Fig. 12.23).

After admission, moxifloxacin and symptomatic support therapy were administered for infection, hemostasis, and expectoration. But the symptoms of cough and hemoptysis persisted, with irregular fever. The highest body temperature reached 39 °C. Electronic bronchoscopy on May 6, 2013, demonstrated fresh blood at the trachea and left and right major bronchus. The left major bronchus was demonstrated with mucosal congestion and edema and obstruction of opening of the left lingual lobe by neoplasm, and its surface was coated by white moss. Around the neoplasm, there was fresh blood. Bronchoscopic brushing of the lingual segment of left upper lung lobe for biopsy. And intraoperative bleeding was in a large volume (Fig. 12.24). Biopsy following

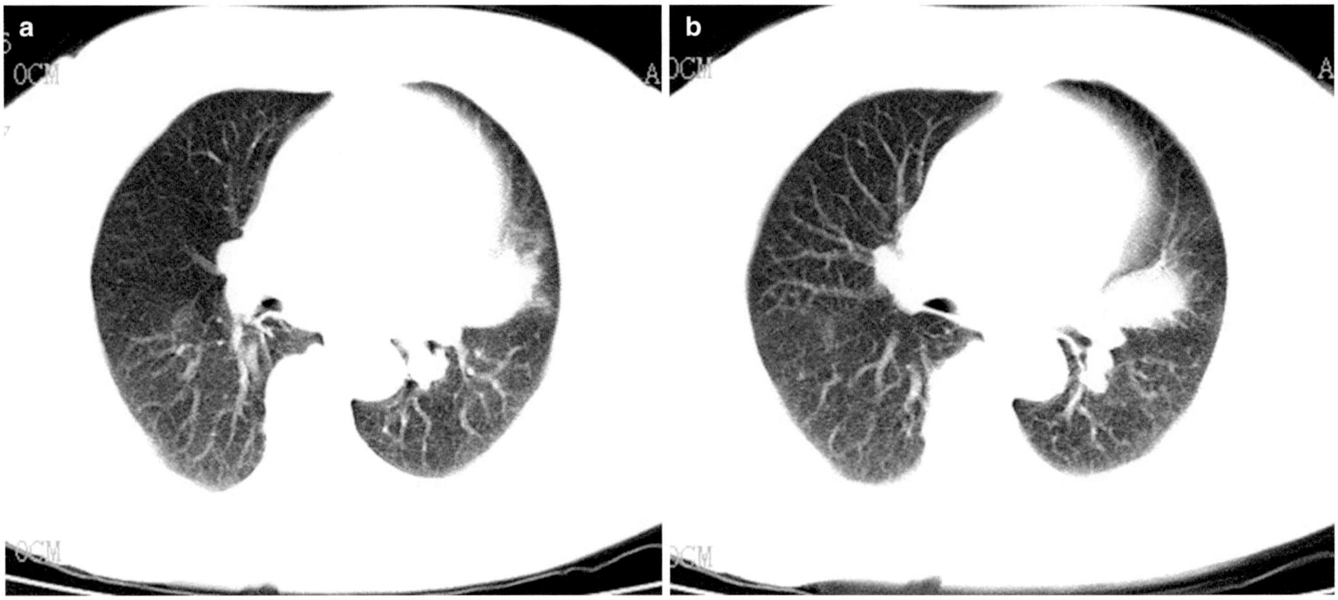

Fig. 12.23 (**a**–**c**) Chest CT scan. (**a**, **b**) The lung window demonstrates mass opacity at the lingual segment of left upper lung lobe in a size of about 36 mm × 25 mm, which is connected medially with the heart opacity. The lung tissue distal to the mass is demonstrated with small flake of blurry opacity. (**c**) The mediastinum window demonstrates mass opacity at the left lung with homogeneous intensity and well-defined margin

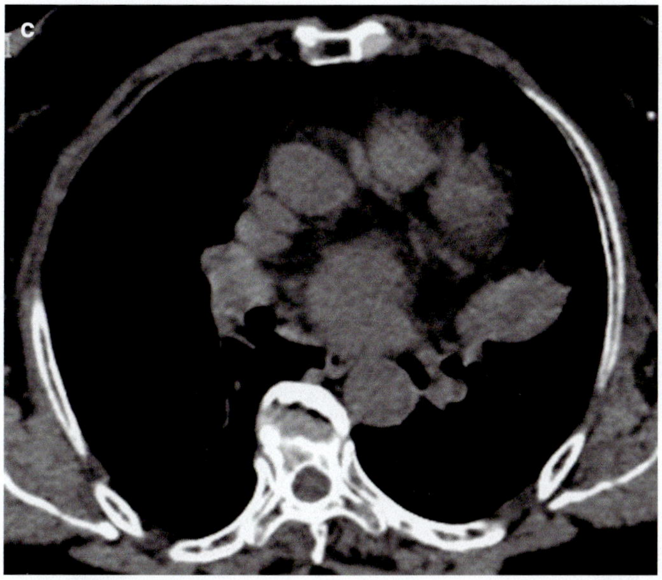

Fig. 12.23 (continued)

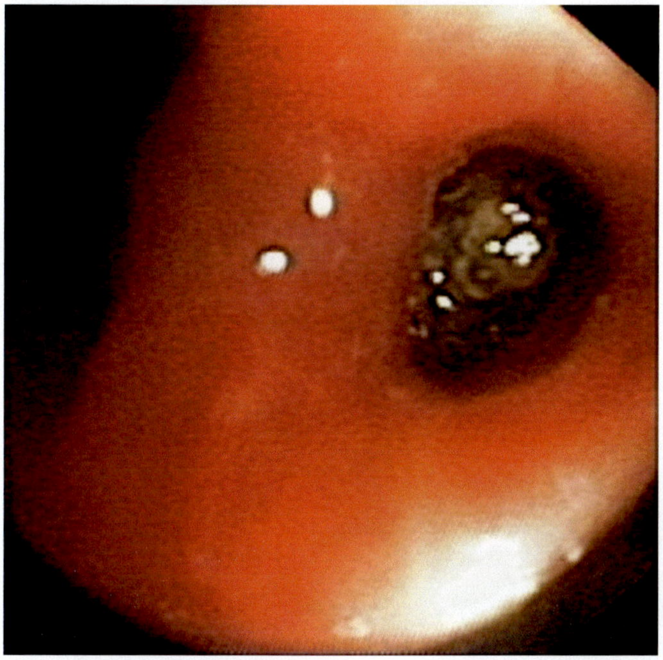

Fig. 12.24 Electronic bronchoscopy. Electronic bronchoscopy demonstrates trachea and carina with no abnormality. The major bronchi of right lung as well as upper, middle, and lower lung lobes are demonstrated with smooth mucosa and unobstructed lumen. There is no neoplasm. The major bronchus at the left lung is demonstrated with smooth mucosa and unobstructed lumen. The lumen of upper lingual lobe is unobstructed. And the lumen of lower lingual lobe is demonstrated with obstruction by yellowish necrotic substances, mucosa swelling, and widened crest

bronchoscopic brushing demonstrated many ciliated columnar epithelial cells and neutrophile granulocytes, with small quantity of hyphae-like substances at local lesion. The pathology of mucosa at the lingual segment of left lung demonstrated aspergillus hyphae with even thickness and transverse septa. The hyphae were demonstrated with branching in sharp angle, and there were small round spores, which were consistent to aspergillus infection (Fig. 12.25).

Intravenous infusion of voriconazole was commenced on May 10, 2013, and her body temperature decreased to around 37.5 °C. And the symptoms of cough and expectoration were improved. But recurrent hemoptysis persisted in a volume of 5–10 ml each day. On May 25, the patient required discharge. And after discharge, oral medication of voriconazole was continued in a dose of 200 mg, twice a day. But hemoptysis persisted, with the largest volume of about 100 ml. On June 10, she was admitted to our hospital again. Enhanced chest CT scan was performed on June 14, 2013 (Fig. 12.26). In multidisciplinary meeting with specialist from the thoracic surgery department, surgery was recommended. On June 22, 2013, thoracoscopic exploration demonstrated adhesion of the left lung with thoracic wall and pericardium, and a tenacious mass with a diameter of 6 cm adjacent to the oblique fissure of the left lower lung, which involved visceral pleura. There were also calcified lymph nodes around the inferior pulmonary artery, absence of anatomical borderline, and adhesion of the inferior pulmonary artery with bronchus, which could hardly be separated. Under the thoracoscope, the pulmonary arteries and bronchus were removed, and a gross specimen was removed (Fig. 12.27).

The final diagnosis was obstructive aspergillus tracheobronchitis.

After surgery, the recovery was favorable. Oral intake of voriconazole was continued for 4 weeks, and the symptoms disappeared. One year after surgery, the lesion did not relapsed (Fig. 12.28).

12.9.4 Discussion

Pulmonary aspergillosis is a group of acute and chronic lung diseases induced by inhalation of aspergillus. Leukemia, radiotherapy and chemotherapy for malignancies, organ transplantation, long-term application of hormones in a large dose, and application of immunosuppressant may increase the risk of aspergillus infection. Pulmonary aspergillosis rarely occurs in immunocompetent populations. Obstructive aspergillus tracheobronchitis (OATB) is a rare type of pulmonary aspergillosis [40], which is believed to be a subtype of invasive aspergillosis (IPA) and closely related to presence of large quantity of aspergillus spores in environment [41]. The clinical manifestations of OATB are non-specific, commonly including cough, expectoration, fever, dyspnea, chest pain, and hemoptysis. The characteristic demonstrations on CT scan include protrusion of neoplasm in bronchial lumen, which induces local luminal narrowness or complete obstruction. In some other cases, the characteristic demonstrations

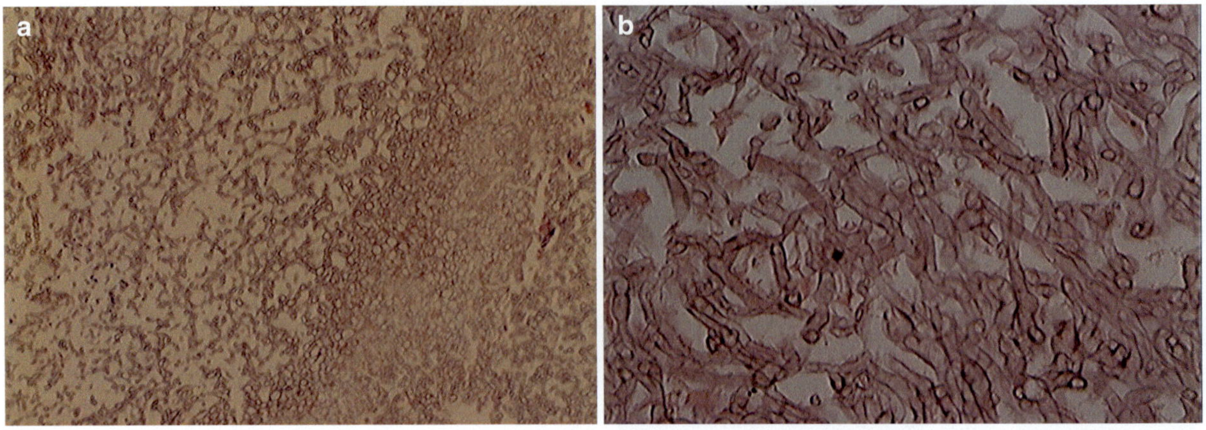

Fig. 12.25 (**a**, **b**) Pathology of lung tissue. (**a**) Biopsy of mucosa at the left lingual lobe demonstrates aspergillus hyphae and spores (H&E staining). (**b**) Biopsy of mucosa at the left lingual lobe demonstrates aspergillus hyphae and spores (H&E staining)

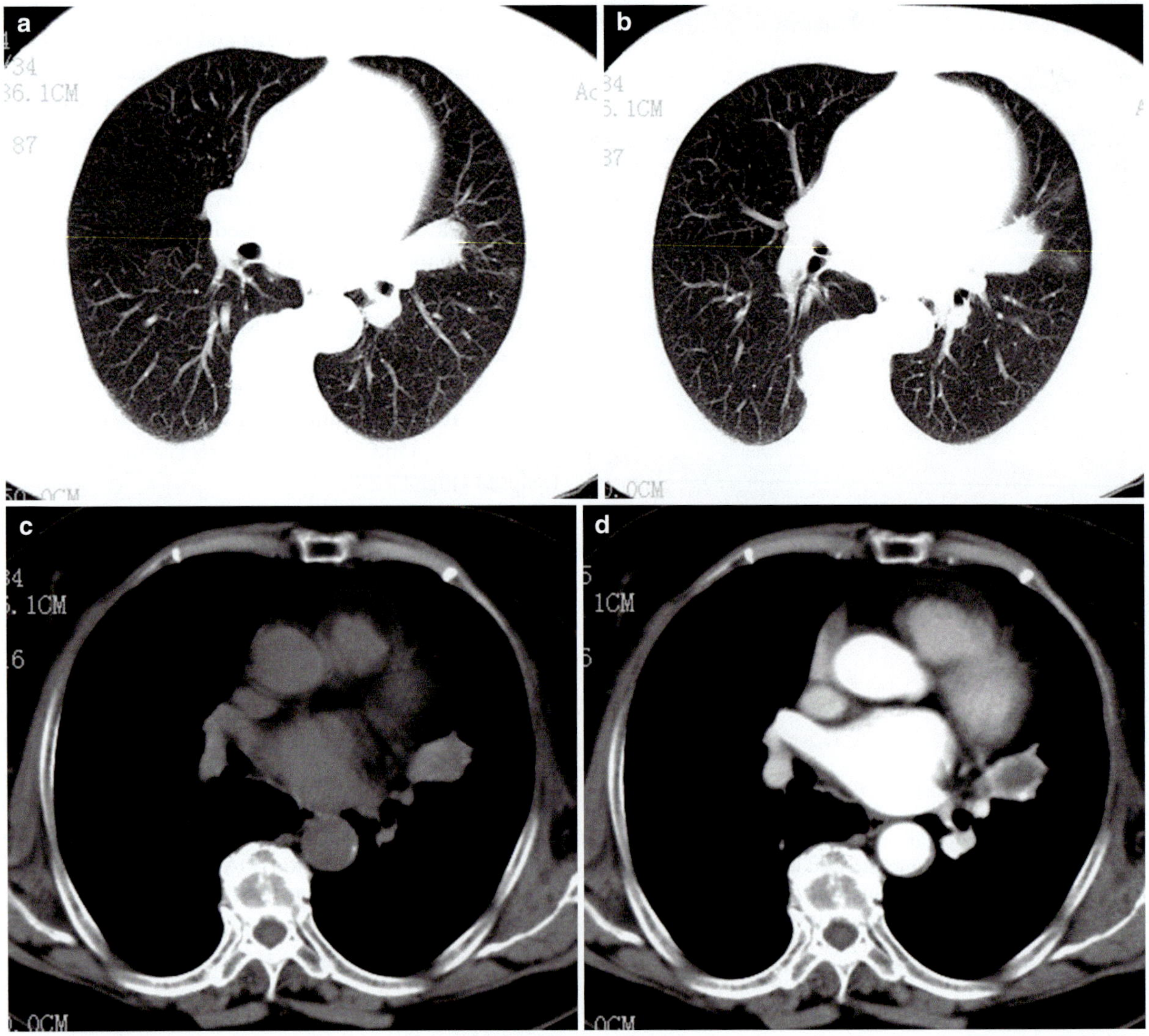

Fig. 12.26 (**a**–**d**) Enhanced chest CT scan. (**a**, **b**) The lung window demonstrates formation of mass at the lingual segment of left upper lung lobe, with the largest section area of about 34 mm × 24 mm. The lung tissue distal to the mass is demonstrated with small flake of blurry opacity. (**c**) The mediastinum window demonstrates heterogeneous intensity of the lesion, with a marginal CT value of 59 Hu and central CT value of 36–45 Hu. (**d**) Enhanced scan demonstrates heterogeneous enhancement in almost ring shape, with obvious marginal enhancement, CT value of 110 Hu, and slight central enhancement, CT value of 40–53 Hu. The mediastinum is demonstrated with enlarged lymph nodes and partial calcification

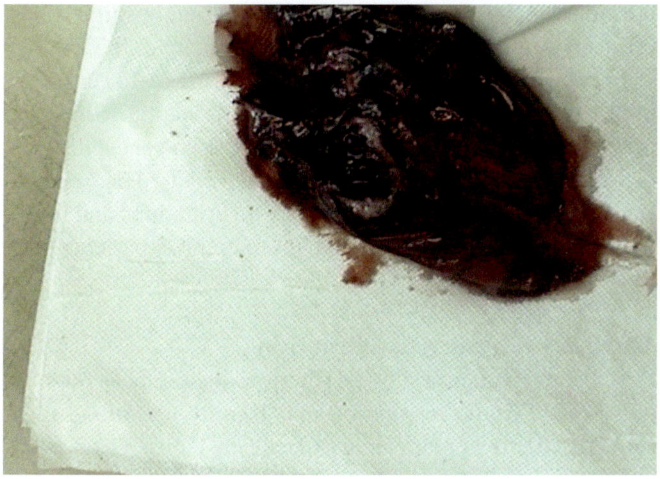

Fig. 12.27 Observation of removed tissue by naked eyes

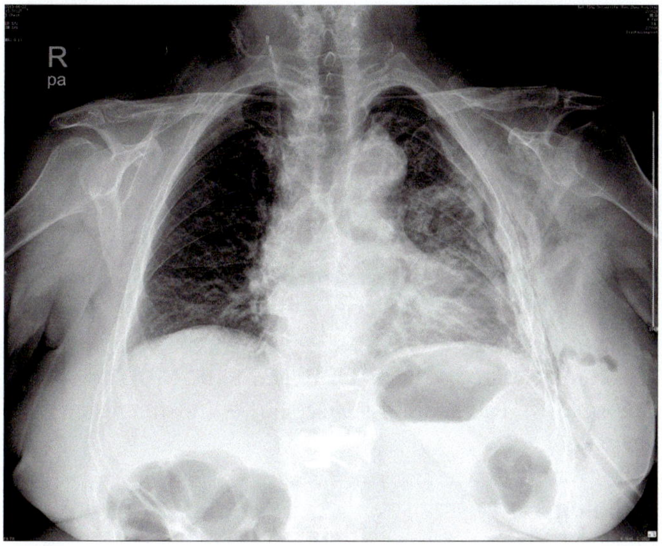

Fig. 12.28 Chest X-ray. Chest X-ray demonstrates patchy and strips of opacity at the left upper lung field and blunted costophrenic angle

on CT scan may include thickening of tracheal wall or mass opacity. Bronchoscopy plays an important role in the diagnosis of OATB, which provides direct observation of luminal lesions and facilitates harvesting specimens via biopsy, aspiration, and irritation for definitive diagnosis. Bronchoscopic biopsy for pathology is the direct and the most effective way for its definitive diagnosis [42]. In this case, the patient was an environmental sanitation worker in a city with subtropical climate. She always worked in early mornings. And it was speculated that the aspergillus infection is possibly related to contacts to rotted and damp plants and soil with aspergillus and their inhalation via respiratory tract. The clinical manifestations were non-specific, and the symptoms included chronic cough and hemoptysis. Antibacterial therapy seemed effective, but the disease was not healed with a prolonged illness course. Chest CT scan demonstrated bronchostenosis at the lingual segment of left upper lung lobe, with accompanying formation of mass. Bronchoscopy demonstrated neoplasm, which may be misdiagnosed as lung carcinoma or obstructive pneumonia.

The therapies for OATB mainly include antifungal therapy, endovascular interventional therapy, or surgery. In this case, the patient received medication of voriconazole for 1 month, but the clinical symptoms were not improved. Recurrent hemoptysis persisted. Reexamination of chest CT scan demonstrated neoplasm, with heterogeneous enhancement by enhanced CT scan, which was considered to be invasion of aspergillus into major pulmonary vascular vessels. Thoracoscopic exploration demonstrated adhesion of the left lung with thoracic wall and pericardium, invasion of the mass into visceral pleura, and close adhesion of the inferior pulmonary artery with bronchus that could hardly be separated. Based on these findings, the condition was considered to be invasion of aspergillus into the inferior pulmonary artery, which may be the pathomechanism of recurrent hemoptysis. The most common symptom of pulmonary aspergillosis is hemoptysis, with an incidence rate of up to 80% and an incidence of life-threatening major hemoptysis up to 30%. Therefore, for patients with poor therapeutic efficacy by medications, persistent hemoptysis, and localized lesion, active surgical removal of lesions is recommended [43]. For patients with small lesions, noninvolvement of pleural cavity, and no obvious adhesion, thoracoscopic removal of lesions is recommended. Postoperative administration of antifungal medication is recommended to reduce the chance of its relapse and prevent intrathoracic secondary aspergillus infection.

12.9.5 Comments

This is a definitively diagnosed case of pulmonary aspergillosis based on pathological findings of aspergillus hyphae at the bronchial mucosa. The diagnosis of invasive pulmonary mycosis can be defined based on microbiological evidence from histology or sterile body fluid investigation regardless of the host factors. In this case, the patient worked as an environmental sanitation worker, and she was repeatedly exposed to large quantity of aspergillus spores, which may be the main reason of her infection. However, the existence of compromised immunity was not clearly defined. On admission, her WBC count was 3.20 × 109/L by routine blood test. And the changes of WBC counts before and after admission were not recorded. And the test for count of lymphocyte subgroups was not performed. Presence of basic disease that may compromise the immunity cannot be excluded. In this case, the patient had a past medical history of percutaneous vertebroplasty of T12 for compression fracture of lumbar vertebra. The relationship of the health status and nourishment in daily life and past medical history of surgery with occurrence and progression of pulmonary disease needs further exploration.

Surgery plays an important role in the treatment of IPA. Patients with lesion adjacent to major vascular vessels or pericardium, hemoptysis induced by singular cavity, or involved thoracic wall can benefit from surgery. In this case, the lesion was morphologically a mass, which induced bronchial obstruction. Medications showed unfavorable therapeutic efficacy, and surgery was indicated. During the surgical operation, adhesion of the lesion with thoracic wall and pericardium, invasion of mass into visceral pleura, and close adhesion of the inferior pulmonary artery with bronchus that could hardly be separated were confirmed. In this case, antifungal medication was continued for 4 weeks after surgical operation. Postoperative follow-ups for 1 year showed no relapse of the disease, indicating successful treatment.

12.10 Case 10: Recurrent Cough, Expectoration and Hemoptysis for More Than 6 Years and Aggravation for 1 Day

Yazhou Cai, Wendi Huang, Ping Xu, Huaisheng Chen, Xueyan Liu, and Budong Chen

12.10.1 Presenting Symptom

Recurrent cough, expectoration, and hemoptysis for more than 6 years and aggravation for 1 day.

12.10.2 Brief Case History

A 49-year-old man from Anhui province of China was admitted to our hospital on August 7, 2013, due to complaints of recurrent cough, expectoration, and hemoptysis for more than 6 years and aggravation for 1 day. Since 2009, the patient began to experience recurrent cough, and expectoration, with no obvious regularity. The sputum was yellowish white. In another hospital, he was diagnosed with bronchiectasis and received medications with unfavorable therapeutic efficacy (specifically unknown). The symptoms then showed repeated onset, with variant times of onset each year and occasional hemoptysis. The symptoms were improved by anti-infection therapy (specifically unknown). In 2012, he received interventional therapy (specifically unknown) in a local hospital due to hemoptysis, and the symptom was improved. On August 6, 2013, the symptoms of cough, expectoration of yellowish white thick sputum, and accompanying hemoptysis of about 10 ml onset again. And he presented in the emergency department of our hospital. Chest CT scan demonstrated mass intensity opacity at the anterior segment of left upper lung lobe and bronchiectasis at the left upper lung, and the patient was then admitted. Since the onset of symptoms, the patient experienced no chest distress, breathlessness, chest pain, and night sweat. His spiritual state and appetite were quite good. The urinations and bowel movements were normal. And the patient experienced no obvious weight loss.

12.10.2.1 Physical Examination

Physical examination showed a body temperature of 36.4 °C, pulse rate 74/min, respiration rate 18/min, and blood pressure BP 102/62 mmHg. He was well conscious. The superficial lymph nodes were unpalpable and not enlarged. The bilateral tonsils were not enlarged. The respiration sounds of both lungs were slightly coarse, with moist rales at the left upper lung. The heartbeat was rhythmic, with no obvious murmur. The abdomen was soft, with no tenderness and rebound pain. The liver and spleen were subcostally unpalpable. The liver and kidney areas were not sensitive to percussion. Both lower limbs showed no edema, and there was no clubbing finger. The nervous system showed no abnormalities.

12.10.2.2 Auxiliary Investigation

Laboratory Test

The routine blood test, hs-CRP, and CPK-MB showed no abnormality. The sputum smear showed no fungi and acid fast bacilli.

Radiology

Chest CT scan on August 6, 2013, is shown in Fig. 12.29.

12.10.2.3 Initial Diagnosis

The initial diagnosis was bronchiectasis complicated by hemoptysis.

12.10.3 Diagnosis and Treatment

After admission, routine blood test, ESR, and (1,3)-β-D glucan showed no abnormality. The alanine transaminase was 67 U/L, total protein 51.8 g/L, and albumin 27.3 g/L. The sputum cultures for fungi and bacteria showed negative. Piperacillin sodium/tazobactam sodium and cefradine were consecutively administered for infection and etamsylate and aminomethylbenzoic acid for symptomatic support. But the symptoms were not improved, and hemoptysis tended to aggravate. To further define the diagnosis for corresponding treatment, surgery was recommended in multidisciplinary meeting with specialist from

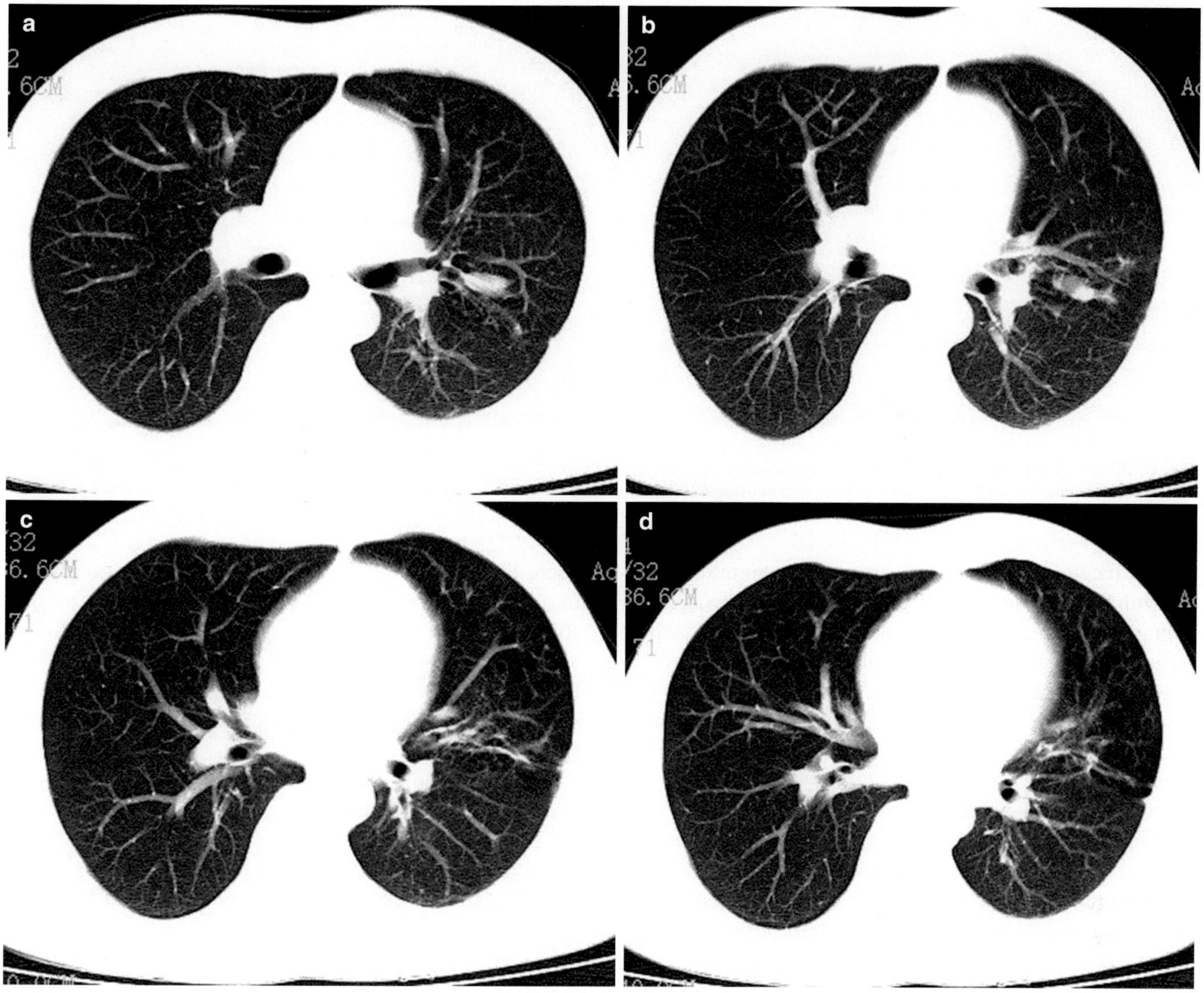

Fig. 12.29 (**a**–**d**) Lung window of chest CT scan. The apicolingual segment of left upper lung lobe is demonstrated with bronchiectasis. The posterior segment of left upper lung lobe is demonstrated with poorly defined nodular opacity with slightly high intensity in size of about 2.3 cm × 1.0 cm

the thoracic surgery department. Thoracoscopic removal of left upper lung lobe and lysis of pleural adhesion were performed under general anesthesia on August 16, 2013. The postoperative pathology (Fig. 12.30) demonstrated partial bronchiolar dilation of the lung tissue specimen, with fungal mass in some bronchiolar lumen. There were also infiltration of lymphocytes around the bronchiolar lumen, vascular dilation and congestion of the surrounding alveolar septa, and bleeding of local alveolar cavity. The inferior layer of bronchial mucosa at the dissected section was congested with slight edema, with infiltration of less lymphocytes. The lesion was consistent to bronchiectasis accompanied by fungal (possibly aspergillus) infection.

The final diagnosis was bronchiectasis complicated by chronic pulmonary aspergillosis.

After operation, combined use of voriconazole, cefotiam, and etimicin was prescribed for infection. The symptoms were greatly improved. Follow-ups after discharge showed no relapse of hemoptysis.

12.10.4 Discussion

Aspergillosis is an opportunistic infection caused by aspergillus and its conidiospores, and the lung is its most common target organ. Aspergillus is a conditional pathogenic fungus, and onset of symptoms is based on interactions between aspergillus and the host [44]. Invasive pulmonary aspergillosis commonly occurs in patients with seriously compromised immunity, including patients

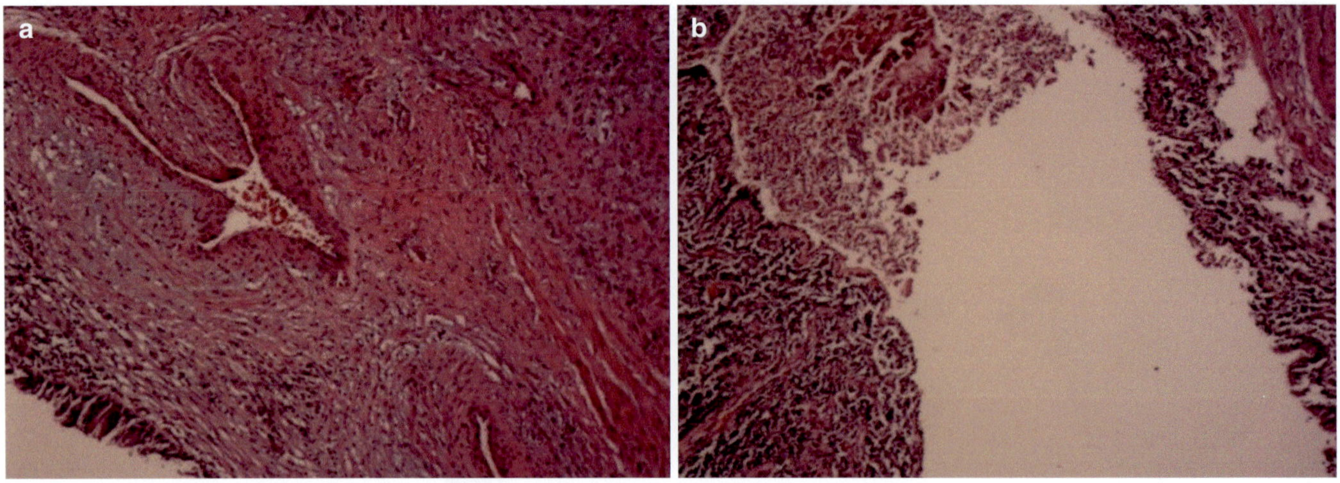

Fig. 12.30 Postoperative pathology after thoracoscopic removal of the lesion. H&E staining demonstrates aspergillus hyphae and spores, with infiltration of many lymphocytes, plasmocytes, and neutrophile granulocytes

with or receiving neutropenia, organ transplantation, critical and serious illness, and glucocorticoid. Chronic pulmonary aspergillosis has a chronic progression, which commonly occurs in patients with lung disease and no or slight immunodeficiency, such as chronic obstructive pulmonary disease, bronchiectasis, sarcoidosis, lung carcinoma, and tuberculosis or nontuberculosis mycobacteria infection [45].

In this case, the patient had a past medical history of bronchiectasis. The clinical manifestations included recurrent cough, expectoration, and hemoptysis. Chest CT scan only demonstrated bronchiectasis of the lingual segment of left upper lung lobe as well as mass and flake of high intensity opacity at the posterior segment of left upper lung lobe. Chest CT scan demonstrated non-specific changes of aspergillus infection. In addition, the G test showed negative. Hemoptysis induced by pulmonary aspergillosis tended to be neglected, and early clinical diagnosis was challenging. The patient received repeated anti-infection therapy, but the symptoms were not improved. Thus complication of opportunistic fungal infection should be considered. In this case, the diagnosis was defined based on surgical removal of the lung lobe and postoperative pathology. The diagnosis indicated that patients with no compromised immunity but chronic lung disease may susceptible to aspergillus infection.

Patients with pulmonary aspergillosis commonly show no systemic symptoms. The most common clinical symptom is hemoptysis. And associate symptoms include chronic cough and dyspnea. Radiology demonstrates lung cavity with or with no aspergilloma, infiltration, nodule, and various degrees of pulmonary or pleural fibrosis. Radiology demonstrates typical pulmonary aspergilloma as spherical or sphere-like opacity as well as crescent-shaped translucent area, namely, crescent sign, superior to the spherical opacity [46]. Pulmonary aspergillosis shows non-specific clinical symptoms. Its overlapping with primary disease presents challenge for its diagnosis. In this case, the initial diagnosis was hemoptysis induced by bronchiectasis, and pulmonary aspergillosis was neglected.

The main reasons for missed diagnosis of chronic pulmonary aspergillosis include:

1. Insufficient knowledge about chronic pulmonary aspergillosis by clinicians and hemoptysis tends to be attributed to the primary disease.
2. Overlapping with the primary disease conceals the characteristic radiological sign of chronic pulmonary aspergillosis.
3. Awareness to chronic pulmonary aspergillosis is not sufficiently high. Especially when appropriate medication shows unfavorable therapeutic efficacy, chronic pulmonary aspergillosis is not considered.

Treatment of pulmonary aspergillosis is intended to improve the symptoms, prevent hemoptysis, and avoid fibrosis. The treatment approaches mainly include medication and surgery. Because antifungal medication seriously affects liver and kidney functions and the therapeutic course is comparatively long, its side effects on the liver and kidney as well as resistance to the medication are the key points during treatment. For patients with simplex or complex aspergilloma and unfavorably controlled hemoptysis, if the lung function permits, surgery is recommended. Surgical removal of lung lobe is the most common surgical approach [3, 47].

12.10.5 Comments

Chronic pulmonary aspergillosis (CPA) refers to chronic aspergillus infection of the lung, with an illness course of more than 3 months. It may be secondary to other respiratory disease. In this case, the patient was admitted due to complaints of recurrent cough, expectoration, and hemoptysis for more than 6 years and aggravation for 1 day. The illness course far exceeded 3 months. During early diagnosis and treatment, chronic pulmonary aspergillosis was not considered. For patients with long-term cough, expectoration, and hemoptysis, chronic pulmonary aspergillosis should be considered based on the diagnostic criteria and differential diagnosis listed in the clinical guideline, which greatly facilitates the diagnosis of CPA.

Based on the current clinical guideline, the diagnosis of CPA should meet all the following conditions:

1. Chest radiology demonstrates characteristic signs, especially chest CT scan.
2. There is direct evidence supporting aspergillus infection or immunoassay for aspergillus shows positive.
3. Other possible diseases are excluded.

In this case, radiology demonstrated poorly defined nodular opacity with slightly high intensity at the posterior segment of left upper lung lobe in a size of about 2.3 cm × 1.0 cm. Based on radiological demonstrations, it is not typical pulmonary aspergilloma, but aspergillus nodule should be suspected. The direct evidence of aspergillus infection can be harvested via biopsy of lung tissue. Because aspergillus nodule is clinically rare, its differentiation from pulmonary tuberculosis, lung carcinoma, lung metastasis, cryptococcus nodule, and coccidioidomycosis can hardly be radiologically made. Therefore, the diagnosis should only be based on histological biopsy. If invasion of fungal hyphae into lung parenchyma is observed under a microscope, a diagnosis of subacute invasive pulmonary aspergillosis can be made. If only aspergillus hyphae observed in respiratory specimen and/or culture for aspergillus positive and/or PCR for aspergillus positive, a diagnosis of CPA cannot be defined. BALF, instead of blood, GM test can improve the diagnostic sensitivity and specificity of CPA.

In this case, the patient continued the medication of triazoles for fungal infection. However, in the current clinical guideline, only regular observation should be performed if aspergillus nodule is completely removed by surgery. Except patients with compromised immunity, antifungal mediation is not necessary for patients with singular aspergillus nodule and its complete removal by surgery. It is recommended that aspergillus IgG quantification, inflammatory indices, and dynamic radiological changes should be monitored every 3 months after the surgery. If necessary, antifungal medication can be administered.

12.11 Case 11: Intermittent Hemoptysis for More Than 4 Months

Hongtao Chen, Dong-Na Su, Xiaojing Guo, Huaisheng Chen, Xueyan Liu, and Junmin Wen

12.11.1 Presenting Symptom

Intermittent hemoptysis for more than 4 months.

12.11.2 Brief Case History

A 42-year-old man was admitted to our hospital on December 2, 2014, due to complaints of intermittent hemoptysis for more than 4 months. Four months ago, the patient began to experience intermittent hemoptysis with no known reasons. At first, he coughed up sputum with blood streak in a small quantity, with no symptoms of chest pain, chest distress, fever, night sweat, poor appetite, and weight loss. He paid no close attention to it. And recurrent hemoptysis occurred, in large or small quantity. When in large quantity, he coughed up blood clot in about 1–2 ml. When in small quantity, he coughed up sputum with blood streak. He presented in another hospital, and the diagnosis was secondary pulmonary tuberculosis of the right upper lung and cavity at the right upper lung. But he received no corresponding therapy. He then presented in our hospital on December 2, 2014, and was admitted to the thoracic surgery department. Since the onset of symptoms, his spiritual state, appetite, strength, urinations, bowel movements, and sleeping were normal. And he experienced no weight loss.

12.11.2.1 Past Medical History

Twenty years ago, he suffered from pulmonary tuberculosis. He then received antituberculosis therapy (specifically unknown) and was cured. And he denied habitual smoking and drinking. The patient also denied medical histories of hypertension and diabetes.

12.11.2.2 Physical Examination

Physical examination showed a body temperature of 36.4 °C, respiration rate 18/min, pulse rate 90/min, and blood pressure 121/73 mmHg. The patient was well conscious, with normal appearance. The tone was coherent, and respirations were smooth. There was no clubbing finger. The systemic superficial lymph nodes were unpalpable and not enlarged. The conjunctiva was not pale. The trachea was on the midline and thorax bilaterally symmetric. The bilateral vocal fremitus was not weakened. Percussion showed clear sounds of both lungs. By auscultation, the right upper lung showed weakened respiration sounds, and the left lung showed clear respiration sounds, with no dry and/or moist rales. The heartbeat was 90/min, rhythmic. And the valvular areas showed no pathological murmur. The abdomen was soft, with no mass, no tenderness, and rebound pain. The liver and spleen were unpalpable. The shifting dullness was negative. And both lower limbs showed no edema.

12.11.2.3 Auxiliary Investigation

Chest CT scan on November 25, 2014, is shown in Fig. 12.31.

12.11.2.4 Initial Diagnosis

The initial diagnosis was aspergilloma of the right upper lung and secondary pulmonary tuberculosis of both lungs (fibrous cavitary type).

12.11.3 Diagnosis and Treatment

After admission, the investigations were ordered. The routine blood test showed WBC 5.1 × 109/L, N 42%, L 41%, and EO 10%, RBC 3.9 × 1012/L, and PLT 126 × 109/L. ESR was 5 mm/h and CRP 11 mg/L. The liver function test, kidney function test, blood sugar, and coagulation function test showed no abnormality. HIV antibody was negative. The sputum smear (including acid fast staining) showed negative.

Thoracoscopic removal of right upper lung lobe, cautery of pleural adhesion, and intercostal nerve block were performed under general anesthesia on December 8, 2014, due to cavity at the right upper lung and obvious right pleural adhesion. By surgical exploration, formation of cavity at the right upper lung was found, with aspergilloma inside. The postoperative pathology demonstrated aspergilloma at the right upper lung (Fig. 12.32).

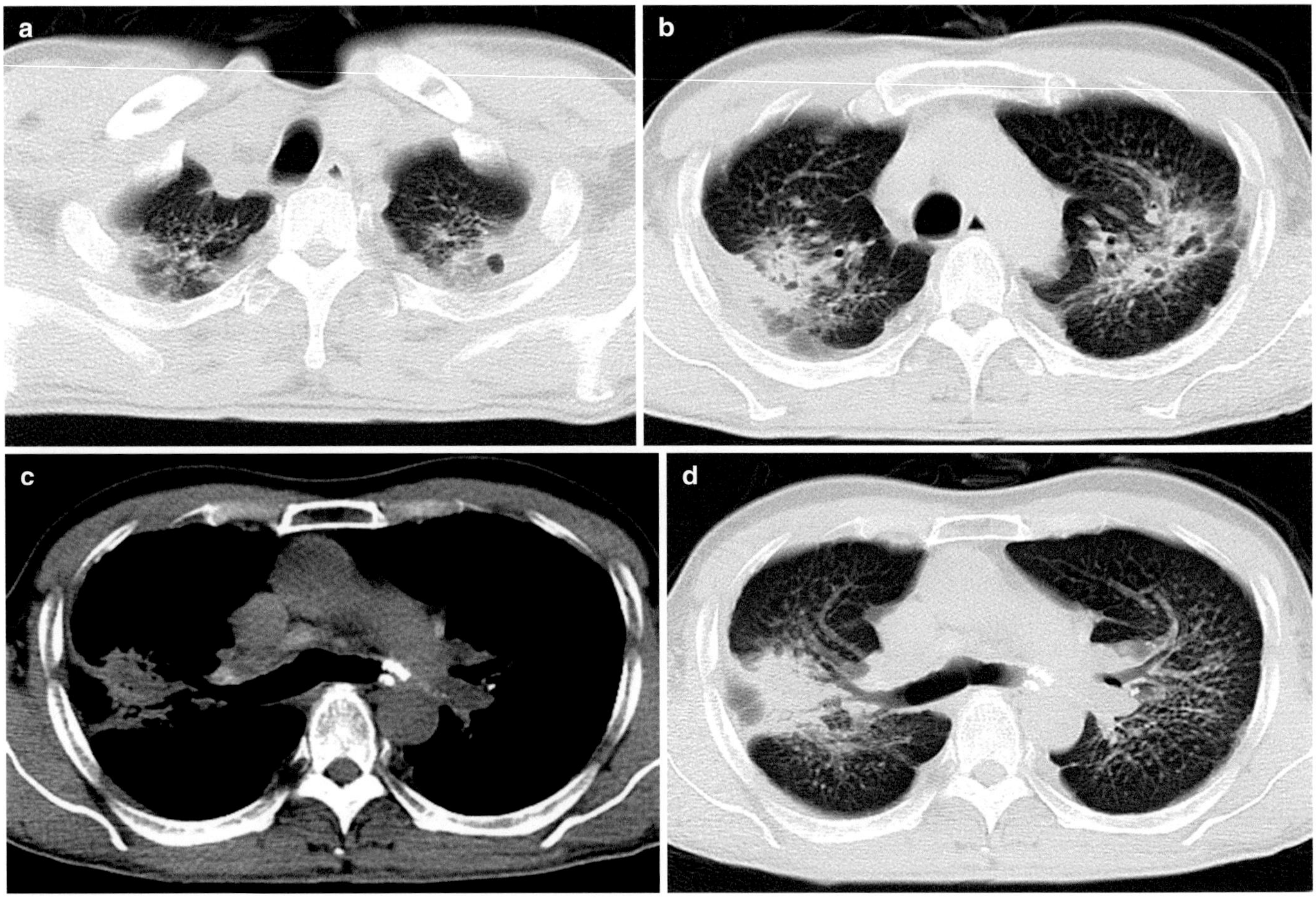

Fig. 12.31 (**a**–**d**) Chest CT scan on November 25, 2014. (**a**, **b**) The lung window demonstrates irregular patchy opacity with increased intensity, translucent areas in different sizes, and bilateral pleural thickening. (**c**, **d**) The bronchial branching level is demonstrated with mass-like opacity at the right upper lung, cavity near pleura at the right upper lung, and adhesion of mass opacity with lateral pleura. There is parallel linear calcification opacity at the opening of left major bronchus

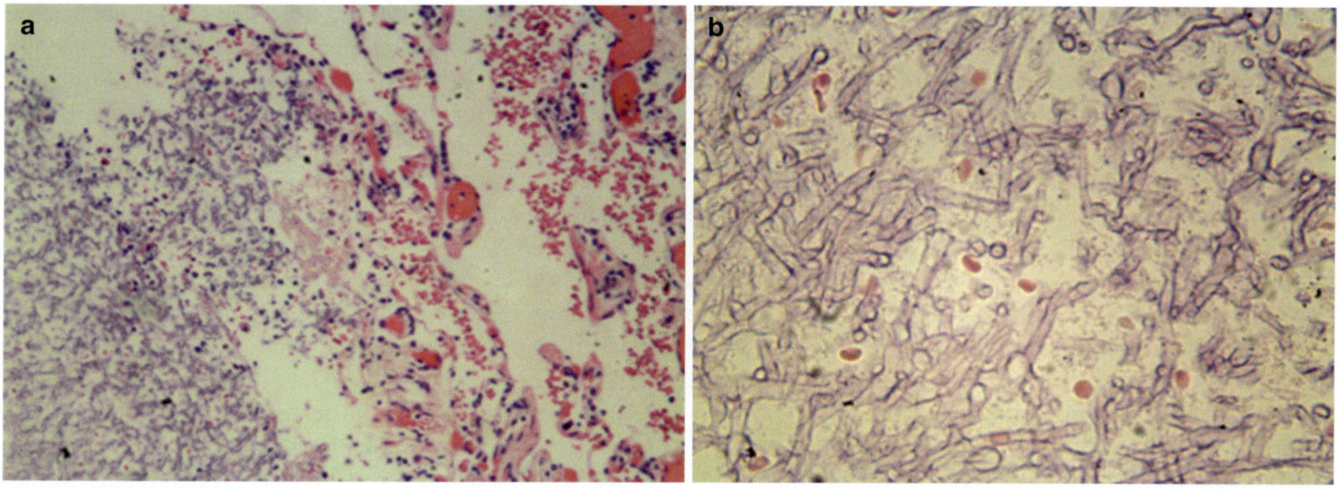

Fig. 12.32 (**a**, **b**) Pathology of lung tissue. (**a**) H&E staining of pulmonary aspergilloma. (**b**) H&E staining demonstrates aspergillus hyphae and spores. The hyphae are uniform in size with septa and branching in 45° angle

After the surgical operation, no medication was administered. And the condition was favorably improved, with no hemoptysis.

The diagnosis on discharge was aspergilloma at the right upper lung and secondary pulmonary tuberculosis of both lungs (fibrous cavitary type).

12.11.4 Discussion

Aspergilloma is the mixture of aspergillus hyphae, fibrin, mucus, and cellular necrotic substance [25], which is the most common type (61.8%) of pulmonary aspergillosis [48]. Aspergilloma is parasitic pulmonary aspergillosis, which occurs in lung cavity and is advanced chronic pulmonary aspergillosis (CPA). In most cases, aspergillus hyphae do not exist in the lung tissue outside of the cavity, which is different from invasive pulmonary aspergillosis (IPA). When the diameter of cavity in the lung exceeds 2 cm, the risk of aspergilloma is 15–20%. Complex aspergilloma is actually chronic cavitary pulmonary aspergillosis (CCPA).

In this case, the basic disease was secondary pulmonary tuberculosis of both upper lungs. CT scan demonstrated fibrous proliferative lesion at both upper lungs, formation of fibrous cavity in the right upper lung near the pleura, and its adhesion with local pleura. There was dense opacity with slightly high intensity in the cavity. Based on this indirect sign, we considered existence of aspergilloma. Actually, the common susceptible factors of pulmonary aspergilloma include pulmonary tuberculosis, bronchiectasis, and bronchial abscess. And pulmonary tuberculosis is the most common basic disease of pulmonary aspergilloma, accounting for 93% [48, 49] in cases of pulmonary aspergilloma. In patients with pulmonary aspergilloma, 42% shows lesion at the right upper lung. Therefore, based on the basic disease and location of cavity, it can be speculated that the patient is more likely to suffer from pulmonary aspergilloma. By literature review, we found that in patients with a past medical history of pulmonary tuberculosis, the incidence of CPA is 15.3% in Manchester of the UK and 93% in Korea [50]. Six months after pulmonary tuberculosis is cured, by chest X-ray, the incidence of cavity in the lung is up to 21% in gold mine workers in South Africa. A research in North America showed that the incidence of cavity in the lung is up to 23.3% [51, 52]. Persistent existence of cavity in the lung is the high-risk factor of pulmonary aspergilloma. A previous research from Britain [53, 54] has demonstrated that in patients with antituberculosis therapy for 1 year and sputum negative, the incidence of pulmonary aspergilloma is 14% and 4 years later, 22%. In patients receiving antituberculosis therapy for 1 year, the incidence of aspergillus precipitin positive is up to 25%. Therefore, in patients with pulmonary tuberculosis, the incidence of pulmonary aspergilloma has been underestimated. These clinical data suggested that in patients with pulmonary tuberculosis, if persistent existence of cavity in the lung is detected, complication of pulmonary aspergilloma should be suspected.

Just like the patient in this case, patients with pulmonary aspergilloma may not show obvious symptoms for many years. Most patients with pulmonary aspergilloma experience hemoptysis of a small quantity. In some serious cases, major hemoptysis occurs, mostly in patients with tuberculous cavity. Hemoptysis is the most common symptom for which the patient presents in hospital. In patients with old tuberculous cavity complicated by aspergilloma, the incidence of hemoptysis is up to 81%. Due to abundant blood vessels and formation of angioma around aspergilloma as well as invasion of blood vessels by aspergillus, bleeding and hemoptysis are common. Without intervention, aspergilloma persists and even threatens the life.

The typical radiological demonstrations of aspergilloma include solitude spherical lesion in cavity or cavum, crescent-shaped translucent area, adjacent pleural thickening, and movable aspergilloma along with body posture (pendulum-like) [55]. Huge or too small aspergilloma may cause difficulty for its diagnosis. In this case, the cavity at the right upper lung showed no obvious spherical lesion and pendulum-like opacity. Based on findings of dense opacity in the cavity, we speculated existence of aspergilloma. Generally speaking, the diagnosis of pulmonary aspergilloma mainly depends on clinical manifestations and radiological demonstrations. Biopsy of the lung may not be harvested. Radiologically, it should be differentiated from pulmonary tuberculosis, lung carcinoma, and hydatidosis. For patients with simplex pulmonary aspergilloma, surgical removal is recommended. For patients with complex pulmonary aspergilloma, such as chronic cavitary pulmonary aspergilloma (CCPA), medications including itraconazole, voriconazole, and posaconazole or surgical removal of lesion can be chosen [56]. For patients with tolerance to surgery, data from postoperative follow-ups for 0.5 to 7 years indicated no relapse and definitive therapeutic efficacy.

12.11.5 Comments

In this case, the patient presented to hospital due to hemoptysis for more than 4 months. Chest CT scan after admission demonstrated mass opacity at right upper lung at the bronchial branching level and cavity at the right upper lung near the pleura. Due to sufficient knowledge about CPA by clinicians, the diagnosis was rapidly made to be pulmonary aspergilloma of the right upper lung. And the patient received timely and appropriate treatment.

CPA usually has an illness course of more than 3 months and is secondary to other respiratory diseases, especially pulmonary tuberculosis. Pulmonary aspergilloma is the advanced stage of CPA due to growth of aspergillus into cavity induced by pulmonary tuberculosis and formation of a sphere there. Because aspergilloma has typical and characteristic radiological demonstrations, its diagnosis can be made based on radiology. And histopathology is not necessary. In this case, the patient received early diagnosis and appropriate treatment due to the typical and characteristic radiological demonstrations.

Concerning treatment, surgical removal of aspergilloma is the optimal choice for patients without pulmonary function. Patients with severe hemoptysis should also be treated surgically. Before the operation, the cardiopulmonary functions of the patients should be carefully assessed, and assistant nutritional support should be given. Although combination of triazoles and other antifungal medication is recommended in the clinical guideline, no evidence has been found supporting surgery and mediations of triazoles for patients with solitude pulmonary aspergilloma. In this case, the patient received surgical removal of lung lobe but no antifungal medication. And the patient showed favorable therapeutic efficacy due to complete surgical removal of the lesion.

In this case, the successful treatment depends on sufficient knowledge about CPA by clinicians and timely surgical removal of the lesion. Early diagnosis was made based on chest CT scan due to sufficient knowledge about CPA by clinicians. And timely surgical removal of the lesion ensured successful treatment of the disease. In this case, in addition to surgical operation for pulmonary aspergilloma, further diagnosis and treatment of pulmonary tuberculosis should also be paid close attention.

12.12 Case 12: Hemoptysis for More Than 2 Years and Aggravation for 1 Day

Guoxin Huang, Mengjie Feng, Shusong Peng, Xiongfei Sun, Xueyan Liu, and Zhijian Yu

12.12.1 Presenting Symptom

Hemoptysis for more than 2 years and aggravation for 1 day.

12.12.2 Brief Case History

A 53-year-old man was admitted to our hospital due to complaints of hemoptysis for more than 2 years and aggravation for 1 day. Two years ago, the patient began to experience intermittent hemoptysis in a small quantity. But he experienced no fever, cough, expectoration, chest pain, and breathlessness. In a local hospital, he received chest CT scan, demonstrating secondary pulmonary tuberculosis of both lungs and formation of cavity at the left upper lung. He then presented in Shenzhen Infectious Disease Hospital, and the diagnosis was aspergillosis of the left upper lung and old pulmonary tuberculosis. Medications for fungal infection and hemostasis were administered (specifically unknown), and the symptoms were improved. One day before his admission to our hospital, he experienced hemoptysis again of fresh red blood in volume of 5 ml, with no chest distress, chest pain, flush, and night sweat. For further diagnosis and treatment, he presented in our hospital and was admitted on April 5, 2014. Since the onset of symptoms, his spiritual state, sleep, appetite, urinations, and bowel movements were normal. And he experienced no recent obvious weight loss.

12.12.2.1 Past Medical History

The patient had a past medical history of radial treatment for gastric cardia carcinoma in 2006, and the postoperative recovery was favorable.

12.12.2.2 Physical Examination

Physical examination showed a body temperature of 36.4 °C, pulse rate 76/min, respiration rate 21/min, and blood pressure BP116/64 mm. The patient was well conscious. The thorax was bilaterally symmetric, with no deformity. The bilateral vocal fremitus was symmetric. By percussion, both lungs showed clear sounds. By auscultation, both lungs showed clear respiration sounds, with no dry and/or moist rales. The heart was not enlarged, with heartbeat of 76/min, rhythmic. The heart sounds were normal.

12.12.2.3 Auxiliary Investigation

Laboratory Test

By routine blood test, WBC was 10.7 × 109/L, N 69.2%, and Hb 132 g/L. The blood electrolytes were normal. CEA was 1.130 ng/ml, CA125 32.4 U/ml, CA19-9 41.26 U/ml, cytokeratin 2.120 ng/ml, and neuron-specific enolase 8.730 ng/ml. The liver and kidney function tests showed no abnormality. The acid fast staining of sputum showed negative. The sputum TB-DNA was negative. And the sputum cultures for common bacteria, fungi, and tuberculosis mycobacteria were negative.

Radiology

Chest CT scan on November 22, 2011, is shown in Fig. 12.33.

Chest CT scan on April 8, 2014, is shown in Fig. 12.34.

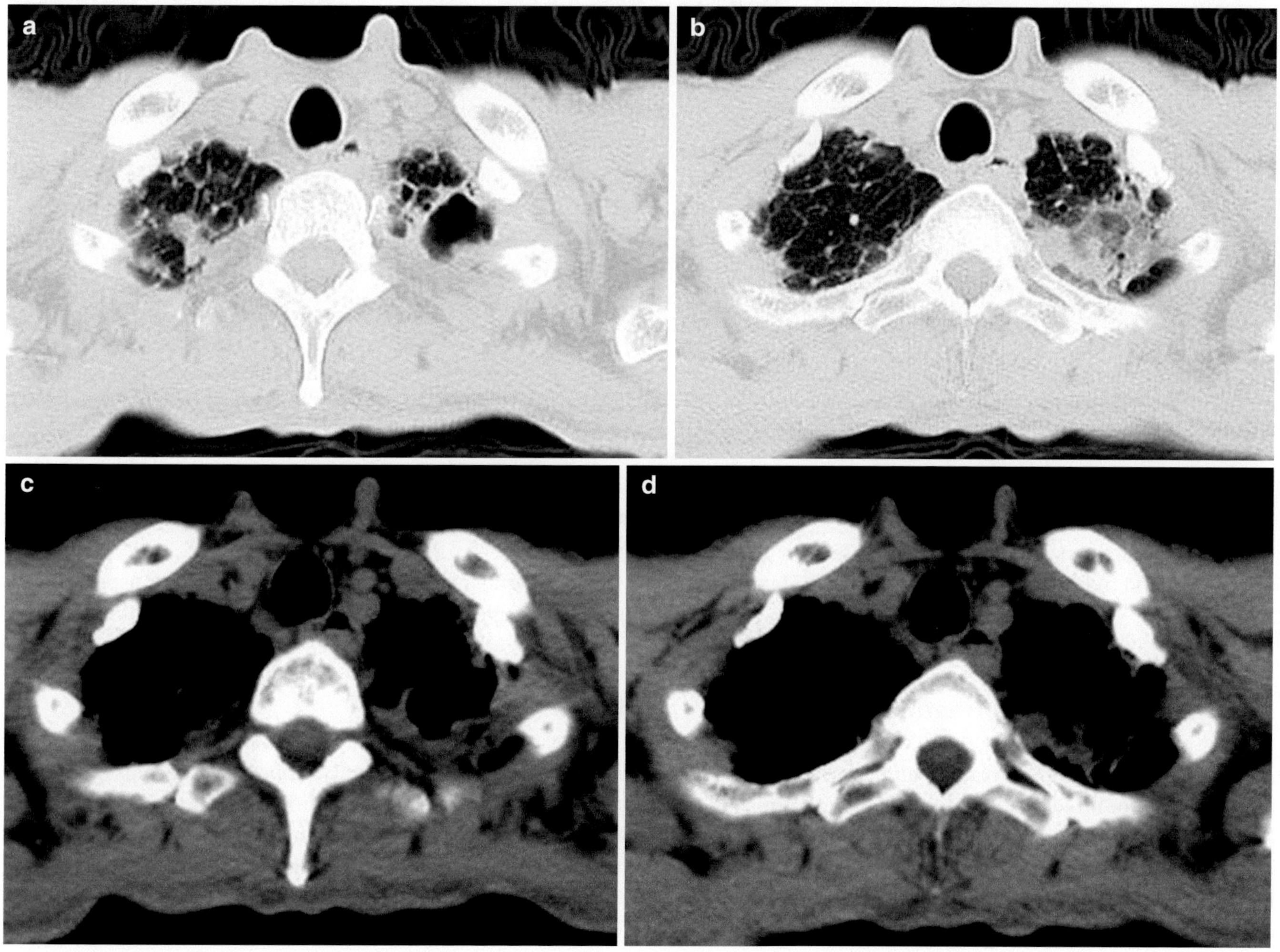

Fig. 12.33 (**a**–**d**) Chest CT scan. (**a**) The bilateral upper lungs are demonstrated with old cords opacity and small nodular opacity. And the apical segment of left upper lung lobe is demonstrated with thin wall cavity opacity. (**b**) A small spherical dense opacity is demonstrated in the dorsal thin wall cavity at the apical segment of left upper lung lobe. (**c**) The bilateral superior pleura are demonstrated to be thickened, and cords opacity with increased intensity is demonstrated at the bilateral lung apices. (**d**) A small nodular opacity is demonstrated in the dorsal thin wall cavity at the apical segment of left upper lung lobe

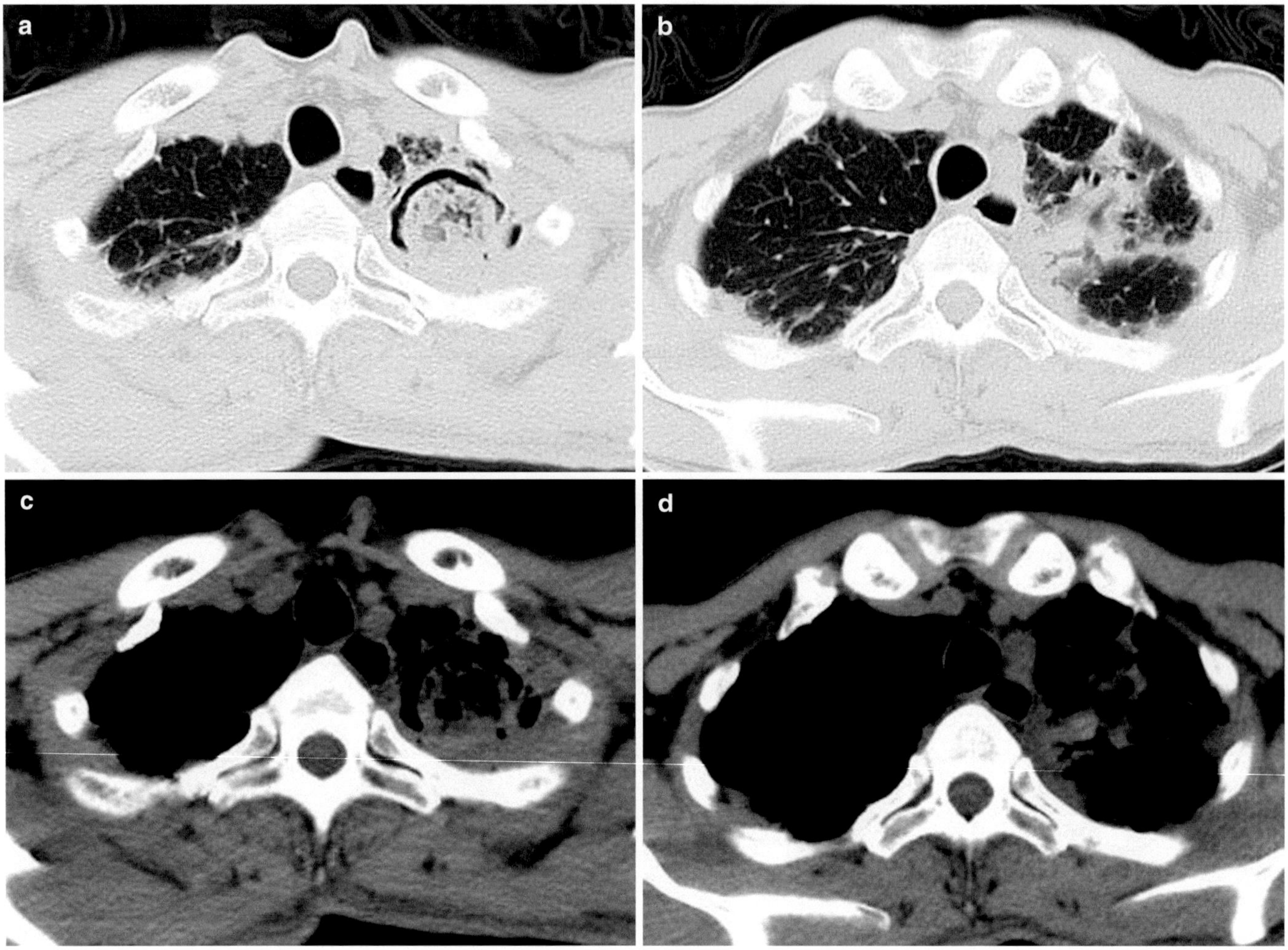

Fig. 12.34 (**a**–**d**) Chest CT scan. Compared to chest CT scan on November 2, 2011, the thin wall cavity at the apical segment of left upper lung lobe is enlarged, and the aspergilloma in the lung is enlarged, with obvious crescent sign. In addition, the scattering nodules in both lungs and nodular patchy opacities at the right middle lung lobe are increased in number

12.12.2.4 Initial Diagnosis

The initial diagnosis was aspergillus infection at the left upper lung and old pulmonary tuberculosis at bilateral upper lungs.

12.12.3 Diagnosis and Treatment

After admission, moxifloxacin and voriconazole were administered for infection, and pituitrin was administered for hemostasis. During his hospitalization, major hemoptysis occurred. And hemoptysis was improved by emergency interventional therapy, and the condition was stabilized. Thoracoscopic removal of left upper lung lobe, cautery of left pleural adhesion, and left intercostal nerve block were performed on July 21, 2014, under tracheal double-lumen intubation and general anesthesia. The postoperative pathology demonstrated fungal hyphae and spores in the specimen, which were morphologically consistent to pulmonary aspergillosis (Fig. 12.35).

The diagnosis on discharge was pulmonary aspergilloma at the left upper lung and old pulmonary tuberculosis.

12.12.4 Discussion

Based on their pathogenicity, fungi can be classified into pathogenic and conditional pathogenic. The pathogenicity of the conditional pathogenic fungi is weak, which cannot infect immunocompetent populations. However, immunocompetent populations can be infected via contacts to conditional pathogenic fungi in a large quantity, and immunocompromised populations are at high risk of their infection. In most cases, aspergillus is conditional pathogenic fungus, which tends to infect patients with lung disease, especially patients with pulmonary tuberculosis.

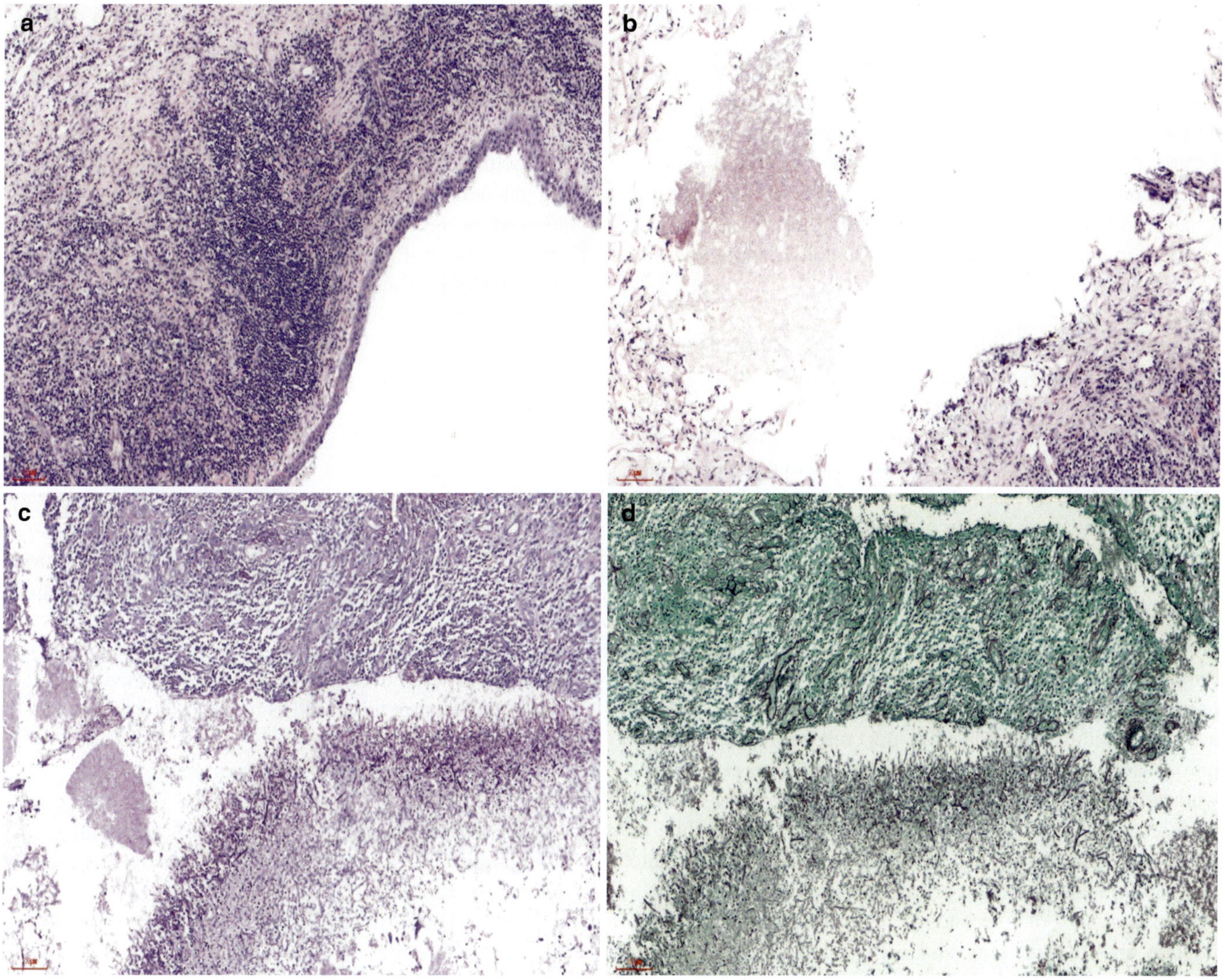

Fig. 12.35 (**a**–**d**) Pathology of lung tissue. (**a**) H&E staining demonstrates infiltration of many inflammatory cells around bronchus. (**b**) H&E staining demonstrates fungal hyphae in the cystic cavity. (**c**) PAS staining. (**d**) PASM staining

In China, the population with pulmonary tuberculosis is large, and the quantity of patients with pulmonary tuberculosis complicated by aspergilloma is considerable. In recent years, the incidence of aspergillosis has been increasing [57]. Aspergillus may invade each organ of human body, and it most commonly invades the bronchus and lung. Aspergillus-related respiratory disease can be approximately classified into three clinical types: allergic aspergillosis, aspergilloma, and invasive aspergillosis.

Patients with pulmonary tuberculosis are susceptible to pulmonary aspergillosis, and pathomechanism is summarized as the following:

1. Pulmonary tuberculosis is a chronic lung disease, with serious destruction of the lung tissue. The pathological change decreases the cleanup effect of the airway, and the fungi at the oropharynx move downward to invade the lung tissue. Most patients with pulmonary tuberculosis show formation of cavity, bronchiectasis, or atelectasis induced by obstruction, which cause obstructed drainage of secretions. The obstructed drainage of secretions provides favorable environment for planting and growth of aspergillus. In a large-scale literature review by Denning et al. [58], the global incidence of chronic pulmonary aspergillosis after pulmonary tuberculosis was estimated. The results showed that the lowest incidence of cavity in patients with pulmonary tuberculosis was 21% in the USA and its highest incidence was 35% in Taiwan, China. And patients with chronic pulmonary aspergillosis account for about 22% in patients with cavity induced by pulmonary tuberculosis.
2. Pulmonary tuberculosis is a chronic consumptive disease whose T-cell count and/or function decreases. The patients thus show compromised cellular immunity,

which causes increasing incidence of aspergillus infection [59].

3. Patients with pulmonary tuberculosis, especially when the condition is complicated by tubercular meningitis, a large dose of glucocorticoid is administered, which compromise the immunity of the patients.
4. Combined use of multiple antituberculosis medications and the use of wide-spectrum antibiotics tend to cause flora imbalance. And the conditional pathogenic fungi tend to take the chance to invade.

Pulmonary aspergillus infection radiologically resembles to pulmonary tuberculosis. Therefore, the diagnosis of pulmonary tuberculosis complicated by aspergillus infection is challenging. And the condition tends to be misdiagnosed. The chest CT scan demonstrations of primary pulmonary aspergillosis are different from those of secondary pulmonary aspergillosis. A research study [60] has demonstrated that the lesion of primary pulmonary aspergillus infection may be singular or multiple nodular or mass-like opacity by chest CT scan, with or with no crescent sign. There are also ground-glass opacity and rare occurrence of mediastinal lymphadenectasis. The lesions are commonly located at the periphery of both lungs [61]. The lesions of primary pulmonary aspergillus infection with no crescent sign are commonly located at the upper lung lobe, presented as well-defined singular nodule or mass. The obvious features include central low intensity of the consolidated nodule or mass and surrounding ground-glass opacity, namely, halo sign, around many nodules or masses. Typical chest CT scan demonstrations of secondary pulmonary aspergillosis include air crescent sign and rolling-ball sign. Enhanced scan demonstrates no obvious enhancement. Air crescent sign is the characteristic demonstration of aspergilloma, which is presented as crescent-shaped translucent area around the nodular opacity or spherical opacity. Rolling-ball sign is demonstrated due to movable aspergilloma along with body postures. Pulmonary aspergilloma should be differentiated from the following pulmonary disease with formation of cavity:

1. Tuberculous cavity with tuberculoma. The content in tuberculous cavity is commonly irregular with heterogeneous density. Without calcification, its density is higher than non-calcified aspergilloma. The average CT value of pulmonary aspergilloma is 2.56 Hu, and in most cases, the CT value is lower than 20 Hu. However, the average CT value in the cases of pulmonary tuberculosis or lung carcinoma is above 35 Hu, and in most cases, the CT value is above 20 Hu. The CT value in the cases of pulmonary tuberculosis and lung carcinoma is obviously higher than that in the cases of pulmonary aspergilloma.
2. Lung carcinomatous cavity. Lung carcinomatous cavity is demonstrated as lobulated mass, eccentric cavity, and short dense spikes at the margin. There are also pleural indentation sign and involved adjacent mediastinum.
3. Cavity induced by pulmonary abscess. There are thick wall with liquid level but no air crescent sign. The radiological demonstrations of pulmonary tuberculosis complicated by pulmonary aspergillus infection are diverse. The radiology of the two diseases resembles, and it tends to be misdiagnosed. The diagnosis should be based on clinical symptoms, radiology, mycological investigations, and biopsy. The characteristic radiological signs are helpful for the definitive diagnosis, which have great clinical significance.

12.12.5 Comments

This is a typical case of pulmonary tuberculosis complicated by pulmonary aspergillosis. And the patient has the following clinical features:

1. The patient was an elderly man, with past medical histories of pulmonary tuberculosis and formation of cavity at the left upper lung.
2. The presenting symptom is recurrent hemoptysis.
3. Chest CT scan demonstrated enlarged thin wall cavity opacity at the apical segment of the left upper lung lobe and spherical dense opacity inside the cavity, with obvious air crescent sign.
4. Pathology demonstrated fungal hyphae and spores in the tissue of left upper lung, which were morphologically consistent to aspergillosis.

Based on the diagnostic criteria in clinical guideline issued by ESCMID/ERS, the diagnosis was defined to be chronic (saprophytic) pulmonary aspergillosis. Chronic (saprophytic) pulmonary aspergillosis mainly includes two clinical types, pulmonary aspergilloma and chronic cavitary pulmonary aspergillosis. It commonly occurs in cavity induced by pulmonary tuberculosis, bronchiectasis, pulmonary abscess, and bronchopulmonary abscess. According to literature report, the incidence of hemoptysis in patients with pulmonary aspergilloma is up to 90%, with a blood volume ranging from a small quantity to fatally large quantity. Therefore, its diagnosis should also be based on differentiation from abovementioned primary diseases.

We failed to obtain the clinical data of his past pulmonary tuberculosis. However, based on chest CT scan in a local hospital, the lung window demonstrated thin wall cavity at the apical segment of left upper lung lobe and a small spherical dense opacity at its dorsal inner part. In addition, the mediastinum window demonstrated a small nodular opacity in dorsal part of a thin wall cavity at the apical segment of left upper lung lobe. Both indicated possible existence of aspergillus infection. But the initial diagnosis in that local hospital was secondary pulmonary tuberculosis of both lungs and formation of cavity in the left upper lung. Pulmonary aspergillus infection was not considered, indicating insufficient knowledge about pulmonary tuberculosis complicated by pulmonary aspergillus infection by the clinicians.

When the patient presented in Shenzhen Infectious Disease Hospital, the diagnosis was considered as aspergillosis of the left upper lung and old pulmonary tuberculosis. And after treatment for fungal infection and hemostasis, the symptoms were improved. It is obvious that the physician suspected the condition as pulmonary aspergillus infection. But the diagnosis was only clinical diagnosis or suspected diagnosis. Microbiology and percutaneous lung puncture for biopsy should be actively performed to define the diagnosis. When the patients are clinically diagnosed with pulmonary aspergillus infection, microbiological and pathological evidence should be actively collected for definitive diagnosis.

In this case, the patient had a definitive past medical history of pulmonary tuberculosis and formation of cavity at the left upper lung. He experienced recurrent hemoptysis for more than 2 years, with obvious clinical symptoms. Chest CT scan demonstrated enlarged cavity and aspergilloma at left upper lung, indicating progressively aggravating condition. These are not consistent to the clinical feature of pulmonary aspergilloma, such as slight clinical symptoms and chronic progression of the condition. Therefore, the authors believe that the diagnosis should be chronic cavitary pulmonary aspergillosis of left upper lung.

It is currently believed that antifungal medication can hardly permeate into the cavity containing aspergilloma and systemic administration of antifungal medication thus shows unfavorable therapeutic efficacy. For the patients with pulmonary aspergilloma but no bleeding, clinical observation should be performed. And for patients with pulmonary aspergilloma as well as frequent or large quantity hemoptysis, surgical removal of the lesion is recommended. For the patients with basic disease or lung dysfunction who are not tolerant to surgery, bronchial artery embolization can be performed for hemostasis. But due to abundant lateral circulation of aspergilloma, hemoptysis may relapse after bronchial artery embolization. Therefore, surgery can still be performed for patients with improved condition but recurrent hemoptysis after bronchial artery embolization. In this case, hemoptysis was gradually decreased after emergency interventional therapy. After the condition was stabilized, surgical removal of left upper lung was performed, and the therapeutic efficacy was favorable.

The analysis of this case is intended to raise clinicians' awareness about aspergilloma that complicates cavity induced by pulmonary tuberculosis, bronchiectasis, pulmonary abscess, and bronchopulmonary abscess.

12.13 Case 13: Recurrent Cough and Hemoptysis for 3 Years and Onset Again for 1 Month

Yuemei Lu, Zhengqiang He, Xia Huang, Xiongfei Sun, Chang'e Jin, and Xueyan Liu

12.13.1 Presenting Symptom

Recurrent cough and hemoptysis for 3 years and onset again for 1 month.

12.13.2 Brief Case History

A 58-year-old man was admitted to our hospital on July 29, 2013, due to complaints of recurrent cough and hemoptysis for 3 years and onset again for 1 month. Three years ago, the patient began to experience recurrent paroxysmal cough and accompanying hemoptysis of fresh red blood in a volume of about 10 ml. He experienced no fever, aversion to cold, chest pain, chest distress, breathlessness, night sweat, and emaciation. In a local hospital, anti-infection therapy and treatment for hemostasis were administered. And the symptoms of cough and hemoptysis were improved but repeatedly onset. One month ago, the patient experienced paroxysmal cough and hemoptysis of fresh red blood in a large quantity again. And he presented in Shenzhen Hospital of Chinese Medicine, and chest CT scan demonstrated bronchiectasis and formation of cavity at the right upper lung, with a round-like soft tissue intensity mass opacity in an inner diameter of about 26 mm inside, and fibrosis at the left upper lung and right middle lung. Therapies for infection, elimination of sputum, and hemostasis were administered. But the symptoms were not improved. For further diagnosis and treatment, he presented in our hospital and was admitted.

He reported no special past medical history and personal history.

12.13.2.1 Physical Examination

Physical examination showed a body temperature of 36.3 °C, respiration rate 20/min, pulse rate 86/min, and blood pressure 110/85 mmHg. The systemic superficial lymph nodes were not enlarged. By palpation, the bilateral thoracic vocal fremitus was symmetric. The sternum showed no tenderness. Respirations were normal. The respiration sounds of both lungs were coarse, and the right upper lung showed less moist rales. The heart was not enlarged. The heartbeat was

86/min, rhythmic. By auscultation, there was no pathological murmur.

12.13.2.2 Auxiliary Investigation

Laboratory Test

Routine blood test showed WBC 4.93 × 109/L, N% 63.9%, and L% 19.5%. Hs-CRP was 17.60 mg/L and ESR 17.00 mm/h. The antibodies against HIV and syphilis showed negative.

Radiology

Chest CT scan on August 1, 2013, is shown in Fig. 12.36.

12.13.2.3 Initial Diagnosis

The initial diagnosis was cavity at the right upper lung with formation of aspergilloma and bronchiectasis.

12.13.3 Diagnosis and Treatment

After admission, the patient was initially diagnosed with formation of cavity at the right upper lung and possible aspergilloma. Because the patient experienced persistent hemoptysis, thoracoscopic removal of the right upper lung was performed on August 5, 2013. The postoperative pathology demonstrated a lung tissue in size of about 12.5 cm × 8 cm × 4.5 cm, with oval-shaped grayish white cavity in size of about 3.5 cm × 2 cm near pleura. The thickness of the cavity wall was 1–5 mm. The cavity wall showed fibrosis and thickening near pleura. Under a microscope, the lung tissue was demonstrated with chronic inflammation and partial proliferation of fibrous tissue. There was formation of cavity, with fungal mass and infiltration of many neutrophile granulocytes inside. The hyphae had uniform thickness, with branching in about 45° angle, many transverse septa, and oriented arrangement. There were also small round spores. By special staining, PAS staining showed positive and methenamine silver staining showed positive (Fig. 12.37).

The final diagnosis was chronic cavitary pulmonary aspergillosis at the right upper lung and bronchiectasis.

Postoperative medication of voriconazole was administered intravenously in a dose of 200 mg, twice a day, for 1 week. And the postoperative recovery was favorable, and the patient was discharged home. After discharge, oral intake of voriconazole was continued as sequential therapy.

12.13.4 Discussion

Pulmonary aspergillosis was firstly reported by Deve in the year of 1938. It is mainly exogenous infection and is mostly caused by inhalation of aspergillus via respiratory tract. The most common pathogenic aspergillus is *Aspergillus fumigatus*. Pulmonary aspergillosis is a clinically rare pulmonary infection. However, due to wide applications of wide-spectrum antibiotics and immunosuppressant as well as increasing patients receiving organ transplantation, the incidence of pulmonary aspergillosis has been increasing in recent years [29, 62, 63]. Clinically, pulmonary aspergillosis is classified into invasive pulmonary aspergillosis, allergic pulmonary aspergillosis, and parasitic pulmonary aspergillosis [64].

Parasitic pulmonary aspergillosis is the most common type of pulmonary aspergillus infection, including aspergilloma and chronic cavitary pulmonary aspergillosis, which is caused by parasitism of aspergillus in the cavity or cavitary lesion of the lung. It commonly occurs based on cured pulmonary tuberculosis, cavitary bronchiectasis, or pulmonary abscess. It also occurs in individuals with no basic disease. The clinical symptoms are non-specific, including common symptoms of cough and hemoptysis and rare symptoms of chest pain and breathlessness. In some cases, accompanying systemic symptoms may occur, such as weight loss and fatigue. The blood that the patients cough up is mostly from rupture and bleeding of bronchial artery, which is commonly intermittent and self-limited. But when the lesion enlarges, major bleeding may occur [65]. In this case, the patient had no basic disease. And during his repeated presentations in hospitals, fungal infection was not considered, and appropriate treatment to control the symptoms was delayed. Therefore, for patients with recurrent cough and hemoptysis, the common reasons such as pulmonary tuberculosis and bronchiectasis should be considered. In addition, investigations for fungal infection should also be performed for early intervention.

Multilayer spiral CT scan is an important technology for the diagnosis of pulmonary aspergillosis. The radiological demonstrations of pulmonary aspergillosis are diverse, including cavity, air crescent sign, nodular and wedge-shaped consolidation, pleural thickening, halo sign, and linear scar opacity. During early stage of invasion by aspergillus, the aspergillus destructs the minor vascular vessels and bronchus of the lung to cause hemorrhagic infarction of the lung. Therefore, within the first 1–2 weeks of pulmonary aspergillosis, CT scan demonstrates characteristic halo sign. And the halo sign and multiple inflammations and nodules in both lungs are commonly demonstrated at the early stage of the lesions. When aspergilloma reproduces and grows in the cavity, a space between aspergilloma and the cavity wall exists to form crescent sign, which is commonly demonstrated at the absorption or advanced stage of the lesions. Air crescent sign is a characteristic CT scan demonstration of chronic (saprophytic) pulmonary aspergillosis [66], which has diagnostic significance for chronic (saprophytic) pulmonary aspergillosis. In this case, the lung CT scan demonstrated

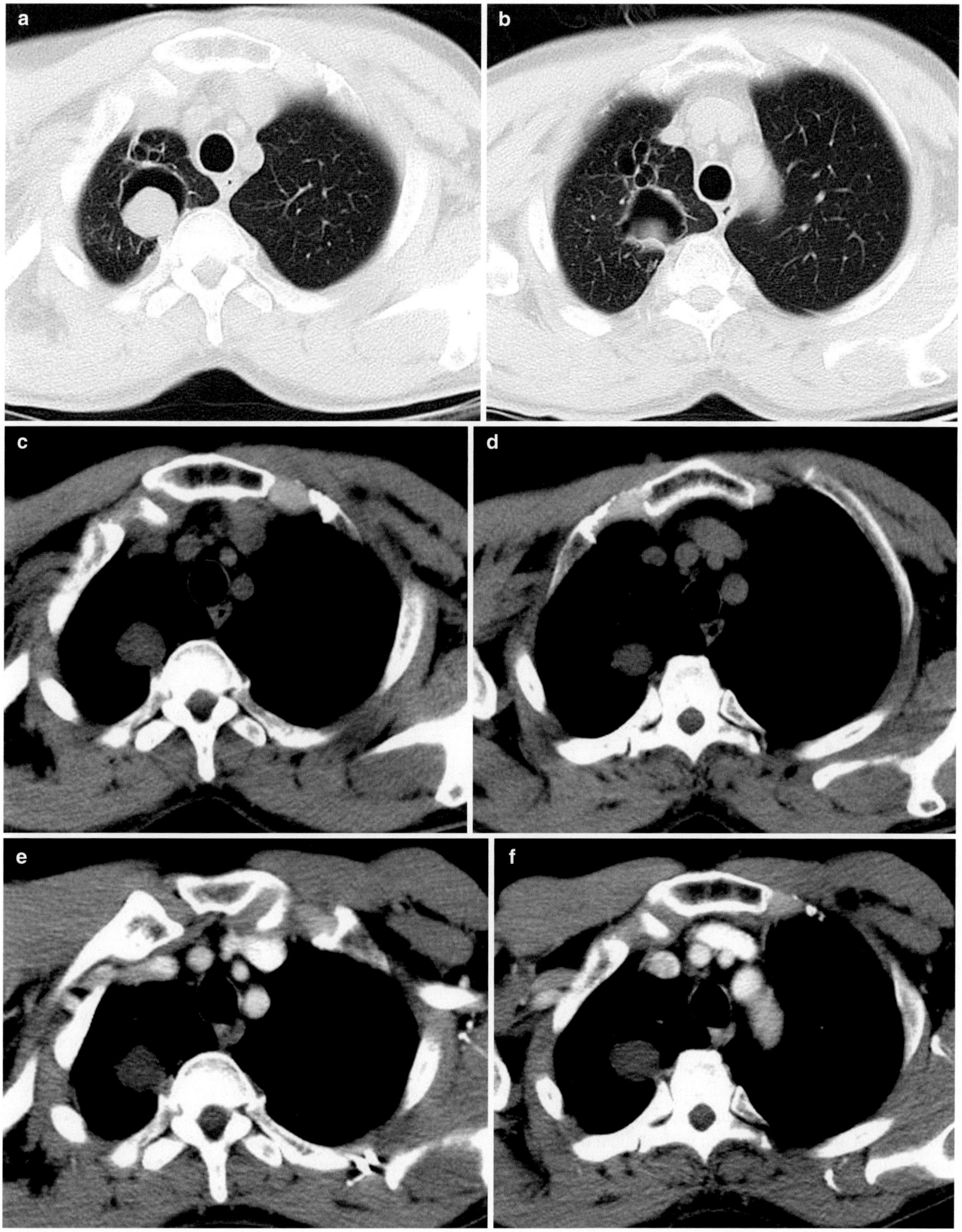

Fig. 12.36 (**a**–**f**) Chest CT scan. (**a**, **b**) The lung window demonstrates cavity opacity at the right upper lung, with a round-like nodular opacity of soft tissue intensity in a diameter of about 26 mm inside. The nodular opacity has a CT value of about 22 Hu. (**c**, **d**) The mediastinum window demonstrates well-marginated nodular opacity of increased intensity at the right upper lung, and its density is homogeneous. (**e**, **f**) Enhanced CT scan demonstrates no obvious enhancement of the lesions

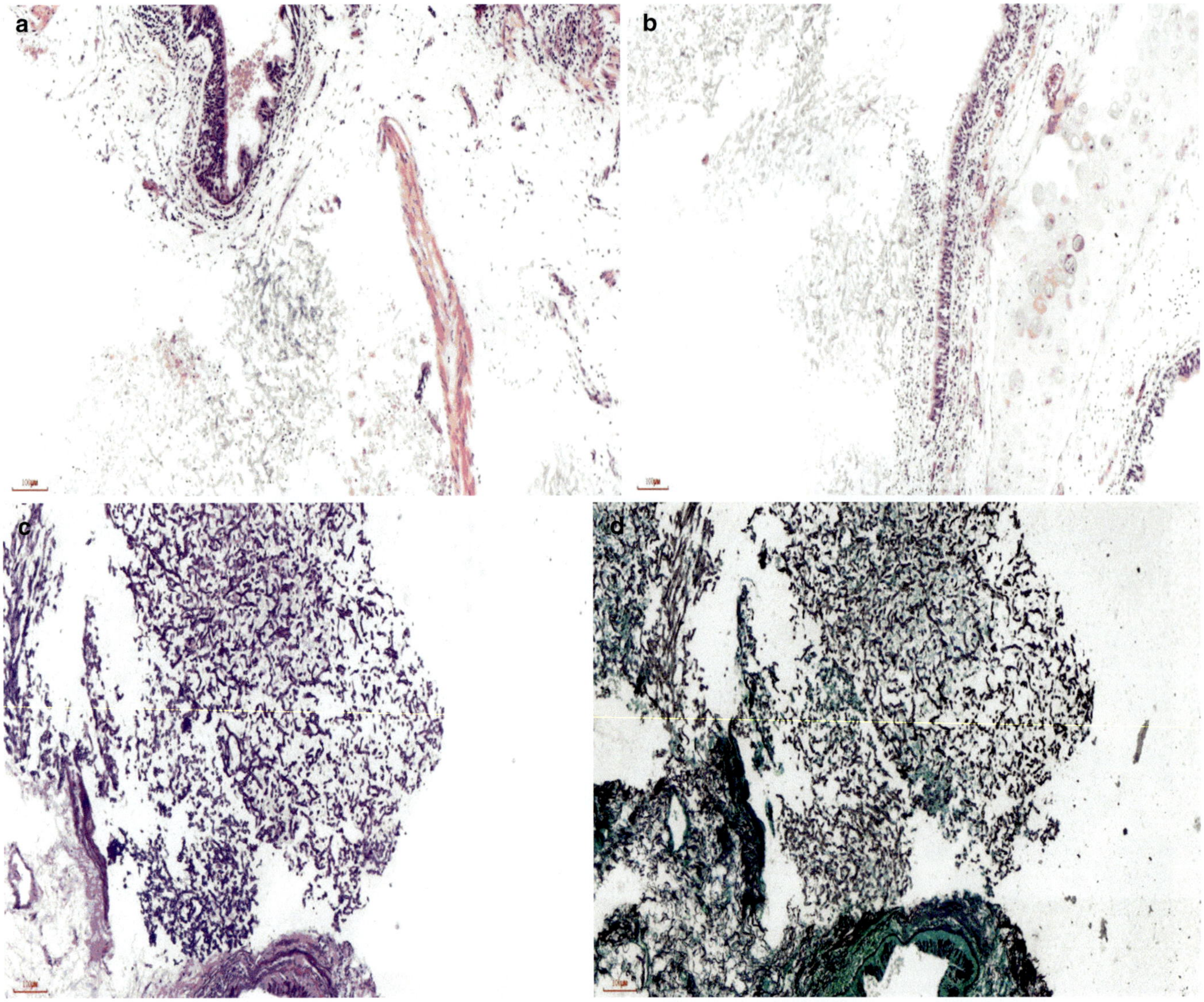

Fig. 12.37 (**a–d**) Pathology of lung tissue. (**a**) H&E staining demonstrates formation of cavity in lung tissue and aspergillus hyphae in the cavity. (**b**) H&E staining demonstrates formation of cavity in lung tissue and aspergillus hyphae in the cavity. (**c**) PAS staining. (**d**) PASM staining

bronchiectasis of the right upper lung with formation of cavity. And there was round soft tissue intensity mass opacity in the cavity, which presented typical demonstrations. Although multilayer spiral CT greatly facilitates the diagnosis of pulmonary aspergillosis, typical and characteristic signs are not always demonstrated due to the diverse radiological demonstrations of pulmonary aspergillosis. The final diagnosis should be based on its combination with clinical data as well as microbiology or histopathology. In this case, the diagnosis was finally defined based on postoperative pathology.

The lesion of chronic (saprophytic) pulmonary aspergillosis by pathology is mixture of aspergillus hyphae, fibrin, mucus, and necrotic cell fragments that is located within the cavity in the lung or dilated bronchus. The cavity wall and surrounding lung tissues are partially destructed, and there is no invasion into deep lung tissue [67]. In addition, histopathology is also golden standard in differentiating chronic necrotizing pulmonary aspergillosis from chronic (saprophytic) pulmonary aspergillosis. Both diseases show aspergillus hyphae with branching in sharp angle and septa. However, in the cases of chronic necrotizing pulmonary aspergillosis, aspergillus may infiltrate the lung tissue to cause tissue bleeding and necrosis as well as formation of microabscess and infiltration of inflammatory cells. And in the cases of chronic (saprophytic) pulmonary aspergillosis, aspergillus only grows in the cavity or cyst. In this case, the pathology of lung tissue demonstrated chronic inflammation, with proliferation of fibrous tissue in some areas, which supported the diagnosis of pulmonary aspergilloma.

In the cases of chronic (saprophytic) pulmonary aspergillosis, the lesion is located within the cavity, and the antifungal medication can hardly permeate into the thick wall of the cavity to achieve favorable therapeutic efficacy. Therefore, the antifungal medication shows limited therapeutic efficacy. In addition to completely eliminating the lesion, surgery can also provide basis for definitive diagnosis. Therefore, surgery is the main way of treatment for chronic (saprophytic) pulmonary aspergillosis [68]. Surgical removal of the lung lobe is the main surgical approach for chronic (saprophytic) pulmonary aspergillosis. It has been indicated in the clinical guideline that surgery is effective for patients with the lesion adjacent to major vascular vessel or pericardium, patients with hemoptysis induced by singular lesion, or patients with involved thoracic wall. In a literature report, scholars believed that for patients who tolerate to surgery or even asymptomatic patients, early surgical removal of the lesion is recommended to avoid major hemoptysis and to provide a chance of permanent cure [69]. However, surgical removal of the lesion may induce serious complications. For patients with accompanying diseases or patient with pulmonary dysfunction, surgery shows limited value. For patients with contraindications of surgery, clinicians can attempt percutaneous injection of antifungal medication into the cavity. But such a therapy has low success rate [8]. In addition, bronchial artery embolization is currently applied to temporarily control hemoptysis. In this case, the lesion is localized, and the patient experienced recurrent hemoptysis. Combination treatment of antifungal medication and surgery was performed. Based on such a therapy, the diagnosis was defined, and the lesion was eliminated. The treatment achieved favorable therapeutic efficacy.

12.13.5 Comments

Cough and hemoptysis are the common clinical symptoms. In clinical practice, differential diagnosis should be carefully made to avoid missed diagnosis and misdiagnosis. In this case, the patient was an elderly man, with presenting complaints of recurrent cough and hemoptysis for 3 years. In a local hospital, therapies for infection and hemostasis were administered, which were inappropriate. For patients with cough and hemoptysis, especially the elderly patients, neoplasm, tuberculosis, and bronchiectasis should be carefully excluded. And chronic pulmonary aspergillosis should also be differentiated. According to literature report, recurrent hemoptysis presents in about 30–90% cases of chronic pulmonary aspergillosis.

In this case, the patient suffered from typical chronic cavitary pulmonary aspergillosis secondary to bronchiectasis. Chest CT after admission demonstrated cystic and spherical dilation of the air containing bronchus in the right upper lung, with clustering of multiple cysts, which are typical demonstration of bronchiectasis. In combination to the case history, the clinical diagnosis of bronchiectasis can be established. Chest CT scan also demonstrated nodular opacity with increased intensity at the right upper lung, which was homogeneous in intensity and well marginated. Around the nodular lesion, there was typical air crescent sign. According to literature report, air crescent sign is the characteristic CT scan demonstration of chronic pulmonary aspergillosis, which has diagnostic significance for chronic pulmonary aspergillosis. In this case, pathology after surgical removal of the right upper lung demonstrated a large quantity of aspergillus hyphae. Based on the comprehensive analysis of clinical data, the diagnosis was defined as chronic cavitary pulmonary aspergillosis. Previous literature report has indicated that chronic cavitary pulmonary aspergillosis is a common type of pulmonary aspergillus infection, which is commonly secondary to bronchiectasis, cavity of pulmonary tuberculosis, pulmonary abscess, bronchopulmonary cyst, or other pulmonary disease.

The treatment of chronic cavitary pulmonary aspergillosis remains controversial. Some scholars believe that asymptomatic patients should be only observed and patients with slight hemoptysis should receive palliative therapy. However, chronic cavitary pulmonary aspergillosis can hardly be self-cured, and about 30% patients with slight hemoptysis may develop fatal major hemoptysis. Therefore, for patients with generally good condition and tolerance to surgery, surgical removal of the lesion remains to be the optimal therapy. Thoracoscopy has advantages of less intraoperative bleeding, noninvasiveness, and rapid recovery. In this case, the patient received thoracoscopy, which facilitated definitive diagnosis and eliminating the lesion. After the surgery, medication of voriconazole was administered as sequential therapy, which achieved favorable therapeutic efficacy.

The analysis and comments of this case is intended to raise clinicians' awareness about the radiological demonstrations and therapies for chronic cavitary pulmonary aspergillosis.

12.14 Case 14: Recurrent Cough and Expectoration for 19 Years and Aggravation with Hemoptysis for 7 Days

Ying-Yun Fu, Wei Gao, Lukun Zhang, Jian Yang, Budong Chen, and Xueyan Liu

12.14.1 Presenting Symptom

Recurrent cough and expectoration for 19 years and aggravation with hemoptysis for 7 days.

12.14.2 Brief Case History

A 46-year-old man was admitted to our hospital on May 20, 2009, due to complaints of recurrent cough and expectoration for 19 years and aggravation with hemoptysis for 7 days. Nineteen years ago, the patient began to experience recurrent cough. In a local hospital, he was diagnosed with pulmonary tuberculosis, and he received standard antituberculosis therapy (specifically unknown) for 1 year. But cough and expectoration onset again and again. Seven days ago, he began to experience aggravating cough and expectoration due to catching a cold, and there was dark red blood streak in the sputum. And in a local hospital, symptomatic support for infection and hemostasis showed unfavorable therapeutic efficacy. And the blood he coughed up was increasing, to 40 ml per day. For further diagnosis and treatment, he presented in our hospital and was admitted to the thoracic surgery department. Since the onset of symptoms, he experienced no fever, night sweat, and flush after noons. His spiritual state, appetite, and sleep were average. His bowel movements were normal. And he experienced weight loss of 2.5 kg during recent 1 week.

12.14.2.1 Past Medical History

He reported no histories of hypertension, coronary disease, and diabetes. The patient denied histories of hepatitis and other infectious diseases. And he had no histories of surgery, trauma, and blood transfusion.

12.14.2.2 Physical Examination

Physical examination showed a body temperature of 36 °C, pulse rate 79/min, respiration rate 21/min, and blood pressure 101/66 mmHg. He was typically developed and well conscious. And he was emaciated, with appearance of chronic disease. He was in active position and well cooperated with the physical examination. The systemic superficial lymph nodes were not palpable and not enlarged. The trachea was at the midline. And the thorax was bilaterally symmetric with no deformity. By percussion, both lungs showed clear sounds. The respiration sounds of left upper lung were weak, and the respiration sounds of the other lung fields were clear. Both lungs showed no dry and/or moist rales. The heartbeat was 79/min, rhythmic. The valvular areas showed no pathological murmur. The abdomen was soft, with no tenderness and rebound pain. The liver and spleen were subcostally unpalpable. Both lower limbs showed no edema. And there was no clubbing finger.

12.14.2.3 Auxiliary Investigation

Chest CT scan on November 3, 2008, demonstrated chronic fibro-cavitary pulmonary tuberculosis with accompanying possible aspergilloma and formation of bullae of the lung (Fig. 12.38).

12.14.2.4 Initial Diagnosis

The initial diagnosis was suspected chronic cavitary pulmonary tuberculosis at the left upper lung, suspected aspergillosis at the left upper lung, and suspected bronchiectasis.

12.14.3 Diagnosis and Treatment

Investigations after admission showed WBC 6.4 × 109/L, N 4.80 × 109/L, E 0.1 × 109/L, RBC 4.55 × 109/L, Hb 144 g/L, and PLT 183 × 109/L. The liver function test showed GPT 25 U/L, GOT 23 U/L, T-BILI 9.5 μmmol/L, TP 68.1 g/L, and ALB 35.4 g/L. The BUN was 5.9 mmol/L and CR 72 μmmol/L. The complement C4 was 0.684 g/L and complement C3 1.11 g/L. The IgA was 1.69 g/L, IgM 0.7 g/L, and IgG 9.75 g/L. The blood coagulation function was normal. The antinuclear antibody was negative. And PPD skin test showed positive. The urine chemical qualification showed protein 0.75 g/L. And 24 h urine protein quantification was 158 mg.

After admission, levofloxacin was given for infection and thrombin for hemostasis. But the symptoms were not obviously relieved, and the patient still experienced intermittent hemoptysis. The sputum smear showed acid fast staining negative, common bacteria negative, and common fungi negative. The sputum culture showed growth of molds in a small quantity. Reexamination of chest CT scan on May 21, 2009, demonstrated chronic fibro-cavitary pulmonary tuberculosis with suspected formation of aspergilloma and bullae of the lung (Fig. 12.39).

To define the diagnosis, fibrobronchoscopy was performed on May 22, 2009. Fibrobronchoscopy demonstrated sharp trachea carina, yellowish white purulent secretions at the trachea as well as left and right bronchus, and mucosal congestion after aspiration of the secretions. The bronchial branches were unobstructed, with no neoplasm and luminal stenosis. The endoscopic diagnosis was mucosal inflammatory changes at trachea and bronchi under fibrobronchoscopy (Fig. 12.40). Fibrobronchoscopic brushing for cytology demonstrated small quantities of ciliated columnar epithelial cells and squamous cells, with many neutrophile granulocytes but no neoplasm cells. The smear showed no bacteria, fungi, and tuberculosis mycobacteria.

Because the patient experienced intermittent hemoptysis, thoracoscopic removals of the left upper lung lobe and dorsal segment of left lower lung lobe were performed on June 2, 2009, under general anesthesia. Pathology of dissected lung tissue demonstrated multiple fungal masses in diameter of about 3–5 cm, with densely arranged hyphae and spores. The hyphae twined into mass to invade the surrounding tissues and thus the mass was poorly defined. There were infiltration of many inflammatory cells, purulent necrosis, and accompanying lung hemorrhage in the surrounding tissue.

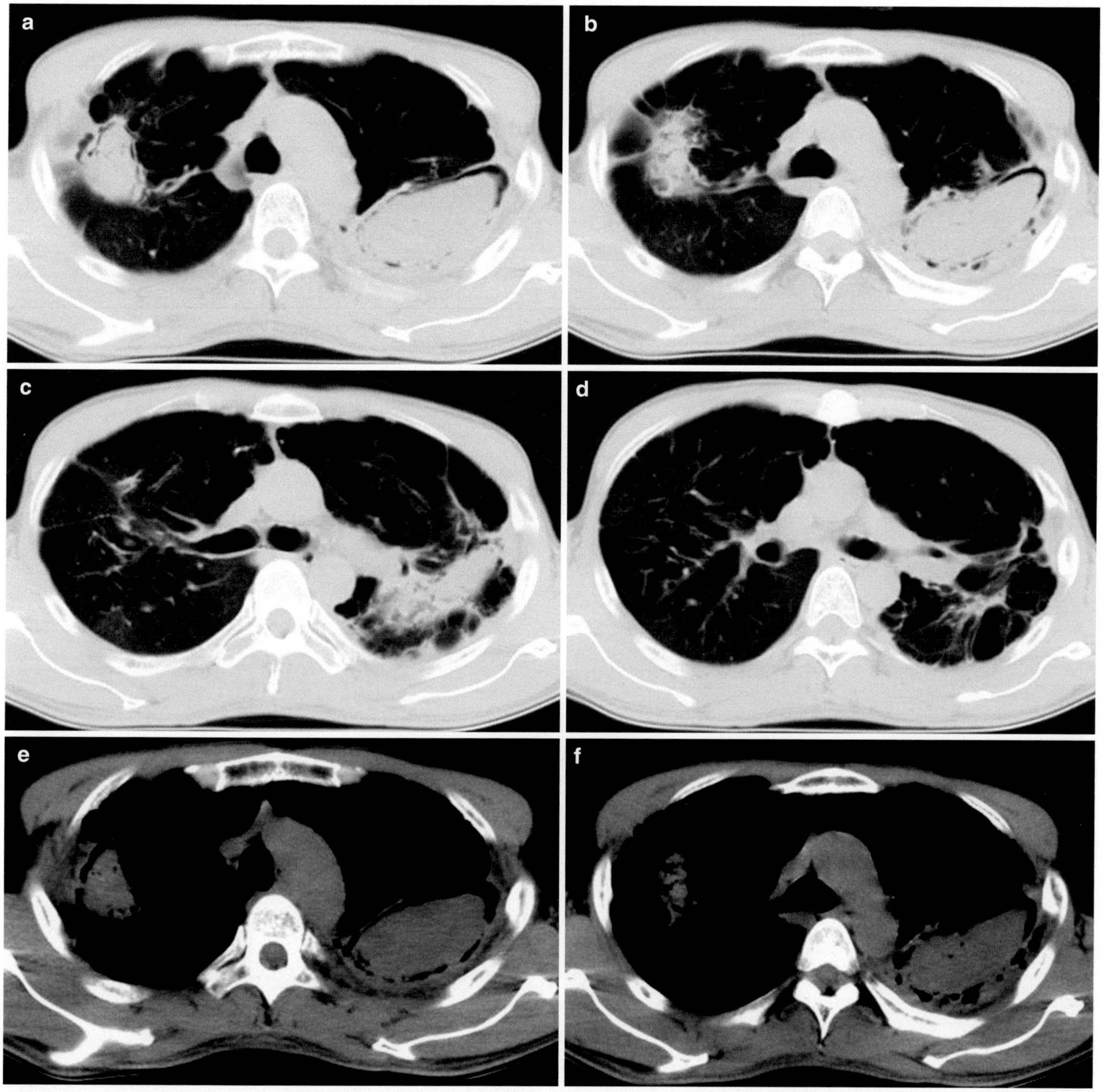

Fig. 12.38 (a–f) Chest CT scan. (**a**) Bilateral upper lungs are demonstrated with large thick wall cavity lesions, with homogeneous soft tissue intensity opacity inside, and air crescent sign. (**b**) Around the cavity lesions in bilateral upper lungs, there are fibrous strips and bundles of lesions. (**c**) The pleura adjacent to lesions at bilateral upper lungs shows thickening and adhesion. (**d**) There is formation of lung bullae at the right middle lung lobe and left lower lung. (**e**, **f**) The mediastinum window demonstrates opacity with increased intensity in both lungs, and irregular small translucent area around the mass soft tissue opacity at the left upper lung

Microscopy after methenamine silver staining demonstrated brownish black hyphae that arranged in filiform or radiating form. The hyphae were even in thickness with a diameter of about 5–7 μm. The bilateral hyphae walls were parallel, and the hyphae have septa and branching in 45° angle. There were scattering spores. By PAS staining, there were reddish purple hyphae walls (Fig. 12.41). In the specimen, there were lung tissues and contents of lung cavity, with many fungal masses. The lung tissue was demonstrated with extensive fibrosis and infiltrations of many plasmocytes and lymphocytes. The lesion was consistent to pulmonary aspergillosis.

After the surgery, oral intake of itraconazole was prescribed for fungal infection. The condition was stabilized, and the patient was discharged on July 14. After discharge,

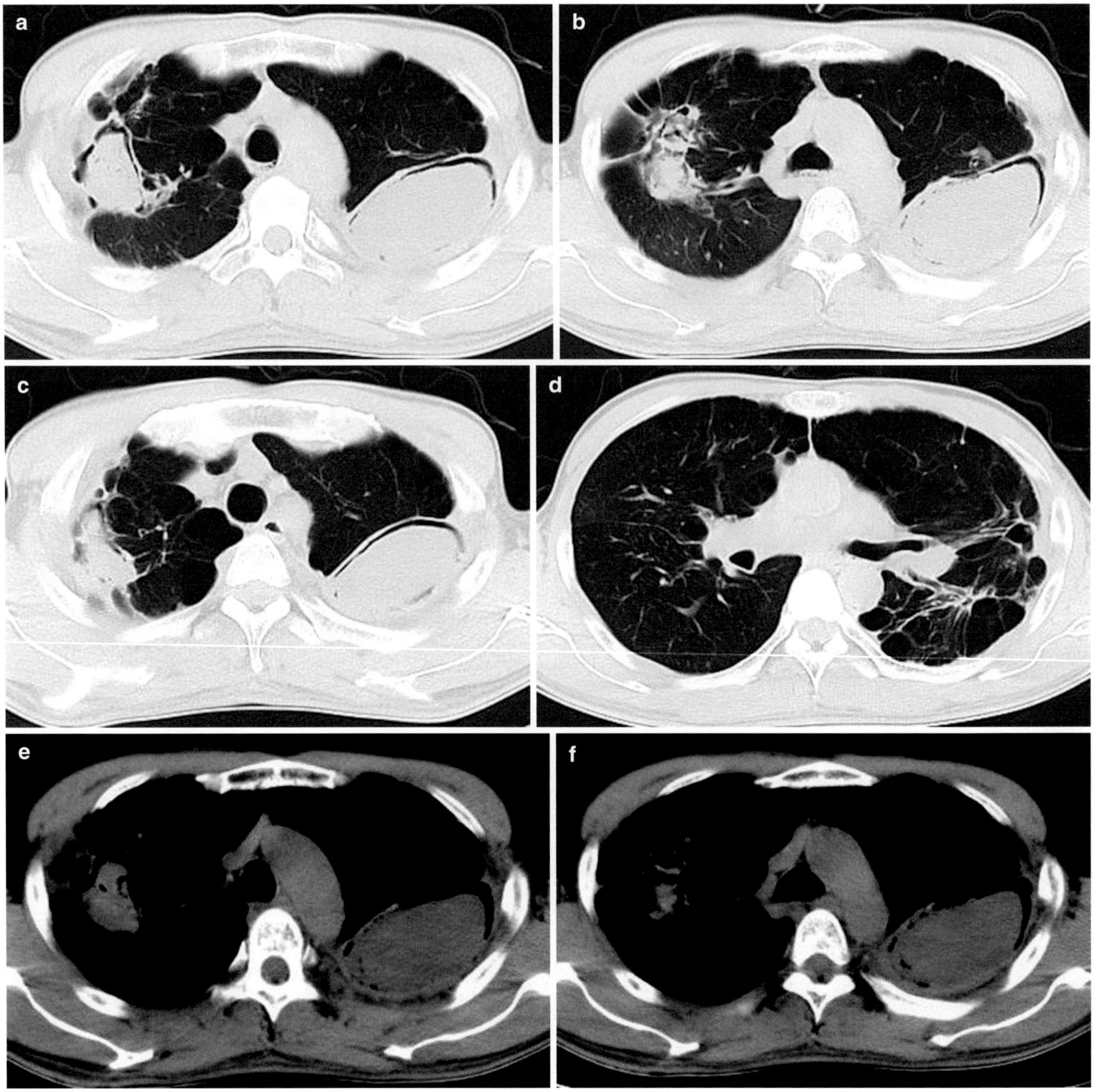

Fig. 12.39 (**a**–**f**) Chest CT scan. (**a**) The bilateral upper lungs are demonstrated with large thick wall cavity lesions, with homogeneous soft tissue intensity opacity inside, and air crescent sign. (**b**) Around the lesions at the bilateral upper lungs, there are fibrous strips and bundles of lesion. (**c**) The pleura adjacent to lesions at bilateral upper lungs shows thickening and adhesion. (**d**) There are bullae of the lung at the right middle lung lobe and the left lower lung, with no change compared to previous chest CT scan. (**e**, **f**) The mediastinum window demonstrates opacity of higher intensity at bilateral lungs, irregular small translucent area around the mass soft tissue opacity at the left upper lung, and no opacity of calcification

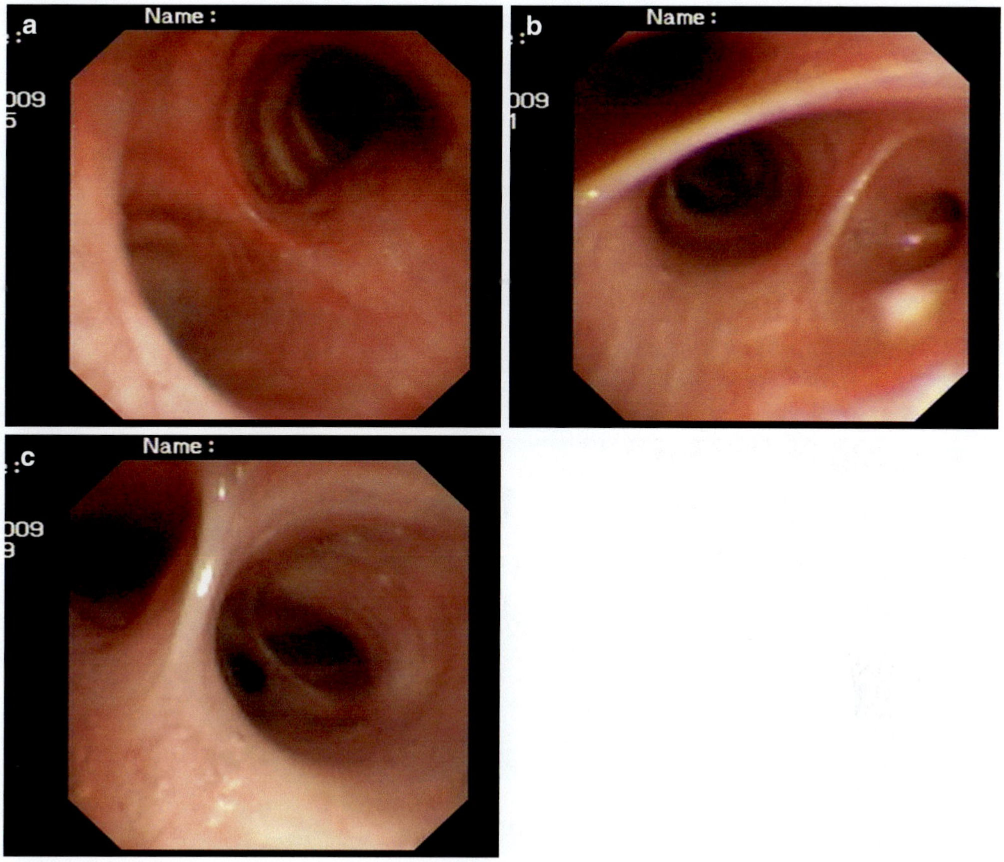

Fig. 12.40 (a–c) Fibrobronchoscopy. (**a**) The trachea carina is congested. (**b**) The middle segment of right bronchus is congested. (**c**) The bronchi at the left upper lung lobe are congested

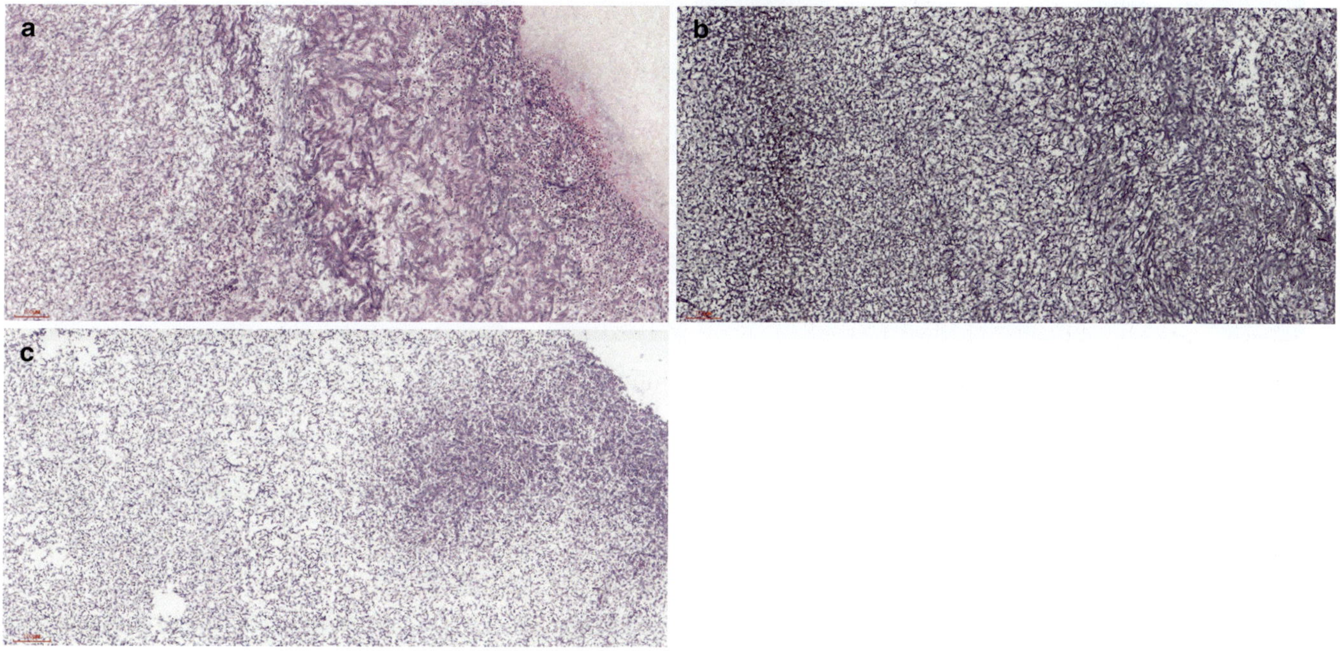

Fig. 12.41 (a–c) Pathology of lung tissue. (**a**) By H&E staining, the aspergillus hyphae is light purplish blue. (**b**) By PASM staining, the hyphae wall and spores are brownish black. (**c**) By PAS staining, the hyphae wall is reddish purple

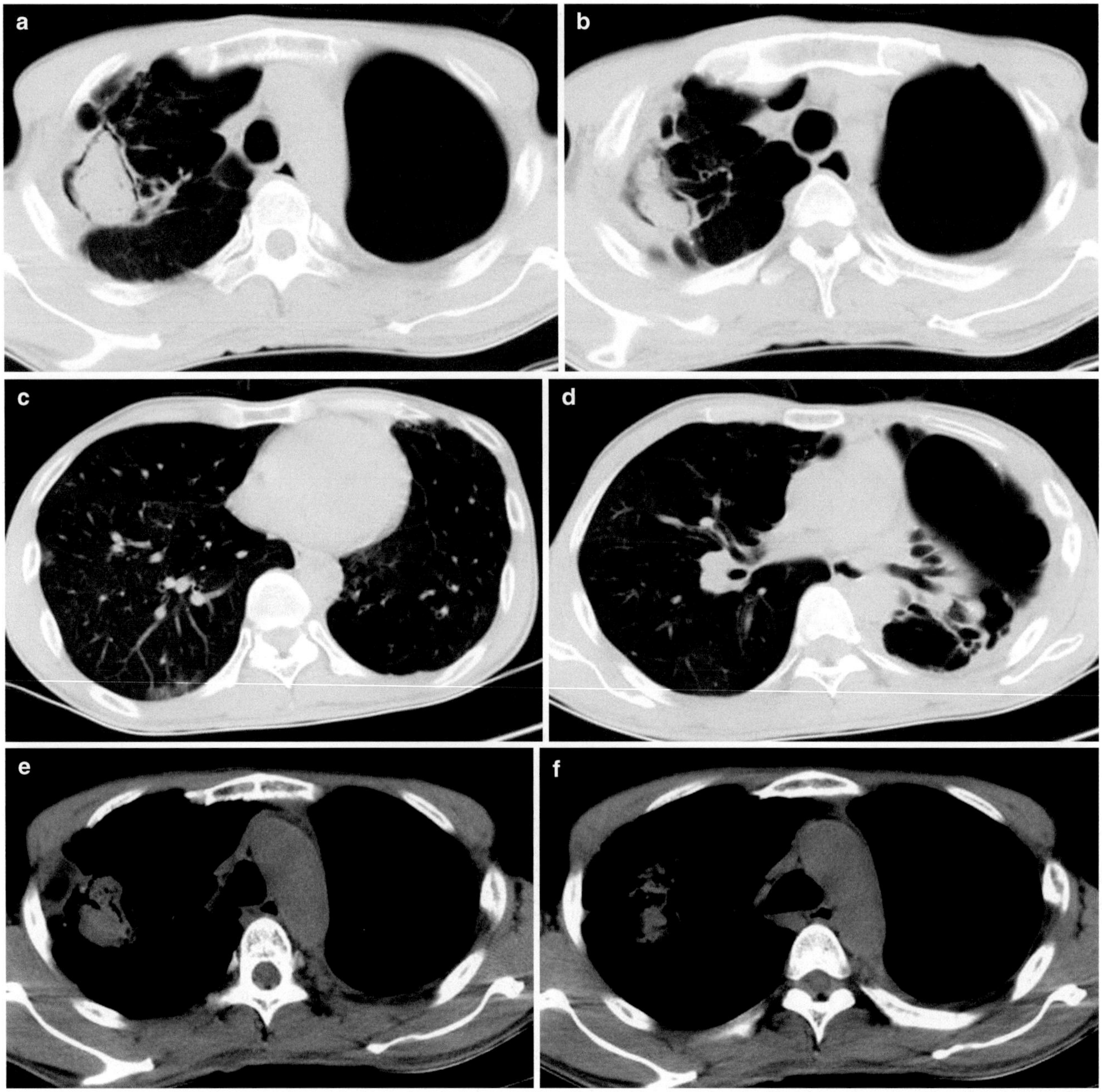

Fig. 12.42 (**a**–**f**) Chest CT scan. (**a**) The right upper lung is demonstrated with large thick wall cavity, with homogenous soft tissue intensity opacity inside, and air crescent sign. There are postoperative changes of the left thorax, and no lung tissue in the left upper thoracic cavity with no opacity of abnormal intensity. (**b**) The pleura adjacent to the lesion at the right upper lung shows thickening and adhesion. (**c**) The right lung is demonstrated with subpleural light flake of opacity. (**d**) The residual left lung is demonstrated with patchy and cords high intensity opacity near the operation area, with pleural thickening, adhesion, and local bronchiectasis due to traction. The residual left lower lung is demonstrated with compensatory dilation. (**e**, **f**) The mediastinum window demonstrates irregular patchy and nodular opacity with increased intensity at the left upper lung

oral intake of itraconazole was continued for fungal infection.

The final diagnosis was aspergilloma of bilateral upper lungs and multiple bullae in both lungs.

After discharge for 1 month, the patient experienced recurrent hemoptysis. And itraconazole was discontinued, but voriconazole was prescribed. The patient discontinued the medication by himself after the symptoms were relieved (Fig. 12.42). The patient was hospitalized in March 2010 and December 2014 due to relapse of hemoptysis. And medication of voriconazole was administered due to a diagnosis of pulmonary aspergilloma. Reexamination of chest CT scan (Figs. 12.43 and 12.44) was performed. G test showed negative, and repeated sputum smears showed acid fast bacilli

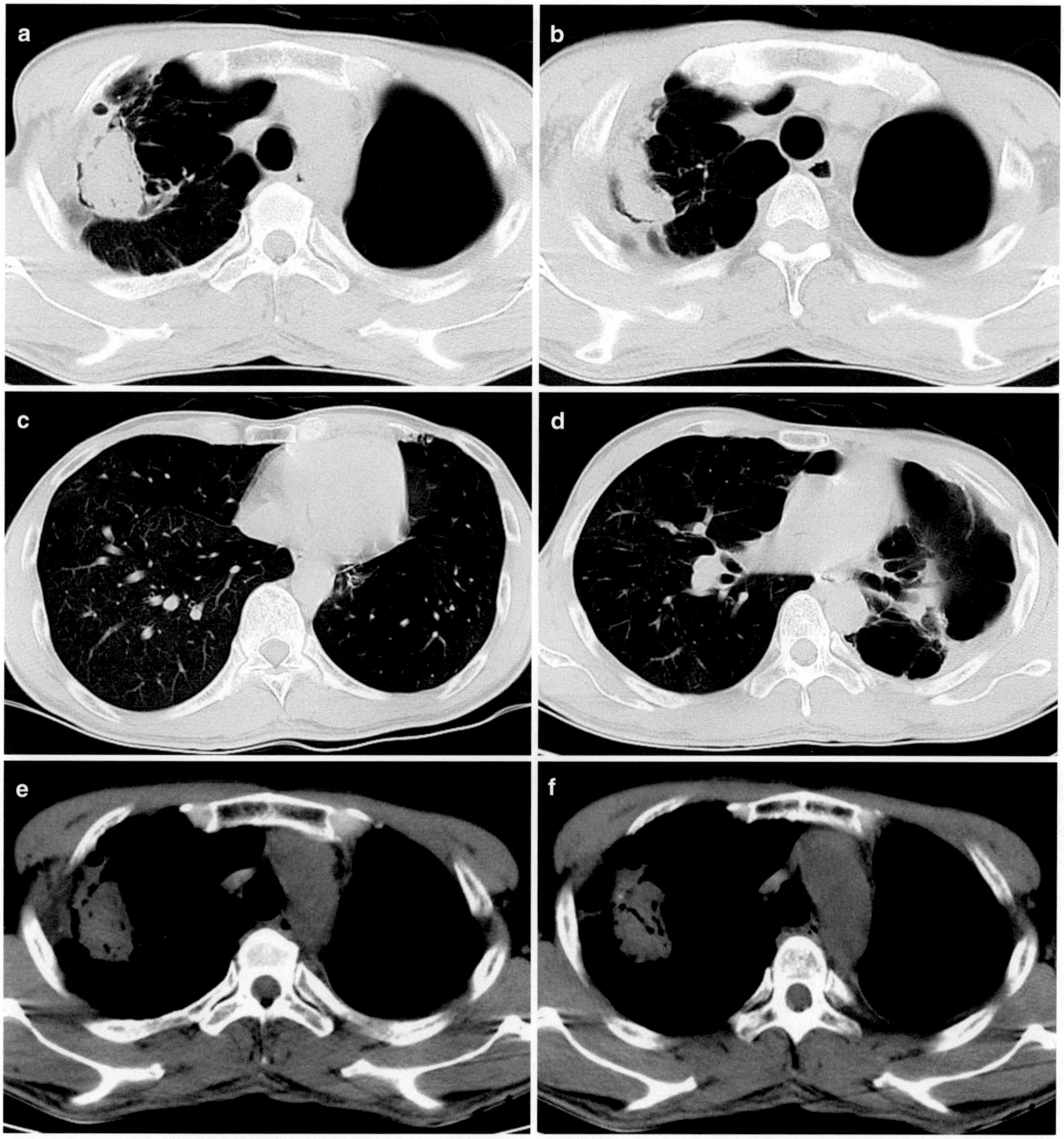

Fig. 12.43 (a–f) Chest CT scan. (**a**) The right upper lung is demonstrated with thick wall cavity, with homogeneous soft tissue intensity opacity. There are no changes compared to the previous chest CT scan. (**b**) The pleura adjacent to the lesion at the right upper lung shows thickening and adhesion. (**c**) The light flake of opacity at the right lung under the pleura is absent. (**d**) The residual left lung near surgical area is demonstrated with patchy and cords high intensity opacity. There are also pleural thickening and adhesion, local bronchiectasis due to traction, and compensatory dilation of the residual left lower lung with more translucent lung field compared to previous chest CT scan. (**e**, **f**) The mediastinum window demonstrates irregular mass-like and nodular opacity with increased intensity at the left upper lung, with small translucent area inside

and fungi negative. Electronic bronchoscopy demonstrated postoperative residual margin of the left upper lung lobe, smooth mucosa, and no neoplasm and hemorrhage (Fig. 12.45). The culture of secretions harvested by fibrobronchoscopy showed no growth of pathogenic bacteria.

12.14.4 Discussion

Based on the clinical characteristic, pulmonary aspergillosis can be classified into invasive pulmonary aspergillosis, chronic pulmonary aspergillosis (CPA), and allergic

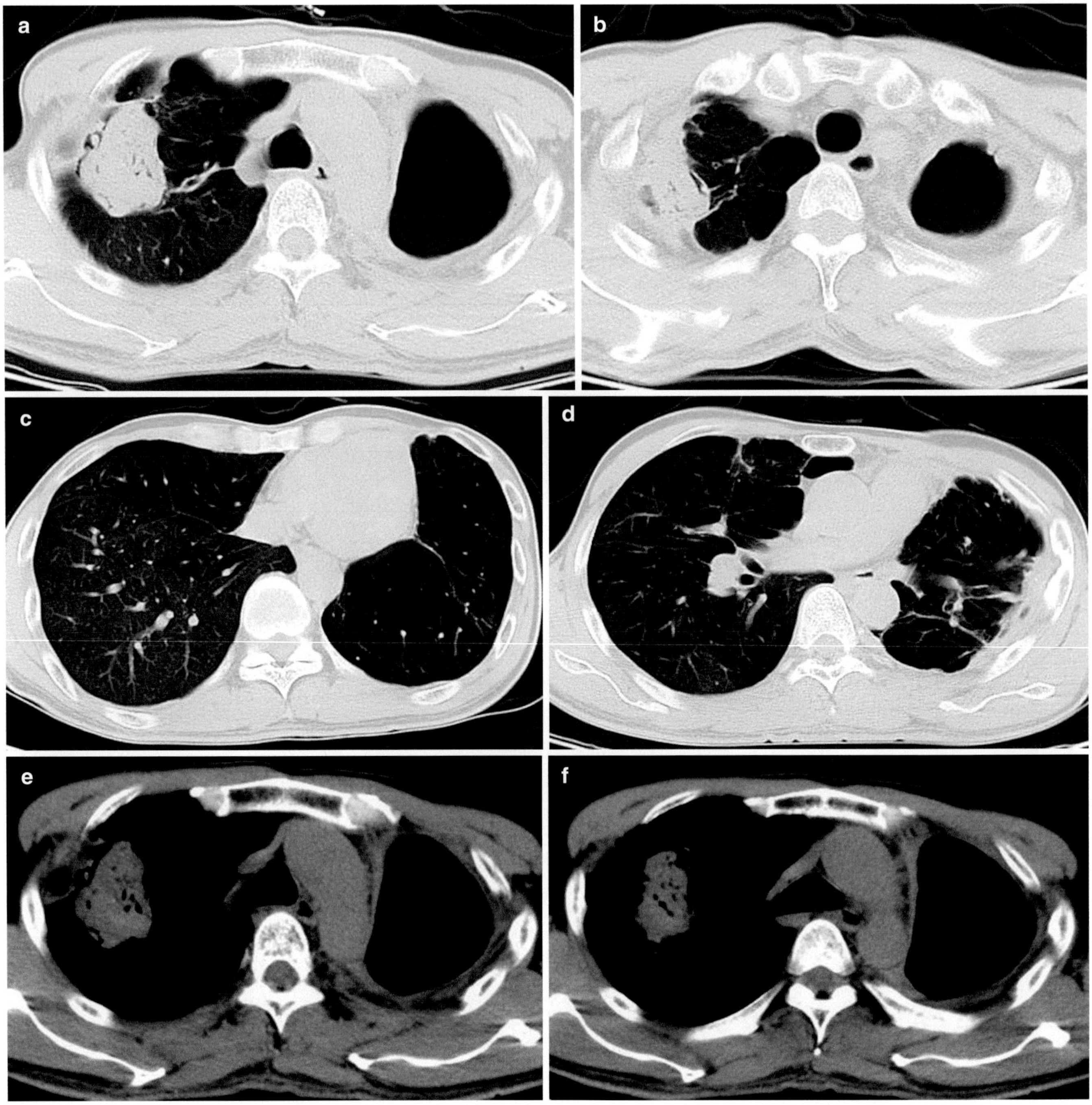

Fig. 12.44 (a–f) Chest CT scan. (**a**) The right upper lung is demonstrated with a large thick wall cavity, with homogeneous soft tissue intensity opacity inside. (**b**) The pleura adjacent to the lesion at the right upper lung shows thickening and adhesion. (**c**) Both lungs are demonstrated with multiple spots of nodular opacity and calcification opacity. (**d**) The right lung is demonstrated with less light opacity. And the right middle lung is demonstrated with less high intensity opacity and fibrous cords opacity. The residual left lung is demonstrated with patchy opacity and cords high intensity opacity near the surgical area. There are also pleural thickening and adhesion, local bronchiectasis due to traction, compensatory dilation of the residual left lower lung, and cords and flakes of opacity near diaphragmatic surface. (**e**, **f**) The mediastinum window demonstrates irregular mass-like and nodular opacity with increased intensity at the left upper lung, with small translucent area inside. The soft tissue opacity is enlarged compared to previous chest CT scan

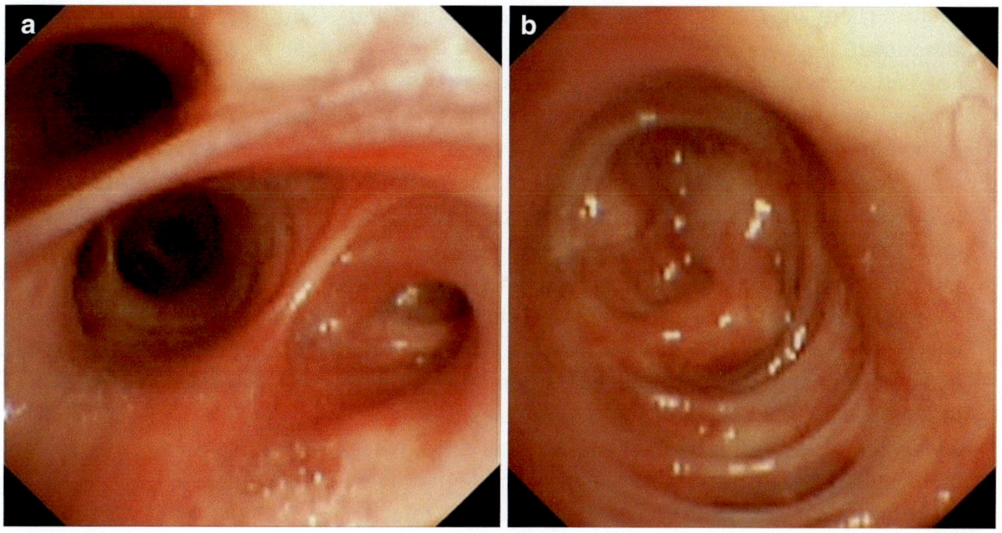

Fig. 12.45 (**a**, **b**) Electronic bronchoscopy. (**a**) The right middle bronchus is unobstructed, with no neoplasm and hemorrhage. The mucosa is smooth. (**b**) Postoperative ends at the left upper lung lobe

bronchopulmonary aspergillosis (ABPA) [25]. Chronic necrotizing pulmonary aspergillosis is also known as subacute invasive pulmonary aspergillosis or semi-invasive pulmonary aspergillosis. Some scholars categorize chronic necrotizing pulmonary aspergillosis into chronic cavitary pulmonary aspergillosis [29, 70].

The common risk factors of chronic necrotizing pulmonary aspergillosis include COPD, nonactive pulmonary tuberculosis, pulmonary cystic fibrosis, and pulmonary sarcoidosis. The clinical manifestations include cough, expectoration, and hemoptysis. The CT scan of the lungs demonstrates unilateral or bilateral round segmental consolidation, with or with no cavity and adjacent pleural thickening. There may be multiple nodular opacities with increased intensity. And it may develop into aspergilloma in cavity with destructed lung tissue around the cavity. Chronic necrotizing pulmonary aspergillosis shows chronic progression [1, 27].

In this case, the patient was a middle-aged man, with a past medical history of pulmonary tuberculosis. He experienced symptoms of cough, expectoration, and hemoptysis. CT scan of the lungs demonstrated aspergilloma in the cavity of bilateral upper lungs with destructed lung tissue around the cavity and adjacent pleural thickening and adhesion. Pathology of lung tissue demonstrated fungal mass in lung cavity, infiltration of many inflammatory cells around the cavity with purulent necrosis, and lung tissue hemorrhage [71]. According to the diagnostic criteria of invasive pulmonary aspergillosis formulated by Chinese Medical Society, the case was definitively diagnosed as pulmonary aspergillosis, and the clinical typing was chronic necrotizing pulmonary aspergillosis. According to the clinical guideline issued by IDSA, for patients with chronic necrotizing pulmonary aspergillosis and low risks of surgery, surgical removal of the lesions provides long-term cure and facilitates avoiding local expansion of the lesion. Thus the survival rate of the patients can be increased [4]. Therefore, in this case, the patient received surgical removal of the serious lesions at the left lung, and postoperative oral medication of itraconazole was administered for fungal infection for 2 months. However, hemoptysis relapsed during antifungal medication due to presence of aspergilloma at the right upper lung. The medication was then changed to voriconazole, and the condition was stabilized.

We summarize the following key points about this case:

1. Hemoptysis in patients with a past medical history of chronic fibro-cavitary pulmonary tuberculosis is commonly considered to be relapse of pulmonary tuberculosis. And other possibilities tend to be neglected. However, chronic necrotizing pulmonary aspergillosis commonly occurs based on COPD, pulmonary tuberculosis, and other pulmonary disease. Relapse of pulmonary tuberculosis thus tends to be confused with chronic necrotizing pulmonary aspergillosis. Therefore, for patients with hemoptysis and a past medical history of chronic fibro-cavitary pulmonary tuberculosis, both relapse of pulmonary tuberculosis and pulmonary aspergillosis should be considered.
2. CT scan demonstrates chronic necrotizing pulmonary aspergillosis as aspergilloma in unilateral or bilateral cavities in the lung with destructed lung tissue around the

cavity. There may be adjacent pleural thickening and adhesion.
3. For patients with hemoptysis and low risks of surgery, surgical removal of the lesions can be performed.
4. Although the lesions at the left lung were surgically removed in this case, postoperative medication for fungal infection was administered due to presence of aspergilloma in the right lung.
5. Oral intake of triazoles, including voriconazole and itraconazole, is the optimal medication for chronic pulmonary aspergillosis. In this case, the patient still experienced recurrent hemoptysis after administration of itraconazole. After the medication was changed to voriconazole, the condition was stabilized. Therefore, when medication of one triazole showed unfavorable therapeutic response, it can be changed to another triazole for fungal infection.

12.14.5 Comments

Chronic pulmonary aspergillosis may occur in individuals with compromised immunity and or weak constitution, such as patients with or receiving diabetes, malnutrition, elderly, long-term immunosuppressant, COPD, connective tissue disease, tuberculosis mycobacteria infection, and HIV infection. In this case, the patient had a medical history of pulmonary tuberculosis. Chest CT scan demonstrated large thick wall cavities in bilateral upper lungs, with homogeneous soft tissue opacity inside, and air crescent sign. A clinical diagnosis of fungal infection was not challenging. Tuberculosis mycobacteria infection may occur before, after, or concurrent with chronic pulmonary aspergillosis. Therefore, chronic cavitary pulmonary tuberculosis should be clinically differentiated from pulmonary tuberculosis complicated by chronic pulmonary aspergillosis. The smear and culture of lung tissues, the nuclear acid amplification of tuberculosis mycobacteria and histopathology are important ways for their differentiation.

Chronic pulmonary aspergillosis can be further classified into chronic cavitary pulmonary aspergillosis (CCPA), chronic fibrotic pulmonary aspergillosis (CFPA), and subacute invasive pulmonary aspergillosis (SAIA). And these three subtypes may be overlapping, and one subtype may progress into another subtype. At the terminal stage of CCPA, fibrosis of CCPA indicate occurrence of CFPA. The clinical manifestations and radiological demonstrations of SAIA resemble to those of CCPA. However, SAIA progresses more rapidly. Without pathological evidence and further tracing during follow-ups, CCPA can be hardly differentiated from SAIA. In this case, the patient was definitively diagnosed as having SAIA based on histopathologic evidence.

Slight, moderate, or even life-threatening hemoptysis may occur in patients with chronic pulmonary aspergillosis and singular aspergilloma. Slight and moderate hemoptysis can be treated by tranexamic acid. For patients with moderate and serious hemoptysis, surgery can be considered. As temporary measure before surgery or therapy, embolization is necessary. In this case, the patient showed lesions of pulmonary aspergillosis in both lungs. Hemoptysis persisted after the surgery. That is to say, the surgery achieved unfavorable therapeutic efficacy.

12.15 Case 15: Intermittent Hemoptysis for 5 Years and Aggravation for 1 Year

Dong-Na Su, Guangsuo Wang, Hongtao Chen, Shi-Ping Wu, Ling-Wei Wang, and Chang’e Jin

12.15.1 Presenting Symptom

Intermittent hemoptysis for 5 years and aggravation for 1 year.

12.15.2 Brief Case History

A 63-year-old woman was admitted to our hospital on May 11, 2006, due to complaints of intermittent hemoptysis for 5 years and aggravation for 1 year. Five years ago, the patient began to experience intermittent hemoptysis with no known reasons. The hemoptysis was irregular, once after several days. At the beginning, the blood that she coughed up was in a small quantity, mostly sputum with blood streak, with accompanying slight cough. But she experienced no fever, chest pain, and breathlessness. The symptom was temporarily relieved after medication of vitamin K1 for hemostasis, but hemoptysis was recurrent. One year ago, hemoptysis was aggravated, with shortened intervals and increased blood that she coughed up. The largest volume of blood was up to about 100 ml a day, and the blood was fresh red, with more blood than sputum. She presented repeatedly to a district hospital specialized in chronic diseases in Shenzhen, China. And the symptoms were relieved after medications for inflammation and hemostasis (specifically unknown). Two months ago, hemoptysis further aggravated. The blood she coughed up was all fresh red blood with clots, and the volume was above 100 ml. She still experienced no aversion to cold, fever, flush after noons, and night sweat. On May 11, 2006, she presented in our hospital and was admitted to the respiratory department. Since the onset of the symptoms, her spiritual state and appetite were quite good. During the recent 4 months, she experienced body weight loss of about 2.5 kg.

12.15.2.1 Past Medical History

She reported a past medical history of pulmonary tuberculosis 13 years ago and received standard antituberculosis therapy for almost 1 year. Then she received follow-up examinations in a district hospital specialized in chronic diseases in Shenzhen, China. And she reported that she was cured. She also reported a past medical history of cerebral infarction 11 years ago. The patient denied histories of hypertension and diabetes. She had no habitual smoking and drinking.

12.15.2.2 Physical Examination

By physical examination, the body temperature was 36.8 °C, pulse rate 85/min, respiration rate 21/min, and blood pressure 116/76 mmHg. She was typically developed with average nourishment. The patient was well conscious, with appearance of chronic disease. She was in active position and well cooperated to the physical examination. The systemic superficial lymph nodes were unpalpable and not enlarged. The respiration sounds of both lungs were clear, with less moist rales at the right lower lung. The heart was not enlarged, with heartbeats of 85/min, rhythmic. By auscultation, the valvular areas showed no pathological murmur. The abdomen was soft, and the liver and spleen were not palpable. The shifting dullness was negative. The liver and kidney were not sensitive to percussion. And the bowel sounds were normal.

12.15.2.3 Auxiliary Investigation

Laboratory Test

Routine blood test showed WBC 4.3 × 109/L, N 46.7%, L 42.7%, RBC 3.79 × 1012/L, and PLT 106 × 109/L. The ESR was 26 mm/h and CRP 1.2 mg/L. By the liver function test, T-Bil was 12.1 μmol/L, ALT 24 U/L, AST 24 U/L, TP 74 g/L, and ALB 40 g/L. By the kidney function test, BUN was 6.3 mmol/L (normal range 2.5–7.5 mmol/L) and Cr 68 μmmol/L (normal range 43 μ–115 μmmol).

Radiology

CT scan of the lungs in another hospital on December 8, 2005, demonstrated patchy opacity at the right upper lung and bronchiectasis of bilateral lower lungs. And the diagnosis was considered to be pulmonary tuberculosis of the right upper lung and bronchiectasis.

12.15.2.4 Initial Diagnosis

The initial diagnosis was hemoptysis possibly induced by pulmonary tuberculosis and bronchiectasis.

12.15.3 Diagnosis and Treatment

After admission, levofloxacin was administered for infection; etamsylate, aminomethylbenzoic acid, and vitamin C were administered for hemostasis. But the symptoms were not obviously relieved, and the patient still experienced intermittent hemoptysis. The repeated sputum smear for three times and acid fast staining on May 12–16, 2005, demonstrated no acid fast bacilli, and repeated sputum cultures for three times for bacteria and fungi showed negative. PPD skin test showed a hard nodule in size of 5 mm × 5 mm. To further define the reason of hemoptysis, chest CT scan was performed on May 12, 2006. And the chest CT scan demonstrated a nodular opacity at the posterior segment of right upper lung lobe, with a dense spherical opacity inside. And there was air crescent sign inferior and lateral to the dense spherical opacity. The right middle lung lobe and the bilateral lower lung lobes were demonstrated with focal bronchiectasis. The diagnosis was considered to be aspergillus infection in the right upper lung lobe and bronchiectasis at the right middle lung lobe and bilateral lower lung lobes (Fig. 12.46).

Because the symptom of hemoptysis persisted, fibrobronchoscopy was performed on May 15, 2006, to further define the reason of hemoptysis. Fibrobronchoscopy demonstrated that mucosal congestion of trachea as well as left and right bronchi, unobstructed bronchi with no neoplasm and stenosis, and no caseous necrosis. There was fresh red blood stain at the opening of bronchus at the right upper lung lobe. And the opening of medial branch of right middle bronchus was demonstrated with yellowish white purulent secretions. After the sputum was aspirated, fresh red blood was demonstrated in a small quantity. Brushing of right middle lobe bronchus and making smear for pathology and bacterial and fungal culture (Fig. 12.47). Bronchial brushing demonstrated many ciliated columnar epithelial cells, with infiltration of many neutrophile granulocytes. The bronchial aspirates were sent for bacterial and fungal cultures, which demonstrated no growth of bacteria and fungi.

Because the patient showed persistent hemoptysis and the blood coughed up was in a large volume, specialist from the thoracic surgery department believed that surgery was indicated for the patient at the multidisciplinary meeting. Thoracoscopic partial removals of the right upper lung lobe and right lower lung lobe as well as removal of right middle lung lobe were performed on May 23, 2006, under general anesthesia. During the operation, the lung tissue at the posteroapical segment of right upper lung lobe was found with partial fibrosis, and moderately hard mass in diameter of about 3 cm was palpable. The postoperative pathology indicated large quantities of hyphae and spores, with hyphae twining into mass and infiltration of many inflammatory cells in surrounding lung tissue. By methenamine silver staining, the hyphae were in brownish black in arrangement of filiform or radiating form. The hyphae were even in thickness in a diameter of about 7–10 μm. And the bilateral hyphae walls were parallel, and the hyphae had transverse septa and branching in 45° sharp angle. There were also scattering spores. By PAS staining, the hyphae wall was reddish purple (Fig. 12.48). The pathological diagnosis was fungal infection, which was morphologically consistent to aspergillus infection, and bronchiectasis.

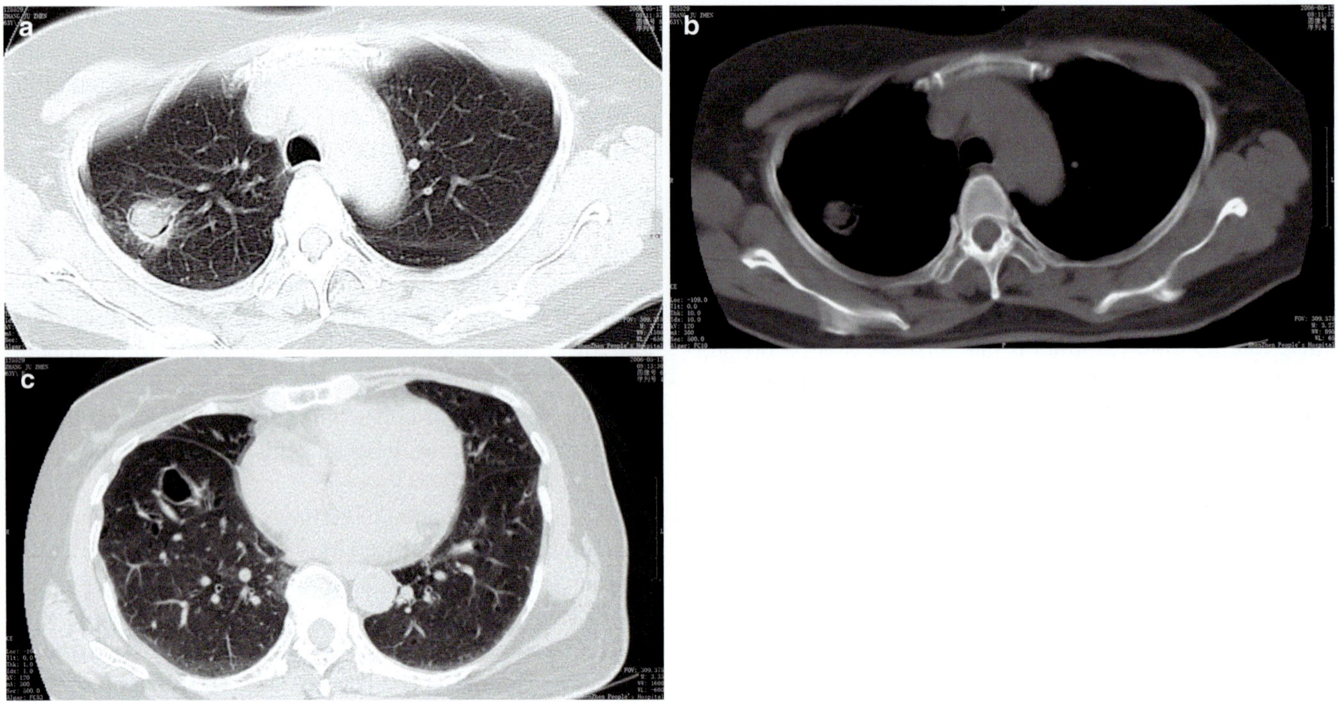

Fig. 12.46 (**a**–**c**) Chest CT scan. (**a**) The lung window at the aortic arch level demonstrates a nodular opacity at the posterior segment of right upper lung lobe, with dense spherical opacity inside, and air crescent sign inferior and lateral to the spherical opacity. There are less ground-glass opacities inferior and lateral to the nodular opacity. (**b**) The mediastinum window at the aortic arch level demonstrates dense spherical density at the posterior segment of right upper lung lobe and air crescent sign inside. (**c**) The lung window at the ventricle level demonstrates cystic bronchiectasis at the inferior basilar segment of right lower lung

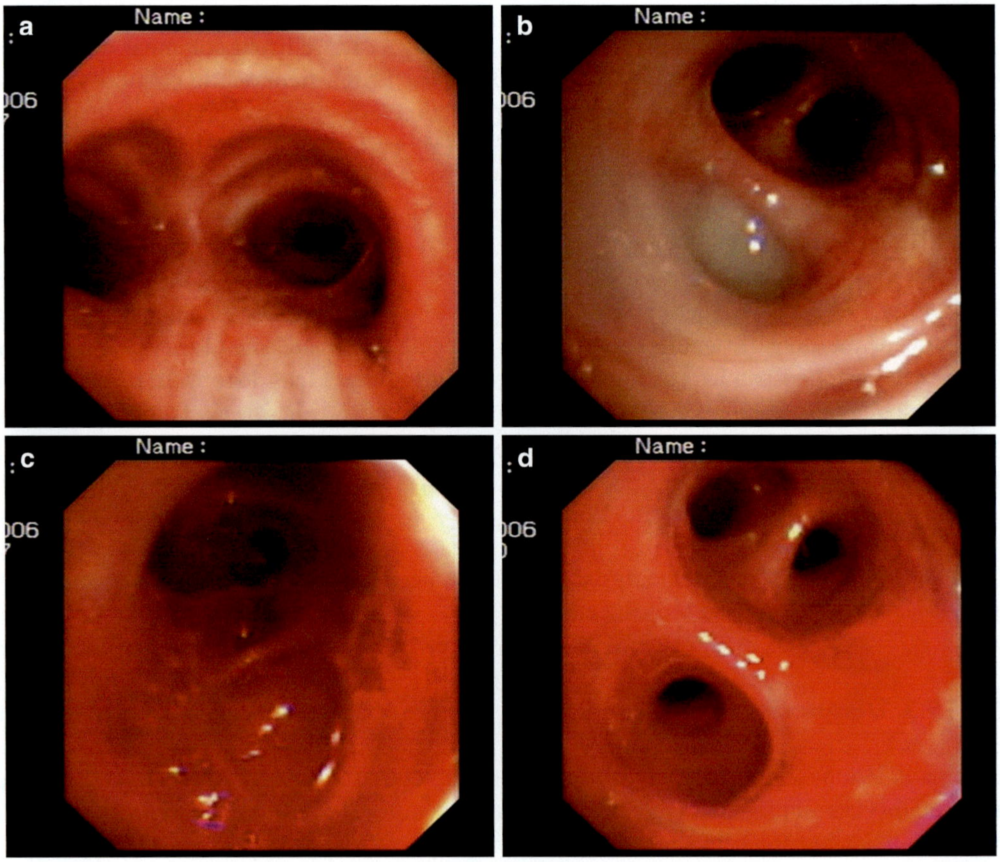

Fig. 12.47 (**a**–**d**) Bronchoscopy: (**a**) The trachea carina is sharp, (**b**) the bronchial opening at the right middle lung lobe is demonstrated with purulent secretions. (**c**) The bronchial opening at the right middle lung lobe is demonstrated with fresh red blood stain. (**d**) The bronchial opening at the right middle lung lobe is demonstrated to be congested

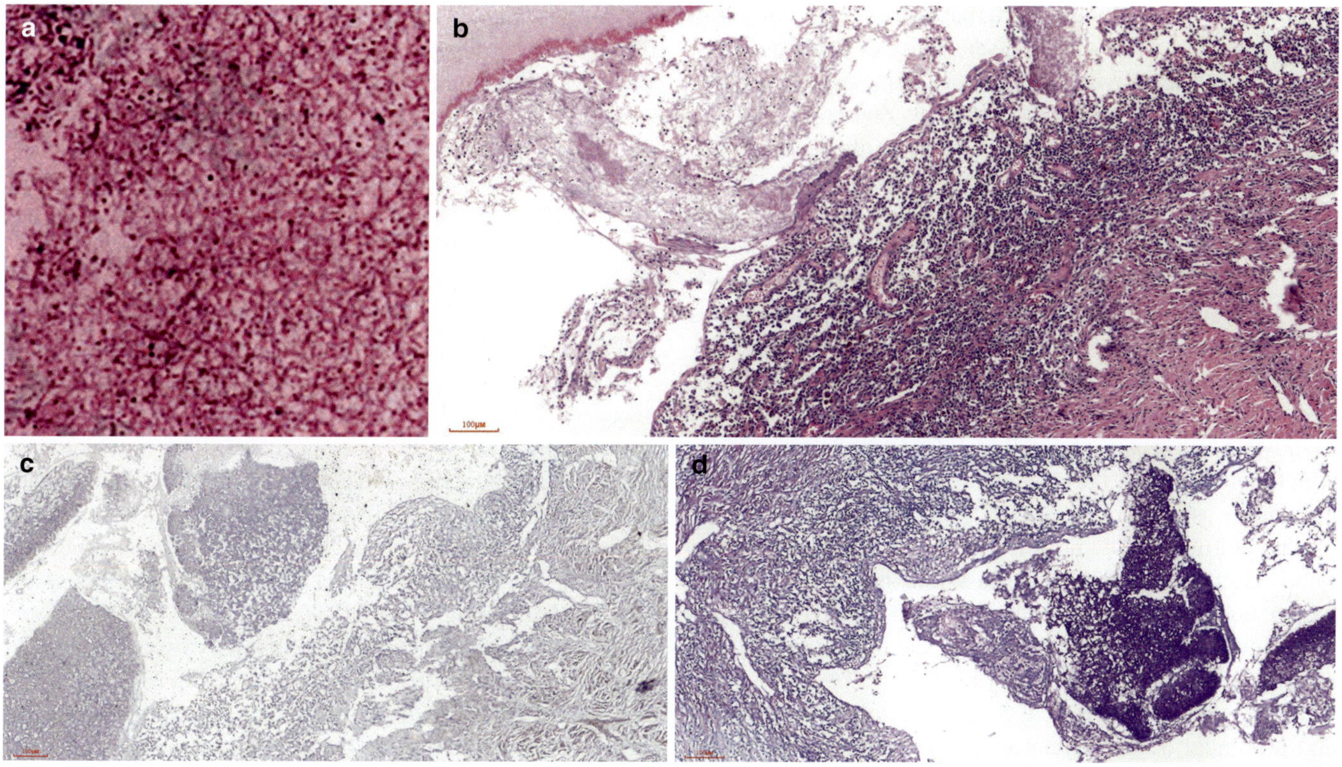

Fig. 12.48 (**a**–**d**) Pathology of lung tissue. (**a**) There are large quantities of hyphae and spores, and the hyphae twine into mass. By H&E staining, there is infiltration of many inflammatory cells in the surrounding lung tissue. (**b**) By H&E staining, the hyphae wall of aspergillus is light purplish blue. (**c**) By PASM staining, the hyphae wall and spores are brownish black. (**d**) By PAS staining, the hyphae wall is reddish purple

After the surgical operation, the patient showed favorable recovery, and hemoptysis was cured. The patient was discharged on June 14, 2006.

The final diagnosis was bronchiectasis complicated by pulmonary aspergilloma at the right upper lung.

After discharge, the condition of the patient was stable. And no hemoptysis occurred during follow-ups.

12.15.4 Discussion

It is commonly believed that pulmonary aspergillosis has a high incidence in immunocompromised populations. But it also occurs in populations with competent immunity but underlying pulmonary disease, such as COPD, bronchiectasis, and cavitary pulmonary tuberculosis. Cavitary pulmonary tuberculosis, bronchiectasis, and other pulmonary structural diseases are always basic disease of aspergilloma. It has been reported that pulmonary aspergilloma occurs in about 10–15% patients with chronic cavitary pulmonary disease. Recent research data indicated that the incidence of pulmonary aspergillosis has been increasing in patients with chronic pulmonary disease, such as COPD and bronchiectasis, which may be related to their use of glucocorticoid [72, 73]. In this case, the patient suffered from pulmonary aspergillus infection based on bronchiectasis. But she had no medical history of using glucocorticoid, which indicated that pulmonary aspergillosis may also occur in populations with competent immunity and structural pulmonary disease.

Patients with pulmonary aspergilloma are commonly asymptomatic, and hemoptysis is the most common symptom. It has been reported that the incidence of hemoptysis with clinical significance is up to 50.3% [37]. The volume of blood that is coughed up ranges from an extremely small quantity to fatally large quantity. Clinically, it should be differentiated from pulmonary tuberculosis, bronchiectasis, and lung carcinoma. In this case, pulmonary tuberculosis or bronchiectasis had been suspected. The underlying mechanism of hemorrhage in the cases of pulmonary aspergilloma is as the following: (1) friction of aspergilloma in the cavity that destructs vascular vessels and (2) invasion of aspergillus into surrounding vascular vessels.

In this case, the serum galactomannan (GM) test was not performed because the hospital was not well equipped for the test. GM test has significant value for the diagnosis of pulmonary aspergillosis. A meta-analysis has demonstrated that the diagnostic sensitivity and specificity of GM test for pulmonary aspergillosis are up to 78% and 81% [74], respectively.

Another research study indicated that the sensitivity of serum GM test is only 38%, while the sensitivity of BALF GM test has improved sensitivity of 92% [45]. A meta-analysis conducted based on 30 research studies by Zou et al. [46] has demonstrated that the sensitivity and specificity of BALF GM test are up to 87% and 89%, respectively. Therefore, for patients with suspected diagnosis of pulmonary aspergillosis, if possible, BALF GM test should be performed to improve the diagnostic positive rate of pulmonary aspergillosis. However, most of these research studies have focused on invasive pulmonary aspergillosis and rare on pulmonary aspergilloma. Park et al. [75] performed serum and BALF GM tests for 48 cases of pulmonary aspergilloma. They found that the sensitivity of BALF GM test is up to 92%, which demonstrated the diagnostic value of BALF GM for pulmonary aspergilloma.

The radiological demonstrations of pulmonary aspergilloma mainly include dense mass-like opacity in cavity, which occupies most of the cavity, and crescent-shaped translucent area in the other part of cavity. The mass-like opacity is movable in the cavity along with body postures. In this case, the radiological demonstrations were typical, and a clinical diagnosis can be made based on the radiological demonstrations. However, in the cases with concurrent COPD, bronchiectasis, and pulmonary cystic diseases, the differentiation of cavity and crescent sign is challenging.

For asymptomatic patients with pulmonary aspergilloma, regular follow-ups for observation of the condition should be performed instead of treatment. But for patients with hemoptysis, treatment is necessary to prevent life-threatening major hemoptysis. Surgical removal of the lesion has definitive therapeutic efficacy [3]. Bronchial artery embolization has poor therapeutic efficacy, which is only performed for emergency therapy treating major hemoptysis. Surgical removal of lung lobe is the most common surgical approach. Thoracoscopy is noninvasive, with less bleeding and rapid recovery. In this case, the patient received thoracoscopy, with rapid recovery and favorable therapeutic efficacy. During follow-ups, no relapse of symptoms was found, indicating successful surgical operation.

12.15.5 Comments

Singular pulmonary aspergilloma occurs in thin wall cavity, while chronic cavitary pulmonary aspergillosis occurs in multiple thick wall cavities, with or with no aspergilloma inside. The surrounding lung parenchyma is subject to pathological changes. In this case, the diagnosis is obviously singular pulmonary aspergilloma.

Hemoptysis is one of the common symptoms of pulmonary aspergilloma. Pulmonary tuberculosis, bronchiectasis, and lung carcinoma are also common reasons of hemoptysis. In the case, based on the experience of diagnosis and treatment, we know that hemoptysis inexplicable or incurable by therapies for pulmonary tuberculosis and bronchiectasis should be considered to be pulmonary aspergillus infection. In this case, the patient suffered from 5 years hemoptysis, which progressively aggravated. In the diagnosis and treatment, the clinicians only considered bronchiectasis instead of aspergillus infection.

Chest CT scan has great diagnostic value for pulmonary aspergilloma. In this case, the radiological demonstrations were typical, and experienced radiologist can make a clinical diagnosis based on radiological findings. CT scan demonstrates typical aspergilloma as air crescent sign, which may also be demonstrated in the cases of bronchopulmonary carcinoma and hematoma. Differential diagnosis is necessary in clinical practice. In the cases with concurrent bronchiectasis, pulmonary cystic diseases, and bullae of the lung, the diagnosis is challenging.

Asymptomatic patients with pulmonary aspergilloma can be observed, and antifungal medication shows unfavorable therapeutic efficacy. For patients with repeated hemoptysis, surgical operation should be considered to prevent life-threatening major hemoptysis. The main indications of surgery include (1) singular aspergilloma; (2) patients with major hemoptysis but good pulmonary functions; (3) repeated hemoptysis; (4) some patients with complex aspergilloma and the primary disease can be treated by surgical operation; and (5) lung carcinoma cannot be excluded. In this case, hemoptysis was cured after surgery, and the patient showed favorable postoperative recovery. The treatment was definitively successful.

12.16 Case 16: Cough and Expectoration for 2 Years and Aggravation with Hemoptysis for 15 Days

Guoxin Huang, Fuqiang Zhu, Fucheng Wu,
Shi-Ping Wu, Hongtao Chen, and Jingshan Gong

12.16.1 Presenting Symptom

Cough and expectoration for 2 years and aggravation with hemoptysis for 15 days.

12.16.2 Brief Case History

A 33-year-old man was admitted to our hospital due to complaints of cough and expectoration for 2 years and aggravation with hemoptysis for 15 days. Two years ago, the patient began to experience cough and expectoration of yellowish white sputum. But he experienced no hemoptysis, fever, night sweat, abdominal pain, and diarrhea. He presented in a local hospital and received chest X-ray. The chest X-ray demonstrated pulmonary tuberculosis (specifically unknown), and he received medications of isoniazid and rifampicin for 2 years. But intermittent cough and expectoration persisted. Fifteen days ago, the symptoms of cough and expectoration aggravated. The volume of sputum increased with hemoptysis of sputum with blood of a small quantity. He also experienced night sweat but no fever and other symptoms. He presented in a hospital, and repeated sputum smears demonstrated no acid fast bacilli. He then presented in a city hospital specialized in chronic diseases, and chest CT scan there demonstrated tuberculosis of both lungs and multiple cavities with aspergilloma in bilateral upper lung lobes. The sputum smear there demonstrated no acid fast bacilli, and PPD test showed strongly positive. The antibody against tuberculosis mycobacteria showed positive. And the sputum culture for fungi showed positive. The diagnosis was pulmonary tuberculosis complicated by aspergillus infection. And levofloxacin, rifapentine, and ethambutol were administered for tuberculosis. The symptoms were obviously relieved. Hemoptysis did not onset again. The patient was transferred to the respiratory department of our hospital on October 29, 2009. Since the onset of symptoms, his spiritual state, sleep, and appetite were average. The urinations and bowel movements were normal. And he experienced no obvious body weight change.

12.16.2.1 Physical Examination

Physical examination showed a body temperature of 37.1 °C, pulse rate 100/min, respiration rate 21/min, and blood pressure 117/86 mmHg. The superficial lymph nodes were not palpable and not enlarged. The trachea was at the midline. The thorax was bilaterally symmetric, with no deformity. And there were no abnormal respirations. The three depressions sign was negative. The sternum showed no tenderness. The vocal fremitus of bilateral lungs was bilaterally symmetric. By percussion, both lungs showed clear sounds. By auscultation, the respiration sounds were coarse, with no obvious dry and/or moist rales. The precordial area showed no protrusion. The apical beats were strong, and the heartbeat was 100/min, rhythmic. The valvular areas showed no pathological murmur by auscultation.

12.16.2.2 Auxiliary Investigation

Laboratory tests showed WBC 9.0 × 109/L and N 64.3%. The blood electrolytes were with normal limits. Hs-CRP was 3.50 mg/L and procalcitonin <0.05 ng/ml. PPD test showed strongly positive and antibody against tuberculosis mycobacteria positive. And the sputum culture for fungi showed positive.

12.16.2.3 Initial Diagnosis

The initial diagnosis was secondary pulmonary tuberculosis of bilateral upper lungs and pulmonary aspergillosis.

12.16.3 Diagnosis and Treatment

After admission, the investigations were performed. The sputum smear demonstrated no acid fast bacilli. PPD test showed strongly positive. The antibody against tuberculosis mycobacteria showed positive. And the sputum culture for fungi showed positive. The chest CT scan was performed on November 3, 2009 (Fig. 12.49).

After admission, levofloxacin, pasiniazide, rifapentine, and ethambutol were administered for tuberculosis. And the symptoms were obviously improved, and the patient experienced no hemoptysis. Thoracoscopic removal of left upper lung lobe, wedge removal of left lower lung lobe, cautery of left pleural adhesion, left intercostal nerve block, and close drainage of the left thorax were performed under general anesthesia. Postoperative pathology demonstrated the cystic content of the left upper lung was fungal hyphae and spores, which were morphologically consistent to aspergillus. There were also infiltration of many chronic inflammatory cells and neutrophile granulocytes in the lung tissue of left upper lung, hyperplasia of fibrous tissue, and chronic purulent inflammation. The diagnosis was aspergillosis of the left upper lung and chronic purulent inflammation of left upper lung (Fig. 12.50).

After the operation, isoniazid, rifampicin, amikacin, voriconazole, and levofloxacin were administered for tuberculosis and fungal infection. The recovery was favorable.

The diagnosis on discharge was pulmonary aspergillosis of the left upper lung, pulmonary tuberculosis of the right upper lung, and tuberculous pleurisy.

12.16.4 Discussion

Pulmonary aspergillosis is an infectious lung disease caused by aspergillus. Clinically, it is classified into invasive pulmonary aspergillosis, chronic and saprophytic pulmonary aspergillosis, and allergic pulmonary aspergillosis. Pulmonary aspergillosis is commonly secondary to primary lung disease or occurs in populations with compromised immunity, with diverse clinical manifestations. Its diagnosis and treatment are challenging [44]. Pulmonary aspergillosis commonly occurs in patients with COPD, bronchiectasis, lung carcinoma, pulmonary tuberculosis, and other lung structural diseases, indicating association of anatomic structural abnormality of lung with pulmonary aspergillosis. Patients with such diseases commonly show compromised immunity and obstructed drainage, which promote the growth of aspergillus in the

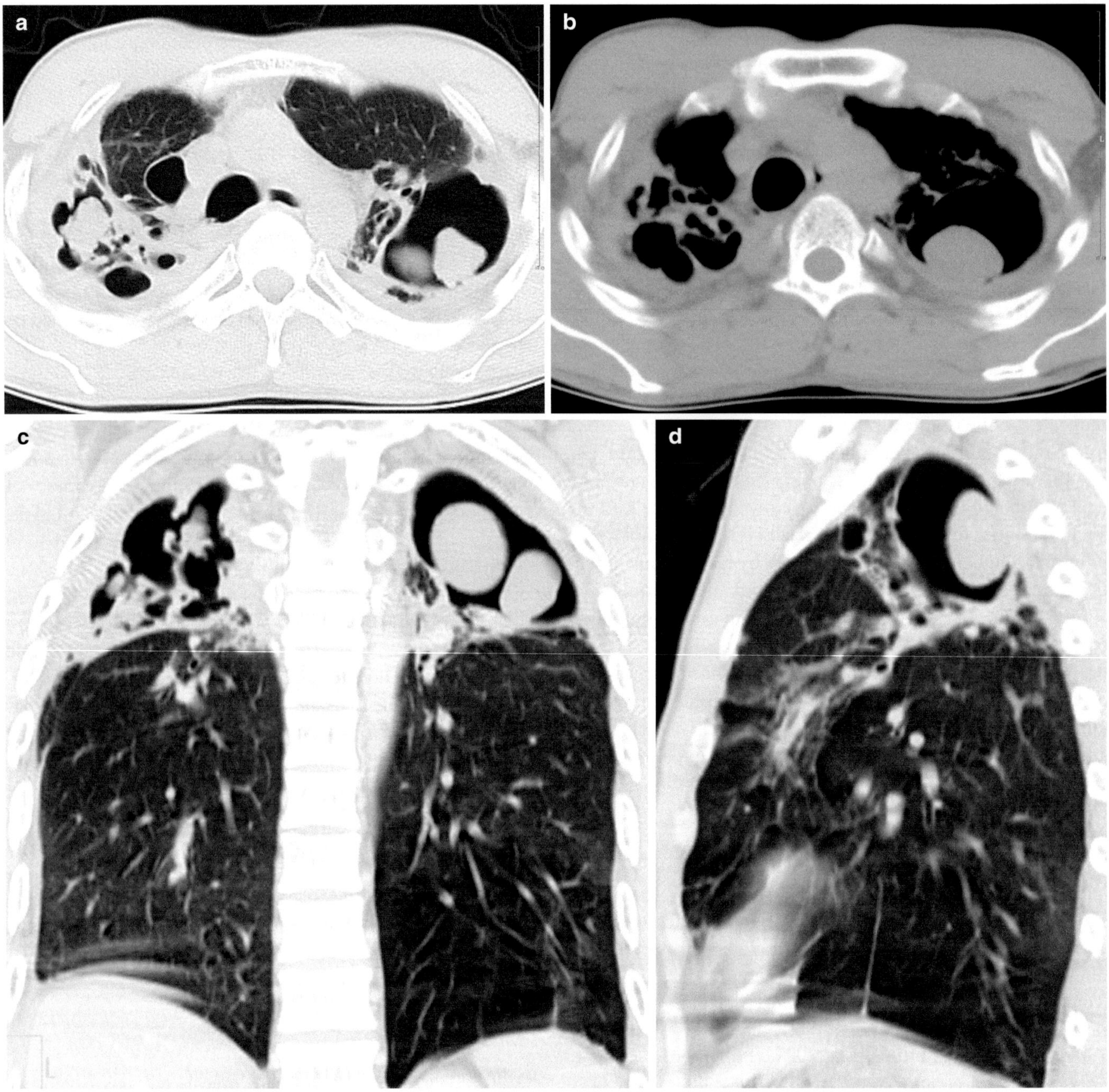

Fig. 12.49 (**a**–**f**) Chest CT scan. (**a**, **b**) Transverse lung window of CT scan demonstrates destructed bilateral upper lung lobes with shrinkage of volumes, local scattering strips and flakes of opacity and irregular nodular soft tissue opacity, and formation of cavity at the left upper lung. There are two spherical soft tissue opacities at the dorsal part of the cavity. The spherical soft tissue opacity has homogeneous intensity, which connects closely with the cavity wall. (**c**, **d**) Coronal lung window of CT scan demonstrates similar changes of the bilateral upper lung lobes to Figs. **a** and **b**. The inferior lingual segment of the left upper lung and bilateral lower lungs is demonstrated with fibrous cords opacity and nodular opacity, some of which are old lesions. (**e**, **f**) Transverse mediastinum window of enhanced CT scan demonstrates slight enhancement of fibrous cords opacity, local pleural thickening and adhesion with slight enhancement, and no obvious enhancement of the two spherical soft tissue opacities in the cavity of left upper lung

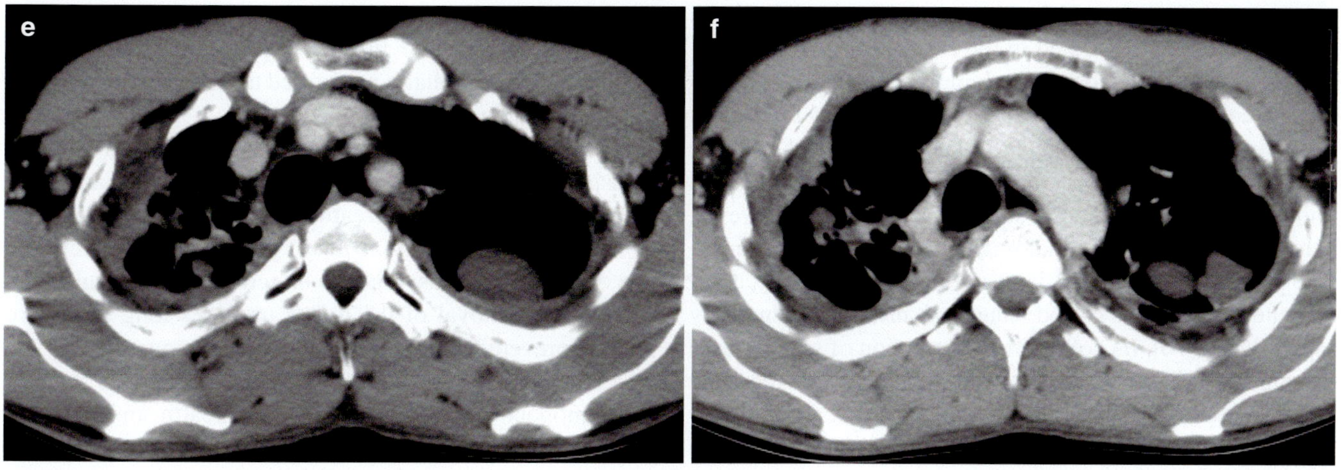

Fig. 12.49 (continued)

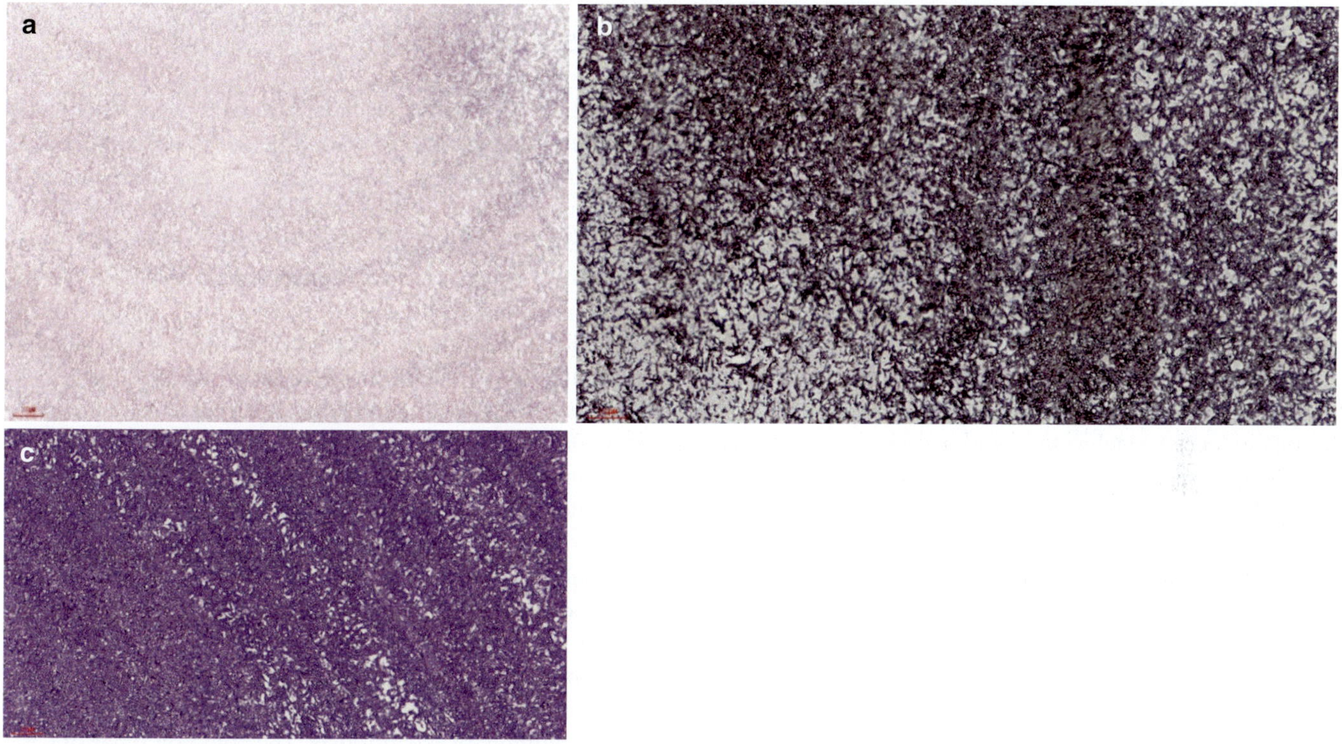

Fig. 12.50 (**a**–**c**) Pathology of lung tissue. (**a**) H&E staining demonstrates light purplish blue hyphae wall of aspergillus. (**b**) PASM staining demonstrates brownish black hyphae wall and spores of aspergillus. (**c**) PAS staining demonstrates reddish purple hyphae wall

cavity. Cough and hemoptysis facilitate aspergillus invading into the surrounding lung parenchyma or blood vessels to cause dissemination of inflammation and infiltration. Long-term aspergillus infection may cause mucous impaction of the airway, bronchiolitis, thickening of the bronchial wall, and even bronchiectasis and atelectasis. And these changes may further aggravate the infection, and the illness course thus prolongs.

The radiological demonstrations of pulmonary aspergillosis are diverse. By chest X-ray, invasive pulmonary aspergillosis is demonstrated as round nodule, infiltration opacity with the pleura as the base (pulmonary infarction), and formation of cavity. Round nodule is the common radiological finding of invasive pulmonary aspergillosis by initial CT scan. Its underlying mechanism is infarction of lung tissue induced by fungal hyphae and slight or moderate obstructive pulmonary infiltration. Halo sign is highly possible to be radiologically demonstrated in the cases of invasive pulmonary aspergillosis, whose underlying mechanism is peripheral alveolar bleeding induced by hemorrhagic infarction. Halo sign is believed to be early demonstration of invasive pulmonary aspergillosis in patients with compromised immunity, indicating active stage of aspergillus. However, halo sign is non-specific radiological demonstration of invasive pulmonary aspergillosis. Cavity is radiologically demonstrated in the advanced stage of invasive pulmonary aspergillosis [76]. Its collapse and formation of solid nodule (aspergilloma in some patients) commonly indicate recovery of the patient's immunity as well as localization and chronicity of the pulmonary lesions. The prognosis is comparatively favorable [77].

Aspergilloma is the most common type of chronic and saprophytic aspergillosis. CT scan may demonstrate early signs of pleural thickening adjacent to aspergilloma and typical air crescent sign. And dynamic X-ray demonstrates movable aspergilloma in the cavity. Chronic cavitary pulmonary aspergillosis, formerly known as complex pulmonary aspergilloma, commonly occurs in patients with bronchial structural diseases. A prior formation of cavity occurs, with or with no aspergilloma inside. The multiple cavities in the lungs are formed by amplification of prior cavities. During the acute progression stage of allergic bronchopulmonary aspergillosis, the lesions may rapidly infiltrate toward the central lung, manifested as thickening of bronchial wall to finger bag-like, lung consolidation, non-caseous bronchial granuloma, and bronchiolitis. Further progression of the lesions induces bronchiectasis and occasional atelectasis of lung lobe or segment. In its advanced stage, it may develop into pulmonary fibrosis and central bronchiectasis. Mucous impaction of the airway is a characteristic change of allergic bronchopulmonary apsergillosis [78]. We found that mucous plug is demonstrated in typical cases of allergic bronchopulmonary aspergillosis, while bud-in-tree sign of lobular central nodule is demonstrated in atypical cases of allergic bronchopulmonary aspergillosis.

In this case, the patient suffered from chronic cavitary pulmonary aspergillosis. And we summarized the following key points about the case:

1. Patients of pulmonary tuberculosis are likely to subject to infection of multiple microorganisms. The cases with multiple nodules and inflammatory changes should be suspected with pulmonary aspergillus infection. Especially when common antibacterial therapy is ineffective, BAL or biopsy should be further performed to define the diagnosis.
2. For the patient with chronic fibro-cavitary pulmonary tuberculosis and chest X-ray demonstration of solid nodule in cavity, chest CT scan should be ordered. If there is air crescent sign or other characteristic signs, aspergillus infection should be highly suspected. Prone CT scan should be additionally performed to demonstrate mobility of the nodule in the cavity.
3. For patients of common populations with pulmonary aspergillus infection, voriconazole and itraconazole are optimal choices for treatment. However, for patients with chronic fibro-cavitary pulmonary tuberculosis complicated by aspergillus infection and aspergilloma, surgical removal of the lesion provides long-term cure and prevents hemoptysis and local expansion of the lesion. However, patients with basic disease, such as pulmonary dysfunction, and poor health and who are elderly, have higher morbidity and mortality after surgery. We should balance the advantages and disadvantages before surgery.

12.16.5 Comments

In this case, two points need further discussion. The first is the differentiation of pulmonary tuberculosis and pulmonary aspergillus infection. In the clinical guideline for the diagnosis and treatment of chronic pulmonary aspergillosis (CPA) jointly issued by ESCMID/ERS in 2015, pulmonary tuberculosis may be before, after, or concurrent with CPA. In this case, the patient had a past medical history of pulmonary tuberculosis. Radiology demonstrated destructed bilateral upper lungs. After admission, PPD test showed strongly positive. Based on these findings, a diagnosis of pulmonary tuberculosis complicated by pulmonary aspergillosis can be established. It should be noted that a definitive diagnosis of tuberculosis mycobacteria infection cannot exclude the possibility of concurrent CPA. In the cases of chronic fibro-cavitary pulmonary tuberculosis, if chest X-ray demonstrates solid nodule in cavity, air crescent sign, or other characteristic sign of pulmonary aspergillosis, aspergillus infection should be considered. The second point is the differentiation of chronic cavitary pulmonary aspergillosis and chronic necrotizing pulmonary aspergillosis. The common types of CPA include chronic cavitary pulmonary aspergillosis (CCPA), chronic fibrosing pulmonary aspergillosis (CFPA), aspergillus nodule, single/simple pulmonary aspergilloma, and chronic necrotizing pulmonary aspergillosis (CNPA) which is also known as subacute invasive aspergillosis (SAIA). The three types of CPA, including CCPA, CFPA, and CNPA, may be overlapping. And along with the progression, the three types can be interchangeable. Without pathological evidence and clinical follow-ups, differentiation of CCPA from CNPA may be challenging. Pathologically, in the cases of CCPA, hyphae can be found in cavity. And there are accompanying chronic inflammatory responses and surrounding fibrosis or its mixture with infiltration of inflammatory cells. In contrast, in the cases of CNPA, histology demonstrates invasion of hyphae into lung parenchyma, with accompanying acute inflammatory responses or necrosis. Clinically, CNPA has a rapid progression, with initial manifestations of singular consolidation and progression into cavity within several days or weeks. During the following 1–3 months, the lesion gradually expands, with accompanying pleural thickening, pneumothorax, and pleural effusion. Air crescent sign may be demonstrated, which may be a sign signaling necrosis. Therefore, the air crescent sign commonly indicates aggravation of the condition. In this case, in combination to clinical diagnosis and treatment as well as pathology, a diagnosis of CCPA can be made. But we should know that CCPA and CNPA may be overlapping. Along with progression, the two diseases are interchangeable.

12.17 Case 17: Recurrent Cough for More Than 10 Years and Intermittent Hemoptysis for 2 Years

Dong-Na Su, Ling-Wei Wang, Hongtao Jin, Shi-Ping Wu, Guangsuo Wang, and Hui Han

12.17.1 Presenting Symptom

Recurrent cough for more than 10 years and intermittent hemoptysis for 2 years.

12.17.2 Brief Case History

A 36-year-old woman was admitted to our hospital on March 22, 2015, due to complaints of recurrent cough for more than 10 years and intermittent hemoptysis for 2 years. More than 10 years ago, the patient began to experience cough and expectoration. But she experienced no fever, night sweat, and breathlessness. She presented in a local hospital, and the diagnosis there was emphysema and bronchiectasis of the left upper lung lobe. Cephalosporin was then administered (specifically unknown) for infection, and the symptoms were relieved. Since then, intermittent cough persisted, which tended to occur when she was tired or caught a cold, but she received no standard treatment. Two years ago, the cough aggravated, occasionally with hemoptysis of sputum with blood streak. But she experienced no fever. In a local hospital, bronchoscopy demonstrated bronchial inflammation of the left upper lung lobe. BALF of the left upper lung lobe was harvested for AFB, TB-DNA, and culture of tuberculosis mycobacteria, all of which showed negative. A diagnosis was then made to be lung infection. And symptomatic therapies for infection and hemostasis were administered, and the symptoms were improved. Hemoptysis was cured. Two months ago, she suffered from bloody sputum again. And she was admitted to a third-grade class-A hospital; chest CT scan there demonstrated irregular mass soft tissue opacity at the anterior segment of left upper lung lobe, which was lobulated with spikes at the margin and poorly defined from the pleura and mediastinum. The diagnosis was mass opacity at the left upper lung lobe, and malignancies were not excluded (Fig. 12.51). The following percutaneous lung puncture for biopsy demonstrated less bronchial mucosa and lung tissue, with infiltration of interstitial inflammatory cells. Thoracoscopic removal of the left upper lung lobe was performed on February 10, 2015. And the postoperative pathology demonstrated a yellowish nodule in the specimen of lung tissue. Under a microscope, the normal lung structure was destructed, with bronchiectasis and well-differentiated

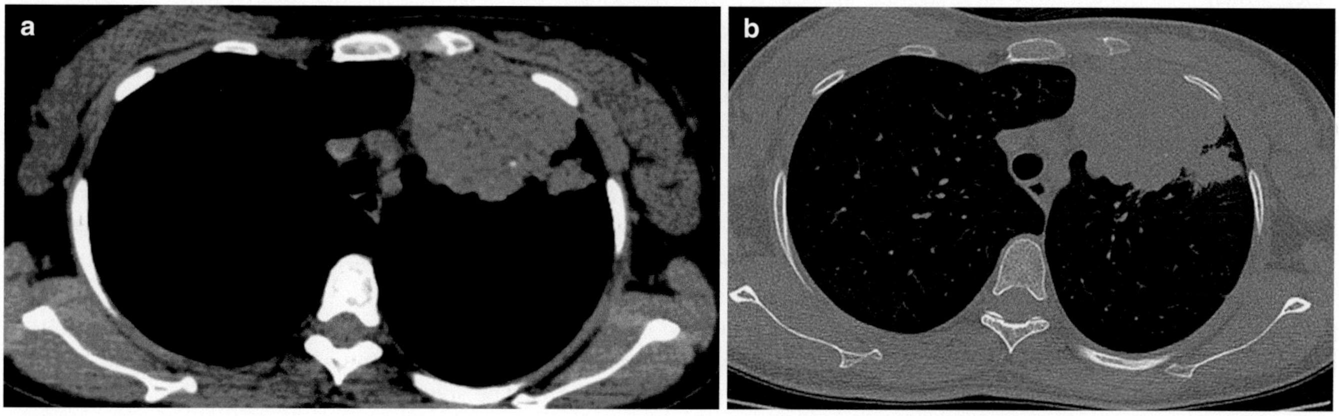

Fig. 12.51 (**a**, **b**) Chest CT scan. (**a**) The mediastinum window demonstrates irregular mass soft tissue opacity at the anterior segment of left upper lung lobe, which has heterogeneous intensity. And its anteromedial part is connected with the mediastinum and pleura. A lateral small nodular opacity is demonstrated to be connected with the mass opacity. (**b**) The lung window demonstrates marginal lobulation of the mass opacity at the left upper lung lobe and spikes around the small nodular opacity

epithelium. There were also hyperplasia of fibrous tissue, with infiltration of many lymphocytes and neutrophile granulocytes. The findings were consistent to bronchiectasis. After the surgery, the symptoms of cough and hemoptysis were relieved. But 1 week ago, she began to experience dry cough again, which gradually aggravated. But she experienced no fever, night sweat, chest distress, breathlessness, and hemoptysis. For further diagnosis and treatment, she was admitted to our hospital.

12.17.2.1 Past Medical History

She reported no special past medical history, personal history, menstruation history, and social history.

12.17.2.2 Physical Examination

Physical examination showed a body temperature of 36 °C, pulse rate 81/min, respiration rate 20/min, and blood pressure 98/58 mmHg. The thorax was bilaterally symmetric, with no deformity. The lateral left thorax showed an operation scar in length of about 6 cm. The sternum showed no tenderness. And the vocal fremitus of both lungs was not weakened. By percussion, both lungs showed clear sounds. By auscultation, both lungs showed clear respiration sounds, with weak respiration sounds at the left upper lung. And there were no obvious dry and/or moist rales. The apical beat of heart was strong, with not enlarged heart. The heartbeat was rhythmic, with no pathological murmur. The abdomen was soft, with no tenderness and no palpable mass.

12.17.2.3 Auxiliary Investigation

Radiology

Chest CT scan was performed on January 18, 2015, in a third-grade class-A hospital. It demonstrated irregular mass soft tissue opacity at the anterior segment of left upper lung lobe, which was lobulated with marginal spikes. It was poorly defined from the pleura and mediastinum. The diagnosis was considered to be mass opacity at the left upper lung lobe, with malignancies not excluded. Enhanced chest CT scan or lung puncture for biopsy were recommended (Fig. 12.51).

Histopathology

Thoracoscopic removal of the left upper lung lobe was performed on February 10, 2015. And the postoperative pathology demonstrated grayish yellow nodule in the lung tissue. Under a microscope, the lung structure was destructed, with bronchiectasis and well-differentiated epithelium. There were also hyperplasia of fibrous tissue, with infiltration of many lymphocytes and neutrophile granulocytes. The lesions were consistent to bronchiectasis (Fig. 12.52).

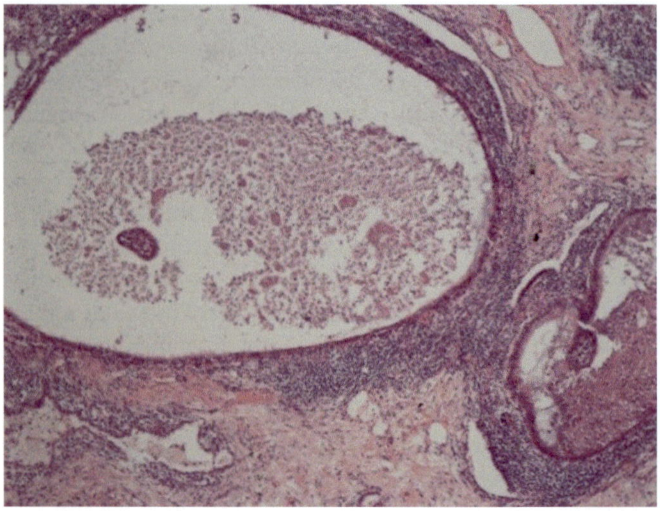

Fig. 12.52 Pathology of lung tissue. H&E staining demonstrates dilation of bronchioles, with surrounding infiltration of many inflammatory cells

12.17.2.4 Initial Diagnosis

The initial diagnosis was space-occupying lesion at the left upper lung which was suspected to be neoplasm and postoperative findings of bronchiectasis at the left upper lung.

12.17.3 Diagnosis and Treatment

After admission, routine blood test showed WBC count 4.40 × 109/L, hemoglobin concentration 142 g/L, neutrophile granulocytes 50.0%, and lymphocytes 39.1%. The liver function test, blood sugar, electrolytes, and myocardial enzymes were within normal limits. The hs-CRP was 0.36 mg/L and procalcitonin <0.05 ng/ml. The ESR was 12.0 mm/h. And the antistreptolysin O test was 44.0 IU/ml. The antibody against tuberculosis mycobacteria showed negative.

Reexamination of chest CT scan was performed on March 24, 2015. It demonstrated postoperative changes after surgical removal of left upper lung lobe, vacuolated exudation at the dorsal segment of left lower lung lobe, and left pleural thickening (Fig. 12.53).

Fibrobronchoscopy was ordered on March 25, 2015, which demonstrated inflammatory changes of the bronchi (Fig. 12.54). The sputum smear and BALF smear were performed for bacteria, fungi, and acid fast bacilli, which showed negative. And the sputum culture showed negative.

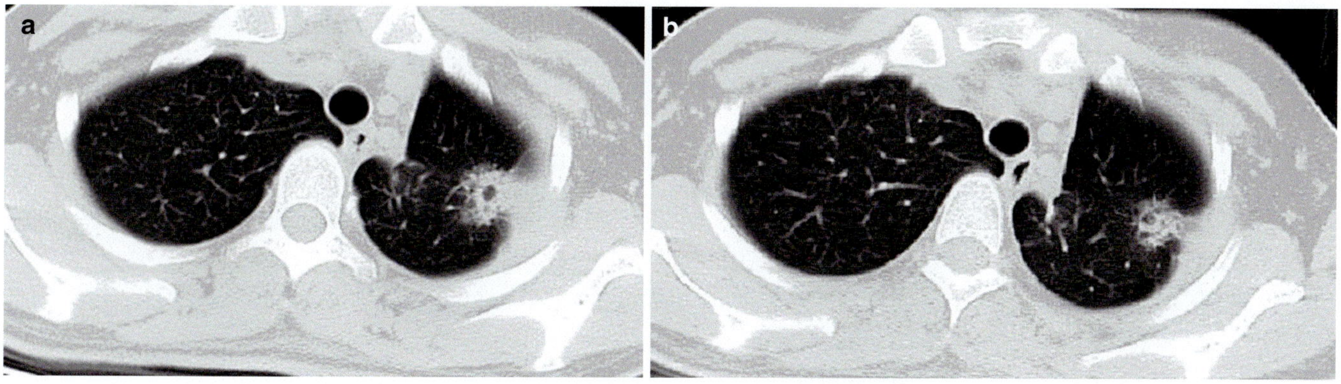

Fig. 12.53 Chest CT scan. (**a**, **b**) Chest CT scan demonstrates postoperative changes after surgical removal of left upper lung lobe, vacuolated exudation at the dorsal segment of left lower lung lobe, and left pleural thickening. There is also irregular small nodule, which is connected with lateral pleura

Fig. 12.54 Fibrobronchoscopy. Fibrobronchoscopy demonstrates inflammatory changes of the bronchi

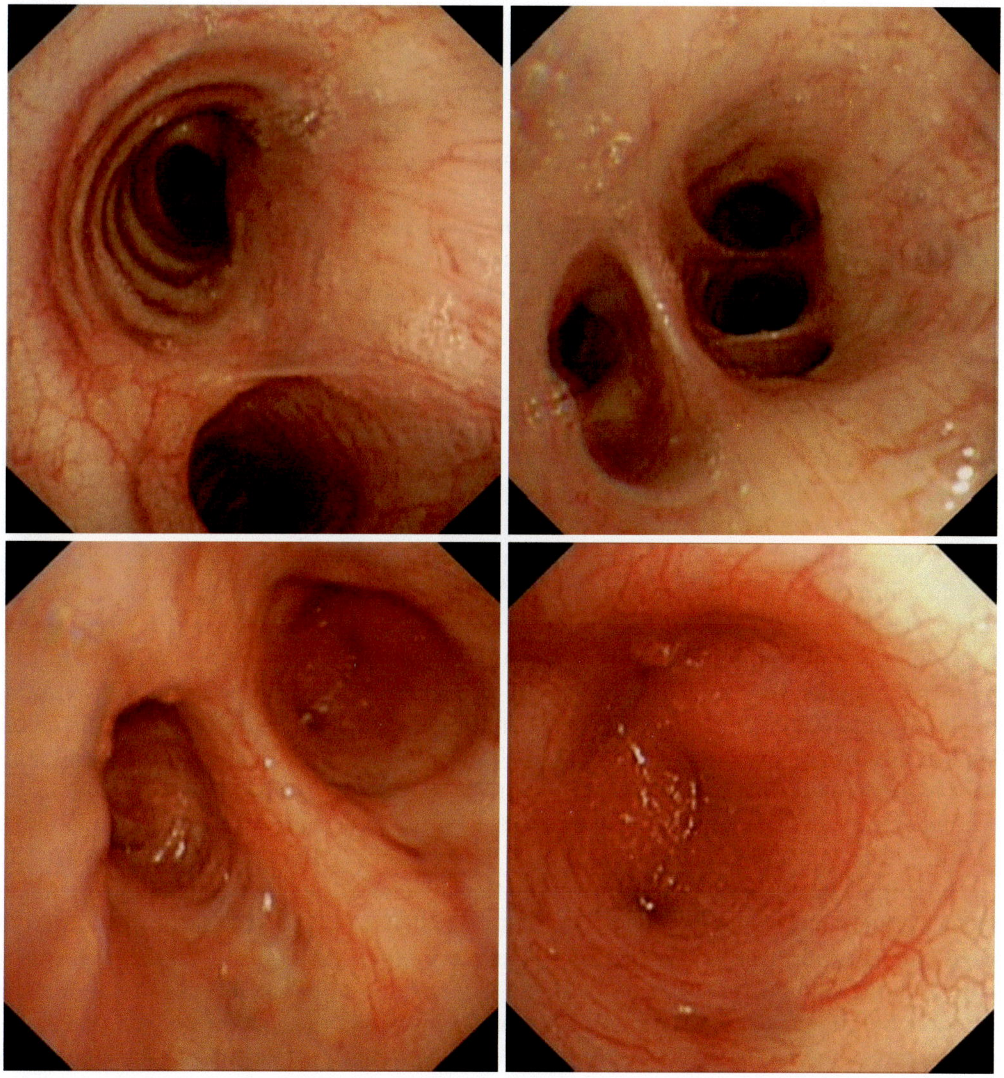

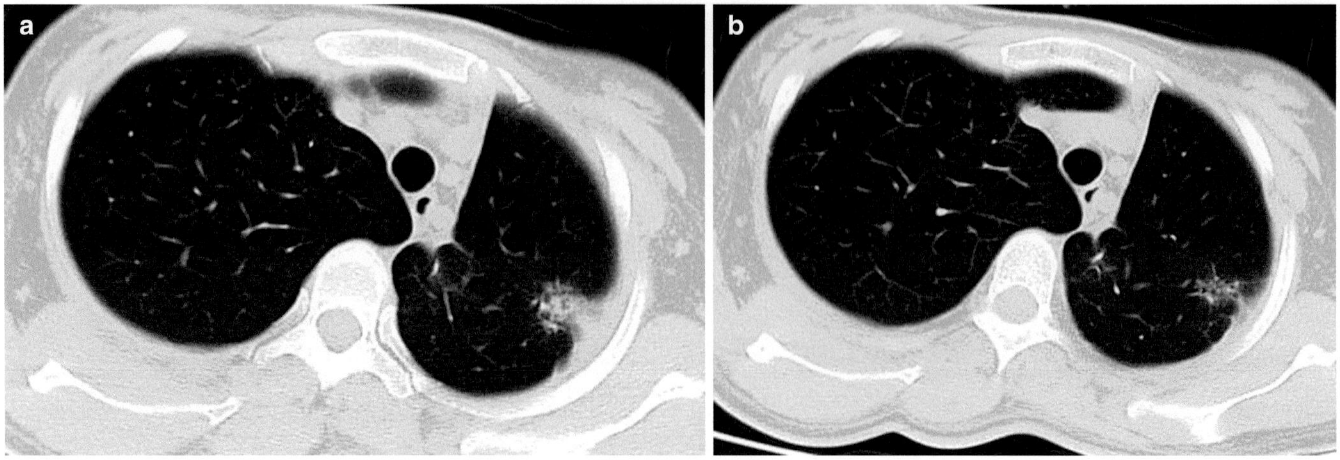

Fig. 12.55 (**a**, **b**) Chest CT scan. (**a**, **b**) Chest CT scan demonstrates postoperative changes after surgical removal of left upper lung and absorption of infection lesions at the left lower lung

The blood G test, GM test, and cryptococcal antigen test showed negative.

After admission, moxifloxacin was administered for infection, but the condition was not obviously improved.

A clinical diagnosis of aspergillus infection was considered. Intravenous infusion of voriconazole was then administered since April 9, 2015. Reexamination of chest CT scan on April 18, 2015, demonstrated absorption of the lesions (Fig. 12.55).

Pathological section of neoplasm at the left upper lung was sent to the superior hospital on April 23, 2015, for multidisciplinary meeting for the case.

On April 29, 2015, the pathology of the superior hospital demonstrated a lung lobe in size of 16 cm × 12 cm × 5 cm, with a quite well-defined grayish yellow nodule at the section in a size of about 9 cm × 6 cm × 5 cm. Under a microscope, the lung tissue showed well-differentiated alveolar epithelium, with bronchiectasis and surrounding infiltration of many lymphocytes and plasmocytes. In the bronchial lumen, there were inflammatory secretions and less fungal hyphae inside. The surrounding lung tissue was destructed, with hyperplasia of fibrous tissue and infiltrations of many lymphocytes and neutrophile granulocytes as well as less multinucleated giant cells.

By special stainings, PAS staining showed positive and methenamine silver staining positive. The pathological diagnosis was bronchiectasis complicated by pulmonary aspergillosis of the left upper lung (Fig. 12.56).

After the diagnosis was defined, intravenous infusion of voriconazole was administered for 2 weeks. And the patient was in a good condition occasionally with cough but no hemoptysis. The patient was discharged on April 29, 2015. And oral intake of voriconazole was continued.

The diagnosis on discharge was chronic necrotizing pulmonary aspergillosis and postoperative changes after surgical operation for bronchiectasis at the left upper lung.

After discharge, the condition of the patient was stable.

12.17.4 Discussion

In this case, the patient was a young woman, with chronic illness course. She experienced recurrent intermittent cough for more than 10 years, which was considered to be caused by bronchiectasis of the left upper lung and emphysema. And the diagnosis can be defined by thoracoscopic pathology. Two years ago, she began to experience bloody sputum, and the condition tended to aggravate. Before her admission to our hospital, a diagnosis of malignancy of left upper lung was considered based on chest CT scan in a third-grade class-A hospital, and further percutaneous lung puncture for biopsy was ordered to define the diagnosis. The condition was suspected to be tuberculosis, fungal infection, and neoplasm. Before her admission to our hospital, she had a past medical history of thoracoscopic removal of the left upper lung lobe, and the condition was improved after the surgery. But 1 week prior to the admission to our hospital, cough aggravated again. Reexamination of chest CT scan demonstrated exudation of the left lung, with vacuole. And the condition was considered to be postoperative relapse. Because the patient was a young woman with no hobby in smoking and relapse of the condition within a short period of time with exudation, neoplasm could be excluded. And possibility of pulmonary aspergillosis or pulmonary tuberculosis should be excluded.

In this case, evidence supporting tuberculosis includes chronic illness course, long-term cough with bloody sputum,

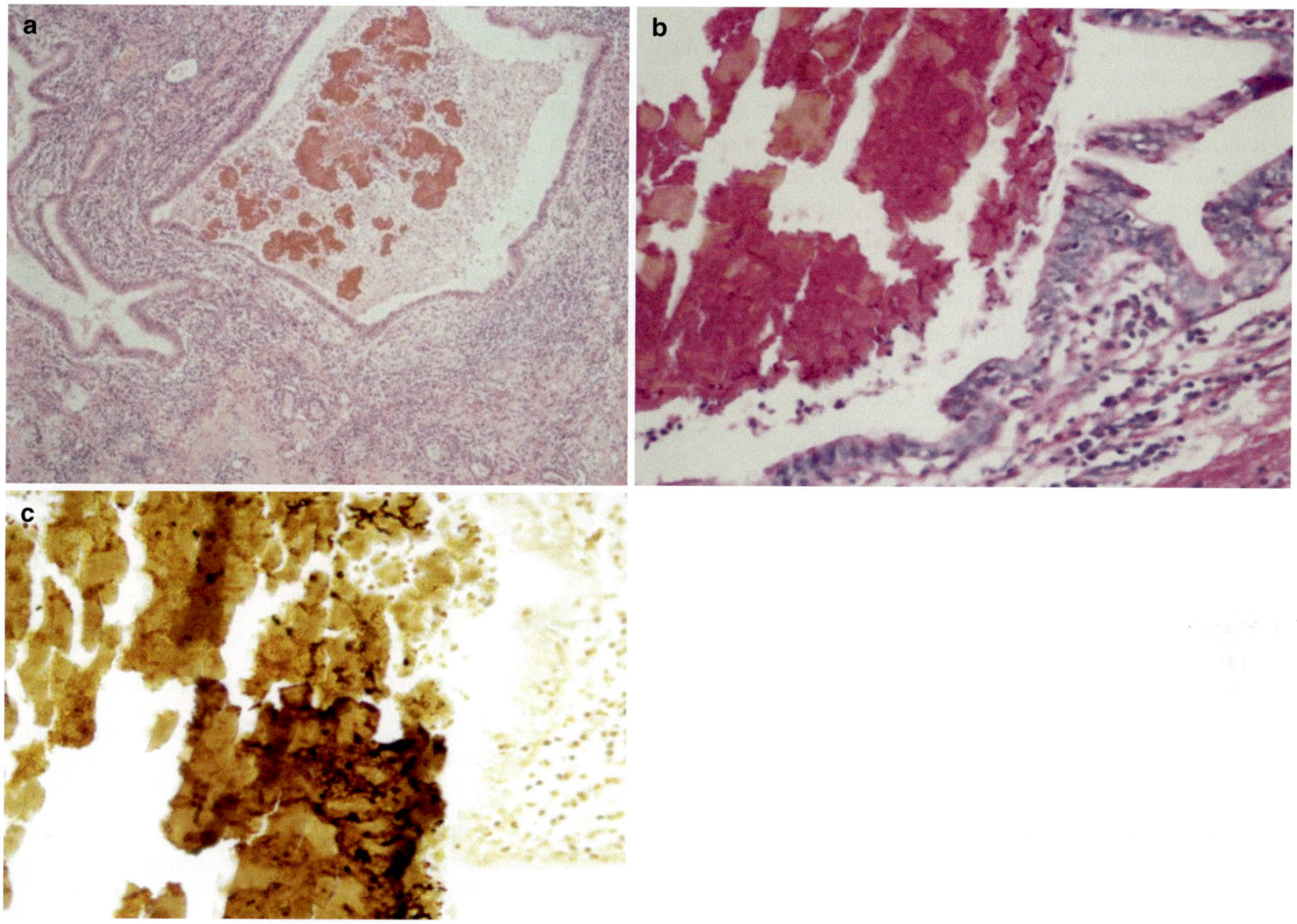

Fig. 12.56 (**a–c**) Pathology of lung tissue. (**a**) H&E staining (H&E × 100) demonstrates fungal hyphae in the bronchi. (**b**) PAS staining showed positive (+). (**c**) Methenamine silver staining showed positive (+)

and location of the lesion at the left upper lung. However, the patient showed no tuberculosis poisoning symptoms of low-grade fever after noons, night sweat, and emaciation. Repeated sputum culture for acid fast bacilli showed negative. All of these did not support the diagnosis of tuberculosis. One month after thoracoscopy, the lesions emerged again, with vacuolation. Compared to tuberculosis or neoplasm, the rapid relapse was more likely to be caused by aspergillus infection. The final diagnosis depended on pathology of lung tissue. And the clinical typing was chronic necrotizing pulmonary aspergillosis. In this case, early pathology did not demonstrated aspergillus infection. And lung tissue section was sent to the superior hospital for multidisciplinary meeting. The diagnosis was finally defined. The course of differential diagnosis was comparatively long.

The condition was clinically considered to be aspergillus infection. Therefore, before the diagnosis was pathologically defined, anti-aspergillus therapy should be administered as early as possible. Favorable therapeutic responses after anti-aspergillus therapy was given support the diagnosis of aspergillus infection. Concerning the administration and therapeutic course of anti-aspergillus therapy, it has been indicated in the clinical guideline for diagnosis and treatment of pulmonary aspergillosis issued by IDSA in 2016. For the cases of highly suspected with invasive pulmonary aspergillosis, if the condition progresses rapidly, antifungal therapy should be administered as early as possible when the diagnostic assessment is performed [79]. Voriconazole is recommended as the medication of first choice [80]. Combined use of polyenes or azoles with echinocandins can exert collaborative or potentiating effect [81]. However, clinical trials have not reached agreement. In the clinical guideline, combined use of voriconazole with echinocandins is recommended for patients with serious invasive pulmonary aspergillosis. Echinocandins is not recommended as the main medication [82]. When azoles and polyenes are contraindicated, echinocandins can be administered for treatment. The therapeutic course for invasive pulmonary aspergillosis is recommended to last for 6–12 weeks [83]. And the therapeutic course is mainly dependent on the immunosuppression and its duration, location of the lesions, and evidence of improvement. When the therapeutic efficacy is not favorable, it is recommended to exclude the possibility of new pathogen infection. And individualized therapy should be given according to the speed of progression, severity, range of infection, and occurrence of complications. The strategies of rescue therapy generally include changing the category of the medication, weakening or reversing immunosuppression if possible, and surgical removal of the lesion [84]. In this case, the patient showed relapse of the symptoms after thoracoscopic removal of the left upper lung lobe. Voriconazole was administered as the rescue therapy. And the condition was stabilized with no relapse, indicating successful treatment.

12.17.5 Comments

This is a case of pulmonary aspergillosis based on bronchiectasis and emphysema. In recent years, the cases of COPD complicated by pulmonary aspergillosis have been increasing. Due to chronic destruction of airway and the lung in patients with COPD, their defense mechanism is decreased, which induces long-term planting of aspergillus in the airway. If the patient receives hormone or wide-spectrum antibiotic for infection at the acute aggravation stage, the systemic and local defense mechanisms further decrease. Thus, occurrence and progression of aspergillus infection are promoted in patients with COPD. In this case, the patient experienced chronic cough for more than 10 years and received anti-infection therapy for several times. The relationship between anti-infection therapy and occurrence of aspergillus infection needs further exploration.

Chest CT scan on January 18, 2015, demonstrated irregular mass soft tissue opacity at the anterior segment of left upper lung lobe, which was lobulated with marginal spikes. Because the mass was large, lung malignancy could not be clinically excluded. And thoracoscopic removal of the left upper lung lobe was appropriate. However, pulmonary aspergillosis was misdiagnosed based on postoperative pathology. It is possibly due to insufficient knowledge and experience about pulmonary aspergillosis.

In this case, the patient experienced relieved symptoms of cough and hemoptysis after surgical operation. But the symptoms rapidly relapsed and aggravated. Reexamination of chest CT scan demonstrated vacuolated exudation at the left lower lung lobe, indicating postoperative relapse of aspergillus infection. Detection of aspergillus antibody titer may have certain value in predicting postoperative relapse of aspergillus infection. Slow decrease of aspergillus antibody titer indicates successful treatment. And rapid increase of aspergillus antibody titer is a sign signaling therapeutic failure or relapse.

Surgical removal of aspergilloma is a good choice for patients with favorable pulmonary functions. However, the success rate of surgery for other types of chronic pulmonary aspergillosis remains low, and postoperative relapse is more likely to occur. According to the clinical guideline for diagnosis and treatment of chronic pulmonary aspergillosis jointly issued by ESCMID and ERS in 2015, patients receiving surgical removal of singular aspergilloma with no intraoperative leakage of fungal substances do not need antifungal medication. But for patients with incomplete removal of the lesion, antifungal medication should be administered to prevent its relapse and aspergillus empyema. Serological quantification of aspergillus IgG can also be performed to monitor its postoperative relapse. Serological quantification of aspergillus IgG, test for inflammatory indices, and radiology should be performed every 3 months to assess necessity of antifungal medication.

References

1. Schweer KE, Bangard C, Hekmat K. Chronic pulmonary aspergillosis. Mycoses. 2014;57(5):257–70.
2. Zhuo S, Luo B. Diagnosis and treatment of pulmonary aspergillosis. Chin J Mod Med. 1998;8(7):31–4.
3. Ba PS, Ndiaye A, Diatta S. Results of surgical treatment for pulmonary aspergilloma. Med Sante Trop. 2015;25(1):92–6.
4. Walsh TJ, Anaissie EJ, Denning DW, et al. Treatment of aspergillosis: clinical practice guidelines of the Infectious Diseases Society of America. Clin Infect Dis. 2008;46:327–60.
5. Khana MA, Dara AM, Kawoosa NU, et al. Clinical profile and surgical outcome for pulmonary aspergilloma: nine year retrospective observational study in a tertiary care hospital. Int J Surg. 2011;9(3):267–71.
6. Ruan J, Zhang T, Duan Y, et al. Surgical treatment of pulmonary tuberculosis complicated by pulmonary aspergilloma. Chin J Med. 2013;93(25):1975–7.
7. Chambon C, Costa JM, Chaumete MT, et al. Galactomannan and polymerase chain reaction for the diagnosis of primary digestive aspergillosis in a patient with acute myeloid leukaemia. J Infect. 2011;43(3):213–4.
8. Limper AH, Knox KS, Sarosi CA, et al. An official American thoracic society statement: treatment of fungal infections in adult pulmonary and critical care patients. Am J Respir Crit Care Med. 2011;183(1):96–128.
9. Takahashi-Nakaguchi A, Muraosa Y, Hagiwara D, et al. Genome sequence comparison of Aspergillus fumigatus strains isolated from patients with pulmonary aspergilloma and chronic necrotizing pulmonary aspergillosis. Med Mycol. 2015;53(4):353–60.
10. Thompson GR 3rd, Patterson TF. Pulmonary aspergillosis: recent advances. Semin Respir Crip Care Med. 2011;32(6):673–81.
11. Denning DW, Pleuvry A, Cole DC. Global burden of chronic pulmonary aspergillosis as a sequel to pulmonary tuberculosis. Bull World Health Organ. 2011;89(2):864–72.
12. Huang Y, Li J, Yue T. CT diagnosis and differential diagnosis of different types of pulmonary aspergillosis. J Med Imaging. 2014;24(4):645–7.
13. Wu Z, Xu Y, Zhang X, et al. Surgical treatment for pulmonary aspergillosis: experience of 36 cases. J Pract Med. 2011;27(2):283–4.
14. Zhang C, Sun C, Cui J. Surgical treatment for 31 cases of pulmonary aspergillosis. Chin J Nosocomial Infect. 2013;23(1):89–90.

15. Zhu J. Diagnosis and treatment of pulmonary aspergilloma: analysis of 28 cases. J Pract Clin Med. 2009;13(5):109–10.
16. Feng C, Lin H, Guo L. Pulmonary aspergillosis: clinical analysis of 17 cases. Chin J Nosocomial Infect. 2006;16(10):1119–21.
17. Zeng D, Wu E, Xue X. Multi layer spiral CT diagnosis of pulmonary aspergillosis. Chin J Med Imaging. 2009;17(5):364–7.
18. Wang Y, Jiang Z, Chan F. CT scan demonstrations of pulmonary aspergillosis. J Huaihai Med. 2011;29(6):478–80.
19. Schulte T, Welcker K, Schatz J, et al. Surgical treatment of pulmonary aspergilloma. Mycoses. 2005;48(Suppl 1):46–50.
20. Massard G. Role of surgery in the treatment of pulmonary aspergillosis. Rev Mal Respir. 2005;22(3):466–72.
21. Cheng X, Liu J, He J, et al. Non-invasive surgery for pulmonary aspergillosis. Chin J Mod Med. 2003;13(24):81–2.
22. Yu X. Etiological analysis of hemoptysis and its therapeutic development. J Asian Pac Tradit Med. 2008;4(8):63–5.
23. Benjelloun H, Zaghba N, Yassine N, et al. Chronic pulmonary aspergillosis: a frequent and potentially severe disease. Med Mal Infect. 2015;45(4):128–32.
24. Hedayati MT, Azimi Y, Droudinia A, et al. Prevalence of chronic pulmonary aspergillosis in patients with tuberculosis from Iran. Eur J Clin Microbiol Infect Dis. 2015;34(9):1759–65.
25. Kosmidis C, Denning DW. The clinical spectrum of pulmonary aspergillosis. Thorax. 2015;70(3):270–7.
26. Karen CP, Mary ES. Diagnosis and treatment of pulmonary aspergillosis syndromes. Chest. 2014;146(5):1358–68.
27. Godet C, Philippe B, Laurent F, et al. Chronic pulmonary aspergillosis: an update on diagnosis and treatment. Respiration. 2014;88(2):162–74.
28. Liu Y, She D, Sun T, et al. Multicentered retrospective survey of clinically defined pulmonary mycosis during 1998 and 2007 in China. Chin J Tuberc Respir. 2012;34(02):86–90.
29. Patterson KC, Strek ME. Diagnosis and treatment of pulmonary aspergillosis syndromes. Chest. 2014;146(5):1358–68.
30. Garnacho-Montero J, Olaechea P, Alvarez-Lerma F, et al. Epidemiology, diagnosis and treatment of fungal respiratory infections in the critically ill patient. Rev Esp Quimioter. 2013;26(2):173–88.
31. Kim SH, Kim MY, Hong SI, et al. Invasive pulmonary aspergillosis-mimicking tuberculosis. Clin Infect Dis. 2015;61(1):9–11.
32. Kim SH, Kim MY, Hong SI. Pulmonary aspergillosis. Thorax. 2015;70(3):270–7.
33. Choo JY, Lee KY, Kim MY, et al. Pulmonary tuberculosis confirmed by percutaneous transthoracic needle biopsy: analysis of CT findings and review of correlations with underlying lung disease. Balkan Med J. 2014;31(3):208–13.
34. Jiang L, Liu X, Zhang X, et al. Misdiagnosis of pulmonary aspergillosis: an analysis of 22 cases. Electron Chin J Diagn. 2015;3(3):208–13.
35. Infection Group, Branch of Respiration of Chinese Medical Society & Editorial Committee of Chinese Journal of Tuberculosis and Respiration. Consensus on diagnosis and treatment of pulmonary mycosis. Chin J Tuberc Respir. 2007;30(11):821–34.
36. Pappas PG, Kauffman C, Andes D, et al. Clinical practice guidelines for the management of candidiasis: 2009 update by the Infectious Diseases Society of America. Clin Infect Dis. 2009;48(5):503–35.
37. Lee JK, Lee YJ, Park SS, et al. Clinical course and prognostic factors of pulmonary aspergilloma. Respirology. 2014;19(7):1066–72.
38. Sharma S, Dubey SK, Kumar N, et al. Monod and air crescent sign in aspergilloma. BMJ Case Rep. 2013; https://doi.org/10.1136/bcr-2013-200936.
39. Moodley L, Pillay J, Dheda K. Aspergilloma and the surgeon. J Thorac Dis. 2014;6(3):202–9.
40. Fernández-Ruiz M, Silva JT, San-Juan R, et al. Aspergillus tracheobronchitis: report of 8 cases and review of the literature. Balt For. 2012;91(5):261–73.
41. Greene RE, Sehlamra lT, Oestmaun JW. CT imaging findings in acute invasive pulmonary aspergillosis: clinical significance of the halo sign. Clin Infect Dis. 2007;44(3):373–9.
42. Tasci S, Glasmacher A, Lentini S, et al. Pseudomembranous and obstructive aspergillus tracheobronchitis: optimal diagnostic strategy and outcome. Mycoses. 2006;49(1):37–42.
43. Danner BC. Surgical treatment of pulmonary aspergillosis/mycosis in immunocompromised patients. Interact Cardiovasc Thorac Surg. 2008;7(5):771–6.
44. Patterson KC, Strek ME. Diagnosis and treatment of pulmonary aspergillosis syndromes. J Chest. 2014;146(5):1358–68.
45. Park SY, Lee SO, Choi SH, et al. Serum and bronchoalveolar lavage fluid galactomannan assays in patients with pulmonary aspergilloma. Clin Infect Dis. 2011;52(7):e149–52.
46. Zou M, Tang L, Zhao S, et al. Systematic review and meta-analysis of detecting galactomannan in bronchoalveolar lavage fluid for diagnosing invasive aspergillosis. PLoS One. 2012;7(8):e43347.
47. Limper AH, Knox KS, Sarosi CA, et al. An official American Thoracic Society statement: treatment of fungal infections in adult pulmonary and critical care patients. Am J Respir Crit Care Med. 2011;183(1):196–28.
48. Liu Y, She D, Sun T, et al. Multi-centered retrospective survey of clinically definitive cases of pulmonary mycosis during 1998 to 2007 in China. Chin J Tuberc Respir. 2011;34(2):85–90.
49. Zhang Z, Chen B. Clinical data analysis of pulmonary aspergillosis in the past 20 years in China. Int J Respir. 2009;29(4):193–6.
50. Smith NL, Denning DW. Underlying conditions in chronic pulmonary aspergillosis including simple aspergilloma. Eur Respir J. 2011;37:865–72.
51. Sonnenberg P, Murray J, Glynn JR, et al. HIV-1 and recurrence, relapse, and reinfection of tuberculosis after cure: a cohort study in South African mineworkers. Lancet. 2001;358:1687–93.
52. Hamilton CD, Stout JE, Goodman PC, et al. The value of end-of-treatment chest radiograph in predicting pulmonary tuberculosis relapse. Int J Tuberc Lung Dis. 2008;12:1059–64.
53. Mohapatra B, Sivakumar P, Bhattacharya S, et al. Aspergilloma and residual tuberculous cavities—the results of a resurvey. Tubercle. 1970;51:227–45.
54. British Tuberculosis Association. Aspergillus in persistent lung cavities after tuberculosis. A report from the Research Committee of the British Tuberculosis Association. Tubercle. 1968;49:1–11.
55. Li X, Xie H, Li S. Clinical typing and radiological demonstrations of pulmonary aspergillosis. Chin J Med Comput Imaging. 2010;16(5):384–8.
56. Thomas JW, Elias JA, David WD, et al. Aspergillus. Clin Infect Dis. 2008;46:327–60.
57. Li Y. CT scan demonstrations of pulmonary tuberculosis complicated by aspergillus infection. J Mod Diagn Treat. 2015;26(1):157–8.
58. Denning DW, Pleuvry A, Cole DC. Global burden of chronic pulmonary aspergillosis as a sequel to pulmonary tuberculosis. Bull WHO. 2011;89(12):864–72.
59. Agarwal AK, Bhagat R, Panchal N, et al. Allergic bronchopulmonary aspergillosis with aspergilloma mimicking fibrocavitary pulmonary tuberculosis. Asian Pac J Allergy Immunol. 1996;14(1):5–8.
60. Yoon SH, Park CM, Goo JM, et al. Pulmonary aspergillosis in immunocompetent patients without air-meniscus sign and underlying lung disease: CT findings and histopathologic features. J Acta Radiol. 2011;52:756–61.
61. Chien WL, Tseng JS. Pulmonary aspergillosis in an immunocompetent patient. Braz J Infect Dis. 2013;17:375–6.
62. Martinez D, Ananda-Rajah MR, Suominen H, et al. Automatic detection of patients with invasive fungal disease from free-text computed tomography (CT) scans. J Biomed Inform. 2015;53:251–60.
63. Oliva A, Flori P, Hennequin C, et al. Evaluation of the Aspergillus Western blot IgG kit for diagnosis of chronic aspergillosis. J Clin Microbiol. 2015;53(1):248–54.

64. Thomas JW, Elias JA. Treatment of aspergillosis: clinical practice guidelines of the Infectious Diseases Society of America. Clin Infect Dis. 2008;46(3):327–60.
65. Chun J-Y, Morgan R, Belli A-M. Radiological management of hemoptysis: a comprehensive review of diagnostic imaging and bronchial arterial embolization. Eur Radiol. 2010;33(2):240–50.
66. Lee YR, Choi YW, Lee KJ, et al. CT halo sign: the spectrum of pulmonary diseases. Br J Radiol. 2005;78(933):862–5.
67. Jeannette G, Mary EB. Histopathologic Diagnosis of Fungal Infections in the 21st Century. Am Soc Microbiol. 2011;24(2):247–80.
68. Farid S, Mohamed S, Devbhandari M, et al. Results of surgery for chronic pulmonary aspergillosis, optimal antifungal therapy and proposed high risk factors for recurrence—a National Centre's experience. J Cardiothorac Surg. 2013;8(1):180.
69. Sagan D, Goździuk K, Korobowicz E. Predictive and prognostic value of preoperative symptoms in the surgical treatment of pulmonary aspergilloma. J Surg Res. 2010;163(2):35–43.
70. Zhang J, Qu J. Disease spectrum of pulmonary aspergillosis and the strategies for their diagnosis. Chin J Tuberc Respir. 2015;38(1):11–3.
71. Editorial Committee of Chinese Journal of Internal Medicine. Diagnostic criteria and therapeutic principles of invasive pulmonary fungal infection. Chin J Intern Med. 2006;45(8):697–700.
72. Bulpa P, Dive A, Sibille Y. Invasive pulmonary aspergillosis in patients with chronic obstructive pulmonary disease. Eur Respir J. 2007;30(4):782–800.
73. Guinea J, Torres-Narbona M, Gijón P, et al. Pulmonary aspergillosis in patients with chronic obstructive pulmonary disease: incidence, risk factors, and outcome. Clin Microbiol Infect. 2010;16:870–7.
74. Leeflang MM, Debets-Ossenkopp YJ, Visser CE, et al. Galactomannan detection for invasive aspergillosis in immunocompromised patients. Cochrane Database Syst Rev. 2008;(4):CD007394.
75. Park SY, Lee SO, Choi SH. Serum and bronchoalveolar lavage fluid galactomannan assay in patients with pulmonary aspergilloma. Clin Infect Dis. 2011;52:e149–52.
76. Shroff S, Shorrf GS, Yust-katz S, et al. The CT halo sign in invasive aspergillosis. J Clin Case Rep. 2014;2(3):113–4.
77. Luo BL, Zhang LM, Hu CP, et al. Clinical analysis of 68 patients with pulmonary mycosis in China. Multidiscip Respir Med. 2011;6(5):278–83.
78. Singh Sehgal I, Agarwal R. Pulse methylprednisolone in allergic bronchopulmonary aspergillosis exacerbations. J Eur Respir Rev. 2014;23(131):149–52.
79. Bozeman S, deShazo R, Stringer S, et al. Complications of allergic fungal sinusitis. Am J Med. 2011;124:359–68.
80. Thompson GR 3rd, Patterson TF. Fungal disease of the nose and paranasal sinuses. J Allergy Clin Immunol. 2012;129:321–6.
81. Tsabouri S, Tseretopoulou X, Priftis K, et al. Omalizumab for the treatment of inadequately controlled allergic rhinitis: a systematic review and meta-analysis of randomized clinical trials. J Allergy Clin Immunol Pract. 2014;2:332–40.
82. Moreira AS, Silva D, Ferreira AR, et al. Antifungal treatment in allergic bronchopulmonary aspergillosis with and without cystic fibrosis: a systematic review. Clin Exp Allergy. 2014;44:1210–27.
83. Howard BE, Lal D. Oral steroid therapy in chronic rhinosinusitis with and without nasal polyposis. Curr Allergy Asthma Rep. 2013;13:236–43.
84. Tanou K, Zintzaras E, Kaditis AG. Omalizumab therapy for allergic bronchopulmonary aspergillosis in children with cystic fibrosis: a synthesis of published evidence. Pediatr Pulmonol. 2014;49:503–7.

Pulmonary Aspergillosis with Presenting Symptom of Breathlessness

13

Wei-Dong Song and Ling-Wei Wang

The clinical typing of pulmonary aspergillosis depends on the immunity of the patients. After aspergillus spores are inhaled, populations with competent immunity may show no adverse consequences. In populations with immunosuppression, invasive pulmonary aspergillosis (IPA) occurs. In populations with slight immunosuppression or competent immunity, chronic pulmonary aspergillosis or aspergilloma occurs. And in populations with hyperreactive immune response, allergic bronchopulmonary aspergillosis (ABPA) occurs. The clinical typing and manifestations of pulmonary aspergillosis are diverse in populations with no immunosuppression. According to a literature report, the incidence rates of breathlessness and wheezing are up to 57.9% and 26.3%, respectively.

In this section, we introduce and analyze four cases of pulmonary aspergillosis with presenting symptom of breathlessness and wheezing. Of the four cases, there is one case of ABPA, one case of IPA, one case of chronic renal inadequacy complicated by IPA, and one case of SAIA. These cases represent different types of pulmonary aspergillosis with presenting symptoms of breathlessness and wheezing.

As the most common type of allergic pulmonary aspergillosis, ABPA commonly occurs in patients with asthma and cystic fibrosis. In recent years, there are also reports of ABPA in patients with COPD and bronchiectasis. The underlying mechanism is allergic inflammation in bronchi, alveoli, and lung interstitium induced by aspergillus (mainly *Aspergillus fumigatus*) antigen instead of aspergillus infection. Its pathomechanism is related to aspergillus-specific IgE-mediated type II allergic responses and specific IgG-mediated type III allergic responses. Breathlessness and wheezing are the most common clinical manifestations, which always show unfavorable therapeutic responses to simple anti-asthma medication. Other clinical manifestations include bronchitis or pneumonia, fever, eosinophilia in peripheral blood or induced sputum, transient pulmonary infiltration, and golden brown jellylike sputum bolt. Obstruction of the bronchus by mucus plug containing aspergillus hyphae and eosinophils may induce bronchiectasis, which is more obvious in patients with chronic condition. No accurate data is available about the incidence of ABPA in populations. And patients with skin test positive for aspergillus antigen account for 28% in patients with asthma, and the incidence of ABPA is about 12.9%. It had been believed that ABPA is a rare disease. However, due to insufficient knowledge about ABPA, most patients with ABPA are misdiagnosed as intractable bronchial asthma. Therefore, some scholars proposed that patients with asthma should routinely receive skin test for aspergillus allergen and regular follow-ups. Those with the skin test positive should further receive test for IgE to exclude ABPA.

Compared to the low incidence of ABPA, the incidence of another pulmonary aspergillosis-related disease, COPD, is far higher. More and more clinical data suggest that COPD is closely related with IPA, and patients with COPD are the high-risk population of subacute invasive pulmonary aspergillosis (SAIA). Based on the statistical data from 11,881 cases of invasive mycosis in more than 1000 medical institutions in the United States, among the populations with basic diseases and secondary invasive fungal infections, COPD is the most common (22.2%) basic disease, followed by diabetes and hematologic malignancy. Persistent wheezing is possibly the most common clinical manifestation (79%) in patients with COPD complicated by IPA, whose incidence is

The corresponding author of section 13.1 is Jiaxuan Zhou, Email: 195137680@qq.com.
The corresponding author of section 13.2 is Wenhui Tang, Email: 13902444613@163.com.
The corresponding author of section 13.3 is Yanwei Chen, Email: 853361654@qq.com.
The corresponding author of section 13.4 is Dandan Chen, Email: chendandan81@163.com.

W.-D. Song (✉)
Shenzhen Hospital of Beijing University, Shenzhen, Guangdong, China

L.-W. Wang
Second Clinical Medical College of Jinan University, Shenzhen, Guangdong, China

C. Qiu et al. (eds.), *Pulmonary Aspergillosis*, https://doi.org/10.1007/978-981-13-3435-1_13

significantly higher than fever (38.5%). The high-risk factors of IPA include the use of wide-spectrum antibiotic, large dose of hormone, and structural abnormality of the lung in patients with COPD. In addition, for patients with acute exacerbation of COPD and persistent wheezing, airway hyperresponsiveness induced by aspergillus should be prevented. The chest CT scan of such patients may only demonstrate thickening of the bronchial wall but no obvious exudation. The clinical manifestation is wheezing that shows unfavorable therapeutic responses to medications of spasmolysis, asthma relieving, and hormones. The diagnosis of COPD complicated by IPA is challenging. The sensitivity of serum GM test was low (20–45.5%). And most patients with COPD complicated by IPA show pulmonary dysfunction and are intolerant to bronchoscopy due to wheezing. Therefore, its diagnosis can be hardly defined. In addition, patients with COPD complicated by IPA may show false positive in serum or BALF GM test due to their simultaneous use of β-lactam antibiotics, such as cefoperazone/sulbactam and piperacillin/tazobactam. In general, patients receiving hormone therapy for serious COPD, if recent aggravation of breathlessness occurs and chest radiology demonstrates ineffectively treated pneumonia by antibiotics within recent 3 months, especially nodule with formation of cavity, should be suspected with COPD complicated by IPA.

The introduction, analysis, and comments of these cases are intended to increase clinicians' knowledge about the diverse clinical manifestation of IPA in populations with no immunosuppression. Breathlessness or wheezing and even dyspnea are presenting symptoms of such patients. The diagnosis mainly depends on clinical diagnosis because the serum GM test shows low positive rate (lower than 50%).

Patients' consents have been obtained for images or other clinical information relating to the cases to be published.

13.1 Case 1: Cough, Expectoration and Wheezing for 26 Years and Aggravation for 2 Weeks

Jiaxuan Zhou, Qingsi Zeng, Xiaoyan Huang, Qin Liu, Dong-Na Su, Hui Zeng, and Ruming Xie

13.1.1 Presenting Symptoms

Cough, expectoration, and wheezing for 26 years and aggravation for 2 weeks.

13.1.2 Brief Case History

A 29-year-old man was admitted to our hospital on July 10, 2013, due to complaints of cough, expectoration, and wheezing for 26 years and aggravation for 2 weeks. Twenty-six years ago, the patient began to experience recurrent cough, expectoration, and wheezing. The cough was paroxysmal, with whitish loose sputum, which commonly occurred when there were major climatic changes. But he experienced no hemoptysis and occasional fever (the body temperature unknown). He presented in a local hospital for several times and the diagnosis was bronchial asthma. And the symptoms were relived after he received asthma relieving therapy and other symptomatic therapies. Six years ago, he was diagnosed with bronchiectasis and infection in another hospital due to complaints of aggravated cough and expectoration of yellowish purulent sputum in a large quantity with blood streak. Medications for infection, spasmolysis, and asthma relieving were administered, and the symptom of wheezing was controlled. However, cough and expectoration of brownish mucus sputum persisted. In recent 2 weeks, the symptoms of cough, expectoration, and breathlessness obviously aggravated. But he experienced no fever, emaciation, and night sweat. For further diagnosis and treatment, he was admitted to our hospital. Since the onset of symptoms, his spiritual state, appetite, and sleep were normal. The urinations and bowel movements were normal. And the patient experienced no obvious body weight change.

13.1.2.1 Past Medical History

He denied histories of hypertension, diabetes, and coronary heart disease. And he had no hobbies in smoking and drinking.

13.1.2.2 Physical Examination

Physical examination showed a body temperature of 36.5 °C, pulse rate 105/min, respiration rate 20/min, and blood pressure 120/70 mmHg. He was typically developed, with average nourishment. The patient was well conscious. And the respirations were smooth. The patient was in active position and can answer to the questions. And he was well cooperated with physical examination. The skin mucosa showed no yellowish stains. The systemic superficial lymph nodes were unpalpable. By auscultation, both lungs showed no dry and/or moist rales. The heart was not enlarged, with a heartbeat of 105/min, rhythmic. By auscultation, the valvular areas showed no pathological murmur. The abdomen was soft. The liver and spleen were not palpable. The shifting dullness was negative. And the liver and kidney were not sensitive to percussion. The bowel sounds were normal. And there was clubbing finger.

13.1.2.3 Auxiliary Investigation

Laboratory Test

Laboratory tests showed WBC 8.12 × 10^9/L, N 59%, E 16%, and E 1.30 × 10^9/L. ESR was 90 mm/h.

Radiology
Chest CT scan in another hospital demonstrated segmental atelectasis at the lingual lobe of the left lung.

13.1.2.4 Initial Diagnosis

The initial diagnosis was bronchiectasis, infection, and asthma.

13.1.3 Diagnosis and Treatment

After admission, investigations were performed. The pulmonary function test showed moderate obstructive dysfunctional ventilation and histamine bronchial provocation test (HBPT) positive. Chest CT scan on July 12, 2013, demonstrated (Fig. 13.1) dilated proximal and middle segments of the bronchi near the hilum in both lungs and thickening of the partial bronchial wall that were more obvious in the right upper lung and lingual segment of the left upper lung. There were also bronchial mucus plug in the apical segment of the right upper lung and lingual segment of the left upper lung, patchy blurry opacity around the bronchi, and subsegmental consolidation and atelectasis at the lingual segment of the left upper lung. The condition was considered to be allergic bronchopulmonary aspergillosis (ABPA).

After admission, the serum total IgE was 1949.99 IU/ml (normal range <100 IU/ml); the titer of specific IgE antibody against *Aspergillus fumigatus* was 35.3 kAu/L (normal range < 0.35 kAu/L); and the cryptococcal antigen was negative. The G test for fungi was lower than 10 pg/ml, aspergillus antigen negative, and candida antigen negative. The TB-DNA was negative, and the sputum culture showed no growth of pathogenic bacteria. The skin test for aspergillus antigen showed rapid positive response.

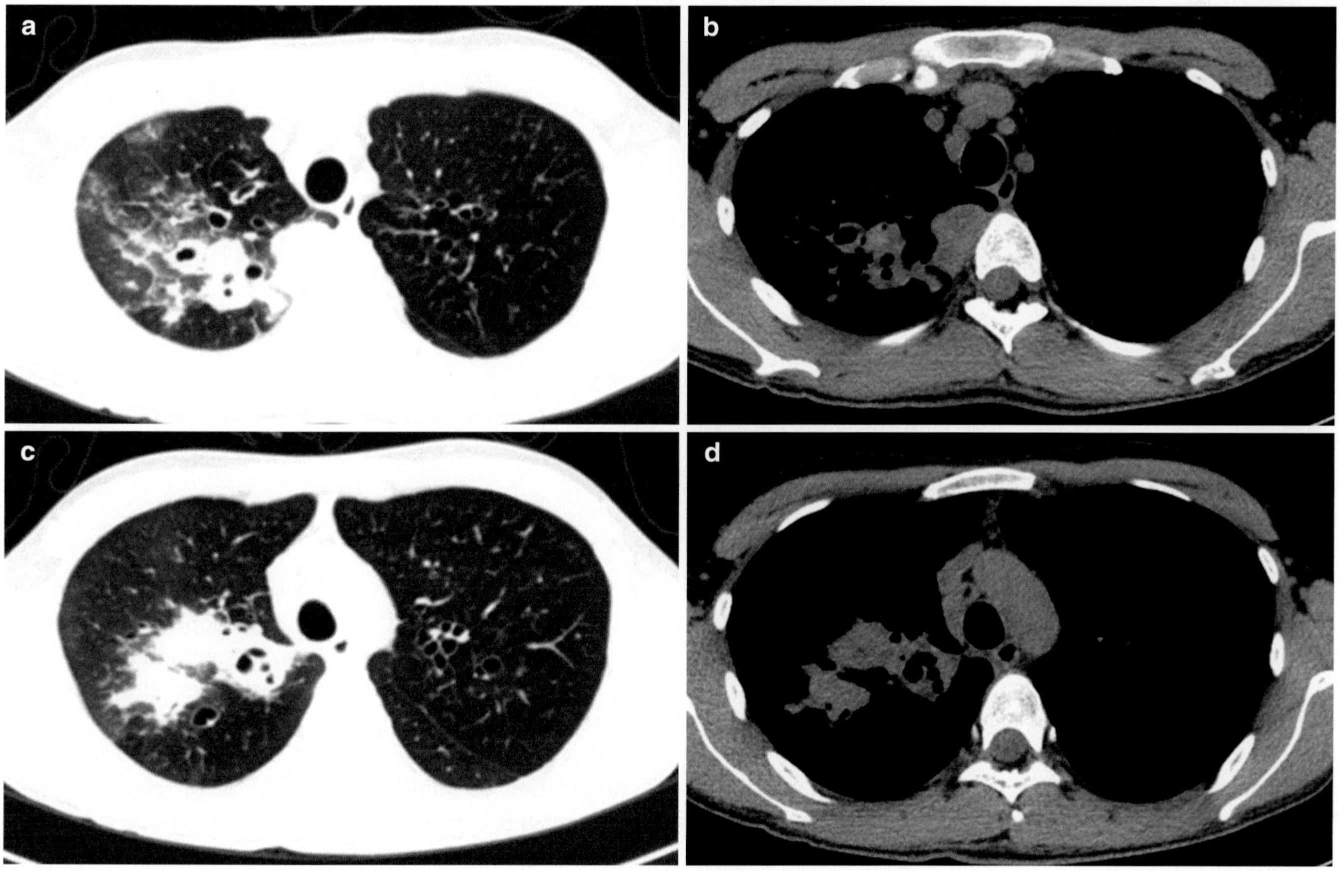

Fig. 13.1 (**a**–**g**) Chest CT scan. (**a**) The lung window demonstrates bronchiectasis at the apical segment of the right upper lung, with poorly defined multiple nodules and surrounding patches of ground-glass opacity. (**b**) The mediastinum window demonstrates multiple nodules. By plain scan, the CT value is about 29 Hu, and partial bronchi are demonstrated with thickening of the bronchial wall. (**c**) The lung window demonstrates central bronchiectasis of the right upper lung, mucus plug in the bronchus (bronchial casting sign), and surrounding blurry consolidation opacity. (**d**) The mediastinum window demonstrates a homogeneous intensity of mucus plug, with an average CT value of about 35 Hu. (**e**) The lung window demonstrates central bronchiectasis of bilateral upper lungs. And the dilated bronchus is mainly located at the inner medial part of the lung field, with thickening of the bronchial wall. There is sputum bolt in the lumen of some bronchi. (**f**, **g**) The lung window and the mediastinum window demonstrate obvious thickening of the bronchial wall at the lingual segment of the left upper lung, local mucus plug, and consolidation and atelectasis of subsegmental lung tissue

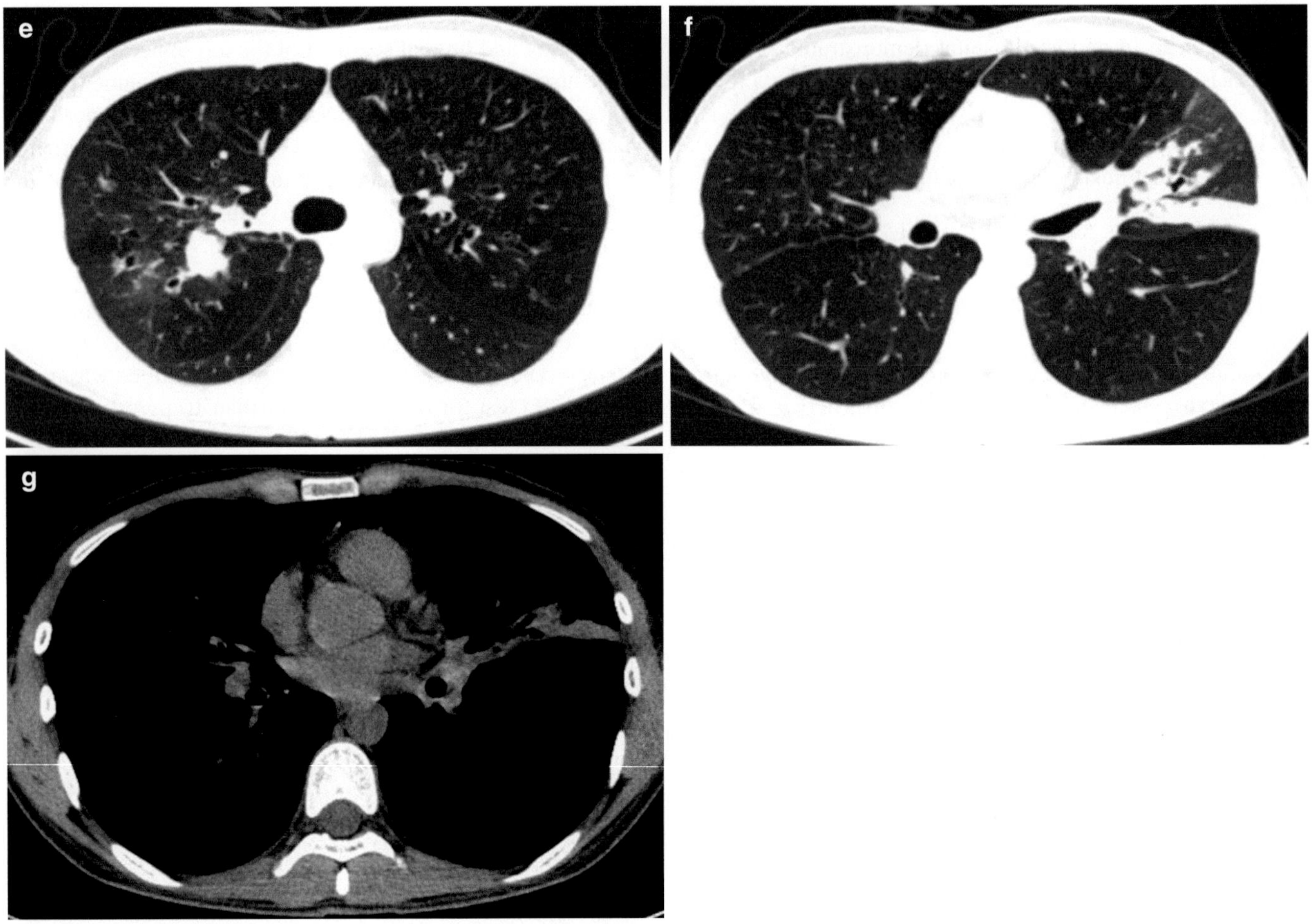

Fig. 13.1 (continued)

Bronchoscopy for biopsy was performed on July 18, 2013. The pathology demonstrated mucus plug in the bronchial lumen at the left upper lung lobe composed of mucus and many eosinophil granulocytes. Some eosinophil granulocytes degenerated and fungal hyphae were observed. The bronchus showed submucosal exudation of lymphocytes and many eosinophil granulocytes. By special staining, acid-fast staining showed negative, methenamine silver staining positive, gram staining negative, and PAS staining positive. The diagnosis was considered to be allergic bronchopulmonary aspergillus (Fig. 13.2).

Because the patient was a young man with chronic illness course and history of asthmatic attacks, along with laboratory, radiological, and pathological findings, the diagnosis was considered to be allergic bronchopulmonary aspergillosis. Glucocorticoid and itraconazole were then administered. Reexamination of chest CT scan 15 days later demonstrated absorption of lesions. However, reexamination of serum total IgE still showed increased level. After discharge, the oral intake of itraconazole and hormone was continued. Reexamination of chest CT scan on October 11, 2013, demonstrated absorption of most lesions (Fig. 13.3).

13.1.4 Discussion

The clinical diagnosis of allergic bronchopulmonary aspergillosis (ABPA) mainly depends on the main diagnostic criteria and secondary diagnostic criteria proposed by Rosenberg-Patterson [1]. The main diagnostic criteria include (1) a history of asthmatic attacks; (2) radiological demonstration of pulmonary infiltration opacity; (3) rapid positive response in the skin test for *Aspergillus fumigatus* (Af), namely, type I allergic response; (4) increased peripheral eosinophil granulocyte count along with pulmonary infiltration opacity; (5) serum precipitated antibody positive to *Aspergillus fumigatus*; (6) increased total serum IgE level (>1000 IU/ml); (7) increased levels of serum IgE-Af and IgG-Af; and (8) central bronchiectasis. The cases with 1–7 items should be diagnosed with serum-positive type of ABPA (ABPA-S), while the cases with all eight items should be

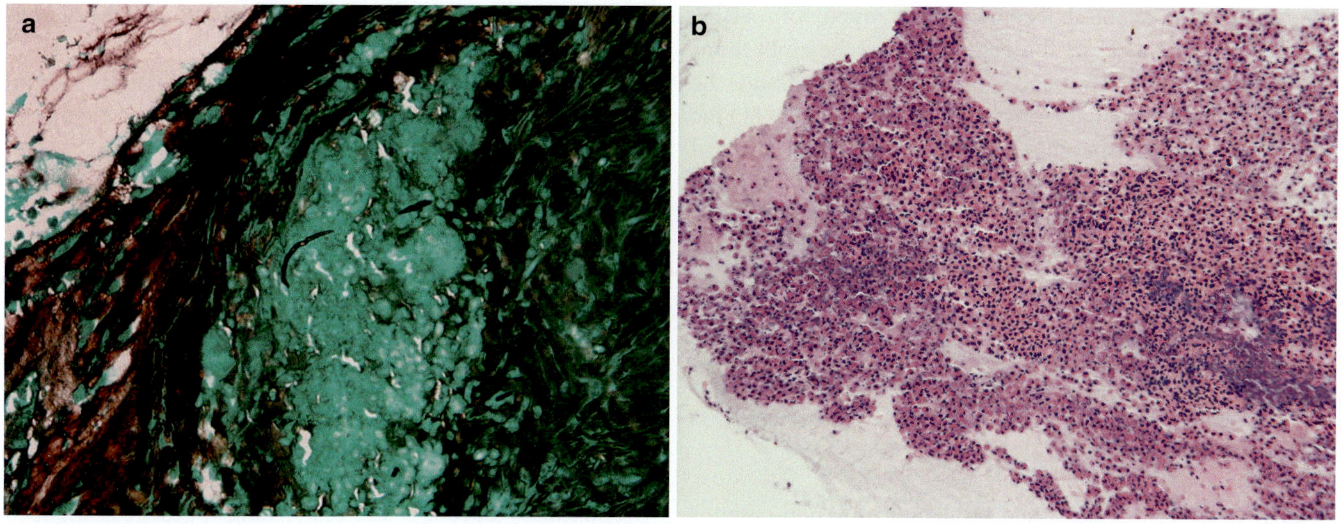

Fig. 13.2 (**a**, **b**) Bronchoscopy for pathology. (**a**) Under a microscope, hyphae and spores are observed to be brownish black by PASM staining. (**b**) There are many eosinophil mucus plug and eosinophil granulocytes by H&E staining

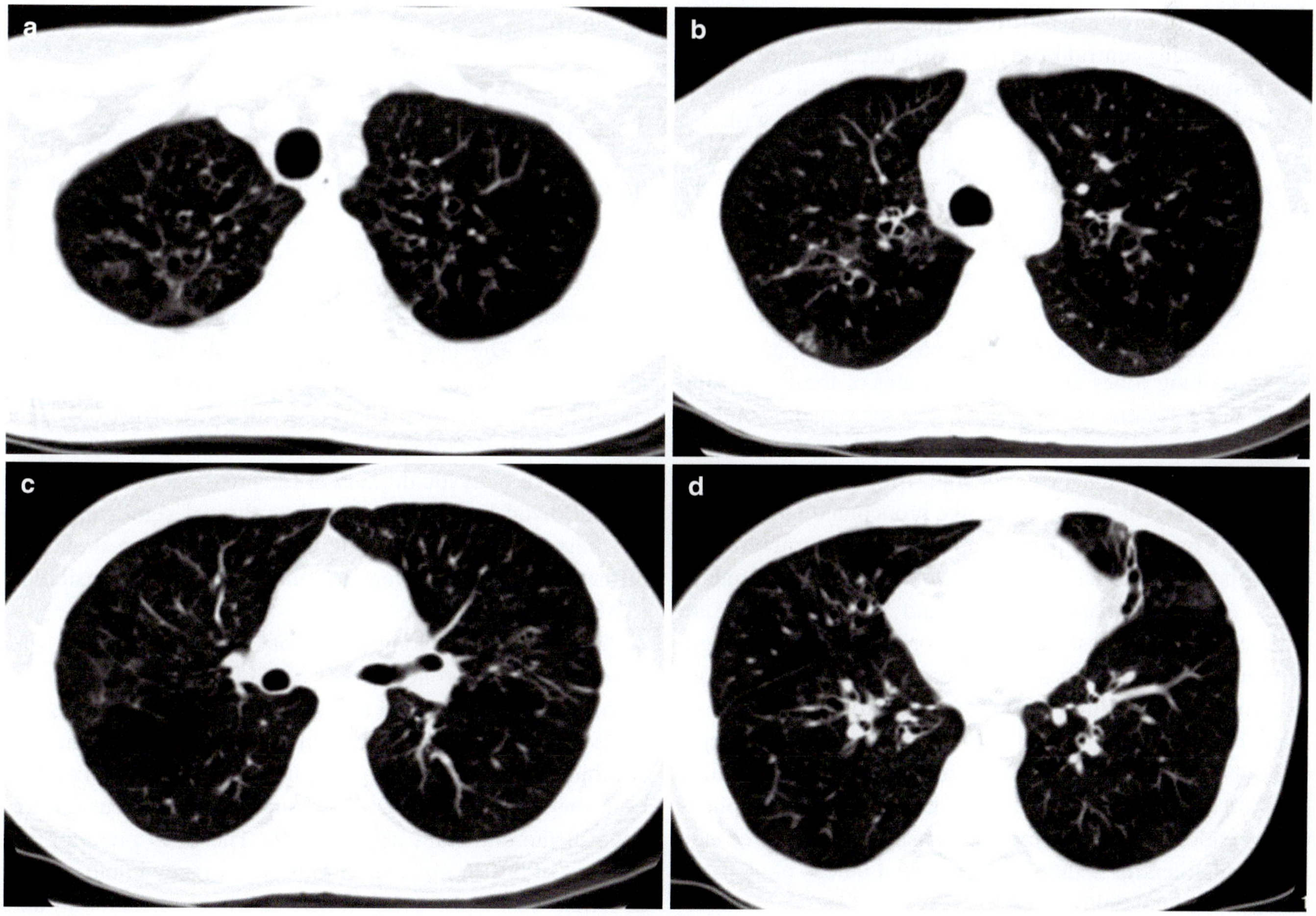

Fig. 13.3 (**a**–**d**) Reexamination of chest CT scan after treatment for 3 months. It demonstrates absorption of most lesions at both lungs. There is no bronchial casting sign and obviously improved bronchiectasis and thickening of the bronchial wall. The patchy exudations are absorbed and decreased compared to previous chest CT scans

diagnosed with central bronchiectasis type of ABPA (ABPA-CB). In this case, the patient met all the eight items of diagnostic criteria, and the diagnosis should be ABPA-CB. The secondary diagnostic criteria include (1) the sputum culture for aspergillus positive; (2) expectoration of brownish or brownish-green sputum bolt; and (3) delayed positive response in the skin test for Af antigen, namely, type III hyperresponse. The typical cases are found in patients with long-term asthma or cystic fibrosis [2, 3]. The most prominent feature of ABPA is bronchiectasis due to obstruction by mucus plug that is composed of aspergillus hyphae and eosinophil granulocytes. And the underlying pathophysiological mechanism is allergic response. Its pathology is characterized by the following:

1. Involvement of bronchi and bronchioles by non-caseous granuloma with abundant eosinophil granulocytes and common lobular central granulomatous inflammation.
2. Formation of mucus plug by increased secretions of mucus and fibrin in the bronchial lumen as well as reproduction of aspergillus hyphae inside, which further induces central bronchiectasis due to segmental or subsegmental bronchial cystic dilation and comparatively normal diameter of distal bronchus, with no invasion of the airway wall and lung tissue by aspergillus hyphae.
3. Possible infiltration of eosinophil granulocytes and mononuclear cells in the bronchus and lung tissue, with surrounding slight vasculitis [4, 5].

Lesions commonly occur at the posteroapical segment of the upper lung lobes and dorsal segment of the lower lung lobes. Some lesions are migratory. The main manifestations include bronchiectasis and formation of bronchial mucus plug, namely, bronchial casting sign. Bronchiectasis mainly occurs as cystic or varicose veinlike bronchial dilation at the segmental or subsegmental major bronchus. Central bronchiectasis is a characteristic sign of ABPA. The bronchial mucus plugs are in rod shape, V shape, and Y shape, which are radiologically demonstrated as tree-branch sign, glove sign, or toothpaste sign, with no enhancement by enhanced scan [6]. Some mucus plugs show high intensity, which may be related to thickness of the mucus and malnutritional calcification [7]. The lung tissue around bronchial mucus plug may show no lesion, slight exudation, or large flakes of consolidation or atelectasis. HRCT may demonstrate buds-in-tree sign and lobular central nodule near bronchial mucus plug, especially distal lung fields.

In this case, the patient suffered ABPA for many years, but the condition was always misdiagnosed as bronchiectasis. The therapeutic efficacy was then unfavorable. Therefore, patients with long-term asthma, if chest HRCT demonstrates central bronchiectasis and migratory mucus impaction of slightly high intensity in the dilated lumen, should be considered with ABPA. In combination with laboratory findings, the diagnosis can be defined.

When ABPA is suspected, a differential diagnosis from the following conditions should be made:

1. Cystic bronchiectasis. Cystic bronchiectasis commonly occurs at the lower lung lobes, and peripheral bronchial dilation is more common. Six months after disappearance of mucus plug in patients with ABPA, the diameter of dilated bronchus commonly returns to normal, which is different from long-term existence of dilated bronchus in patients with common bronchiectasis. However, in the cases of recurrent ABPA, the diameter of dilated bronchus cannot return to normal.
2. Tuberculous bronchiectasis. Tuberculous bronchiectasis commonly occurs at the upper lung lobes. It is induced commonly by the destruction of smooth muscle and elastic fibers at the bronchial wall and traction of surrounding scar tissues. There are satellite lesions around the dilated bronchus but rare mucus plugs in the dilated bronchial lumen.

13.1.5 Comments

In this case, the lesions are mainly located at the proximal and middle segments of the bronchi near the hilum of both lungs, especially at the right upper lung and lingual segment of the left upper lung. Chest HRCT demonstrated central bronchiectasis, mucus plugs, and exudation opacity around the lesions. The laboratory, radiological, and pathological findings met all the eight items of the main diagnostic criteria. And the diagnosis can be defined as ABPA-CB. The characteristic central bronchiectasis is mainly manifested as column-like or cystic dilation of the proximal bronchus, and normal distal bronchus, which has clinical significance for the diagnosis of ABPA. In this case, the condition should be differentiated from severe asthma with fungal sensitation (SAFS).

In this case, in a long period of time, the condition was misdiagnosed as bronchiectasis and infection. The treatment then showed unfavorable therapeutic efficacy. The misdiagnosis is related to the chronic illness course of ABPA and the common symptoms of chronic pulmonary diseases. In addition, the misdiagnosis is also related to insufficient knowledge of the clinicians about ABPA. The early pathological changes of ABPA include infiltrations of many mononuclear cells and eosinophil granulocytes in the bronchial wall and no invasion of lung tissue. Then mucus impaction, central bronchiectasis, and eosinophilic pneumonia occur, which further progress into chronic bronchiolitis and non-caseating bronchial granuloma. In its advanced stage, extensive pulmonary fibrosis occurs. Therefore, patients with long-term asthma, if chest HRCT demonstrates central bronchiectasis and migratory mucus impaction of slightly high intensity in the dilated bronchial lumen, should be considered with ABPA. For such patients, the skin test for Af, serological test, and bronchoscopy should be timely performed. The skin test for Af positive is a necessary condition for the diagnosis of ABPA. If negative, ABPA can be excluded. If positive, further serological test should be ordered.

13.2 Case 2: Cough and Breathlessness for More Than 4 Months and Aggravation for 1 Month

Wenhui Tang, Senquan Wu, Ping Zhang, Dong-Na Su, Xuemei Han, and Xiongfei Sun

13.2.1 Presenting Symptom

Cough and breathlessness for more than 4 months and aggravation for 1 month.

13.2.2 Brief Case History

A 53-year-old man from Guangdong province of China was admitted to our hospital on February 25, 2014, due to complaints of cough and breathlessness for more than 4 months and aggravation for 1 month. Four months ago, the patient began to experience irritating dry cough occasionally with whitish mucus sputum and accompanying breathlessness after physical activities. The breathlessness was more obvious when he lied supine during nights and did morning exercise. And contacts to oil fume as well as cold and hot air may also induce the aggravation of breathlessness. In a local hospital, the chest CT scan demonstrated emphysema, and inhalation of ipratropium bromide was administered. But the therapy showed no effectiveness. Reexamination of chest CT scan 1 week ago demonstrated honeycomb-like opacity at the posterior segment of the right upper lung, right middle lung, and right lower lung. For further diagnosis and treatment, he presented in our hospital and was admitted due to breathlessness. Since the onset of the symptoms, his spiritual state, appetite, and sleep were average. The urinations and bowel movements were normal. And he experienced a recent weight loss of about 3 kg.

13.2.2.1 Past Medical History

He had been in a good health. And he denied histories of hypertension, coronary heart disease, and diabetes.

13.2.2.2 Physical Examination

Physical examination showed a body temperature of 36.5 °C, pulse rate 93/min, respiration rate 20/min, and blood pressure 131/81 mmHg. The blood oxygen saturation was 99% when oxygen was inhaled at 2 L/min. The thorax was bilaterally symmetric. And the respirations were smooth, with normal intercostal space. The respirations were bilaterally symmetric, with normal vocal fremitus. By percussion, both lungs showed hyperresonant note. By auscultation, both lungs showed low respiration sounds, with moist rales at the right lower lung and no dry rales at both lungs.

13.2.2.3 Auxiliary Investigation

Laboratory Test

Routine blood test showed WBC 5.96 × 10^9/L, neutrophil granulocytes 62.8%, eosinophil granulocytes 2.9%, and platelets 372 × 10^9/L. The procalcitonin was <0.05 ng/ml. C-reactive protein was 1.62 mg/dl. And ESR was 65 mm/h.

Radiology

Chest CT scan on February 17, 2014, demonstrated a honeycomb-like opacity at the posterior segment of the right upper lung, the right middle lung, and the right lower lung.

13.2.2.4 Initial Diagnosis

Lesions at the right lung with the reason to be detected, and suspected acute exacerbation of chronic obstructive pulmonary disease.

13.2.3 Diagnosis and Treatment

After admission, the fungal G test was above 1000 pg/ml, and the fungus antigen test for aspergillus, candida, and cryptococcus was negative. The sputum culture and smear for common bacteria, fungi, and tuberculosis mycobacteria were negative. The lung ventilation test, bronchodilation test, diffuse function test, residual volume determination, and forced oscillation airway resistance determination showed severe mixed ventilation dysfunction, bronchodilation test positive (inhalation of Ventolin 400 μg, elevation of FEV1 above 12%, and increase of absolute value above 200 ml), severely decreased diffuse function, normal total lung capacity, increased residual volume and total residual ratio, and airway resistance within normal limits. Pulmonary arteriography and reconstruction as well as plain and enhanced scans on February 26, 2014, demonstrated a heterogeneous increase of transparency of both lungs and thickened and deranged lung markings. There were also flakes and patches of high-intensity opacity and cystic translucent area at the posteroapical segment of the right upper lung, which were honeycomb-like flakes of opacity with heterogeneous intensity. Enhanced scan demonstrated heterogeneous enhancement, with patches of liquefied necrotic area inside (Fig. 13.4). The right lower lung was demonstrated with patches, cords, and flakes of high-intensity opacity. And

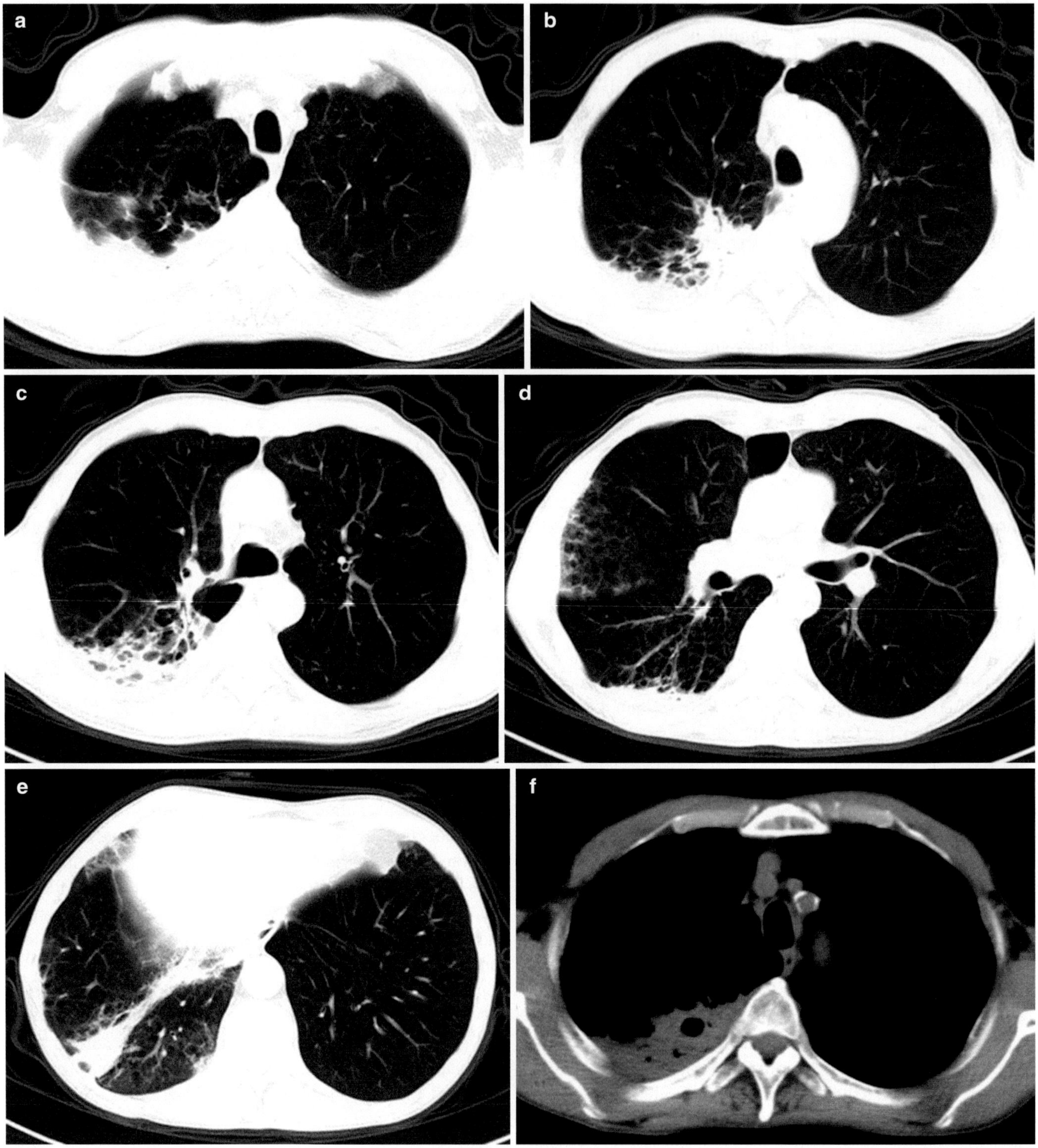

Fig. 13.4 (**a**–**i**) Chest CT scan. (**a**–**c**) The lung window demonstrates flakes and patches of high heterogeneous intensity opacity, cystic opacity, and honeycomb-like opacity at the posteroapical segment of the right upper lung. (**d**, **e**) The right lower lung is demonstrated with patches, cords, and flakes of high-intensity opacity. (**f**, **g**) The mediastinum window demonstrates irregular cavity opacity at the right upper lung lobe and right lower lung lobe. (**h**–**i**). Enhanced scanning demonstrates heterogeneous enhancement and patches of liquefied necrotic area in flaky opacity

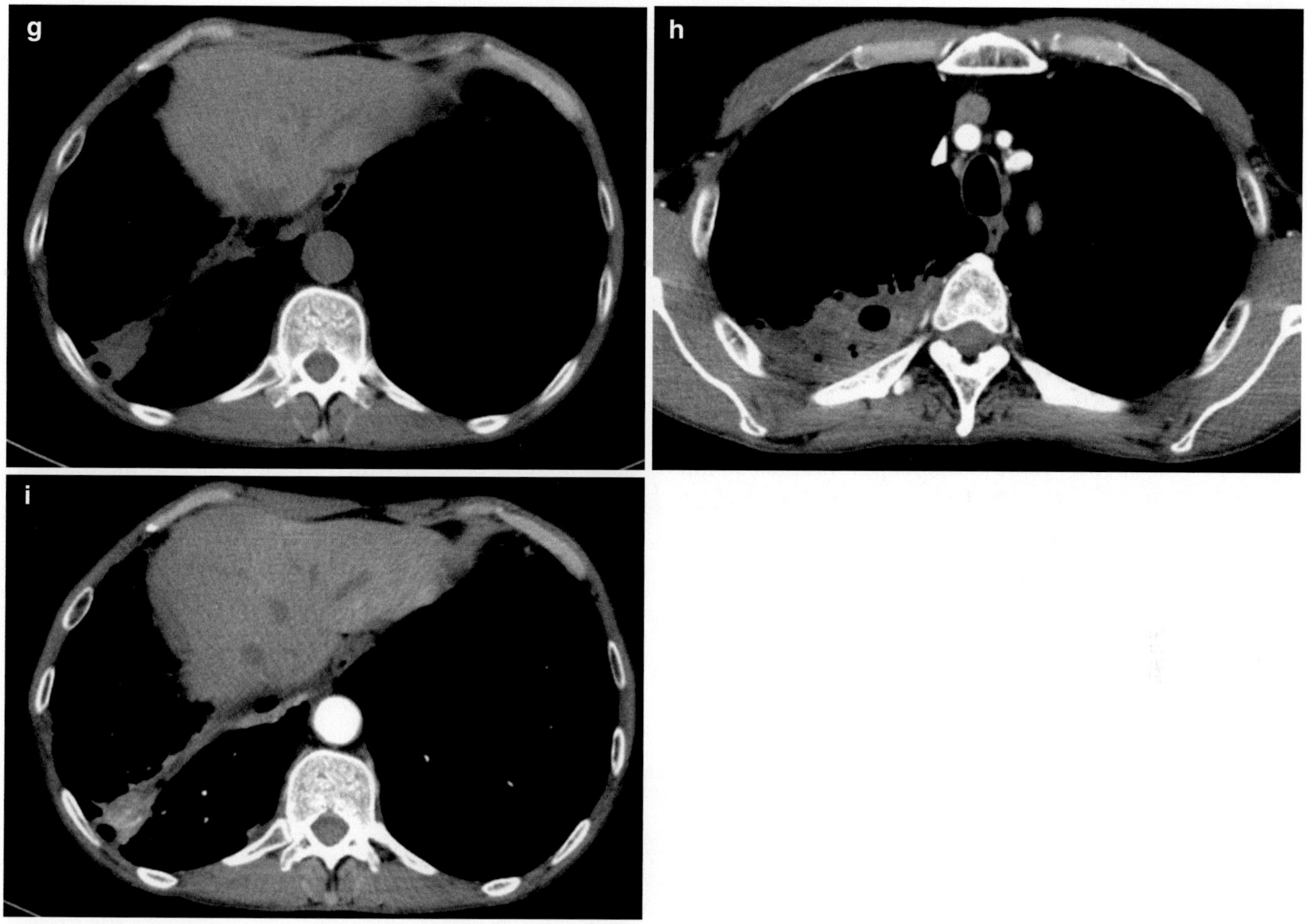

Fig. 13.4 (continued)

there was a strip of opacity with liquid intensity between the flakes of opacity at the posterior basilar segment of the right lower lung and pleura (Fig. 13.4). The posteroapical segment of the left upper lung was demonstrated with a well-marginated solid small nodular opacity with size of about 1.0 cm × 0.6 cm, which showed surrounding fine and long spikes (Fig. 13.4). Both lungs were demonstrated with multiple thin-walled cavities in different sizes, the largest one with size of about 3.3 cm × 2.3 cm, and unobstructed saber-sheath trachea (Fig. 13.4). The right hilum was demonstrated with enlarged lymph nodes with a short diameter of about 1.5 cm, and the left hilum was not enlarged. The mediastinum was demonstrated with multiple small lymph nodes, with a short diameter of less than 1.0 cm. And the right thoracic cavity showed encapsulated effusion in a small quantity (Fig. 13.4). Pulmonary arteriography and reconstruction demonstrated no stenosis, dilation and filling defect of the pulmonary artery, and no abnormal vascular mass. The radiological diagnosis was:

1. Chronic bronchitis, pulmonary emphysema, and multiple bullae in both lungs.
2. Multiple infections at the posteroapical segment of the right upper lung as well as the right lower lung, with pulmonary abscess of the right upper lung, organized pneumonia of the right lower lung, and right hilar lymphadenectasis not excluded.
3. Solid small nodule at the posteroapical segment of the left upper lung, which was more likely to be inflammatory granuloma, and regular reexaminations recommended.
4. Right pleural encapsulated effusion in a small quantity and slight focalized thickening of the right upper pleura.
5. No definitive embolism of subsegmental and above pulmonary artery by pulmonary arteriography.

Because of the suspected diagnosis of infection at the right lung, piperacillin sodium/tazobactam sodium was administered. But the therapeutic efficacy was unfavorable. Bronchoscopy for biopsy was then performed on February 28, 2014 (Fig. 13.5).

The pathology demonstrated granuloma at the lateral basilar segment of the right lower lung lobe and less organized lesions in alveolar cavity. There were also epithelial lesions, which were well marginated with central hyphae and spore-like substances. Hyphae were uniform in thickness, with branching in sharp angle. By special staining, acid-fast staining showed negative, methenamine silver staining positive, AB staining negative, and PAS staining positive. Histological changes were consistent with pulmonary aspergillosis (Fig. 13.6). Caspofungin was then administered for fungal infection. At day 1, one injection of 70 mg loading dose was administered and 50 mg in the following days. After treatment for 2 weeks, the clinical symptoms were relieved, indicating effective antifungal therapy. On discharge, oral liquid of itraconazole was prescribed for oral intake twice a day.

Compared to chest CT scan on February 26, 2014, reexamination of plain chest CT scan on March 24, 2014, demonstrated (Fig. 13.7) heterogeneously increased transparency of both lungs, with thickened and deranged lung markings. There were also flakes and patches of high-intensity opacity and cystic translucent area at the posteroapical segment of the right upper lung, which were honeycomb-like flakes of opacity with heterogeneous intensity. In the honeycomb-like flakes of opacity, there was a patchy liquefied necrotic area (**a**–**b**), which shrank compared to the previous chest CT scan. The right lower lung was demonstrated with decreased patches, cords, and flakes of high-intensity opacity (**c**–**e**) compared to the previous chest CT scan. The posteroapical segment of the left upper lung was demonstrated with a solid small nodular opacity, which was the same as the previous chest CT scan. Both lungs were demonstrated with scattering multiple thin-walled cavities in different sizes, which were the same as the previous chest CT scan. The right hilum was demonstrated with enlarged lymph nodes, which were the same as the previous chest CT scan. And the mediastinum was demonstrated with multiple small lymph nodes, which

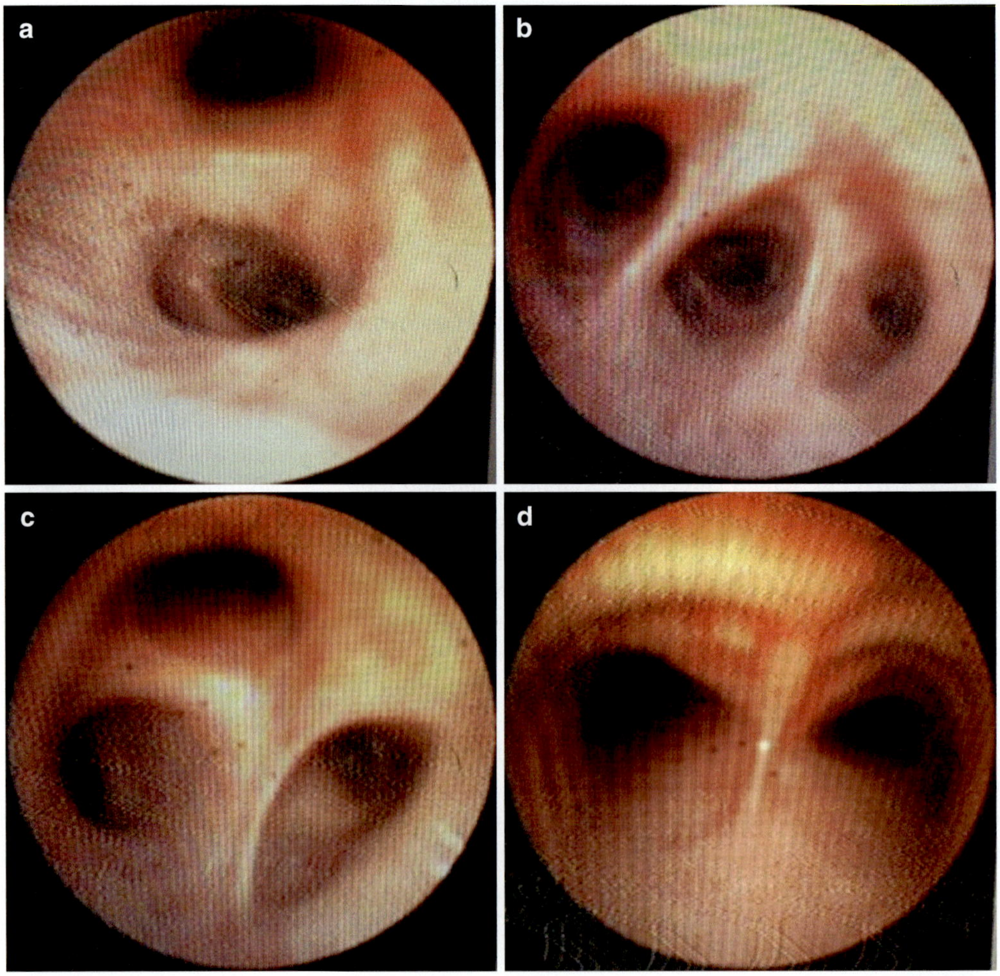

Fig. 13.5 (**a**–**d**) Fibrobronchoscopy. Fibrobronchoscopy demonstrates smooth bronchial mucosa, unobstructed bronchial lumen, and no neoplasm in the bronchial lumen. And the lung tissue at the lateral basilar segment of the right lower lung is harvested under fibrobronchoscopy for biopsy

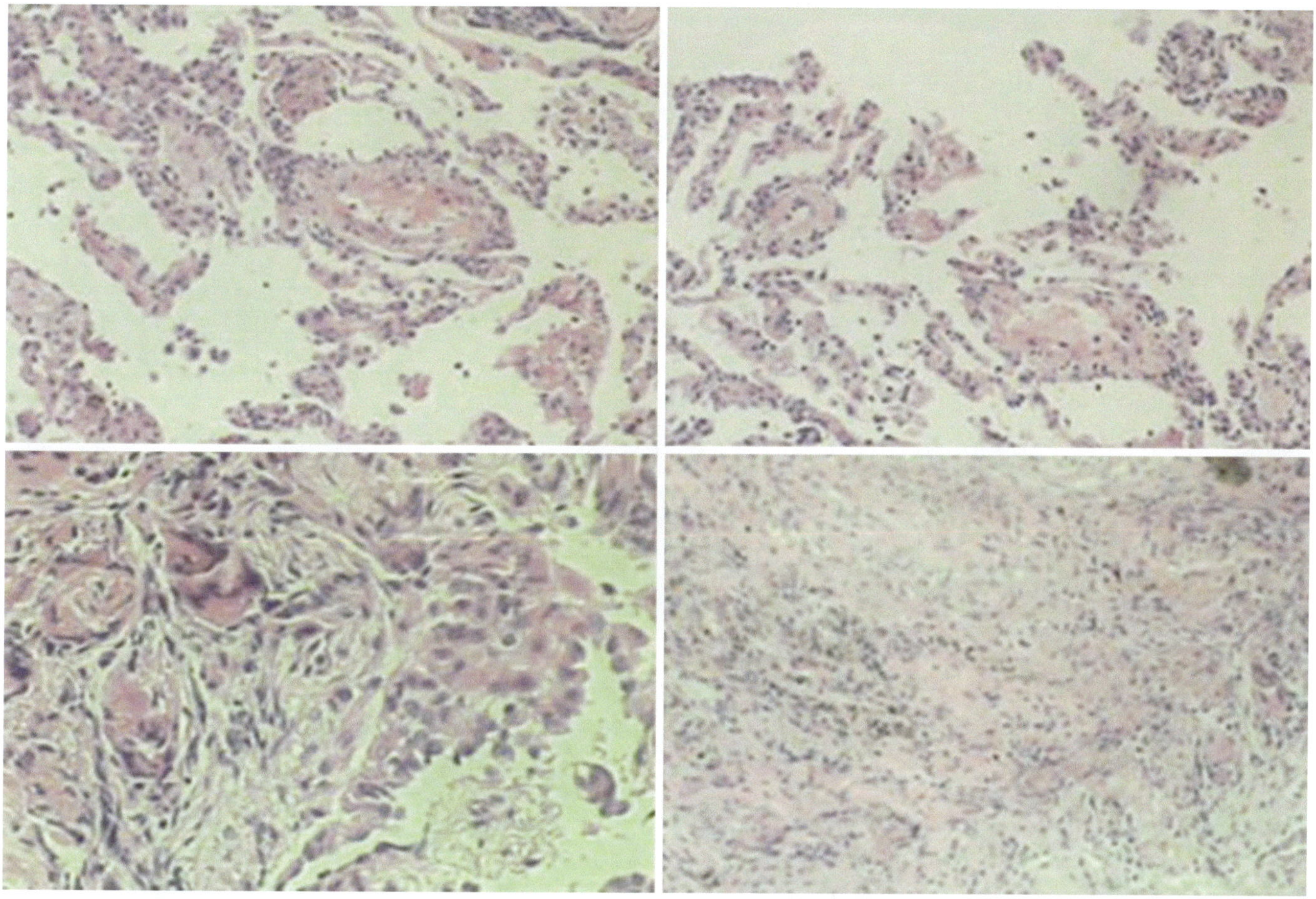

Fig. 13.6 Pathology of harvested lung tissue. Hyphae and spores are observed, with infiltration of many inflammatory cells (H&E staining)

were the same as the previous chest CT scan. There were also right pleural encapsulated effusion in a decreased quantity and focalized slight pleural thickening. The radiological diagnosis was the following:

1. Chronic bronchitis, emphysema, and multiple bullae in both lungs.
2. Decreased multiple infections at the posteroapical segment of the right upper lung and the right lower lung, with pulmonary abscess at the right upper lung not excluded, and right hilar lymphadenectasis.
3. Solid small nodule at the posteroapical segment of the left upper lung, which was considered to be inflammatory granuloma, and regular reexaminations were recommended.
4. Right pleural encapsulated effusion in a decreased quantity and focalized slight thickening of the right upper pleura.

Chest CT scan demonstrated absorption and shrinkage of lesions at the right lower lung, indicating effective antifungal therapy.

The final diagnosis was invasive pulmonary aspergillosis of the right lower lung and acute exacerbation of chronic obstructive pulmonary disease.

After discharge, the condition of the patient was stable. Reexamination of chest CT scan 2 weeks after discharge demonstrated shrinkage of lesions at the right lower lung.

13.2.4 Discussion

Invasive pulmonary aspergillosis (IPA) is commonly secondary to immunodeficiency. The recognized high-risk factors include serious agranulocytosis, hematologic malignancies, post-hematopoietic stem cell transplantation, and post-solid organ transplantation. In recent years, incidence of IPA in patients with pulmonary disease but no above high risk factors has been increasing. These pulmonary diseases include COPD, bronchial asthma, and cystic pulmonary fibrosis. Patients with COPD commonly receive long-term administration of hormone and antibiotic, and most of them are elderly who suffer from concurrent basic diseases. Therefore, patients with COPD are the high-risk population of

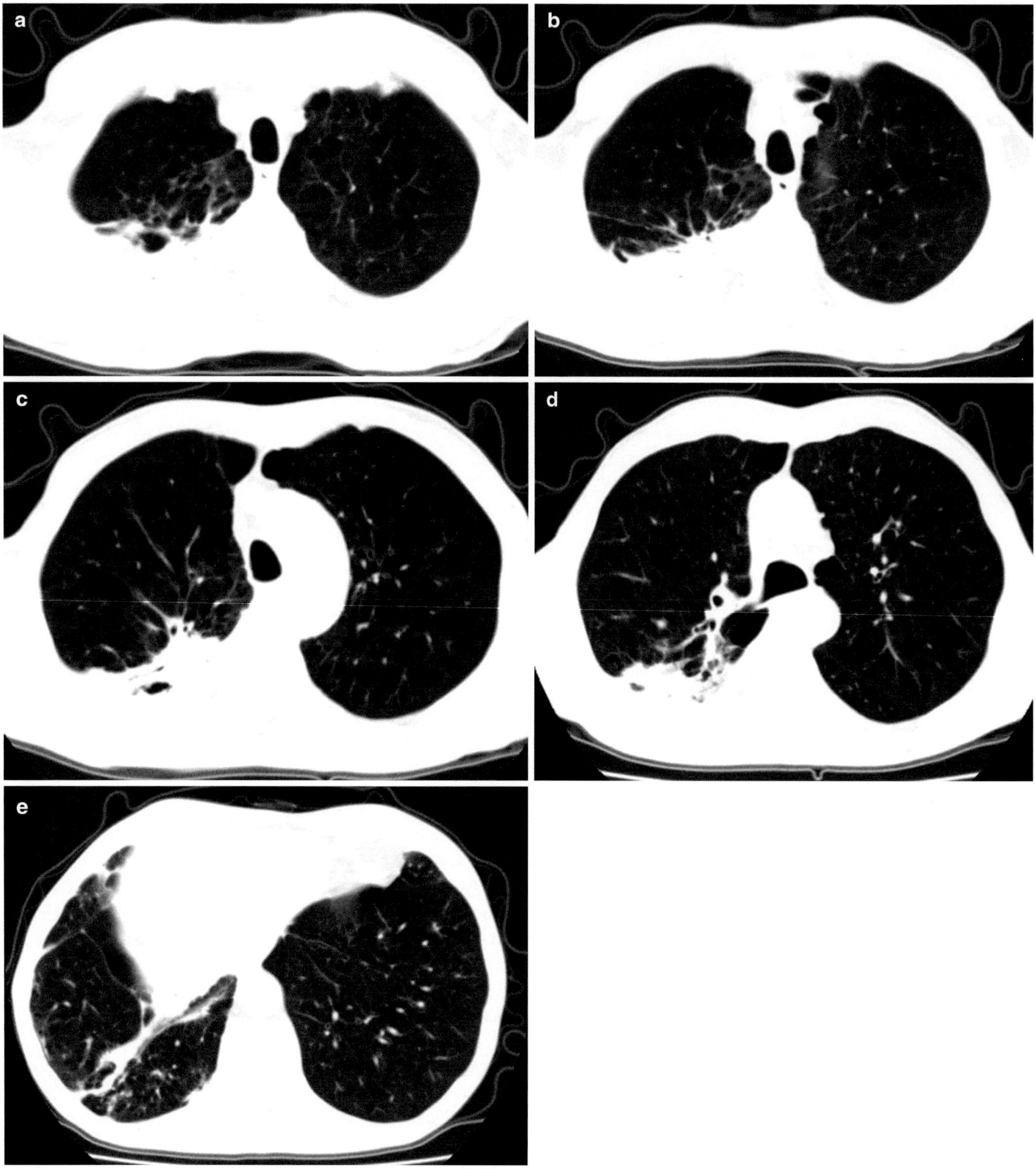

Fig. 13.7 (**a**–**e**) Chest CT scan. (**a**–**d**) The posteroapical segment of the right upper lung is demonstrated with flakes and patches of high-intensity opacities as well as cystic translucent area, which are honeycomb-like flakes of opacities with heterogeneous intensity. There is a patchy liquefied necrotic area inside, which is absorbed compared to the previous chest CT scan. (**e**) The right lower lung is demonstrated with patches and cords opacity, which are absorbed compared to the previous chest CT scan

pulmonary aspergillus infection. And aspergillus infection exacerbates the condition of patients with COPD, which results in poorer prognosis of COPD. The global mortality of COPD complicated by IPA is up to 50–100% [8].

More and more clinical data indicated that COPA is associated with the occurrence of IPA. In patients with COPD, the lung structures change, destruction of airway mucosa and ciliary function, application of glucocorticoids and broad spectrum antibiotics can lead to the impairment of local and systemic immune function, which provides for pulmonary aspergillus infection.

Evidence supports that admission to ICU, chronic cardiac insufficiency, use of antibiotic 3 months before hospitalization, accumulative dose of glucocorticoid above 700 mg (calculated based on prednisone) within 3 months before hospitalization or from admission to hospital to detection of aspergillus infection are independent risk factors of IPA. Some scholars believe that inhalation of glucocorticoid by certain patients may also impair their systemic immunity and therefore increase the risks of IPA and other opportunistic infections.

In the standards jointly issued by EORTC and MSG, halo sign, air crescent sign, and cavity with consolidation opacity are radiological evidence supporting the diagnosis of IPA. These signs are commonly demonstrated in patients with agranulocytosis complicated by IPA, but rarely demonstrated in patients with COPD complicated by IPA. Chest X-ray and chest CT scan demonstrate COPD complicated by IPA as no abnormality in its early stage. Radiology commonly demonstrates signs of airway invasion, such as lesions at minor airway, peribronchial consolidation, and bronchiectasis [10]. Specifically, there are increased lung markings, light flakes of exudation, and consolidation, which may be related to damages of airway barrier in patients with COPD. Patients with COPD show squamous mucosal epithelium and decreased cilia with impaired function. Therefore, aspergillus spores that are inhaled into airway cannot be eliminated via defense mechanism. Instead, they invade the airway and gain their access to the terminal bronchi and alveoli. The atypical radiological demonstrations are also caused by inhibition of inflammatory responses due to the use of hormone by patients with COPD.

In this case, the clinical manifestations were atypical, and his radiological demonstrations were also atypical. The diagnosis was initially suspected to be pneumonia of the right lung. But piperacillin/tazobactam sodium for infection showed unfavorable therapeutic efficacy. The diagnosis was finally defined by fibrobronchoscopy for biopsy. And caspofungin for fungal infection for 2 weeks showed therapeutic response. Reexamination of chest CT scan demonstrated shrinkage of lesions at the right lower lung.

In recent years, knowledge about COPD complicated by IPA has been increasing. Early clinical manifestations of COPD complicated by IPA can hardly be differentiated from acute exacerbation induced by other pathogens. In clinical practice, when patients with COPD show unfavorable therapeutic response to hormone and antibacterial medication, aspergillus infection should be suspected. If aspergillus infection is not considered and larger dose of hormone or wider-spectrum antibiotic is administered, the immunity of the patient is then further suppressed. Consequently, aspergillus infection rapidly progresses.

13.2.5 Comments

In this case, the patient was a middle-aged man, with subacute onset of symptoms. Radiology demonstrated multiple cavities in the lungs. And the pathology demonstrated formation of inflammatory granuloma. The clinical illness course lasted for 4 months, with aggravation for 1 month. As for the clinical typing, the condition should be categorized into chronic pulmonary aspergillosis (CPA). The progression was comparatively rapid, which should be differentiated from acute invasive pulmonary aspergillosis (IPA). The illness course of IPA commonly lasts for less than 1 month. Clinically, the cases with pathological demonstration of granuloma and an illness course of more than 1 month can be categorized as chronic. CPA commonly occurs in patient with basic pulmonary disease, especially patients with COPD. In this case, radiology demonstrated solid small nodule at the posteroapical segment of the left upper lung, which was considered to be inflammatory granuloma. Both the lung window and mediastinum window demonstrated multiple cavities. The pathology indicated granulomatous lesion at the lateral basilar segment of the right lower lung and less organized lesion in alveolar cavity. The clinical typing was chronic necrotizing pulmonary aspergillosis. In the clinical guideline for diagnosis and treatment of chronic pulmonary aspergillosis issued in 2015, patients with chronic necrotizing pulmonary aspergillosis and compromised or failed immunity can be diagnosed with invasive pulmonary aspergillosis. Compared to acute invasive pulmonary aspergillosis, chronic necrotizing pulmonary aspergillosis shows chronic progression, with an illness course of 1–3 months. In the cases of chronic necrotizing pulmonary aspergillosis, serum aspergillus antigen and antibody are commonly positive, and histology demonstrates invasion of hyphae into the lung parenchyma.

In this case, the condition was initially diagnosed as pneumonia, but active antibacterial medication showed unfavorable therapeutic response. The following bronchoscopy demonstrated aspergillus infection. If long-term wide-spectrum antibiotic had been administered, the risk of fungal infection definitively increased. In this case, radiology demonstrated honeycomb-like multiple small cavities, which should be considered as an aspergillus infection as early as possible. In this case, early medication of caspofungin was administered for 2 weeks, and the medication was then changed to oral intake of itraconazole. The treatment of chronic necrotizing pulmonary aspergillosis is the same as that of acute invasive pulmonary aspergillosis. A cohort study has demonstrated that long-term oral medication of itraconazole is effective in the treatment of chronic necrotizing pulmonary aspergillosis. And a prospective multicentered research study has come to a preliminary conclusion that voriconazole shows more favorable therapeutic efficacy in the treatment of chronic necrotizing pulmonary aspergillosis than in the treatment of chronic cavitary pulmonary aspergillosis. The treatment of chronic necrotizing pulmonary aspergillosis is intended to cure, and the recommended therapeutic course is 3–6 months, preferably 6 months. For patients with immunosuppression, the treatment should be prolonged. During the treatment, blood concentration of azoles should be monitored for possible drug interactions and toxicity.

13.3 Case 3: Dull Pain at the Left Lower Back for 3 Years, Chest Distress and Breathlessness for More Than 2 Months

Yanwei Chen, Zhijian Yu, Qiwen Deng, Shi-Ping Wu, Minjie Yang, and Jiaxuan Zhou

13.3.1 Presenting Symptom

Dull pain at the left lower back for 3 years, chest distress, and breathlessness for more than 2 months.

13.3.2 Brief Case History

A 49-year-old man was admitted to our hospital due to complaints of dull pain at the left lower back for 3 years as well as chest distress and breathlessness for more than 2 months. Three years ago, the patient showed dull pain at the left lower back with no known reasons. And he experienced no frequent, painful, and urgent urinations and no aversion to cold and fever. In the outpatient department of our hospital, laboratory tests showed serum creatinine 407.3 μmol/L and cystatin 5.38 mg/L. The color Doppler ultrasound of the abdomen demonstrated enlarged volumes of both kidneys, with multiple cystic lesions and the largest with size of 35 mm × 34 mm, which were consistent with the polycystic kidney. And the condition was diagnosed as stage IV of chronic kidney disease and polycystic kidney. Kangshen particles and Corbin capsules were administered for treatment. Multiple reexaminations of blood creatinine showed a gradual increase. More than 2 months ago, he began to experience chest distress and breathlessness, which were more obvious after walking and climbing stairs and were relieved after rest. During nights, he could lie flat in bed but the sleeping was poor. He experienced no cough, expectoration, and fever. And he was admitted to our hospital due to aggravation of the symptoms. After admission, laboratory tests showed blood BUN 32.3 mmol/L, Cr 949.3 μmol/L, and CysC 4.78 mg/L. Abdominal color Doppler ultrasonography showed enlarged bilateral kidney volume with multiple cystic space-occupying lesions, which was considered to be polycystic kidney. After admission, anti-infection therapy and blood pressure control therapy were administered. And the condition was stabilized and the patient was discharged. Ten days ago, he showed chest distress, breathlessness, inability to lie flat in bed, and expectoration of pinkish-red sputum. In a local hospital, the chest X-ray indicated pulmonary edema. Since February 2, 2014, the patient began to receive hemodialysis, which relieved the symptom of breathlessness. For further diagnosis and treatment, he was admitted to our hospital again. During the illness course, night urination obviously increased, 4–5 times per night. And he experienced no recent weight loss.

13.3.2.1 Family History

His younger brother had a history of polycystic kidney.

13.3.2.2 Physical Examination

Physical examination showed a body temperature of 36.6 °C, pulse rate 80/min, blood pressure 140/90 mmHg, and respiration rate 20/min. He was well conscious, with appearance of chronic illness and anemia. The face and eyelid showed no edema. And the systemic skin and sclera showed no yellowish stain. The superficial lymph nodes were not enlarged. The pharynx was not congested. And the bilateral tonsils were not enlarged. The respiration sounds of both lungs were clear, with no dry and/or moist rales. The heart was slightly enlarged leftwards, and the heart beats 80/min, rhythmic. The valvular areas showed no pathological murmur. The abdomen was soft, with no tenderness. The liver and spleen were subcostally unpalpable. The bilateral ureters showed no tenderness, and the bilateral kidneys were not sensitive to percussion. Both lower limbs showed no edema. The left forearm showed an A-V fistula with fremitus palpated and vascular buzzing heard.

13.3.3 Diagnosis and Treatment

After admission, the routine blood test showed WBC 4.4×10^9/L, N 79.5%, RBC 1.53×10^{12}/L, HGB 45 g/L, and PLT 108×10^9/L. Routine urine test showed WBC 54×10^9/L, urine protein (++). The liver function test showed TP 53.5 g/L and ALB 25.0 g/L. And the kidney function test showed BUN 26.2 mmol/L, Cr 728.1 μmol/L, and CysC 6.06 mg/L. The 24 h M-TP was 2941 mg. The hemopoietin was 35.63 IU/L. And 5-hydroxy vitamin D was 11.59 ng/ml. The parathyroid hormone was 48.50 pmol/L. The sputum culture showed the growth of *Pseudomonas aeruginosa* in a small quantity. And the color Doppler ultrasound of the liver, gallbladder, spleen, and kidneys showed signs of multiple cysts in the liver, bilateral polycystic kidneys, and ascites in a small quantity. Chest X-ray on February 12, 2014, demonstrated enlarged hilar opacity of the right lung (Fig. 13.8).

After admission, active anti-infection therapy and symptomatic support were administered for about 1 week. Reexamination of anterior-posterior and lateral chest X-rays on February 19, 2014, demonstrated no change of right hilar space-occupying opacity, and chest CT scan was recommended (Fig. 13.9). Plain chest CT scan was then performed on February 19, 2014. And it demonstrated lesions in both lungs, which were considered to be infection, bilateral pleural effusion in small quantities, polycystic liver, and polycystic kidneys (Fig. 13.10).

To further define the diagnosis, fibrobronchoscopy was performed on February 21, 2014, and the harvested tissue was sent for biopsy. The pathology demonstrated a clamped tissue from the right upper lung lobe with necrotic tissue and acute inflammatory exudates in a small quantity. There seemed to be necrotic fungal hyphae near the necrotic tissue. And the diagnosis should be made based on exclusion of fungal infection. The cytological smear of bronchial brushing demonstrated many neutrophil granulocytes, less pseudostratified ciliated columnar epithelia, and no neoplasm cells. By methenamine silver staining, less aspergillus was found (Fig. 13.11).

Based on the findings of fibrobronchoscopy and pathology, the clinical diagnosis was initially made to be pulmonary aspergillosis, polycystic kidneys, stage V of chronic kidney disease, renal anemia, renal hypertension, secondary hyperparathyroidism, uremic heart disease, and polycystic liver. Itraconazole was then administered in a dose of 0.1 g, twice a day, for fungal infection. And maintenance hemodialysis was given three times a week. The symptoms were gradually improved. Reexamination of chest X-ray on March 5, 2014, demonstrated shrinkage of hilar space-occupying lesion in the right lung (Fig. 13.12). Reexamination of chest X-ray on March 6, 2015, demonstrated absorption of lesions in the lungs (Fig. 13.13).

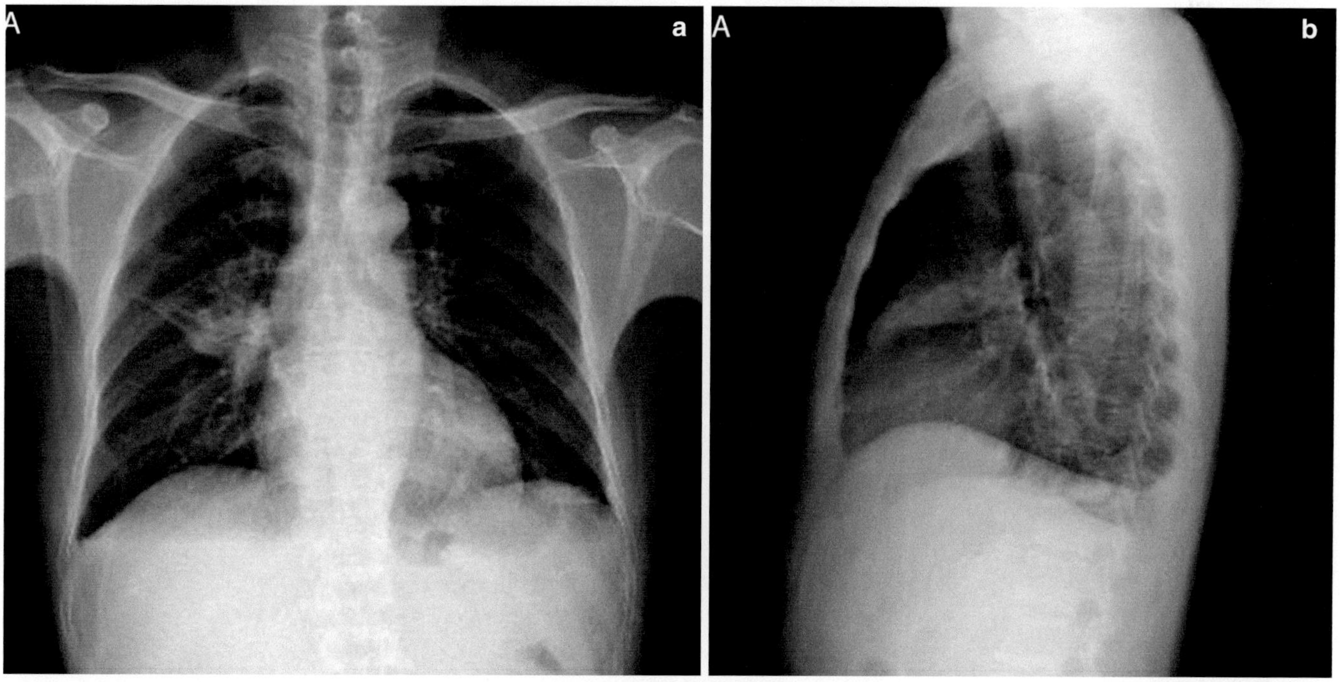

Fig. 13.8 (**a**, **b**) Chest X-ray. (**a**) Chest X-ray demonstrates enlarged hilar opacity of the right lung, with unclearly defined structure. (**b**) The right middle lung lobe is demonstrated with strips of consolidation opacity

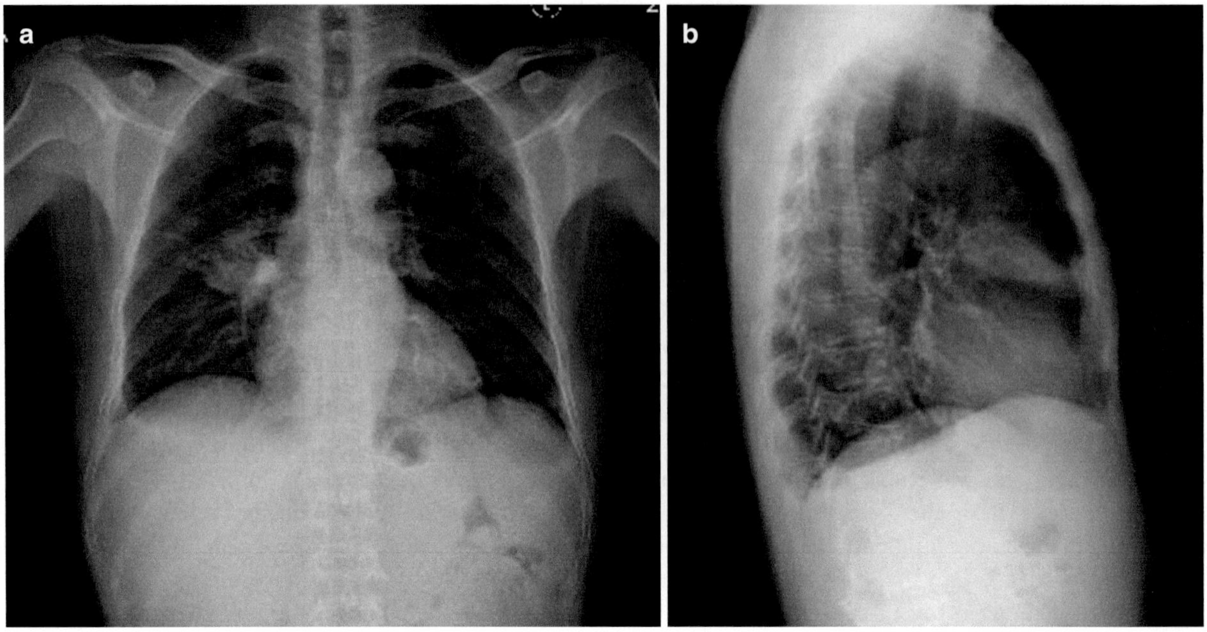

Fig. 13.9 Anterior-posterior and lateral chest X-rays. (**a**, **b**) The hilar opacity at the right lung is demonstrated to be enlarged, and the right middle lung lobe is demonstrated with consolidation opacity. The lesions show no change compared to previous chest X-ray 1 week ago

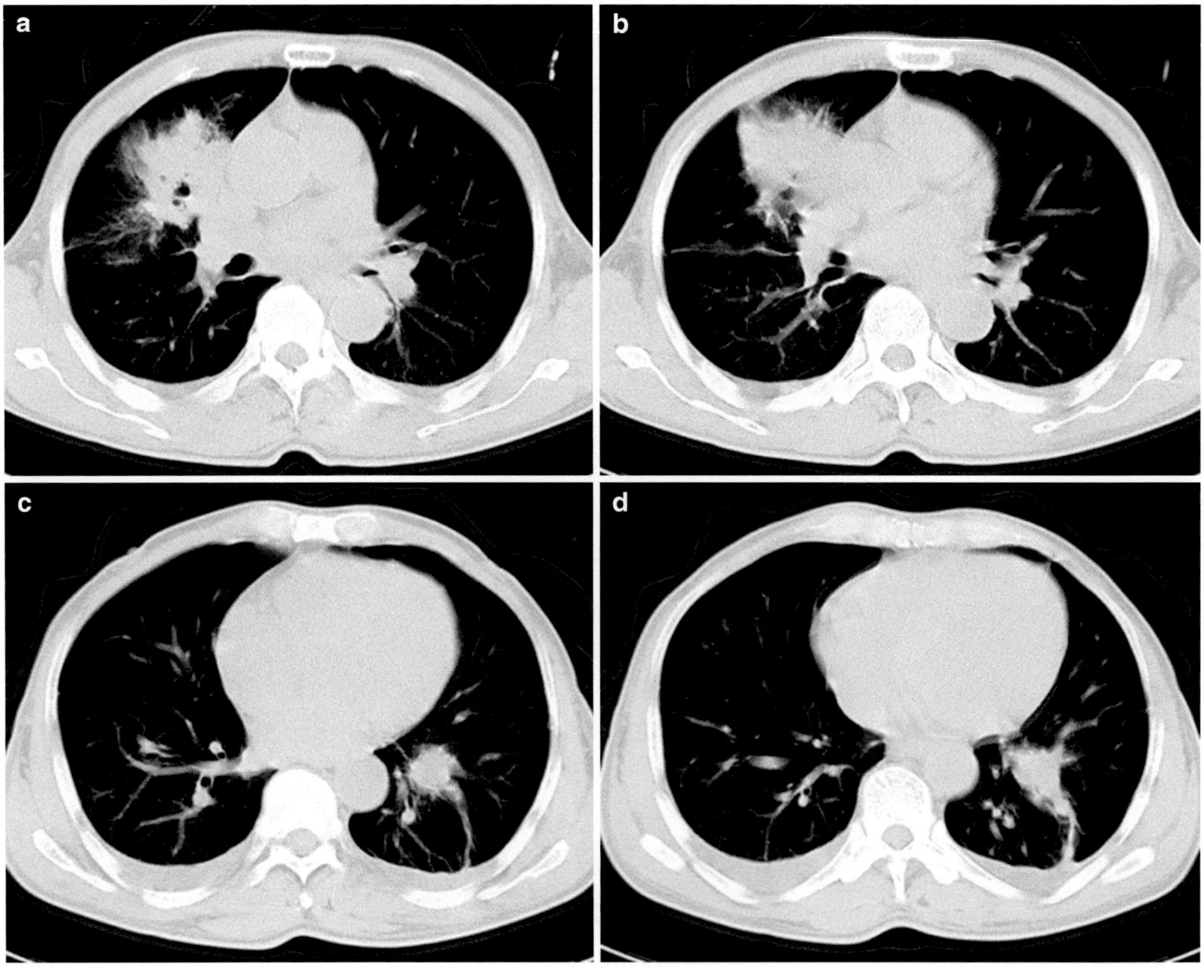

Fig. 13.10 (**a**–**d**) Plain chest CT scan. (**a**, **b**) The lung window demonstrates mass-like consolidation opacity with coarse margin and small flakes of ground-glass opacity in the right middle lung lobe. (**c**, **d**) The left lower lung is demonstrated with nodular high-intensity opacity. There are also strips of opacity that connect with the left pleura and bilateral pleural effusion in small quantities

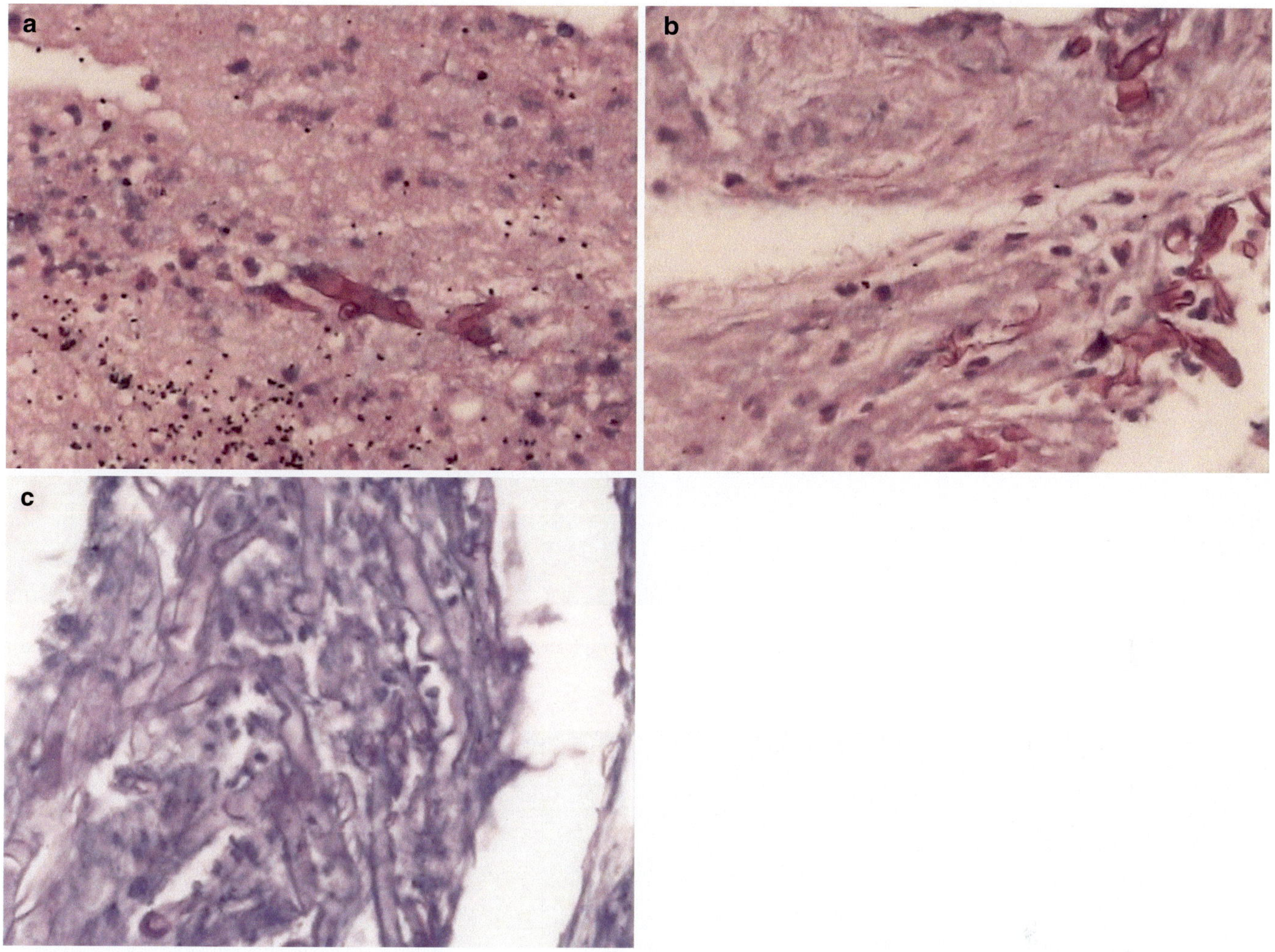

Fig. 13.11 (**a**–**c**) Pathology of lung tissue. (**a**) H&E staining demonstrates possible necrotic aspergillus hyphae near the necrotic tissue in the clamped specimen from the right upper lung lobe. (**b**) H&E staining demonstrates possible necrotic aspergillus hyphae near the necrotic tissue in the clamped specimen from the right upper lung lobe. (**c**) Methenamine silver staining demonstrates a small quantity of aspergillus (PASM staining)

13.3.4 Discussion

Polycystic kidney is also known as congenital cyst of kidney, benign multilocular cystoma of the kidney, polycystic disease, Potter (I) syndrome, Perlman syndrome, cytosolic kidney, and bilateral renal dysplasia syndrome [11]. In China, it was firstly reported in the year 1941 by Xianli Song. Polycystic kidney is common clinically and can be classified into two types. One is the autosomal recessive inheritance type (infant type), which occurs during infancy and is clinically rare. And the other is the autosomal dominant inheritance type (adult type), which is commonly detected in young or middle-aged adults and may occur at any age. The etiology of polycystic kidney is gene deletion. The adult type of polycystic kidney is commonly caused by gene deletion on chromosome 16 and occasionally on chromosome 4. The infant polycystic kidney disease is an autosomal recessive inheritance. Only when both parents have genetic changes of the disease, their children can develop the disease. The incidence of the disease is 25%.

Pulmonary aspergillosis commonly occurs in populations with immunodeficiency whose diagnosis is challenging and mortality is high [12, 13]. In this case, the patient presented in the hospital due to kidney disease, but the initial symptom was chest distress and breathlessness. The patient was immunocompromised and belonged to the high-risk population of invasive pulmonary aspergillosis. Bronchoscopy for biopsy demonstrated fungal hyphae, which supported the diagnosis of pulmonary aspergillosis. After administration of itraconazole for fungal infection, the respiratory symptoms were rapidly improved, and the lesions in the lungs were gradually absorbed. Reexamination of chest X-ray after treatment for 1 year demonstrated complete absorption of lesions in lungs, indicating a long period of time for treatment. We summarize the following key points of this case: (1) Patients with polycystic kidney complicated by renal inadequacy show

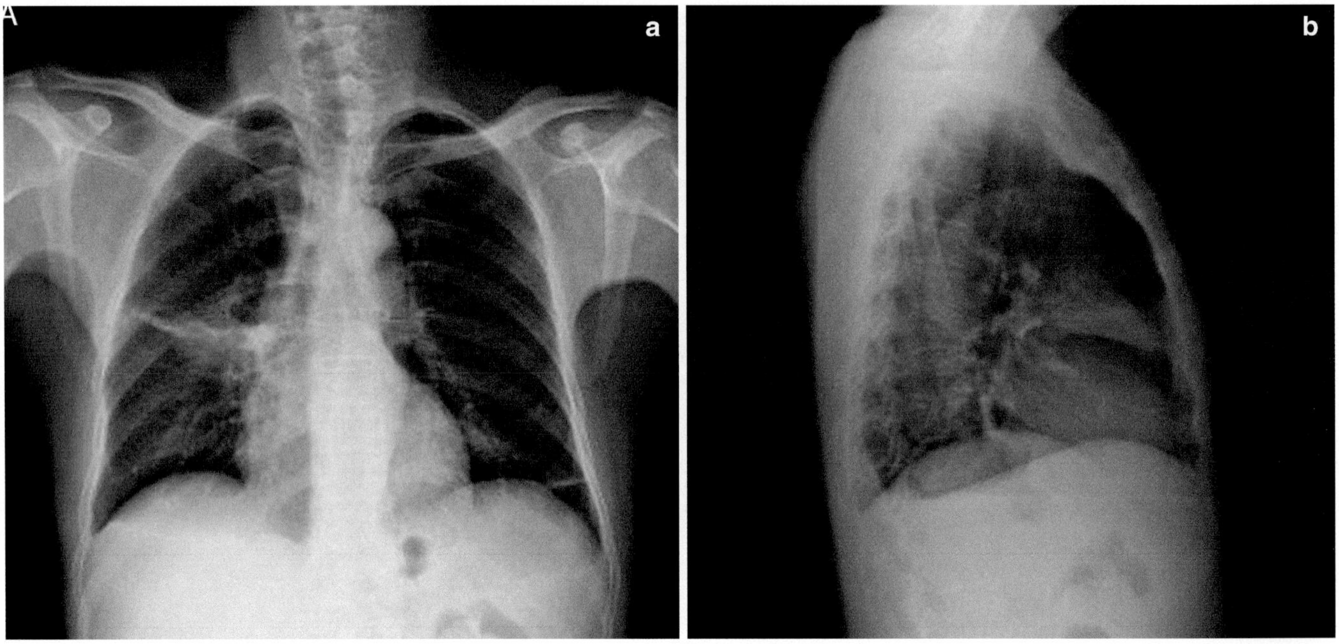

Fig. 13.12 (**a**, **b**) Chest X-ray. The right hilum is demonstrated with strip of high-intensity opacity, with shrinkage compared to the previous chest X-ray on February 19, 2014

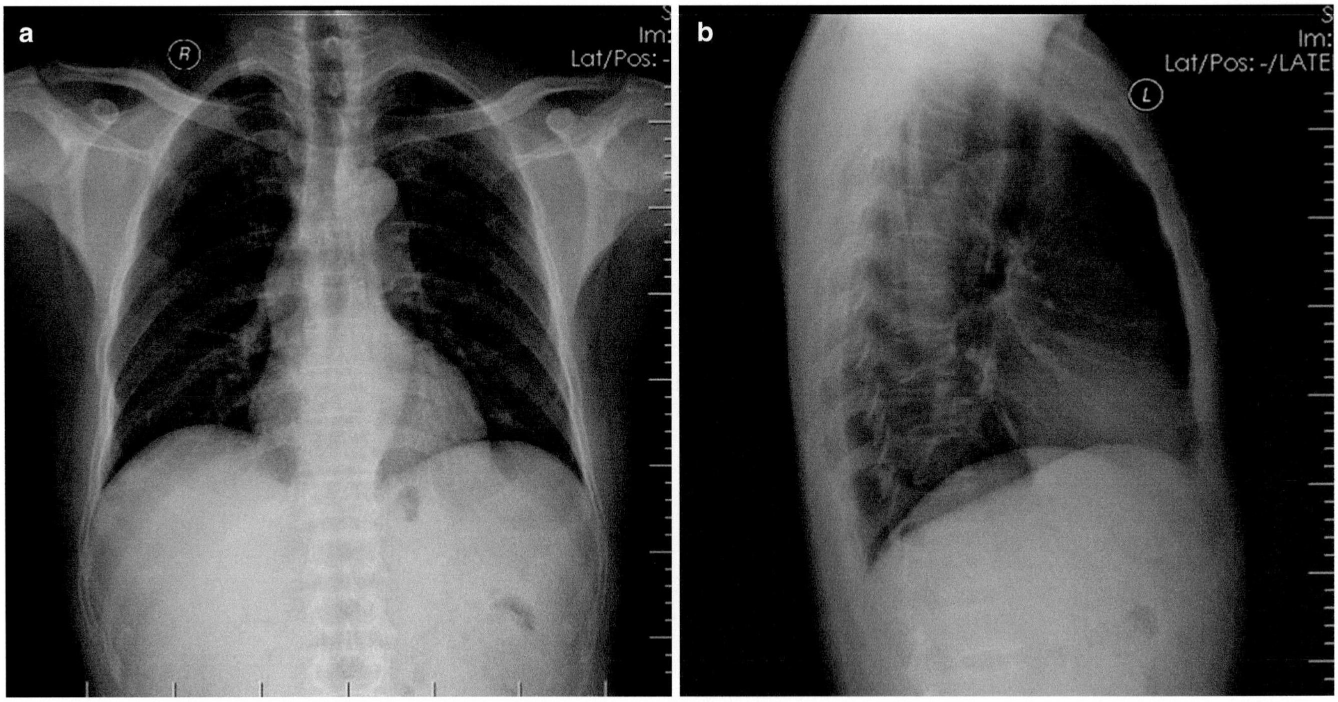

Fig. 13.13 (**a**, **b**) Chest X-ray. The right hilar opacity is basically normal, with absorption compared to the previous chest X-ray on February 19, 2014

compromised immunity. Therefore, they are possibly a susceptible population of pulmonary aspergillosis. (2) Chest CT scan demonstrated a cavity-like change and halo sign in lungs, and the radiologists should first suspect pulmonary aspergillosis. Halo sign is one of the CT signs of pulmonary aspergillosis, which is demonstrated as ground-glass opacity around nodule or mass opacity and is a sign of peripheral bleeding due to invasion of aspergillus. Halo sign is non-specific, which may also be demonstrated in the cases of other diseases with hemorrhagic nodule or focal pulmonary infiltration of neoplasm, such as adenocarcinoma of the lung and bronchioloalveolar carcinoma. However, the incidence of halo sign in the cases of pulmonary aspergillosis is high. And chest CT scan demonstration of halo sign should be firstly considered to be pulmonary aspergillosis. (3) Renal inadequacy complicated by pulmonary aspergillosis is an intractable problem in antifungal treatment. The adverse effect of antifungal medication to renal function is the problem in antifungal treatment.

13.3.5 Comments

In this case, the diagnosis of primary disease was definitive. And the primary disease was diagnosed as polycystic kidney complicated by chronic renal failure. Based on the dynamic changes by chest radiology, histopathology of lung tissue, and therapeutic efficacy of antifungal treatment, the diagnosis of pulmonary aspergillosis was also definitive.

Patients with chronic renal failure are hosts of immunodeficiency, and they are susceptible to secondary infection with no obvious systemic responses. The underlying mechanism is complex, possibly including the following: (1) Research study had found that the number of T lymphocyte in patients with chronic renal failure was significantly reduced, especially in CD4 subgroup with auxiliary function and induction effect, which was significantly lower than that in normal subjects. The change is significantly related to serum creatinine value. (2) Patients with chronic renal failure show glucose metabolism disorders of peripheral neutrophil granulocytes, with impaired motion and phagocytosis. (3) Malnutrition in patients with chronic renal failure is one reason for their compromised immunity. (4) Recent research studies on erythrocyte immune function in patients with chronic renal insufficiency indicated obvious decrease of erythrocyte CD35. In addition, there is a decrease of erythrocyte immune adherence, and the tendency of decrease is related to the condition of the patients. The above reasons induce compromised immunity in patients with chronic renal insufficiency. Therefore, they are susceptible to various fungal infections.

The medication of choice for invasive pulmonary aspergillosis is intravenous infusion or oral intake of voriconazole. For some patients, amphotericin B liposomes can be administered as the initial therapy. After the symptoms are improved, the medication can be changed to oral intake of voriconazole or itraconazole. If the initial therapy is ineffective, caspofungin, posaconazole, or itraconazole can be administered as rescue therapy. Antifungal treatment in patients with chronic renal insufficiency is intractable. In this case, the patient received itraconazole and the therapeutic efficacy was favorable. The excipient in injection of itraconazole, 2-hydroxypropyl-beta-cyclodextrin, is metabolized via kidneys. Therefore, injection of itraconazole is contraindicated in patients with a creatinine clearance rate of lower than 30 ml/min. The protein binding rate of itraconazole is 99%, and hemodialysis has no effects on half-value period and clearance of itraconazole given by intravenous infusion or oral intake. However, 2-hydroxypropyl-beta-cyclodextrin can be cleared along with hemodialysis. Therefore, itraconazole should be given at the same dosage before hemodialysis for clearance of beta-cyclodextrin. In this case, the physician chose an oral intake of 0.2 g/day of itraconazole. His/her knowledge about pharmacokinetics facilitates the clinical medication. Data about oral intake of itraconazole by patients with renal dysfunction has been limited. The successful treatment in this case definitively provides reference for the clinical management of such patients.

13.4 Case 4: Chest Upset and Palpitation with Accompanying Breathlessness After Physical Acitivities for More Than 1 Month

Dandan Chen, Guan-Xun Cheng, Chen Qiu, Xiongfei Sun, Xueyan Liu and Chang'e Jin

13.4.1 Presenting Symptom

Chest upset and palpitation with accompanying breathlessness after physical activities for more than 1 month.

13.4.2 Brief Case History

A 48-year-old woman, a housewife, was admitted to our hospital on May 6, 2013, due to complaints of chest upset and palpitation with accompanying breathlessness after physical activities for more than 1 month. One month ago, the patient began to experience chest upset, burning of the chest, palpitation, and accompanying breathlessness after physical activities. But she experienced no fever, chest pain, cough, expectoration, nausea, and vomiting. In a local hospital, chest CT scan demonstrated a solid space-occupying lesion at the apex of the right lung with marginal fissure-like cavity. Cefoperazone sulbactam was then administered for infection. And reexamination of chest CT scan demonstrated no absorption of the lesion. Then the patient was transferred to our hospital for further diagnosis and treatment. Since the onset of symptoms, her spiritual state, appetite, and sleep were average. The urinations and bowel movements were normal. And she experienced no obvious recent weight loss.

13.4.2.1 Past Medical History

She denied past medical histories of hypertension, diabetes, hepatitis, and tuberculosis. And she denied histories of surgical operation and trauma. The patient had no hobbies in smoking and drinking.

13.4.2.2 Family History

Her daughter was diagnosed with pulmonary tuberculosis 1 year ago. And reexamination of chest X-ray demonstrated cure after antituberculosis treatment for 1 year.

13.4.2.3 Physical Examination

Physical examination showed a body temperature of 37.4 °C, pulse rate 83/min, respiration rate 18/min, and blood pressure 137/76 mmHg. She was typically developed and well conscious, with favorable nourishment and normal appearance. The patient was in active position and well cooperated during physical examination. The systemic superficial lymph nodes were not palpable and not enlarged. The thorax was normal. And the respiration sounds at both lungs were coarse, with no dry and/or moist rales. The heart was not enlarged, with a heartbeat of 83/min, rhythmic. The valvular areas showed no pathological murmur. The abdomen was soft. The liver and spleen were unpalpable. The shifting dullness was negative. And the liver and kidneys were not sensitive to percussion. The bowel sounds were normal.

13.4.2.4 Auxiliary Investigation

Chest CT scan in another hospital on April 23, 2013, demonstrated a solid space-occupying lesion at the apex of the right lung, with marginal fissure-like cavity. Reexamination of chest CT scan in another hospital on May 3, 2013, demonstrated the same space-occupying lesion at the apex of the right lung as the previous chest CT scan (Fig. 13.14).

13.4.2.5 Initial Diagnosis

The initial diagnosis was a space-occupying lesion at the right lung, which was suspected to be neoplasm, fungal infection, or pulmonary tuberculosis.

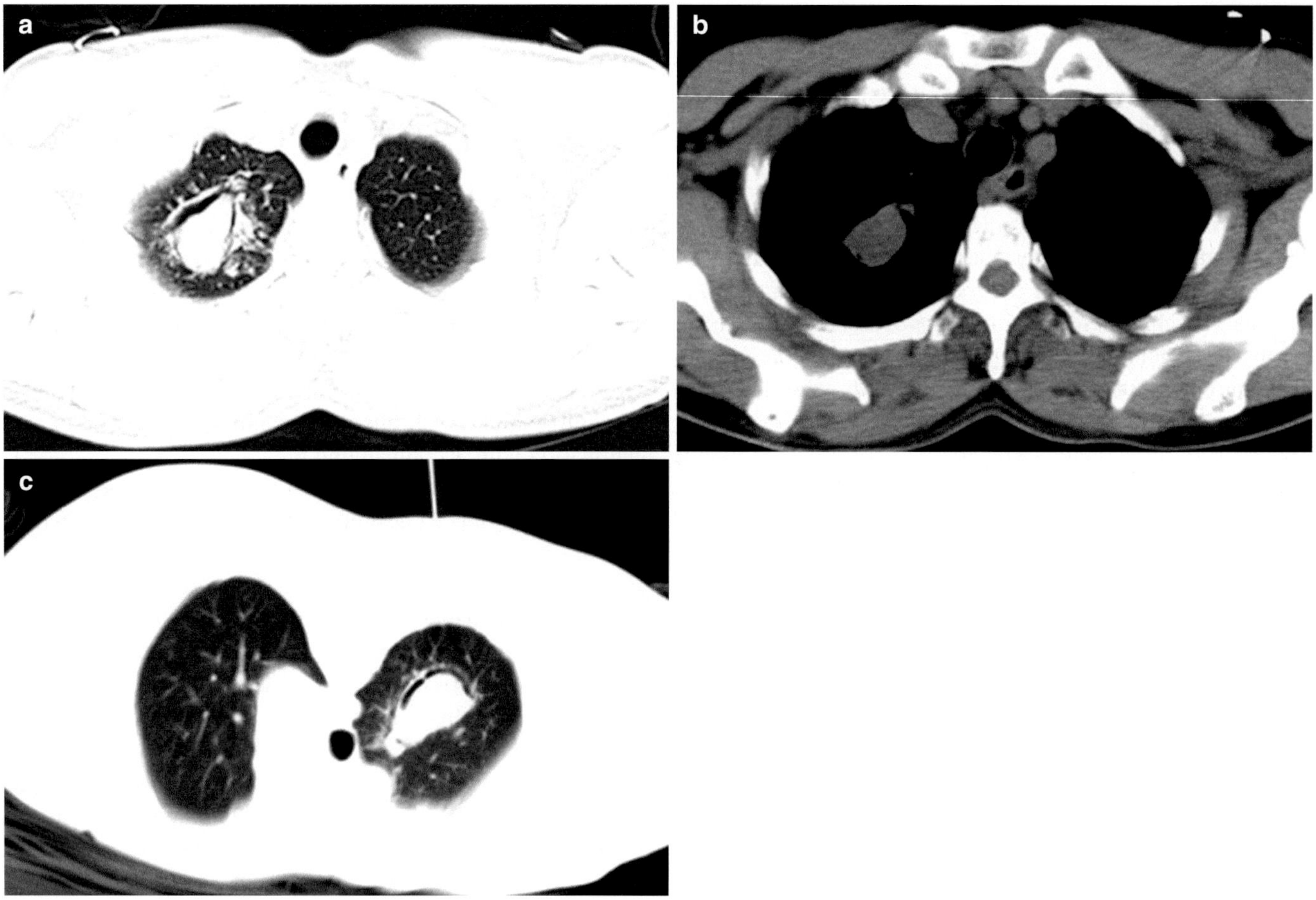

Fig. 13.14 (a–c) Chest CT scan. (**a**) The lung window demonstrates a nodular opacity at the right upper lung lobe, with spherical dense opacity and air crescent sign inside. Around the nodular opacity, less exudation opacity is demonstrated inferior and lateral to the nodular opacity. (**b**) The mediastinum window demonstrates nodular opacity and air crescent sign at the right upper lung lobe. (**c**) After the patient changes her posture from supine to prone, the low-intensity nodular opacity in the lesion is demonstrated to be movable. And the crescent sign is at the dorsal part of the lesion

13.4.3 Diagnosis and Treatment

After admission, levofloxacin was administered for infection. But the patient still experienced chest upset but no fever, breathlessness, and hemoptysis. During her hospitalization, the fungal G test was lower than 10 pg/ml. And *Cryptococcus neoformans* capsule antigen was negative. On May 9, 2013, the CEA was 0.45 μg/L. And repeated sputum smears for four times showed no bacteria, fungi, and acid-fast bacilli. The sputum culture showed no bacteria and fungi. Bronchoscopy demonstrated inflammatory changes in the trachea and bronchi, with thin secretions but no neoplasm and bleeding. Bronchoscopic brushing showed no cancer cells as well as no bacteria, fungi, and acid-fast bacilli. Chest X-ray on May 8, 2013, demonstrated mostly well-marginated mass opacity with slightly high intensity at the right upper lung lobe, with short spikes. The mass was about 5.1 cm × 3.7 cm in size (Fig. 13.15), which was considered to be a space-occupying lesion at the right upper lung lobe. CT scan in another hospital demonstrated a solid space-occupying lesion at the apex of the right lung, with marginal crescent sign. CT-guided percutaneous lung puncture for biopsy was recommended. At day 3 after her hospitalization, percutaneous lung puncture for biopsy was performed. And the pathology demonstrated fungal hyphae and spores in large quantities in the specimen of lung tissue. The hyphae showed branching in sharp angle, with septa but no other structure. The pathological diagnosis was fungal mass in the right lung, which was morphologically consistent with aspergillus.

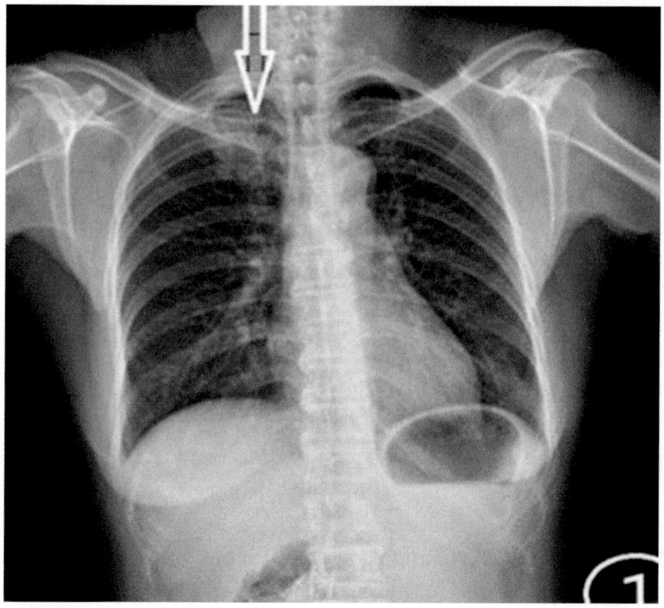

Fig. 13.15 Anterior-posterior chest X-ray. The right upper lung lobe the size of about 5.1 cm × 3.7 cm is demonstrated with a mass-like opacity with slightly high intensity. Most of the mass is well marginated with short spikes. And the mass opacity is irregular

The patient suddenly experienced hemoptysis of fresh red blood in a volume of about 100 ml on May 13, 2013. Treatment for hemostasis was administered, followed by her admission to the critical care department. After antifungal therapy and hemostasis therapy were administered, her condition was stabilized. On May 22, 2013, thoracoscopic wedge removal of the space-occupying lesion at the right upper lung was performed. During the operation, a singular nodule at the right upper lung was palpated, which was movable with size of 2 cm × 3 cm × 4 cm with no adhesion with surrounding tissue. The pathology demonstrated fungal hyphae and spores in large quantities, the branching of hyphae in sharp angle with septa, and fungal mass in the right lung, which was morphologically consistent with aspergillus. The pathological diagnosis was aspergillus infection of the right upper lung (Fig. 13.16).

The postoperative recovery was favorable and the patient was discharged on May 27, 2013. The final diagnosis was pulmonary aspergilloma with hemoptysis. After discharge, the condition of the patient was stable, and she showed no hemoptysis during follow-ups.

13.4.4 Discussion

Pulmonary aspergillosis is a comparatively rare pulmonary infection. But along with wide application of antibiotic, glucocorticoid, immunosuppressant, and anti-neoplasm drugs, its incidence has been increasing. Clinically, pulmonary aspergillosis can be classified into aspergilloma, allergic bronchopulmonary aspergillosis (ABPA), and invasive pulmonary aspergillosis (IPA). And pulmonary aspergilloma (PA) is the most common and best known type of pulmonary aspergillosis. It commonly occurs in the lung cavity, and its most common occurrence is based on pulmonary tuberculosis. Parasitic pulmonary aspergillosis only induces slight inflammatory responses, but it tends to cause vascular damages around the lesion [14].

The clinical manifestations of PA are non-specific, commonly including chronic cough, systemic upset, weight loss, and hemoptysis. In some cases, the patients remain to be asymptomatic. Hemoptysis is the common symptom of PA, and the volume of blood that the patient coughs up ranges from a small quantity to life-threatening large quantity [15]. The reasons of hemoptysis mainly include the following: (1) Abundant vascular network or even angioma forms around the lesion of PA due to inflammatory irritations. The mechanical stimulation induced by respiratory movement may cause vascular rupture. (2) The endotoxin and protease produced by aspergillus cause necrosis and lysis of tissue. (3) Bleeding is induced by primary disease [16]. In this case, the patient initially experienced only chest upset, palpitation, and breathlessness. But during the illness course, hemoptysis

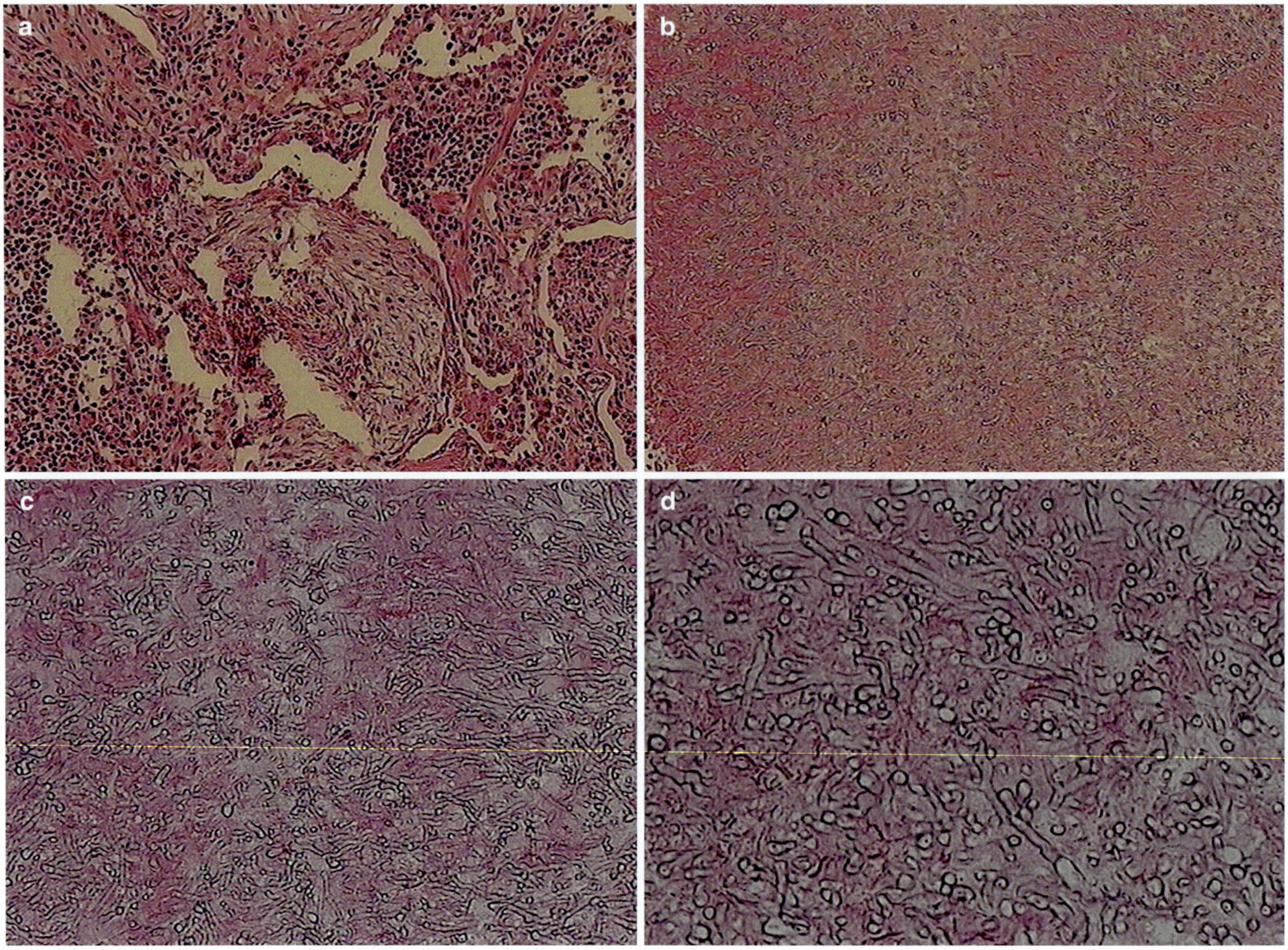

Fig. 13.16 (**a**–**d**) Pathology after thoracoscopic wedge removal of the space-occupying lesion at the right upper lung. (**a**) H&E staining demonstrates aspergillus filamentum membrane. (**b**) H&E staining demonstrates hyphae and spores of aspergillus. (**c**) H&E staining demonstrates hyphae and spores of aspergillus. (**d**) H&E staining demonstrates hyphae and spores of aspergillus in large quantities and branching of hyphae in sharp angle

occurred and the volume of blood was large, which were consistent with the literature report. The lesion of PA is commonly singular at the upper lung lobe. It may also show multiple lesions at multiple lung lobes. Its radiological demonstrations are diverse. Apart from typical pulmonary aspergillosis, it can hardly be differentiated from tuberculosis mycobacteria infection and viral infection due to existence of mixed infection. Chest X-ray demonstrates mass opacity in primary chronic cavity, which is movable in cavity-like pendulum. Chest CT scan plays an important role in the diagnosis of pulmonary aspergillosis. In this case, chest X-ray demonstrations were atypical, showing no obvious crescent-shaped translucent area due to effects of projection position. In addition to demonstrations of marginal spikes and its adjacency to pleura, it tended to be misdiagnosed as peripheral lung carcinoma. Aspergilloma is movable in the cavity along with changes of body postures, which can sometimes be hardly demonstrated by chest X-ray. Chest CT scan is necessary. In this case, chest CT scan demonstrated typical air crescent sign. And when the patient received puncture in a changed body posture, aspergilloma moved in the cavity-like pendulum. When the patient received puncture for biopsy, she was in prone position. The low-intensity opacity in the lesion changed its position accordingly, and the crescent-shaped space was at the dorsal part of the lesion.

For patients with pulmonary aspergilloma, surgical operation, if the patient is tolerant to, is an effective way for treatment [17]. Antifungal medication can hardly reach the lesion, and therefore, it can hardly be effective. For all patients with pulmonary aspergilloma and serious hemoptysis, surgical operation should be considered. Surgical removal of affected lung lobe is the most common surgical approach. Thoracoscopy is noninvasive with less bleeding and rapid recovery. In this case, the patient received thoracoscopy, which showed rapid recovery and favorable therapeutic efficacy. Postoperative follow-ups showed no relapse, which confirmed the efficacy of surgical operation.

13.4.5 Comments

In this case, the combination of clinical manifestations, lung radiology, and pathology defined the diagnosis of pulmonary aspergilloma at the right upper lung. Pulmonary aspergilloma commonly occurs in patients with compromised immunity or basic pulmonary disease. According to literature report, pulmonary aspergilloma commonly complicates cavity of chronic pulmonary abscess, bronchiectasis, bronchopulmonary abscess, or tuberculous cavity. However, there have also been literature reports demonstrating an incidence of aspergillus infection in patients with no basic pulmonary disease to be 18%. The onset of pulmonary aspergillosis is commonly insidious with no obvious clinical manifestations. Therefore, it tends to be misdiagnosed.

In this case, chest CT scan in a local hospital demonstrated a space-occupying lesion at the apex of the right lung with marginal fissure-like cavity, which was actually an air crescent sign. Reexamination of chest CT scan in the hospital demonstrated a space-occupying lesion at the apex of the right lung, which was the same as the chest CT scan demonstrations in the local hospital. The lung window demonstrated a nodular opacity at the right upper lung lobe, with spherical dense opacity inside and air crescent sign. The mediastinum window demonstrated a nodular opacity at the right upper lung lobe and air crescent sign. When the patient changed her posture from supine to prone, the low-intensity nodule in the lesion moved with the crescent-shaped space at its dorsal part. Air crescent sign and pendulum or rolling-ball sign are typical CT scan demonstrations of pulmonary aspergilloma. If further enhanced chest CT scan demonstrated no obvious enhancement, the diagnosis of pulmonary aspergilloma is further supported. Herein, we know that insufficient knowledge about pulmonary aspergillus infection caused the misdiagnosis of infection. And the subsequent medication of cefoperazone sulbactam for infection showed unfavorable therapeutic response.

In this case, the diagnosis was finally defined by pathology. After admission, percutaneous lung puncture for biopsy was performed. And the pathology demonstrated fungal hyphae and spores in large quantities in the specimen. The hyphae branch in sharp angle and there were septa on the hyphae. The pathological diagnosis was fungal mass at the right lung, which was morphologically consistent with aspergillus. The clinicians had sufficient knowledge about pulmonary aspergillus infection.

The treatment of pulmonary aspergilloma remains controversial. In some research studies, it has been demonstrated that antifungal medication can hardly permeate into the cavity containing aspergilloma, and the systemic use of antifungal medication shows unfavorable therapeutic efficacy. For the cases with pulmonary aspergillosis and frequent or major hemoptysis, surgical operation is recommended. For patients with basic pulmonary disease or pulmonary dysfunction who are intolerant to surgery, bronchial artery embolization can be performed for hemostasis. But hemoptysis may relapse. In this case, thoracoscopic wedge removal of the space-occupying lesion at the right upper lung was performed. The surgery is noninvasive with rapid postoperative recovery and definitive therapeutic efficacy, which deserves wider application.

The case analysis and comments are intended to raise clinicians' awareness about pulmonary aspergilloma in patients with no compromised immunity and no basic pulmonary disease. The clinicians should know well about chest CT scan demonstrations of pulmonary aspergilloma to avoid misdiagnosis.

References

1. Patterson R, Greenberger PA, Radin RC, et al. Allergic bronchopulmonary aspergillosis: staging as an aid to management. Ann Intern Med. 1982;96(3):286–91.
2. Eaton T, Garrett J, Milne D, et al. Allergic bronchopulmonary aspergillosis in the asthma clinic. A prospective evaluation of CT in the diagnostic algorithm. Chest. 2000;118(1):66–72.
3. Bains SN, Judson MA. Allergic bronchopulmonary aspergillosis. Clin Chest Med. 2012;33(2):265–81.
4. Hu H, Zhang L, Yu D, et al. Allergic bronchopulmonary aspergillosis: analysis of 7 cases. Chin J Tuberc Respir. 2012;35(1):37–41.
5. Chen B, Jin E, He W, et al. Radiological demonstrations of allergic bronchopulmonary aspergillosis. J Clin Exp Med. 2011;5(11):811–4.
6. Yu H, Li B, Tian K, et al. Misdiagnosis of allergic bronchopulmonary aspergillosis and its differential diagnosis. Chin J Radiol. 2011;45(6):592–4.
7. Zong X, Wang H, Yu T. CT scan demonstration of allergic bronchopulmonary aspergillosis: analysis of 17 cases. Chin J Mycol. 2013;8(3):156–9.
8. Song N, Shi J, Yang X, et al. Radiological analysis of acute exacerbation stage of chronic obstructive pulmonary disease complicated by invasive pulmonary aspergillosis. J Clin Misdiagn Mistreat. 2012;25(2):20–2.
9. Kousha M, Tadi R, Soubani AO. Pulmonary aspergillosis: a clinical review. Eur Respir Rev. 2011;20(121):156–74.
10. Park SY, Lin C, Lee SO, et al. Computed tomography findings in invasive pulmonary aspergillosis in non-neutropenic patients, and their prognostic value. J Infect. 2011;63(6):447–56.
11. Sweeney WE Jr, Avner ED. Pathophysiology of childhood polycystic kidney diseases: new insights into disease-specific therapy. Pediatr Res. 2014;75(1–2):148–57.
12. Kosmidis C, Denning DW. The clinical spectrum of pulmonary aspergillosis. Thorax. 2015;70(3):270–7.
13. Godet C, Philippe B, Laurent F, Cadranel J. Chronic pulmonary aspergillosis: an update on diagnosis and treatment. Respiration. 2014;88(2):162–74.

14. Group of Infection in Respiration Branch of Chinese Medical Society, Editorial Board of Chinese Journal of Tuberculosis and Respiration. Consensus on diagnosis and treatment of pulmonary mycosis. Chin J Tuberc Respir. 2007;30(11):821–34.
15. Patterson KC, Strek ME. Diagnosis and treatment of pulmonary aspergillosis syndromes. Chest. 2014;146(5):1358–68.
16. Franquet T, Müller NL, Giménez A, et al. Spectrum of pulmonary aspergillosis: histologic, clinical, and radiologic findings. Radiographics. 2001;21:825–37.
17. Farid S, Mohamed S, Devbhandari M, et al. Results of surgery for chronic pulmonary aspergillosis, optimal antifungal therapy and proposed high risk factors for recurrence – a National Centre's experience. J Cardiothorac Surg. 2013;8:180.

14 Pulmonary Aspergillosis with Presenting Symptoms of Cough and Expectoration

Ying-Yun Fu and Shi-Ling Song

Cough and expectoration are the most common clinical symptoms. Based on the illness course, cough can be classified into acute cough (<3 weeks), subacute cough (3–8 weeks), and chronic cough (>8 weeks). The etiology of cough is complex and widely involved. And the diseases that induce chronic cough include nasal cavity and sinus abnormalities, asthma, gastroesophageal reflux disease, non-asthmatic eosinophilic bronchitis, and allergic cough. And along with the development of medical technologies, the clinicians have known that pulmonary aspergillosis with presenting symptoms of cough and expectoration is not rare.

At different immunity status, the clinical manifestations of respiratory aspergillus infection are diverse. Pulmonary aspergillus infection in patients with non-compromised immunity manifests as allergic and invasive. At its early stage, respiratory allergic responses occur, with manifestations of dry cough, wheezing, and breathlessness. Patients with invasive infection may present fever, cough, and expectoration. Literature reports from China have demonstrated that incidences of cough and expectoration as presenting symptom in 115 cases of invasive pulmonary aspergillosis are 50.4% and 32.2%, respectively. A research study conducted by the National Aspergillus Research Center in Britain retrospectively reviewed 30 cases of pulmonary aspergillosis treated by surgery during September 1996 and September 2011. The clinical manifestations of these patients are commonly cough (40%) and hemoptysis (43%). Data indicated that pulmonary aspergillosis with presenting symptoms of cough and expectoration is common. But due to its non-specificity, including non-specific radiological demonstration, non-specific microbiology, and non-specific pathology, the early diagnosis rate of pulmonary aspergillosis remains low.

In this section, we analyze and comment on five cases of patients with pulmonary aspergillosis aged 35–65 years. Their presenting symptoms include chronic cough and expectoration. The duration of cough ranged from 2 months to 3 years, in different severity. Two cases had chronic airway disease, and the patients showed no definitive exposure history to aspergillus and no evidence supporting compromised immunity. Four cases had been misdiagnosed and mistreated. In them, one case had chest X-ray demonstration of mass opacity at the right upper lung, which was misdiagnosed as pulmonary *Candida albicans* infection. And the corresponding treatment lasted for up to 6 months. In the total five cases, four cases were defined with pulmonary aspergilloma, and the other one case was defined with invasive pulmonary aspergillosis. All the cases were definitively diagnosed via BALF culture for aspergillus or histopathology.

The diagnosis and treatment of the five cases are enlightening. And we summarized the key points as the following: (1) Pulmonary aspergillosis with presenting symptoms of cough and expectoration is not rare. (2) Pulmonary aspergillosis with presenting symptoms of cough and expectoration overlaps with basic pulmonary disease. Thus, it tends to be misdiagnosed or missed diagnosed. (3) In the etiological diagnosis and differential diagnosis of chronic cough, respiratory specimens should be harvested for corresponding investigations, including BALF GM test, nuclear acid detection for aspergillus, fungal culture, and histopathology, for early diagnosis.

Patients' consents have been obtained for images or other clinical information relating to the cases to be published.

The corresponding author of section 14.1 is Na Li, Email: lanying5204@sina.com.
The corresponding author of section 14.2 is Jiaxuan Zhou, Email: 195137680@qq.com.
The corresponding author of section 14.3 is Fei Shi, Email: shifei2003@126.com.
The corresponding author of section 14.4 is Wei Ma, Email: 1021962751@qq.com.
The corresponding author of section 14.5 is Jiezhu Ding, Email: jiezhuding@163.com.

Y.-Y. Fu (✉) · S.-L. Song
Second Clinical Medical College of Jinan University, Shenzhen, Guangdong, China

C. Qiu et al. (eds.), *Pulmonary Aspergillosis*, https://doi.org/10.1007/978-981-13-3435-1_14

14.1 Case 1: Cough for 6 Months

Na Li, Songming Zhuo, Shusong Peng, Chang'e Jin, Hui Wang, and Xueyan Liu

14.1.1 Presenting Symptom

Cough for 6 months.

14.1.2 Brief Case History

A 35-year-old man was admitted to our hospital on September 18, 2011, due to complaints of cough for 6 months. The patient began to experience slight paroxysmal cough 6 months ago. But he experienced no expectoration, fever, chest distress, chest pain, night sweat, and fatigue. Chest X-ray in a local hospital demonstrated a mass opacity at the right upper lung, which was considered to be *Candida* infection. Oral intake of fluconazole was prescribed for about 6 months, and the symptom was not obviously improved. One month ago, reexamination of chest X-ray in a community hospital in Shenzhen, China, demonstrated enlarged high-intensity mass opacity at the right upper lung, crescent-shaped translucent area, and scattering nodular opacities in both lung fields. The condition was considered to be fungal infection of both lungs, and the patient was transferred to our hospital.

14.1.2.1 Past Medical History

Three years ago, he was diagnosed with pulmonary tuberculosis due to symptoms of cough and expectoration of yellowish sputum. And he was cured and discharged.

14.1.2.2 Physical Examination

By physical examination, his body temperature was 36.6 °C, pulse rate 78/min, respiration rate 20/min, and blood pressure 130/76 mmHg. He was well conscious, with smooth respirations. The superficial lymph nodes were not enlarged. The oral lips showed no cyanosis. And the pharynx was not congested. The jugular vein showed no distension and the trachea was on the midline. The thorax showed no deformity. And the vocal fremitus of both lungs was not weakened or increased. By percussion, both lungs showed clear sounds. And the respiration sounds were coarse, with no dry and/or moist rales. The heartbeat was 78/min, rhythmic, and there was no pathological murmur. The abdomen was soft, with no tenderness and rebound pain. The liver and spleen were subcostally unpalpable. Both lower limbs showed no edema.

14.1.2.3 Initial Diagnosis

There were nodules at both lungs, and the condition was considered to be pulmonary aspergillus infection.

14.1.3 Diagnosis and Treatment

After admission, the investigations were performed. The routine blood test on September 22, 2011, showed no abnormality. The sputum smear showed no fungi. And the sputum culture for acid-fast bacilli showed negative. Bronchoscopy on September 23, 2011, demonstrated slight congestion of bronchial mucosa at the right upper lung. The culture of BALF harvested at the right upper lung lobe showed predominant growth of *Aspergillus fumigatus*. Fibrobronchoscopic brushing demonstrated no fungal hyphae and spores. And bronchoscopic brushing demonstrated no acid-fast bacilli. The repeated sputum cultures for three times demonstrated growth of normal flora in the respiratory tract.

Chest CT scan on September 21, 2011, demonstrated a mass-like solid opacity at the apical segment of the right upper lung lobe, with a CT value of about 25 Hu. There were also surrounding ring-shaped high- and low-intensity opacity, thickening and traction of adjacent pleura, and no mediastinal and hilar lymphadenectasis (Fig. 14.1). The radiological diagnosis was mass opacity at the right upper lung lobe and multiple high-intensity opacities in both lungs, which was considered to be pulmonary aspergillosis. There were also less old tuberculosis lesions at bilateral upper lung lobes and right pleural thickening.

After admission, BALF culture indicated predominant growth of *Aspergillus fumigatus*, and a diagnosis of pulmonary aspergillosis was made. Due to predictions that antifungal medication may show unfavorable response due to the large volume of the lesion, surgical removal of the lesion was recommended. The patient was then transferred to the thoracic surgery department on September 26, 2011. Thoracoscopic removal of the right upper lung lobe was performed under general anesthesia on October 8, 2011. The postoperative pathology demonstrated grayish red lung tissue of the right upper lung in size of about 10 cm × 8 cm × 4 cm and a cyst in size of 4 cm × 3.5 cm after incision, which was filled with yellowish green necrotic-like tissue. Under a microscope, fungal hyphae were observed with uniform thickness and ordered arrangement. Some hyphae branched in sharp angle. Morphologically, it was consistent to aspergillosis of the deep lung tissue (Fig. 14.2). Since October 26, 2011, the patient began to experience severe cough, with expectoration of less yellowish mucous sputum and fever. And the leakage of the right thoracic duct aggravated.

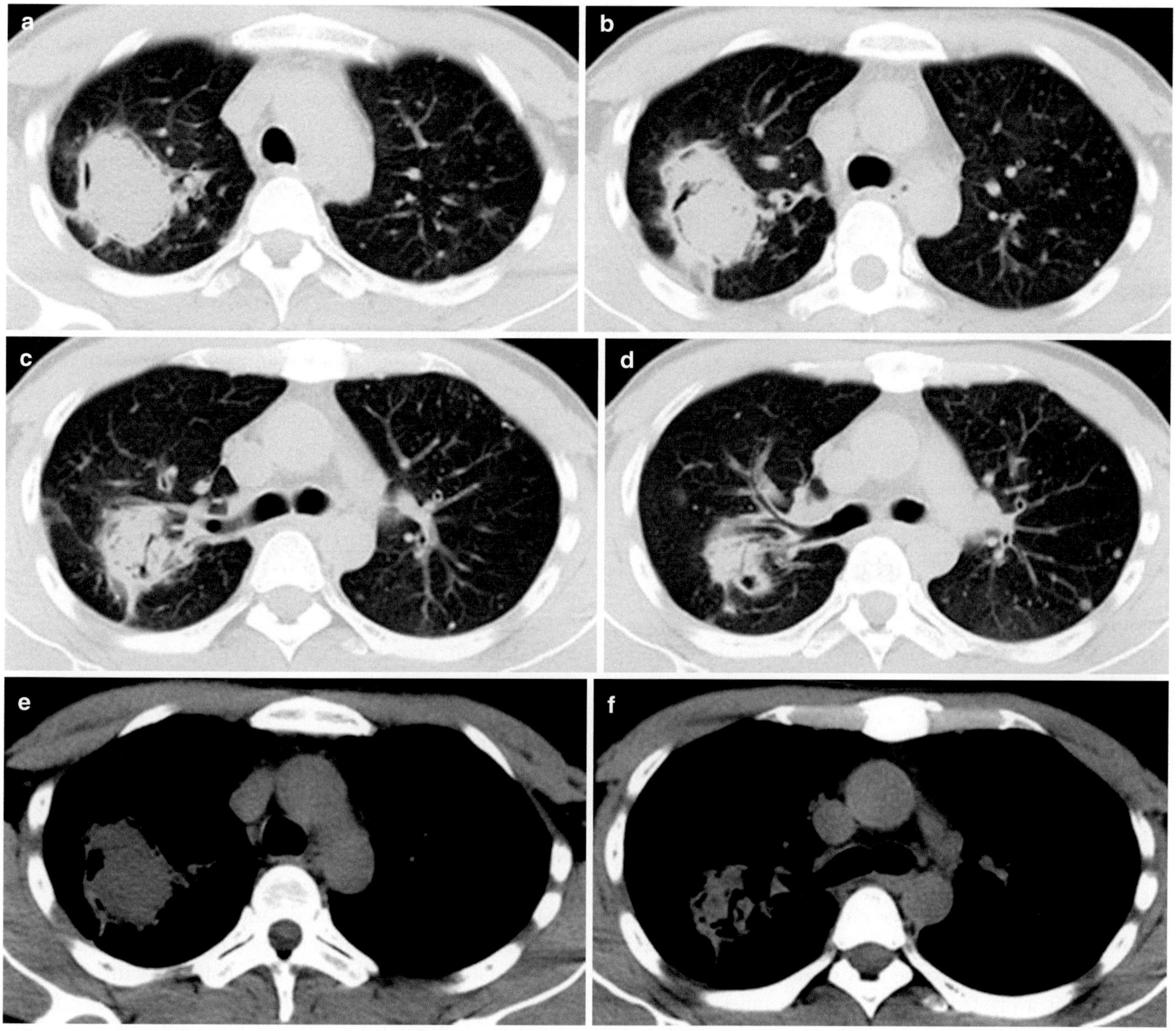

Fig. 14.1 (**a**–**f**) Chest CT scan. (**a**, **b**) The lung window demonstrates a mass-like dense opacity at the apical segment of the right upper lung lobe with a CT value of about 25 Hu. There are also surrounding ring-shaped high- and low-intensity opacities and thickening and traction of adjacent pleura. (**c**, **d**) The lung window at trachea branching level demonstrates a mass opacity at the right upper lung, with arch-shaped and round-translucent area inside. There are also scattering small nodular opacities at the left upper lung, with calcification of some nodules. (**e**, **f**) The mediastinum window demonstrates translucent area lateral and posterior to the mass opacity at the right upper lung and no hilar and mediastinal lymphadenectasis

The condition was suspected to be right bronchopleural fistula, and medications of ceftriaxone and voriconazole were prescribed. But the therapeutic response was unfavorable. On November 4, 2011, he was transferred to a superior hospital for further diagnosis and treatment.

The diagnosis on discharge was pulmonary aspergillosis of the right upper lung, right bronchopleural fistula, and old pulmonary tuberculosis. On January 14, 2016, follow-up by telephone showed no upsets during recent years, and he could manage himself in daily life activities and work.

14.1.4 Discussion

In this case, the patient presented symptom of cough for 6 months. Chest X-ray and CT scan demonstrated air crescent

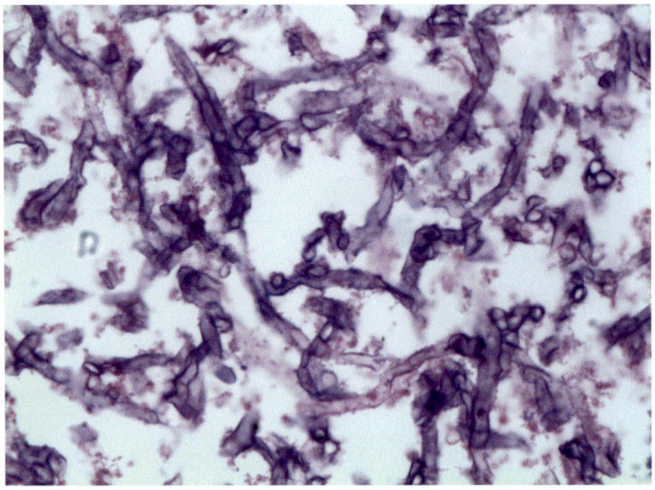

Fig. 14.2 Microscopy. Microscopy demonstrates hyphae and spores. The hyphae are uniform in thickness with branching in 45° angle (H&E staining)

sign in the lesion of the right upper lung. The culture of BALF harvested by fibrobronchoscopy demonstrated predominant growth of aspergillus. And pathology confirmed the diagnosis of pulmonary aspergillosis, and the diagnosis of pulmonary aspergillosis of the right upper lung was established.

In this case, radiology demonstrated mass opacity in the lung, which should be differentiated from neoplasm, infection, congenital developmental abnormality, vascular disorder, and connective tissue disease. The key points for differential diagnosis were the following [1, 2]:

1. The lesion of neoplasm commonly shows coarse margin, with lobulation or spinous processes. The lesion commonly has heterogeneous intensity, with eccentric cavity far away from the hilum. The inner wall of the lesion is commonly unsmooth or nodular, and some lesions show noncentral or marginal calcification. Enhanced CT scan demonstrates obvious enhancement. Around the lesion, there were depression, thickening, and adhesion or vascular aggregation near the pleura. In this case, the lesion showed high intensity, with no lobulation and marginal spinous processes. The inner wall of the cavity was smooth. These findings were not consistent to neoplasm.
2. Tuberculoma is formed by encapsulate of fibrous tissue around caseous necrosis in the lung, which is commonly singular at the upper and middle lung fields. There are satellite lesions around the lesion, which are fibrous proliferations with high heterogeneous intensity. Within the lesion, there are small cavity and calcification. The subcapsular fissure-like cavity, especially near the hilum, is the characteristic demonstration of tuberculoma. In this case, the lesion was large, which is far different from the lesion of tuberculoma. There were no satellite lesions around the lesion and no obvious calcification. The intensity of the lesion was comparatively homogeneous. The radiological demonstrations were not consistent to those of tuberculoma.
3. Aspergilloma is commonly located at the upper lung, with homogeneous sphere and crescent-shaped translucent area superior to it. The sphere is movable along with body posture, with smooth or slightly coarse margin. In this case, the patient had a past medical history of pulmonary tuberculosis, which is one of the high-risk factors of aspergilloma [3]. Before his admission to the hospital, medication of fluconazole had been taken for 6 months, but the cough failed to be improved. Reexamination of chest X-ray demonstrated enlarged lesion at the right upper lung, compared to the previous chest X-ray. Fluconazole is ineffective to aspergillus, which should be paid close attention by clinicians.

In this case, the patient had a past medical history of pulmonary tuberculosis 3 years ago, and chest CT scan demonstrated calcification, pleural thickening, and cords high-intensity opacity about the bilateral upper lungs. And the condition was considered to be old pulmonary tuberculosis. A past medical history of pulmonary tuberculosis is one of the high-risk factors of aspergillosis [4]. In such patients, bronchopleural fistula may occur after surgical removal of the lung lobe due to pleural adhesion and other factors [5]. Surgery is the optimal treatment for pulmonary aspergillosis. Some scholars believed that thoracoscopy is superior to thoracotomy due to its noninvasiveness. Pre- or postoperative antifungal medication has not reached consensus. Preventive use of antifungal drugs for 2 weeks after resection of solitary lesions. For patients with extensive lesions, rupture of cavity, or compromised immunity, medication for above 8 weeks should be administered. And its withdrawal should be based on radiological demonstrations. In this case, factors inducing bronchopleural fistula as well as appropriateness of pre- and postoperative antifungal medication need to be explored.

14.1.5 Comments

The main risk factors of pulmonary *Candida* infection include the administration of wide-spectrum antibiotic, application of central venous catheter, total gastrointestinal nutrition, admission to ICU, and neutropenia. In this case, the patient was a young man with no exposure or experience of the above risk factors, and he showed no suppressed immunity. In a local hospital, chest X-ray demonstrated a mass opacity at the right upper lung, which was considered to be *Candida* infection. And fluconazole was administered for 6 months. The patient was misdiagnosed and mistreated.

After his admission to our hospital, chest CT scan demonstrated a mass opacity at the right upper lung, with arch- and round-shaped translucent area inside and crescent sign, which were typical radiological demonstrations of aspergilloma. Meanwhile, there were radiological demonstrations of scattering small nodular opacities at the bilateral upper lungs, and calcifications of some nodules were radiological changes of old pulmonary tuberculosis. Pulmonary aspergillosis commonly occurs in the cavity induced by bronchopulmonary cyst, bronchiectasis, pulmonary abscess, or pulmonary tuberculosis. In this case, pulmonary aspergilloma occurred based on pulmonary tuberculosis. The diagnosis was considered to be chronic pulmonary aspergillosis, and the clinical typing was pulmonary aspergilloma.

Concerning the treatment of aspergilloma, surgery is the treatment of choice for patients with favorable pulmonary functions. A successful surgery depends on the complete removal of aspergilloma with no leakage of fungal substances in the pleural cavity. In this case, the patient experienced aggravated leakage of the right thoracic tube, which was considered to be a right bronchopleural fistula. Its etiological factors may include pleural adhesion due to tuberculosis and intraoperative leakage of fungal substances in the pleural cavity. According to clinical guideline jointly issued by ESCMID and ERS in 2015, preoperative antifungal medication can be administered for several weeks if the surgical operations are complex and overflow of fungal substances is possible. For patients with intraoperative overflow of fungal substances, amphotericin B deoxycholate should be applied to irrigate the thoracic cavity.

14.2 Case 2: Recurrent Cough, Expectoration and Breathlessness for More Than 3 Years and Aggravation for 1 Month

Jiaxuan Zhou, Qingsi Zeng, Xiaoyan Huang, Qin Liu, Xueyan Liu, Yulin He, and Xuemei Han

14.2.1 Presenting Symptoms

Recurrent cough, expectoration, and breathlessness for more than 3 years and aggravation for 1 month.

14.2.2 Brief Case History

A 54-year-old man was admitted to our hospital on September 10, 2013, due to complaints of recurrent cough, expectoration, and breathlessness for more than 3 years and aggravation for 1 month. More than 3 years ago, the patient began to experience recurrent paroxysmal cough with breathlessness that were more obvious when briskly walking or heavily exerting and occasional expectoration of whitish mucous sputum. But he could manage himself in daily life activities. And he experienced no hemoptysis, flushes after noons, and night sweat. In a local hospital, he received treatment (specifically unknown). But the symptoms relieved and aggravated, which were more serious when the weather turned cold. On August 10, 2013, the above symptoms occur again when he was tired, with increased coughs and expectoration of yellowish mucous sputum. On August 12, he was admitted to a local hospital, and the diagnosis was chronic obstructive pulmonary disease. Anti-infection therapy, aerosol inhalation of oxygen, phlegm-reducing therapy, and breathlessness-relieving therapy were administered, but the condition was not improved. And he showed low-grade fever, with his body temperature fluctuating around 37.8 °C. The sputum smear showed fungal spores and fluconazole was administered. But the condition was not improved. He was then transferred to our hospital for further diagnosis and treatment. Since the onset of symptoms, his spiritual state and appetite were normal. And he experienced weight loss of about 3 kg during the recent 6 months.

14.2.2.1 Past Medical History

He denied histories of hypertension, diabetes, renal disease, tuberculosis, and hepatitis. And he reported hobbies in smoking for more than 30 years, 20 cigarettes per day.

14.2.2.2 Physical Examination

Physical examination showed a body temperature of 36.7 °C, pulse rate 106/min, respiration rate 23/min, and blood pressure 144/86 mmHg. He was typically developed with moderate nourishment. He showed slight shortness of breath. And he was in active position and well cooperated with the physical examination. The systemic superficial lymph nodes were not palpable and not enlarged. By percussion, both lungs showed hyperresonant note. By auscultation, the respiration sounds of both lungs were weakened, with inspiratory fine moist rales. The heart was not enlarged, with a heartbeat of 106/min, rhythmic. And the valvular areas showed no pathological murmur. The abdomen was soft, with the liver and spleen unpalpable. The shifting dullness was negative. The liver and kidneys were not sensitive to percussion. The bowel sound was normal.

14.2.2.3 Auxiliary Investigation

Laboratory Test

During hospitalization in a local hospital, routine blood test showed WBC 31 × 10^9/L. And the sputum smear showed fungal spores.

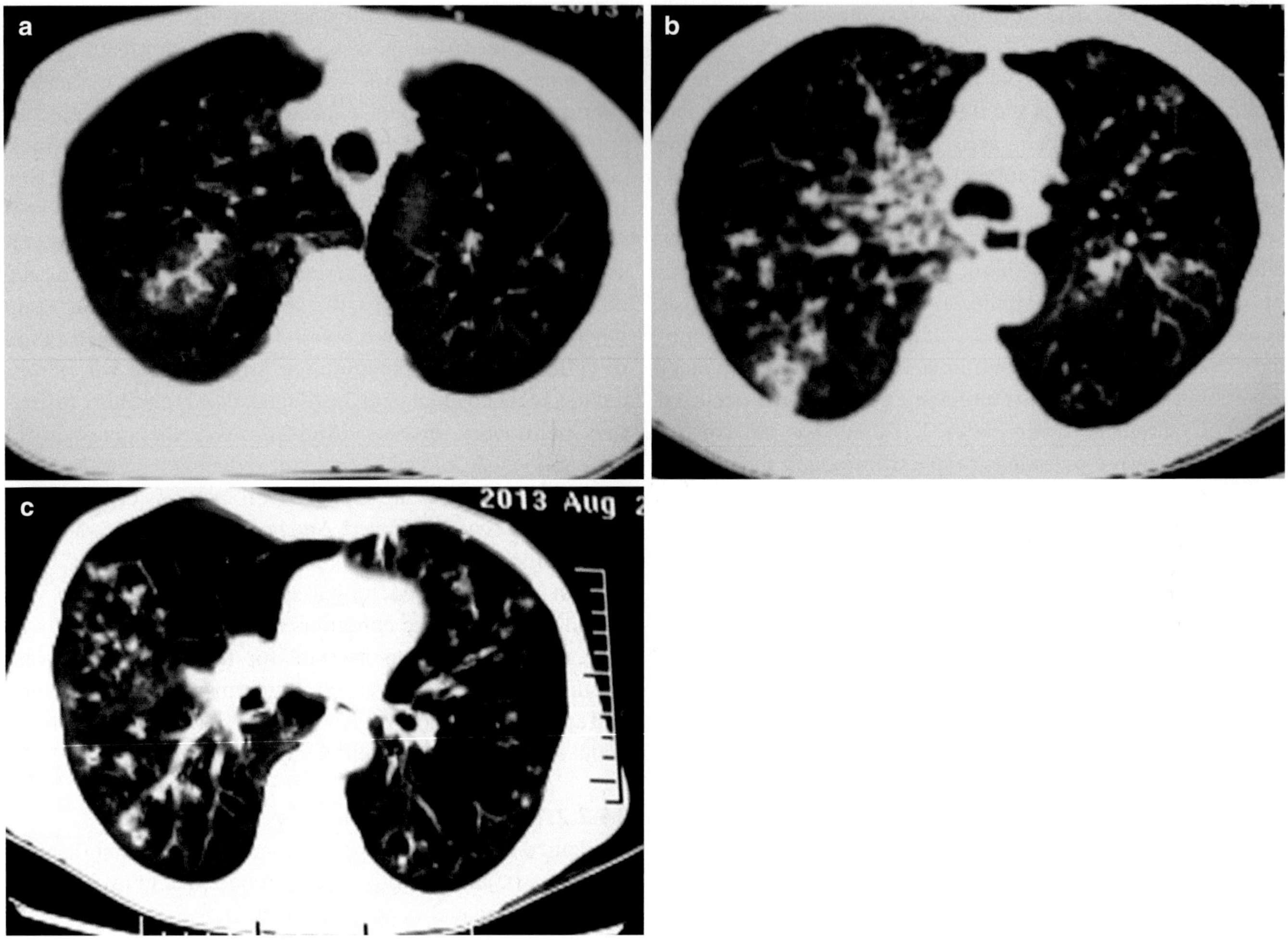

Fig. 14.3 (**a–c**) Chest CT scan in a local hospital. (**a**) The lung window demonstrates patchy opacity and ground-glass opacity at the apical segment of the right upper lung, with marginal halo sign. (**b, c**) The lung window demonstrates multiple small nodular opacities that distribute along the bronchial vascular bundle and halo sign around most of the nodules

Radiology

Chest CT scan on August 25, 2013, in a local hospital demonstrated (Fig. 14.3) multiple patchy opacities and ground-glass opacities in both lungs, which were poorly defined with a halo sign. There were also multiple small nodular opacities in both lungs and marginal halo sign of some small nodules that mainly distributed along the bronchial vascular bundle. The lingual segment of the left upper lung and the subpleural area of the left lower lung were demonstrated with poorly defined consolidation opacity.

14.2.2.4 Initial Diagnosis

The initial diagnosis was lung infection which was suspected to be fungal infection or tuberculosis and acute exacerbation of chronic obstructive pulmonary disease.

14.2.3 Diagnosis and Treatment

After admission, the investigations were performed. The WBC was 24.0×10^9/L and neutrophile granulocytes 86.1%. The procalcitonin was 6.01 ng/ml (normal value 0.05 ng/ml). The ESR was 112 mm/h. And D-dimer was 3410 ng/ml (normal value 494 ng/ml). The antigens of candida and cryptococcus were negative. And the G test showed negative. Various immunological assays for antibody against tuberculosis mycobacteria showed negative. The TB-DNA in sputum was negative. The sputum smear showed no acid-fast bacilli. The sputum culture showed no growths of pathogenic bacteria and fungi.

Piperacillin/tazobactam sodium was clinically administered for infection. Chest CT scan on September 13, 2013,

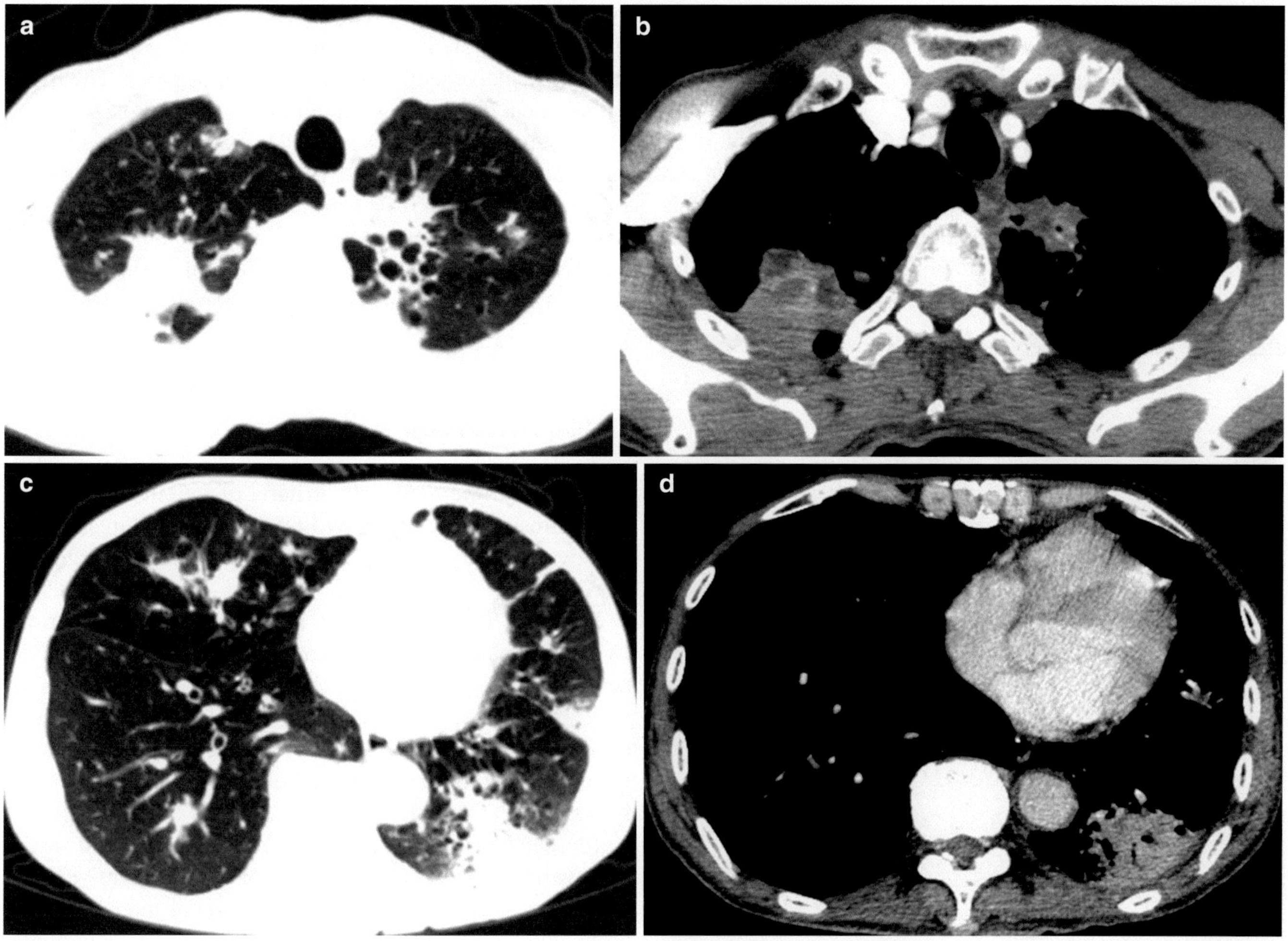

Fig. 14.4 Chest CT scan. (**a**) The lung window of CT scan demonstrates mass and flake of consolidation opacity at the apical segment of the right upper lung and multiple small cavities in the consolidation opacity at the apical segment of the left upper lung. (**b**) The mediastinum window of enhanced CT scan demonstrates low-intensity area with no enhancement in the consolidation opacity at the apical segment of the right upper lung. (**c**, **d**) The lung window of CT scan and the mediastinum window of enhanced CT scan demonstrate the lingual segment of the left upper lung and the basilar segment of the left lower lung with subpleural wedge-shaped consolidation opacity, with air bronchogram inside

demonstrated (Fig. 14.4) progression of the lesions at both lungs. Some patchy opacities and ground-glass opacities progressed into consolidation opacities. There were multiple consolidation opacities at the right upper lung, lingual segment of the left upper lung, and subpleural part of the left lower lung. And air bronchogram was demonstrated in some consolidation opacities. The lesions increased in number and enlarged compared to previous CT scans. Enhanced CT scan demonstrated obvious enhancement of the consolidation opacity. And the CT value before and after enhanced CT scan was about 45/90 Hu. There was no enhanced necrotic area in the consolidation opacity at the apical segment of the right upper lung, but there were multiple cavities at the posteroapical segment of the left upper lung. Some bronchial wall was demonstrated to be thickened, with slight dilation of some bronchial lumen. The left thorax was demonstrated with pleural effusion in a small quantity. And the diagnosis was considered to be pulmonary aspergillosis.

Fibrobronchoscopy on September 13, 2013, demonstrated unobstructed trachea; sharp tracheal carina; unobstructed right major bronchus; unobstructed bronchi; segments and subsegments at the upper lung lobe, middle lung lobe, and lower lung lobe; smooth mucosa; and whitish secretions in a small quantity. The left major bronchus was demonstrated to be unobstructed, unobstructed bronchi, segments and subsegments of upper and lower lung lobes, smooth mucosa, and whitish secretions in a small quantity. The fibrobronchoscope was inserted into the posterior segment of the right upper lung lobe for biopsy and brushing (Fig. 14.5).

Pathology demonstrated (Fig. 14.6) exudation of large quantities of neutrophile granulocytes, lymphocytes, and plasmocytes in the bronchial lumen, thickening and fibrosis of bronchial wall, and large quantities of hyphae and spores in a dilated bronchus with exudation of neutrophile granulocytes in a large quantity. By special staining, methenamine silver staining showed positive, PAS staining positive, AB staining negative, and acid-fast staining negative. The histopathological diagnosis was pulmonary aspergillosis.

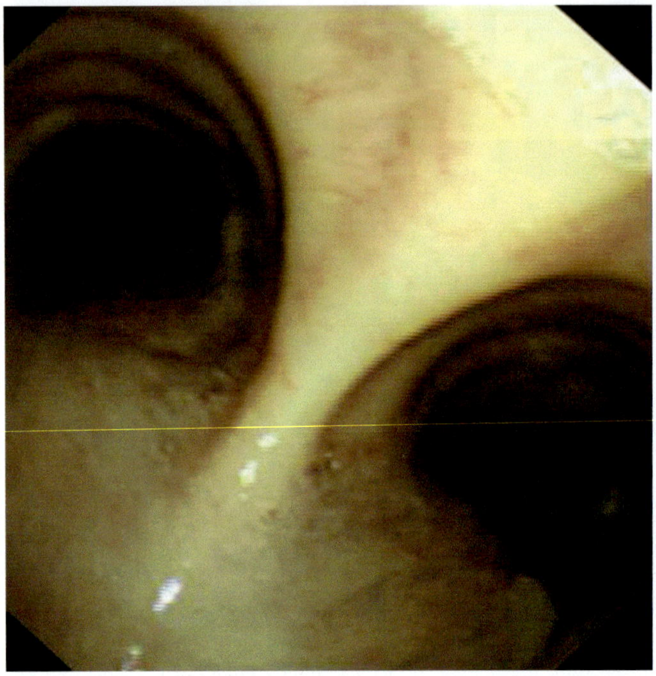

Fig. 14.5 Fibrobronchoscopy. Fibrobronchoscopy demonstrates sharp tracheal carina and whitish secretions in small quantities in bilateral major bronchi

The final diagnosis was COPD complicated by invasive pulmonary aspergillosis. After the diagnosis of IPA was established, voriconazole was administered for fungal infection. And the symptoms were gradually improved. After 48 days of treatment, reexamination of chest CT scan (Fig. 14.7) demonstrated obvious absorption of lesions at both lungs.

14.2.4 Discussion

According to the diagnostic criteria of invasive pulmonary aspergillosis jointly issued by EORTC and MSG in 2008, the case was diagnosed with invasive pulmonary aspergillosis (IPA) [6].

Recently, the incidence of IPA in patients with serious COPD and patients admitted to ICU due to other serious illnesses has been increasing. The changes of bronchopulmonary structures, repeated use of hormone, repeated hospitalization, and use of wide-spectrum antibiotic in patients with COPD have been believed to be the main reasons of COPD complicated by IPA [7, 8].

IPA can be classified into airway invasive type and vascular invasive type [9]. In the cases of airway invasive type, aspergillus invades the basilar membrane of the airway and bronchioles to cause tracheobronchitis, bronchopneumonia, and bronchiolitis [10]. CT scan demonstrates patchy blurry opacity, ground-glass opacity, and multiple lobular central nodules distributing along the bronchial vascular bundle. The pathological change of vascular invasive type is

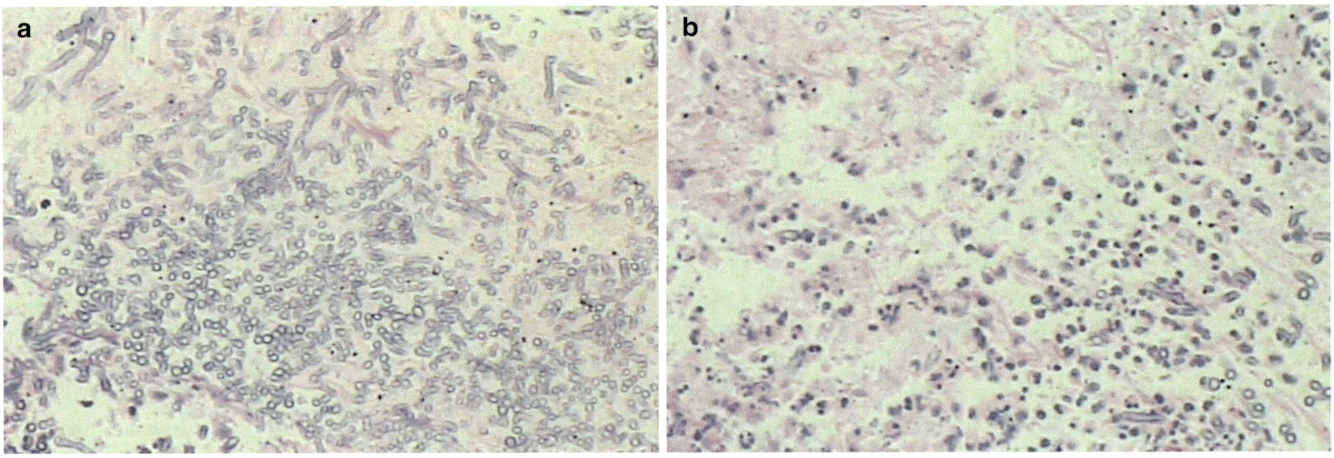

Fig. 14.6 (**a**, **b**) Pathology of lung tissue. (**a**, **b**) Large quantities of hyphae and spores are demonstrated in bronchial necrotic tissue. The hyphae branches in sharp angle, with septa. The bronchial mucosa is demonstrated with exudation of neutrophile granulocytes, lymphocytes, and plasmocytes in large quantities (H&E staining)

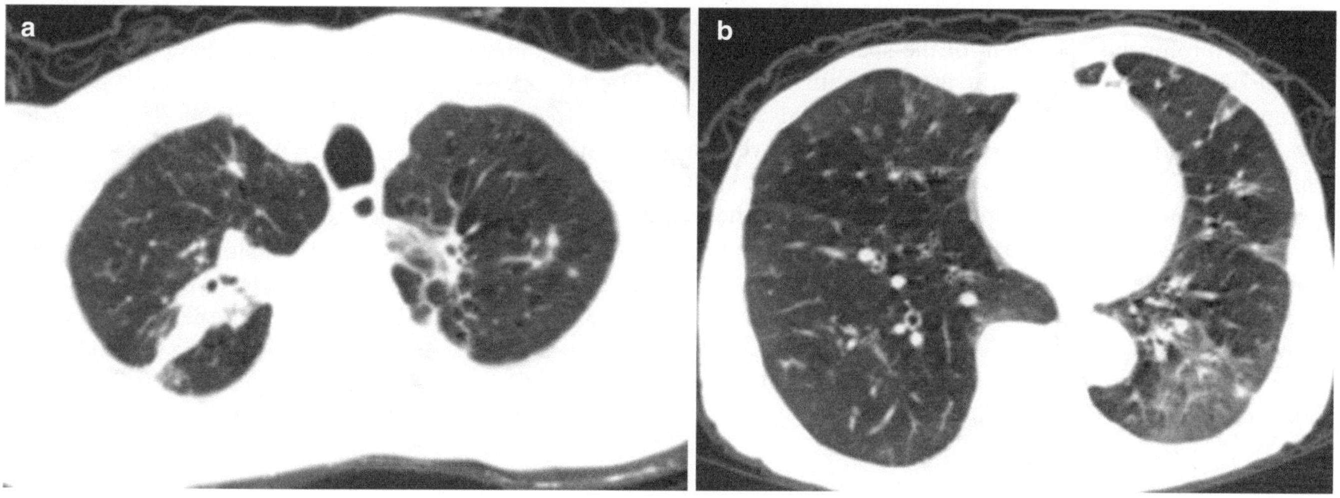

Fig. 14.7 (**a**, **b**) Chest CT scan. Reexamination of chest CT scan after antifungal treatment for 48 days demonstrates obvious absorption of lesions at both lungs

obstruction of local pulmonary vascular vessels by aspergillus hyphae to cause local pulmonary infarction, followed by infarction and necrosis of lung parenchyma to form cavity. CT scan demonstrates multiple subpleural consolidation opacities or nodule/mass opacities, with accompanying halo sign and cavity. The two types are not absolutely independent, and their overlapping is common, which is demonstrated as the mixed type. In this case, the patient mainly presented as the airway invasive type, with multiple small nodules and patchy blurry opacities at both lungs, which distributed along bronchial vascular bundle, as well as ground-glass opacity. It has been pointed out in literature report that patchy ground-glass opacity is CT scan demonstration of early IPA whose underlying pathomechanism is alveolar exudation induced by aspergillus bronchopneumonia or alveolar bleeding induced by damaged pulmonary minor vascular vessels by aspergillus hyphae. Along with the progression of the disease, the lesions of flaky consolidation with cavity and pleural effusion progressed into vascular invasive type, indicating the airway invasion and the vascular invasion are manifestations of different stages of IPA.

At the early stage of IPA, radiology demonstrates ground-glass opacity, nodule with halo sign, and consolidation opacity. At the middle and advanced stage of IPA, radiology demonstrates low-intensity sign, cavity, air crescent sign [11], and cavity separation sign [12]. The distribution of multiple nodular opacities in the cases of IPA is regular, with distribution around the bronchial vascular bundle. Subpleural consolidation is more common and is subject to necrosis (low-intensity sign) and formation of cavity. By CT scan, there may be patchy blurry opacity around the consolidation opacity, with halo sign around most nodules.

In this case, the patient suffered from COPD, initially with multiple patchy exudative blurry opacities at both lungs. Anti-infection therapy showed no therapeutic efficacy. By CT scan, the lesions were enlarged, with necrosis and small cavity. The complication of IPA should be considered. However, it should be differentiated from COPD complicated by pulmonary tuberculosis. The lesions of infiltrating tuberculosis are more commonly located at the posteroapical segment of the upper lung lobe and dorsal segment of the lower lung lobe. But patients with COPD may also present multiple infiltrations at both lungs with diverse CT scan demonstrations, including ground-glass opacity, centilobular nodule, tree-in-bud sign, pulmonary consolidation, necrosis, thick-wall cavity, and thickening of bronchial wall. In this case, pulmonary tuberculosis cannot be excluded based only on radiology. But the clinical manifestations did not support the diagnosis of tuberculosis.

14.2.5 Comments

The risk factors of IPA are classified into high-risk factors, moderate-risk factors, and low-risk factors. And COPD is one of the moderate-risk factors of IPA. In 2007, Bulpa et al. proposed the diagnostic criteria of COPD complicated by IPA, and they especially emphasized the host factors of patients with COPD who receive treatment by glucocorticoid and patients with serious and critical COPD. Therefore, when the condition of COPD exacerbates and shows no therapeutic efficacy to appropriate therapies, the complication of IPA should be suspected. At this time, the patient should be inquired for the medical history of receiving glucocorticoid.

G test can be applied to diagnose multiple fungal infections such as candida infection, aspergillus infection, and *Pneumocystis carinii* infection. In this case, G test performed after admission showed negative, which may be caused by prolonged placement of the specimen and formation of immune complex. In patients with clinically diagnosed candida infection, G test may show false negative for *Candida parapsilosis* infection, and the reason remains to be unclear. Some antifungal medication, such as caspofungin, can noncompetitively inhibit the synthesis of (1,3)-β-D-glucan, which may cause false negative in G test.

Based on the diagnosis and treatment of the patient, we know that patients with acute exacerbation of COPD may suffer from common bacterial infection, fungal infection, and other opportunistic infections.

14.3 Case 3: Recurrent Cough and Expectoration for More Than 1 Year

Fei Shi, Yuemei Lu, Dong-Na Su, Shi-Ping Wu, Xiongfei Sun, and Zhiqiang Cheng

14.3.1 Presenting Symptom

Recurrent cough and expectoration for more than 1 year.

14.3.2 Brief Case History

A 65-year-old woman, housewife, was admitted to our hospital on March 16, 2012, due to complaints of recurrent cough and expectoration for more than 1 year. More than 1 year ago, the patient began to experience recurrent irritable cough and expectoration of yellowish mucous sputum in a small quantity. The expectoration was more obvious in mornings when she got up. But she experienced no hemoptysis, chest pain, breathlessness, fever, and night sweat. In a local hospital, she received anti-infection therapy (specifically unknown). And the symptoms were improved but sometimes relapsed. One week before her admission to our hospital, cough and expectoration aggravated. Chest CT scan in our hospital demonstrated mass opacity at the left upper lung lobe and was admitted then to the thoracic surgery department of our hospital. Since the onset of symptoms, her spiritual state was average and her appetite was good. She experienced no obvious weight change.

14.3.2.1 Past Medical History

She denied medical histories of hypertension and diabetes. And she ever worked in a cotton factory for more than 20 years. And she had no hobbies in smoking and drinking.

14.3.2.2 Physical Examination

Physical examination showed a body temperature of 36.0 °C, pulse rate 72/min, respiration rate 20/min, and blood pressure 111/82 mmHg. She was typically developed and moderately nourished. And she was well conscious in an average spiritual state. The patient was in active position and well cooperated in the physical examination. The skin showed no yellowish stain. The superficial lymph nodes were not palpable and not enlarged. The sclera showed no yellowish stain and the oral lips showed no cyanosis. The neck was soft, with no distension of the jugular vein. The trachea was at the midline. Bilateral vocal fremitus was symmetric. By percussion, both lungs showed clear sounds. And the respiration sounds were clear, with no moist and/or dry rales. The heart was not enlarged, with a heartbeat of 72/min, rhythmic. The valvular areas showed no pathological murmur. The abdomen was soft, with no tenderness and rebound pain. The liver and spleen were not palpable under the ribs. The liver and kidney areas were not sensitive to percussion. The shifting dullness was negative. And both lower limbs showed no edema. No clubbing finger was detected.

14.3.2.3 Auxiliary Investigation

Routine blood test showed WBC 14.72×10^9/L, N% 92.9%, Hb 101 g/L, CRP 3.6 mg/L, and ESR 28 mm/h. 1,3-Beta-D-glucan was 234.0 pg/ml.

The cultures of sputum for bacteria, fungi, and tuberculosis mycobacteria were negative.

14.3.2.4 Initial Diagnosis

The initial diagnosis was space-occupying lesion at the left lung, which was suspected to be pulmonary aspergillosis, pulmonary tuberculosis, or lung carcinoma.

14.3.3 Diagnosis and Treatment

After admission, the investigations were performed. The liver and kidney function tests showed no abnormalities. The levels of CEA, CA125, CA19-9, Cyfra21-1, and NSE were within normal limits. The blood coagulation was normal.

After admission, cefoperazone/sulbactam was administered for infection and ambroxol for resolving phlegm. But the symptoms of cough and expectoration were not improved. Chest CT scan demonstrated cavity at the left upper lung lobe with soft tissue mass, which was suspected to be infection, such as cavity with aspergilloma (Fig. 14.8).

Because the anti-infection therapy was ineffective, thoracoscopic removal of the left lung, cautery for pleural adhesion, and closed thoracic drainage were performed on March 20, 2012. The postoperative pathology demonstrated formation of aspergilloma. Under a microscope, several fungal masses were observed, with dense arrangements of hyphae

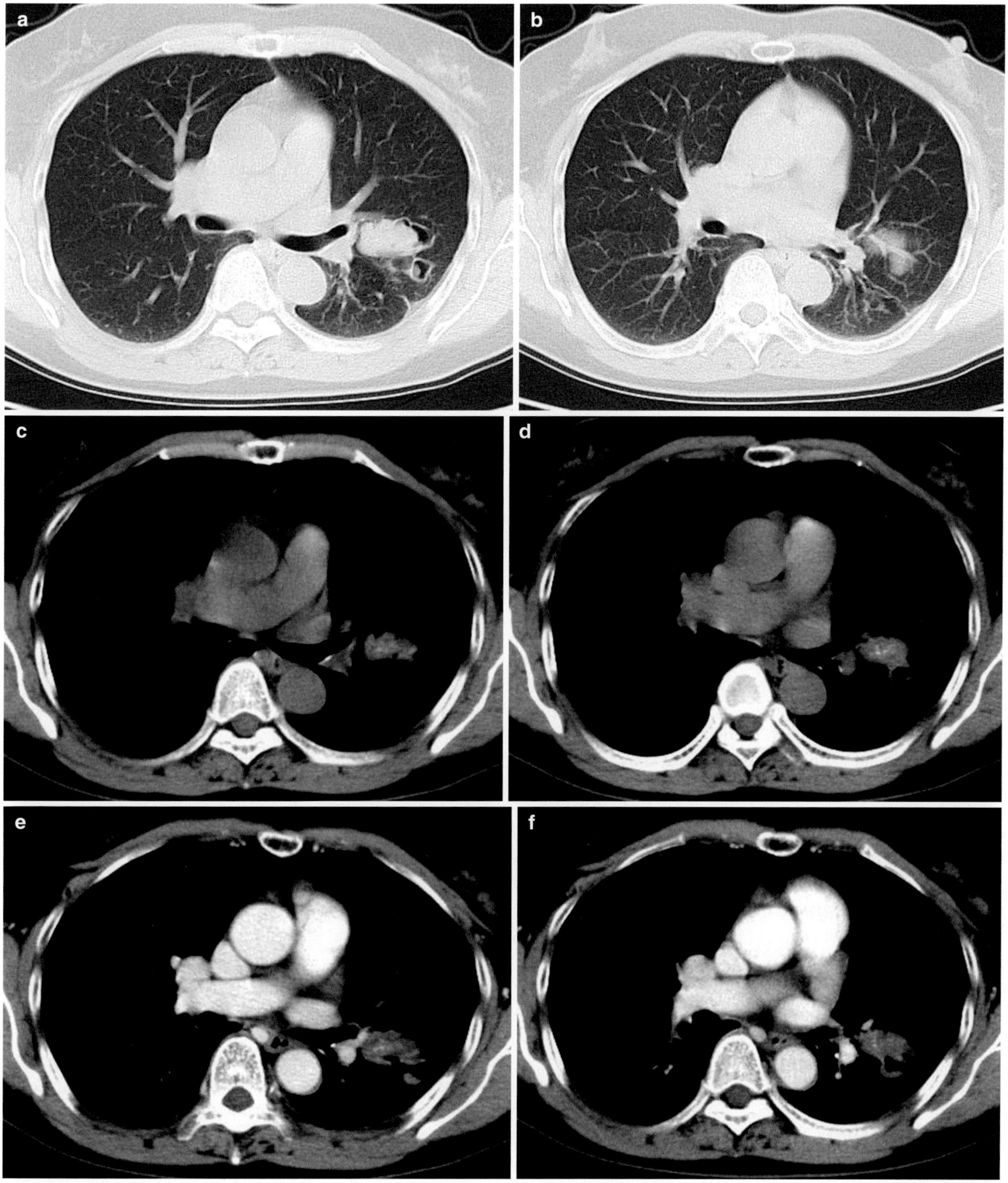

Fig. 14.8 (**a**–**f**) Chest CT scan. (**a**, **b**) The lung window demonstrates cavity at the left upper lung lobe with soft tissue mass, a small cavity opacity beside the large cavity opacity, and its adhesion with the lateral pleura. (**c**, **d**) The mediastinum window demonstrates central spot of calcification at the mass opacity of the left upper lung, which resembles to cavity with aspergilloma. (**e**, **f**) Enhanced CT scan demonstrates no obvious enhancement of the lesion at the left upper lung

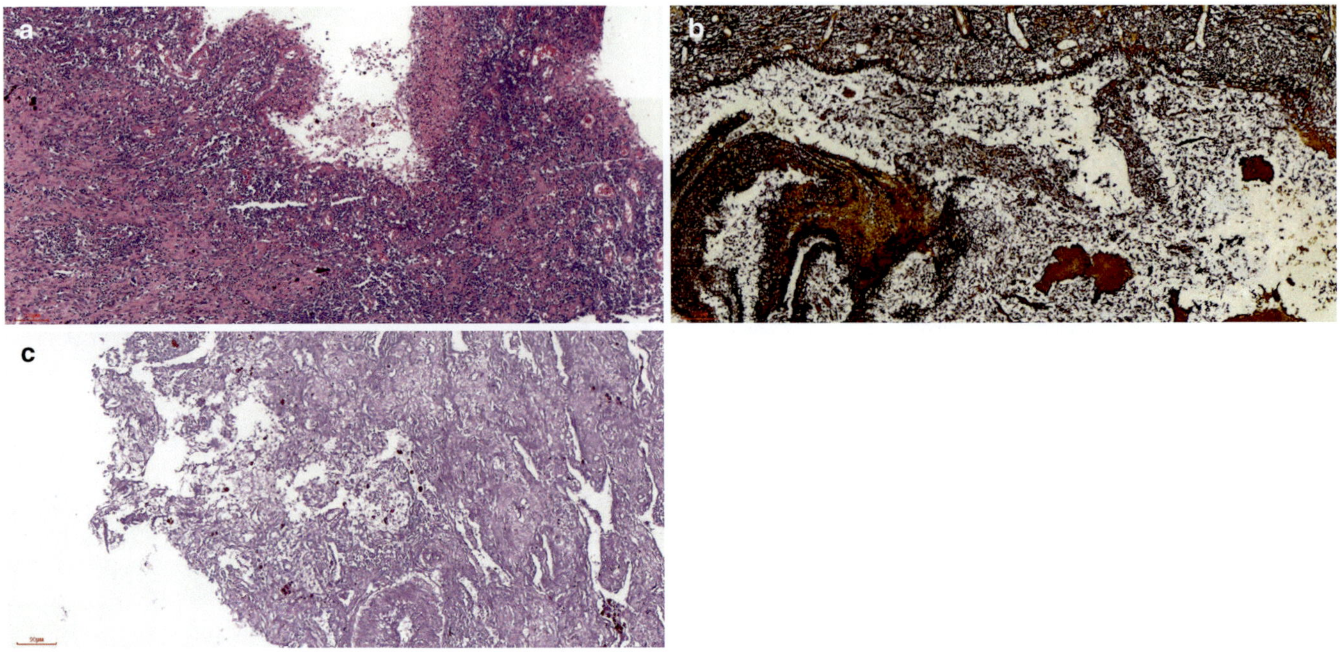

Fig. 14.9 (**a**–**c**) Pathology of lung tissue. (**a**) H&E staining demonstrates light purplish blue hyphae wall of aspergillus. (**b**) PASM staining demonstrates brownish black hyphae wall and spores of aspergillus. (**c**) PAS staining demonstrates reddish purple hyphae wall of aspergillus

and spores in large quantities. The hyphae twined into mass to invade the surrounding tissue and their interface were poorly defined. The surrounding tissue showed infiltration of many inflammatory cells. There was also organizing necrosis with pulmonary bleeding, vasculitis, and eosinophilic pneumonia. By special staining, PAS staining showed positive, and methenamine silver staining showed positive. The pathological diagnosis was fungal infection at the left lung, which was morphologically consistent to aspergillosis (Fig. 14.9).

The postoperative recovery was favorable. Meanwhile, intravenous infusion of voriconazole was administered. And the medication was changed to oral intake of voriconazole since March 23, 2012.

The final diagnosis was aspergilloma at the left lung.

After discharge, the condition of the patient was stable. Follow-ups showed no relapse of cough and expectoration.

14.3.4 Discussion

Invasive pulmonary aspergillosis (IPA) commonly occurs in immunocompromised populations. However, in recent years, reports of IPA have been increasing in patients with non-granulocytic deficiency [13]. Such patients are subject to long-term exposure to the environment with a large quantity of aspergillus spores, such as feeding pigeons, drying grains, processing animal fur, living in poorly ventilated houses, and dismantling old houses. Once the inhaled aspergillus spores exceed body defense load, IPA occurs. Generally, the clinical manifestations are non-specific respiratory symptoms, such as cough, expectoration, chest pain, hemoptysis, breathlessness, and wheezing. In some cases, systemic poisoning symptoms occur, such as fever, systemic fatigue, night sweat, and poor appetite. The clinical manifestations are associated with the position of invasion by aspergillus, the endotoxin produced by aspergillus, and the effects of hemolytic proteinase.

In this case, the patient was an immunocompetent elderly with no past medical histories and no special contact history. Her initial symptoms were chronic cough and expectoration of yellowish mucous sputum. In a local hospital, her condition was diagnosed as bacterial pneumonia, and intravenous infusion of antibiotic was administered. But the therapeutic efficacy was unfavorable. Then, her cough and expectoration aggravated, and she was admitted due to chest CT scan demonstration of mass opacity at the left upper lung. Although laboratory test showed increased WBC and neutrophile percentage as well as increased level of 1,3-beta-D-glucan, the mass opacity at the left upper lung was not defined due to low diagnostic specificity of G test to IPA [14]. The following enhanced chest CT scan demonstrated cavity in the mass opacity, and fungal mass was possible. Finally, pathology of surgical specimen confirmed the diagnosis of aspergillus infection at the left upper lung.

Based on the diagnosis and treatment of this case, we summarize the following key points:

1. In immunocompetent population, if cough, expectoration, and other respiratory symptoms recur, standard anti-infection therapy shows unfavorable therapeutic efficacy, and radiology demonstrates cavity in mass opacity, pulmonary aspergillus infection should be suspected. Further CT-guided lung puncture for pathology or thoracoscopic pathology should be performed to define the diagnosis [15].
2. CT scan may show halo sign in early stage of pulmonary aspergillus infection [16] and crescent sign in advanced stage of pulmonary aspergillus infection. However, these radiological signs are temporary. In 75% of patients with pulmonary aspergillus infection, the halo sign may disappear within 1 week. And not all patients with pulmonary aspergillus infection show characteristic CT sign. Therefore, differentiation of pulmonary aspergillus infection based only on CT scan is limited.
3. IPA commonly occurs in immunodeficient individuals, and semi-invasive pulmonary aspergillosis commonly occurs in patients with slight immunosuppression. However, aspergilloma commonly occurs in immunocompetent individuals. Therefore, for immunocompetent patients with nodular opacity at lung, especially cavity in nodule, lung neoplasm and pulmonary aspergillosis should be suspected. And the diagnosis can be defined based on percutaneous puncture for biopsy or surgical removal for pathology.

14.3.5 Comments

This is a case of pulmonary aspergillosis in an immunocompetent individual. Aspergillus widely exists in the natural world, such as soil, stable, cattle pen, and barn. Aspergillus may also parasitize in healthy human skin and upper respiratory tract. It is a conditional pathogenic fungus. Inhalation of aspergillus by an immunocompetent healthy human is not pathogenic. But when the immunity is compromised or pulmonary disease occurs, inhalation of aspergillus causes aspergillosis. The main risk factors of aspergillus infection include neutropenia, long-term use of hormone and wide-spectrum antibiotic, organ transplantation (such as bone marrow transplantation), and chronic diseases (such as diabetes, hepatocirrhosis, and acquired immunodeficiency syndrome). Pulmonary aspergillosis is commonly secondary to bronchiectasis, cavitary pulmonary tuberculosis, lung carcinoma, and other chronic pulmonary diseases. In this case, the experience of diagnosis and treatment expands past knowledge about pulmonary aspergillosis. That is, the possibility of pulmonary aspergillosis does exist in patients with competent immunity and no basic disease.

In this case, the condition was not complex and the treatment was successful. The postoperative recovery was favorable. But perioperative administration of voriconazole needs further exploration. A research study has found that postoperative administration of antifungal medication does not improve the prognosis of pulmonary aspergillosis. In the clinical guideline for chronic pulmonary aspergillosis jointly issued by ESCMID and ERS in 2015, it has been pointed out that postoperative antifungal medication is not necessary after complete removal of simplex aspergilloma and no evidence supporting leakage of fungal substances. Therefore, the effects of postoperative antifungal medication still need exploration.

14.4 Case 4: Cough for More Than 2 Months

Wei Ma, Qing Yu, Peifen Chen, Shi-Ping Wu, Zhiqiang Cheng, and Guofang Deng

14.4.1 Presenting Symptom

Cough for more than 2 months.

14.4.2 Brief Case History

A 43-year-old woman was admitted to our hospital on March 20, 2013, due to complaint of cough for more than 2 months. More than 2 months ago, the patient was admitted to the hospital for surgical removal of kidney stones. At day 3 after admission, she caught a cold and showed fever, with the highest body temperature of 38.6 °C. She also experienced dry paroxysmal cough but no expectoration and hemoptysis. The fever was improved after symptomatic treatment (specifically unknown) for 2 days, but the cough persisted, even after she was discharged. She then presented in another hospital on March 5, 2013, and the chest CT scan demonstrated cystic dilation of basilar segment at the right lower lung lobe, with accompanying nodular opacity, which was considered to be aspergilloma. For further diagnosis and treatment, the patient presented in our hospital and was admitted to the respiratory department. Since the onset of symptoms, her spiritual state was good. Diet and sleep were normal. And the urinations and bowel movements were normal.

14.4.2.1 Past Medical History

She reported a medical history of kidney stones for more than 10 years.

14.4.2.2 Physical Examination

Physical examination showed a body temperature of 36.3 °C, pulse rate 93/min, respiration rate 19/min, and blood pressure 120/76 mmHg. She was typically developed and moderately nourished. And she was well conscious, in an average spiritual state. The patient was in active position and well cooperated with the physical examination. The skin showed no yellowish stain, with no skin rash and subcutaneous bleeding. The systemic superficial lymph nodes were not palpable and not enlarged. The sclera showed no yellowish stain, and the oral lips were ruddy. The oral mucosa showed no abnormality. The pharynx was not congested. The bilateral tonsils were not enlarged. The neck was soft, with no distention of the jugular vein. The trachea was at the midline. And the thorax was bilaterally symmetric with no deformity. The bilateral vocal fremitus was symmetric. By percussion, both lungs showed clear sounds. By auscultation, the respiration sounds of both lungs were clear, with no dry and/or moist rales. The precordial area showed no protrusion, and no tremble was palpated. The heart was not enlarged, with a heartbeat of 93/min, rhythmic. The heart sound was normal, and the valvular areas showed no pathological murmur. The abdomen was soft, with no tenderness and rebound pain. The liver and spleen were not palpable under the ribs. The liver and kidney areas were not sensitive to percussion. The shifting dullness was negative. And the bowel sounds were four times per minute. Both lower limbs showed no edema. And no clubbing finger was detected. The nervous system showed no abnormality.

14.4.2.3 Auxiliary Investigation

Laboratory Test

Routine blood test showed WBC 11.8×10^9/L, N 8.8×10^9/L, N 74.7%, L 17.7%, Hb 96 g/L, and PLT459 $\times 10^9$/L. The ESR was 58 mm/h and CRP 18.6 mg/L. The IgE was 363 kIU/L. The D-glucan test was 655 μg/L. And the three-item antigen test for fungus showed no abnormality.

Radiology

Lung CT scan on March 5, 2013, demonstrated cystic dilation of basilar segment at the right lower lung lobe, with accompanying nodular opacity, which was considered to be aspergilloma.

14.4.2.4 Initial Diagnosis

The initial diagnosis was aspergilloma at the right lower lung lobe.

14.4.3 Diagnosis and Treatment

After admission, the investigations were performed. The sputum culture for common bacteria showed no growth of pathogenic bacteria within 48 h. The sputum smear showed gram-positive cocci but no fungal hyphae and spores. The sputum culture for fungi showed no growth of fungi within 5 days. To define the diagnosis, CT-guided puncture of the lesion was performed on March 20, 2013 (Fig. 14.10). The pathology demonstrated mostly fungal flora, and the hyphae

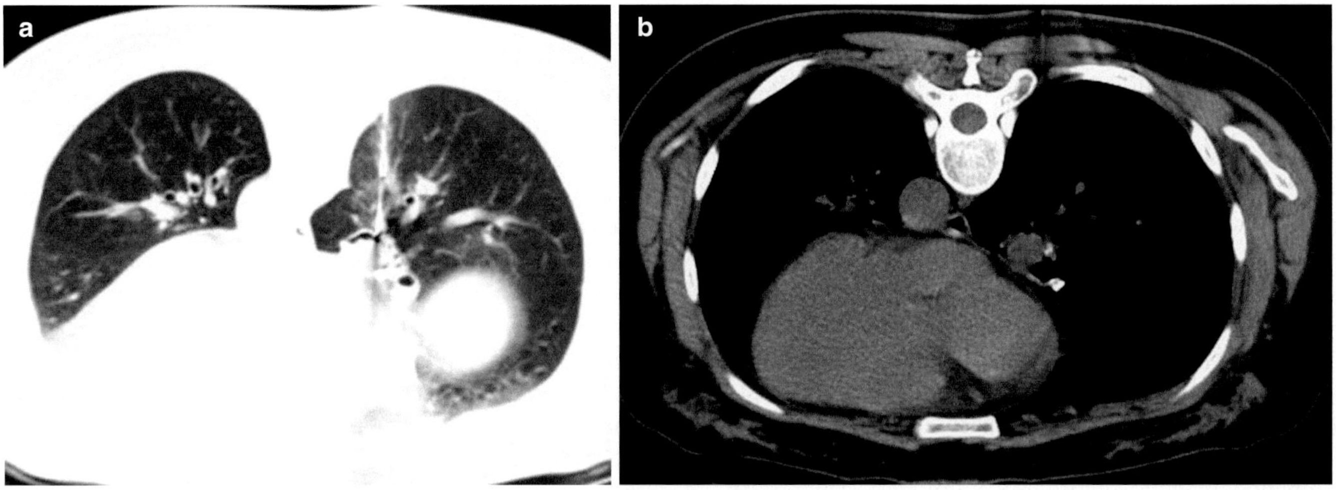

Fig. 14.10 (**a**, **b**) CT-guided percutaneous lung puncture. (**a**) The lung window at prone position demonstrates nodule at the basilar segment of the right lower lung lobe and air crescent sign superior to it. (**b**) The mediastinum window at prone position at the level of cardiac ventricle demonstrates nodule with homogeneous intensity in size of about 2 cm × 1.2 cm

have branch in sharp angle, with septa. There were also less alveolar epithelium, inflammatory exudates, and hyperplasia of alveolar epithelium. By special staining, the methenamine silver staining was positive and PAS staining positive (Fig. 14.11). The pathological diagnosis was aspergillosis at the right lower lung. Amphotericin B and voriconazole were then administered for fungal infection, and cough was obviously improved. The patient then was discharged. Reexamination of chest CT scan 2 months later demonstrated no change of the lesion (Fig. 14.12). After consultation to specialist from the thoracic surgery department, the patient was transferred to the cardiothoracic surgery department on May 18, 2013, due to unfavorable therapeutic efficacy of the antifungal therapy. Thoracoscopic removal of the right lower lung lobe was performed on May 31, 2013. During the operation, a nodule in cyst was detected at the basilar segment of the right lower lung lobe, which was dark brown in color and was soft with a diameter of about 15 mm. The postoperative pathology demonstrated large quantities of hyphae, spores, and necrotic substances in dilated bronchus. The hyphae had branch in sharp angle, with septa. The mucosal interstitium showed edema, with infiltration of many lymphocytes and eosinophile granulocytes. No neoplasm was detected. By special staining, methenamine silver staining was positive, and PAS was positive (Fig. 14.13). The pathological diagnosis was aspergillosis at the right lower lung and bronchiectasis.

The postoperative recovery was favorable, and the patient was discharged on June 23, 2013. The final diagnosis was bronchiectasis at the basilar segment of the right lower lung lobe with accompanying aspergilloma. After discharge, the condition of the patient was stable.

14.4.4 Discussion

Pulmonary aspergilloma is a saprophytic type of pulmonary aspergillosis. When aspergillus enters the primary cavity in the lung, the mycelium of aspergillus is mixed with fiber, mucus and cell fragments into a mass, which is aspergilloma. It occurs in cavity induced by pulmonary tuberculosis, lung carcinoma, pulmonary abscess, bronchiectasis, lung bullae, pulmonary cyst, and other chronic pulmonary diseases and is most common in cavity induced by pulmonary tuberculosis. The clinical symptoms of pulmonary aspergilloma are commonly atypical, and the patients commonly show symptoms of primary pulmonary disease, such as chronic cough, expectoration, hemoptysis or sputum with blood streak, and other non-specific symptoms. In some cases, the patients may even be asymptomatic. According to literature report [17, 18], the most common symptoms include recurrent intermittent hemoptysis or sputum with blood streak, which are also presenting symptoms. In this case, the patient only experienced dry cough with no sputum and blood.

Due to low positive rate of aspergillosis in sputum investigations and existence of aspergillus in the respiratory tract of healthy human, finding of aspergillus in sputum cannot define the diagnosis of aspergillus infection. Fibrobronchoscopy may detect congestion, edema, and polyp-like hyperplasia of tracheal mucosa, and findings of

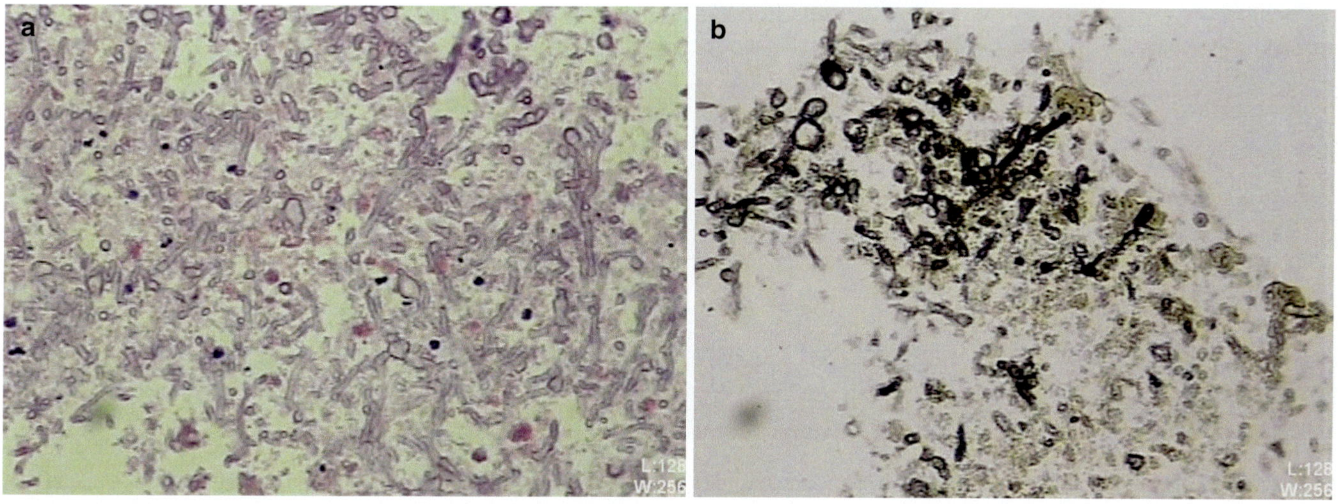

Fig. 14.11 (**a**, **b**) Microscopy of the tissue harvested via percutaneous lung puncture. (**a**) H&E staining demonstrates large quantities of rod-shaped hyphae and spores, with surrounding infiltration of many inflammatory cells. (**b**) PASM staining demonstrates brownish black hyphae wall and spores

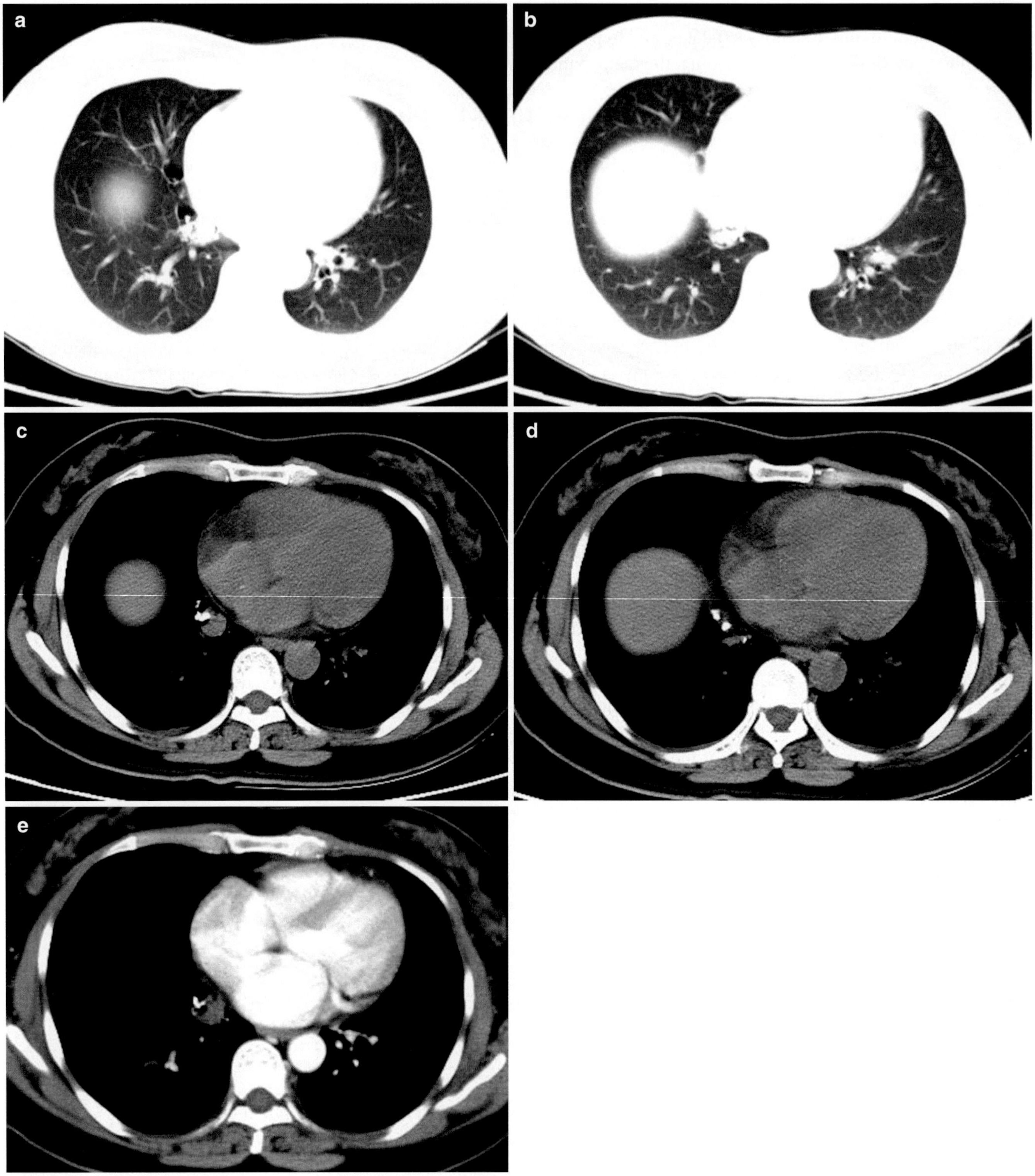

Fig. 14.12 (**a**–**e**) Lung CT scan. (**a**, **b**) The lung window demonstrates a nodular opacity adjacent to the mediastinum at the medial basilar segment of the right lower lung lobe, with surrounding bead-shaped translucent area (beads sign). (**c**, **d**) The mediastinum window demonstrates nodule with homogeneous intensity in size of about 2 cm × 1.2 cm and calcification lesion at the right hilum. (**e**) The mediastinum window of contrast-enhanced CT scan demonstrates no enhancement of the nodule, which is almost the same as the previous CT scan

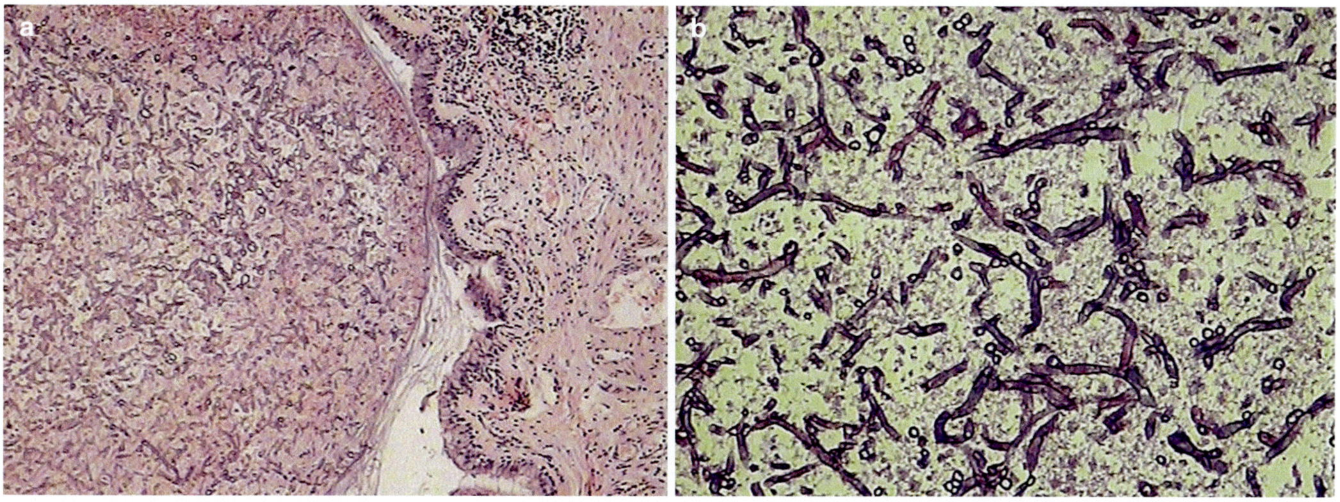

Fig. 14.13 (**a**, **b**) Pathology of lung tissue harvested via thoracoscopic removal of the right lower lung lobe. (**a**) H&E staining demonstrates large quantities of hyphae and spores, with the hyphae twining into mass that is surrounded by infiltration of many inflammatory cells. (**b**) PAS staining demonstrates reddish purple hyphae wall

aspergillus hyphae by biopsy or BALF culture can define the diagnosis of aspergillosis. Fibrobronchoscopy plays a certain role in diagnosing pulmonary aspergillus infection. However, in this case, fibrobronchoscopy in a local hospital only demonstrated chronic inflammation of mucosa. According to literature report, serum and BALF GM test by ELISA have high sensitivity and specificity to IPA, but it has been rarely applied for the diagnosis of localized pulmonary aspergilloma.

Radiological demonstrations of pulmonary aspergilloma are characteristic, which play an important role in indicating diagnosis. Typical CT scan demonstrations of pulmonary aspergilloma include spherical content in lung cavity or cavitary lesion, with crescent-shaped or ring-shaped translucent opacity between the spherical content and the cavity wall, namely, the crescent sign and air-ring sign. In some cases, there is cords opacity between the spherical content and the cavity wall, forming bead-like translucent area, namely, beads sign. And in some other cases, there is opacity of gas intensity in the spherical content, namely, gas-containing sphere sign, which may be a residual space between aspergillus hyphae, fiber, and cell debris. The spherical content is movable due to gravity. If the above sign is demonstrated by CT scan, initial diagnosis of aspergilloma can be made. If CT scan at prone position demonstrates movable spherical content along with body posture, a diagnosis of aspergilloma can be defined. Pulmonary aspergilloma generally has homogeneous intensity, and calcification may occur. In addition, according to literature report [19], aspergilloma is avascular and contrast-enhanced scan demonstrates no enhancement. In this case, contrast-enhanced scan demonstrated no enhancement, which is consistent to literature report. In this case, the clinical manifestations are typically aspergilloma. CT-guided puncture for biopsy demonstrated aspergillus hyphae, which further confirmed the diagnosis.

Pulmonary aspergilloma should be differentiated from the following conditions:

1. Tuberculoma. The cavity containing tuberculoma is commonly located near the hilum, and tuberculoma does not move along with body posture.
2. The mural nodule in cavity induced by lung carcinoma. The structure of mural nodule is the same as the cavity wall of lung carcinoma. By contrast-enhanced CT scan, the CT value of mural nodule shows the same enhancement as the cavity wall of lung carcinoma. The inner wall of cavity induced by lung carcinoma is commonly irregular.

According to literature report [20], once aspergilloma forms, antifungal medication can hardly reach the effective drug concentration in the cavity. Therefore, the palliative medication shows unfavorable therapeutic efficacy. In addition, the therapeutic course of antifungal medication is prolonged, with high cost and serious adverse effects. Therefore, most scholars recommend [21], if not contraindicated, surgical operation. Surgical operation is especially indicated to patients with focalized lesion and recurrent hemoptysis. Thoracoscopic surgery is noninvasive, which is a safe and applicable surgical approach for patients with no serious adhesion and simplex aspergilloma. In this case, the patient received thoracoscopy. The postoperative recovery was favorable, and the patient experienced no postoperative complications.

14.4.5 Comments

Pulmonary aspergilloma is a common type of pulmonary aspergillosis, which is also a parasitic (saprophytic) aspergillosis. Patients with aspergilloma commonly suffer from basic pulmonary disease, such as cavitary pulmonary tuberculosis, cavity of lung carcinoma, bronchial cyst, lung bullae, and bronchiectasis. Recently, along with increasing incidence of pulmonary tuberculosis and wide use of immunosuppressants, the incidence of pulmonary aspergilloma has been increasing. In this case, pulmonary aspergilloma occurred based on bronchiectasis.

Radiology plays an important role in the diagnosis of aspergilloma. The typical CT scan demonstration of aspergilloma is air crescent sign. In this case, the patient received chest CT scan in a local hospital on March 5, 2013, and the diagnosis was considered to be aspergilloma. That is to say, the diagnosis of aspergilloma with typical radiological sign is not challenging for experienced radiologist. For patients with atypical radiological demonstrations, bronchoscopy, percutaneous lung puncture, culture of respiratory secretions, and detection of serum precipitated antibody can be performed for diagnosis. In this case, the patient received CT-guided puncture of the lesion on March 20, 2013. And the pathological diagnosis was finally obtained.

In this case, after the diagnosis was defined, amphotericin B and voriconazole were administered for fungal infection for more than 2 months. But the medications were ineffective. Herein, we summarized the following two points:

1. The therapeutic efficacy and safety of combined use of antifungal medications have not been sufficiently supported by data from clinical trials. In the clinical guideline for aspergillosis issued by IDSA, it has been pointed out that combined use of medications is not recommended for initial medication. It is believed that when single medication is ineffective, there is commonly no other choice but addition of second medication of different antifungal mechanisms.
2. Currently, there has been no sufficient evidence supporting effectiveness of antifungal medication for aspergilloma, which may be related to the difficulty of achieving effective drug concentration in the cavity. Therefore, for asymptomatic patients with aspergilloma, treatment is not necessary, and the patient should be regularly observed. For the symptomatic patients with aspergilloma, especially serious hemoptysis, treatment is necessary. Most scholars believe that surgical operation is the best treatment for hemoptysis. In this case, the patient received surgical operation, and the postoperative recovery was favorable. It indicated that if not contraindicated, surgical operation should be performed. We believe that the clinical treatment for pulmonary aspergilloma should be further standardized to avoid drug toxicity and high cost of antifungal medication.

14.5 Case 5: Cough for More Than 3 Months

Jiezhu Ding, Li Tu, Yazhou Cai, Jiezhu Ding, Li Tu, and Yazhou Cai

14.5.1 Presenting Symptom

Cough for more than 3 months.

14.5.2 Brief Case History

A 41-year-old man from Guangdong province of China, an administrator, was admitted to our hospital on September 3, 2013, due to complaint of cough for more than 3 months. More than 3 months ago, the patient began to experience paroxysmal cough with no known causes. He experienced no expectoration, hemoptysis, chest distress, breathlessness, fever, and night sweat. He presented in the outpatient department of our hospital due to recent severe cough. The lung function test showed slightly impaired ventilation and histamine bronchial provocation test positive. Chest CT scan demonstrated infection at the left upper lung lobe with cystic lesion and fibrous lesion at the right upper lung with adjacent pleural thickening and adhesion. For further diagnosis and treatment, the patient was hospitalized. Since the onset of symptoms, his spiritual state, appetite, and sleep were quite good. The urinations and bowel movements were normal. He experienced no recent obvious weight change.

14.5.2.1 Past Medical History

No past medical history was reported.

14.5.2.2 Physical Examination

By physical examination, the body temperature was 37.3 °C, pulse rate 100/min, respiration rate 20/min, and blood pressure 138/86 mmHg. He was well conscious. The superficial lymph nodes were not palpable and not enlarged. The respiration sounds of both lungs were coarse, with scattering dry rales at the left middle and lower lung and no moist rales. The heartbeat was rhythmic, with no obvious pathological murmur. The abdomen was soft, with no tenderness and rebound pain. The liver and spleen were not palpable under the ribs. And the liver and kidney areas were not sensitive to percussion. Both lower limbs showed no edema. There was no clubbing finger. The nervous system showed no abnormalities.

14.5.2.3 Auxiliary Investigation

Laboratory Test

Routine blood test showed WBC 6.21 × 10^9/L, neutrophile granulocytes 49%, hemoglobin 114 g/L, and platelets 344 × 10^9/L.

The sputum smear showed no fungi and acid-fast bacilli.

The lung function test showed slightly impaired ventilation and histamine bronchial provocation test positive.

Radiology

Chest X-ray was performed on August 28, 2013 (Fig. 14.14).

Chest CT scan was performed on August 29, 2013 (Fig. 14.15).

14.5.2.4 Initial Diagnosis

The initial diagnosis was suspected to be bronchial asthma or lung infection.

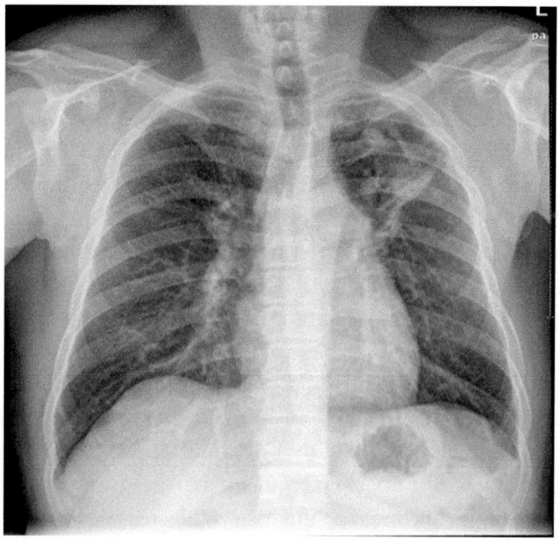

Fig. 14.14 Chest X-ray. The left middle and upper lung fields are demonstrated with patchy and strips of opacity with increased intensity, which are poorly marginated

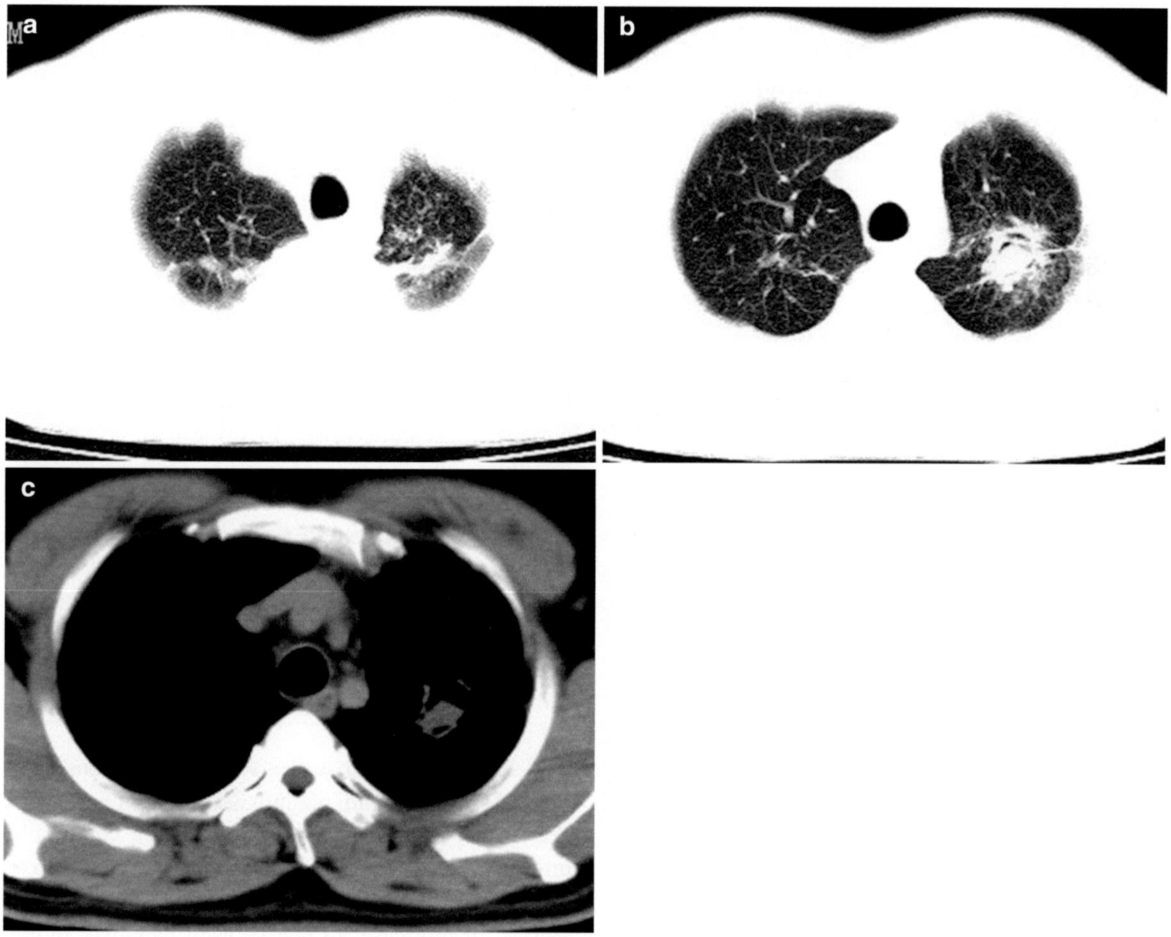

Fig. 14.15 (**a**–**c**) Chest CT scan. (**a**) The lung window demonstrates multiple well-marginated patchy and cords opacity with high-intensity and spots calcification opacity inside. There are also adjacent pleural thickening and adhesion. (**b**) The lung window demonstrates thick-wall cavity at the posteroapical segment of the left upper lung lobe, with coarse and poorly defined outer margin and smooth inner wall. There are also surrounding cords opacity with high-intensity, multiple patchy opacity with increased intensity, and pleural traction. (**c**) The mediastinum window demonstrates thick-wall cavity at the posteroapical segment of the left upper lung lobe, with coarse and poorly defined outer margin and smooth inner wall. There are also surrounding cords opacity with high-intensity, multiple patchy opacity with increased intensity, and pleural traction

14.5.3 Diagnosis and Treatment

After admission, the investigations were performed. The ESR was 2 mm/h, and C-reactive protein was 3.7 mg/L. The carcinoembryonic antigen, AFP, squamous cell carcinoma antigen, carbohydrate antigen, and prostate specific antigen were all within normal limits. The antibody against tuberculosis was negative. And the fungal D-glucan was lower than 10 pg/ml.

After admission, moxifloxacin was administered for infection, but the symptoms were not improved. For further diagnosis and treatment, fibrobronchoscopy was performed on September 5, 2013 (Fig. 14.16). It demonstrated normal trachea and carina, smooth bronchial mucosa and unobstructed lumen with no neoplasm in the right lung, and smooth major bronchial mucosa with less whitish thick secretions in the left lung. There were also whitish necrotic substances at the anterior segment of the left upper lung lobe, which obstructed the lumen and were irrigated and brushing for biopsy. The endoscopic diagnosis was whitish necrotic substances at the anterior segment of the left upper lung lobe, which was suspected to be fungal infection.

BALF culture for fungi demonstrated filiform fungi. Brushing and BALF smear for acid-fast bacilli showed negative. Fibrobronchoscopic brushing for pathology is shown in Fig. 14.17. There were many ciliated columnar epithelial cells and neutrophile granulocytes in BALF smear, with degenerated hyphae-like substances in a small quantity. Fibrobronchoscopic pathology is shown in Fig. 14.18. It showed even thickness of fungal hyphae, with septa and branching in sharp angle. Methenamine silver staining showed positive. The diagnosis was likely to be aspergillus infection.

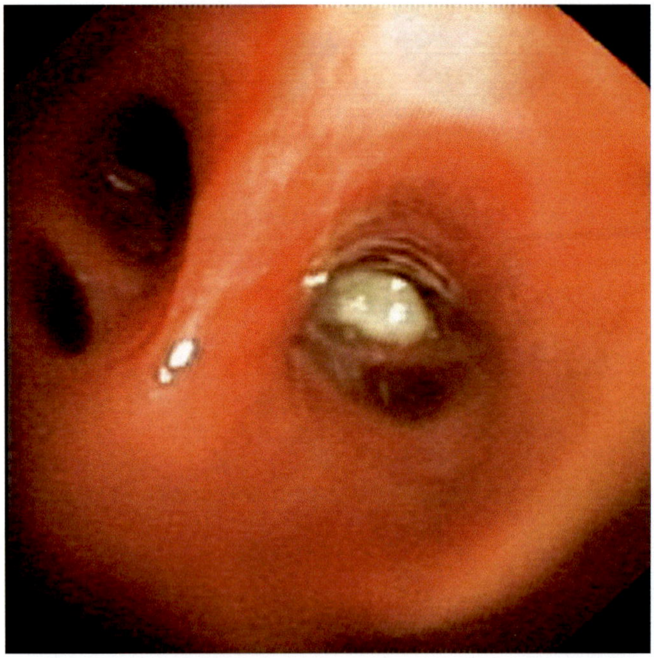

Fig. 14.16 Fibrobronchoscopy. Fibrobronchoscopy demonstrates whitish necrotic substances at the anterior segment of the left upper lung lobe, which obstruct the lumen

After pathological diagnosis was made, voriconazole was added for fungal infection for 2 weeks, and the symptoms were obviously improved. The patient was discharged, and oral intake of voriconazole was prescribed as sequential therapy.

The final diagnosis was pulmonary aspergilloma at the left upper lung. After discharge, the condition of the patient was stable, and the symptom of cough was obviously alleviated.

14.5.4 Discussion

Aspergilloma commonly occurs in the previously existing lung cavity that may be induced by pulmonary tuberculosis, bronchiectasis, pulmonary cyst, and lung carcinoma. It occasionally occurs in pleural cavity, especially in septum induced by surgical scar or pleural adhesion. In this case, the patient had no past medical history of pulmonary disease that may induce cavity, indicating pulmonary aspergilloma may also occur in patients with no lung cavity.

Patients with aspergilloma commonly have no systemic symptoms, and the most common symptom is hemoptysis whose incidence rate is 50–90%. The other common symptoms include chronic cough and rarely body weight loss. In cases with complication of bacterial infection, the patients may show fever. In some patients, the disease is insidious, and the patient remains asymptomatic for many years. The patients with presenting symptom of cough should be differentiated from those with asthma, cough-variant asthma, and chronic bronchitis. In this case, the patient showed positive in histamine bronchial provocation test, and the condition was suspected to be asthma or cough-variant asthma. Pulmonary aspergilloma with presenting symptom of cough is commonly neglected in clinical practice.

1–3-Beta-D-glucan test (G test) is a recently developed technology for rapid diagnosis of fungal infection. It has been mainly applied for the diagnosis of *Candida* blood flow infection. And it also has diagnostic value for aspergillus infection [22], with a sensitivity of 63.0% and a specificity of 74.0%. In this case, G test showed negative, indicating its limited value in the diagnosis of aspergillosis.

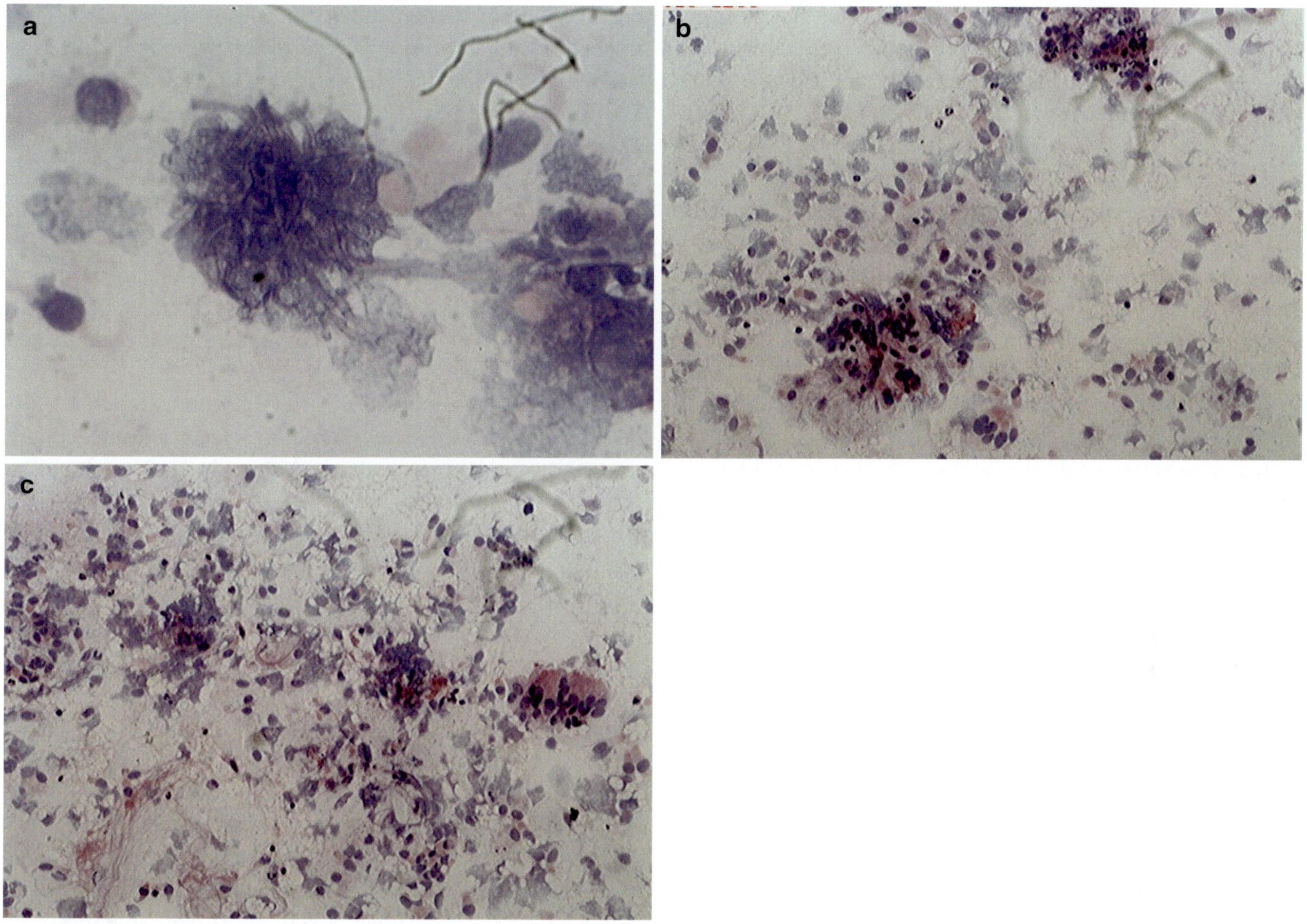

Fig. 14.17 (**a–c**) Fibrobronchoscopic brushing and smear for biopsy. Fibrobronchoscopic brushing and smear demonstrate many ciliated columnar epithelial cells and neutrophile granulocytes. In some focal lesion, there are degenerated hyphae-like substances in a small quantity (H&E staining)

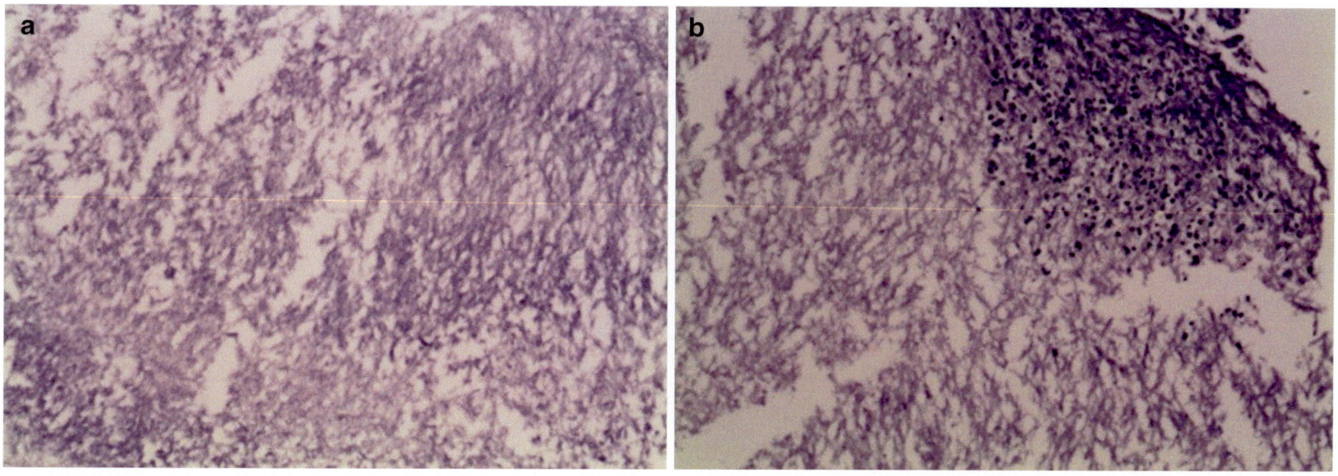

Fig. 14.18 (**a**, **b**) Fibrobronchoscopic biopsy of the necrotic substances. Microscopy demonstrates even thickness of the fungal hyphae, with septa and branching in sharp angle (PASM staining)

Aspergillus galactomannan antigen test (GM test) plays a significant role in the early diagnosis of aspergillosis. According to research study, serum GM test shows a sensitivity of 70–90% and a specificity of 70–90% [23]. The reasons of false positive in GM test include administration of piperacillin sodium/tazobactam sodium, dietary cereal that contains GM antigen, and regular access to blood circulation of aspergillus. BALF GM test shows higher diagnostic sensitivity than serum GM test, BALF culture, and pathological section for biopsy [24]. If the condition permits, GM test should be performed to improve the diagnostic positive rate of pulmonary aspergillosis.

Chest CT scan, especially high-resolution CT scan, facilitates the diagnosis of pulmonary aspergillosis. Chest CT scan demonstrates a halo sign at the early stage of pulmonary aspergillus infection. Along with the progression of the disease, the consolidation opacity is subject to necrosis to form crescent-shaped translucent area (crescent sign) within 10–15 days. The disadvantage of CT scan is that the halo sign and other characteristic signs are temporarily demonstrated and the halo sign may disappear within 1 week in 75% of the cases [25]. Pulmonary aspergilloma is demonstrated as movable mass in cavity, with arch-shaped superior margin to form air crescent sign with its surrounding tissue. The location of aspergilloma is changeable along with body posture. Not all patients with aspergillus infection are demonstrated with characteristic CT scan signs. The halo sign and crescent sign may also be induced by infection of other microorganisms or non-infections [26]. In this case, radiology demonstrated typical crescent sign. But differential diagnosis from cavitary pulmonary tuberculosis and other diseases was still necessary.

If patients with pulmonary aspergilloma show frequent hemoptysis or cough up blood in a large volume, surgical removal of the lesion is recommended. If surgery is contraindicated due to basic disease or lung dysfunction, bronchial artery embolization can be performed for hemostasis. The therapeutic efficacy of systemic use of anti-aspergillus medication is not certain. In this case, the presenting symptom was cough. After administration of voriconazole, the symptom was obviously improved, indicating favorable therapeutic efficacy.

14.5.5 Comments

Pulmonary aspergilloma is a clinical type of pulmonary aspergillosis. It is a chronic pulmonary aspergillosis with no clinical manifestation or only some non-specific respiratory symptoms, such as chronic cough and hemoptysis. And it commonly occurs in patients with COPD, non-active pulmonary tuberculosis, pulmonary cystic fibrosis, pulmonary sarcoidosis, and other basic pulmonary diseases. In this case, chest CT scan demonstrated thick-wall cavity at the left upper lung lobe, with a nodule of heterogeneous intensity inside. And around the nodular lesion, there was air crescent sign. Based on the typical air crescent sign by radiology, a diagnosis of pulmonary aspergillosis was not challenging. But in this case, chest CT scan still demonstrated multiple well-defined patchy and cords opacities of high intensity at the posterior segment of the right upper lung, with spots of calcification opacity inside. There were also adjacent pleural thickening and adhesion. Based on these findings, the condition was likely to be old pulmonary tuberculosis complicated by pulmonary aspergilloma.

The patient presented with cough, which should be differentiated from diseases that may cause chronic cough, especially cough-type asthma. Although the lung function test showed histamine bronchial provocation test positive, the condition cannot be diagnosed as bronchial asthma. And the clinicians should know about asthma-like episodes induced by aspergillus.

(1–3)-β-D-Glucan test (G test) and aspergillus galactomannan antigen test (GM test) are important ways for diagnosis of fungal infection. Especially, GM test plays an important role in the early diagnosis of pulmonary aspergillosis, with a specificity of up to 70–90%. However, serum G test and GM test show low positive rate in the diagnosis of chronic pulmonary aspergillosis. The main reason is that aspergillus antigen does not invade into the blood flow in the cases of chronic pulmonary aspergillosis. But BALF GM test shows a sensitivity and specificity of up to 90% in the diagnosis of chronic pulmonary aspergillosis. Therefore, fibrobronchoscopy can be performed along with BALF GM test to improve the diagnosis of pulmonary aspergillosis.

References

1. Pena TA, Soubani AO, Samavati L. Aspergillus lung disease in patients with sarcoidosis: a case series and review of the literature. Lung. 2011;189(2):167–72.
2. Panjabi C, Sahay S, Shah A. Aspergilloma formation in cavitary sarcoidosis. J Bras Pneumol. 2009;35(5):480–3.
3. Hedayati MT, Azimi Y, Droudinia A, et al. Prevalence of chronic pulmonary aspergillosis in patients with tuberculosis from Iran. Eur J Clin Microbiol Infect Dis. 2015;34(9):1759–65.
4. Yuan Y, Ma X, Zhou P, et al. Surgical treatment for 26 cases of pulmonary aspergilloma. Chin J Mycol. 2014;9(2):93–5.
5. Rummens P, Bruyneel M, Lungarella M, et al. Aspergillus tracheobronchitis, bronchopleural fistula and empyema after lobectomy for aspergilloma. Med Mycol Case Rep. 2014;6(7):25–8.
6. De Pauw B, Walsh TJ, Donnelly JP, et al. Revised definitions of invasive fungal disease from the European Organization for Research and Treatment of Cancer/Invasive Fungal Infections Cooperative Group and the National Institute of Allergy and Infectious Diseases Mycoses Study Group (EORTC/MSG) Consensus Group. Clin Infect Dis. 2008;46(12):1813–21.

7. He H, Jiang S, Zhang L, et al. Aspergillus tracheobronchitis in critically ill patients with chronic obstructive pulmonary diseases. Mycoses. 2014;57(8):473–82.
8. Ader F, Nseir S, Le Berre R, et al. Invasive pulmonary aspergillosis in chronic obstructive pulmonary disease: an emerging fungal pathogen. Clin Microbiol Infect. 2005;11(6):427–9.
9. Park SY, Lim C, Lee S, et al. Computed tomography findings in invasive pulmonary aspergillosis in non-neutropenic transplant recipients and neutropenic patients, and their prognostic value. J Infect. 2011;63(6):447–56.
10. Walsh TJ, Petraitis V, Petraitiene R, et al. Diagnostic imaging of experimental invasive pulmonary aspergillosis. Med Mycol. 2009;47(s1):S138–45.
11. Xu S, Dong X, Bahetnisa, et al. Initial CT scan demonstrations of invasive pulmonary aspergillosis. Chinese Crit Care Med. 2013;25(4):229–32.
12. Chen H, Wu X, Li X, et al. Radiological demonstrations of pulmonary aspergillosis in immunocompetent patients. Chin J Med Imag Technol. 2013;29(04):557–60.
13. Prattes J, Flick H, Prüller F, et al. Novel tests for diagnosis of invasive aspergillosis in patients with underlying respiratory diseases. Am J Respir Crit Care Med. 2014;190(8):922–9.
14. Sulahian A, Porcher R, Bergeron A, et al. Use and limits of (1-3)-β-D-glucan assay (Fungitell), compared to galactomannan determination (Platelia Aspergillus), for diagnosis of invasive aspergillosis. J Clin Microbiol. 2014;52(7):2328–33.
15. Desoubeaux G, Bailly É, Chandenier J. Diagnosis of invasive pulmonary aspergillosis: updates and recommendations. Med Mal Infect. 2014;44(3):89–101.
16. Shroff S, Shroff GS, Yust-Katz S, et al. The CT halo sign in invasive aspergillosis. Clin Case Rep. 2014;2(3):113–4.
17. Yuan P, Wang Z, Bao F, et al. Is video-assisted thoracic surgery a versatile treatment for both simple and complex pulmonary aspergilloma? J Thorac Dis. 2014;6(2):86–90.
18. Guo L, Chen S, Xu D, et al. Thoracoscopic removal of whole lung for pulmonary aspergilloma: analysis of 41 cases. Chinese J Minim Invasive Surg. 2014;14(9):809–11.
19. Park Y, Kim TS, Yi CA, et al. Pulmonary cavitary mass containing a mural nodule: differential diagnosis between intracavitary aspergilloma and cavitating lung cancer on contrast-enhanced computed tomography. Clin Radiol. 2007;62:227–32.
20. Ichinose J, Kohno T, Fujimori S. Video-assisted thoracic surgery for pulmonary aspergilloma. Interact Cardiovasc Thorac Surg. 2010;10(6):927–30.
21. Aydoğdu K, İncekara F, Şahin MF, et al. Surgical management of pulmonary aspergilloma: clinical experience with 77 cases. Turk J Med Sci. 2015;45(2):431–7.
22. Onishi A, Sugiyama D, Kogata Y, et al. Diagnostic accuracy of serum (1–3)-β-D glucan for pneumocystis jiroveci pneumonia, invasive candidiasis, and invasive aspergillosis: systematic review and meta-analysis. J Clin Microbiol. 2012;50(1):7–15.
23. Gangneux JP, Camus C, Philippe B. Epidemiology of invasive aspergillosis and risk factors in non neutropaenic patients. Rev Malad Res. 2010;27(8):e34–46.
24. Hage CA, Knox KS, Davis TE, et al. Antigen detection in bronchoalveolar lavage fluid for diagnosis of fungal pneumonia. Curr Opin Pulmon Med. 2011;17(3):167–71.
25. Leventakos K, Lewis RE, Kontoyiannis DP, et al. Fungal infections in leukemia patients: how do we prevent and treat. Clin Infect Dis. 2010;50(3):405–15.
26. Chandrasekar P. Diagnostic challenges and recent advances in the early management of invasive fungal infections. Eur J Haematol. 2010;84(4):281–90.

Asymptomatic Pulmonary Aspergillosis

15

Guan-Xun Cheng and Ling-Wei Wang

The type of pulmonary aspergillosis that occurs after inhalation of aspergillus spores via the respiratory tract depends on the immunity of the host. The more serious the immunity is compromised, the more likely the occurrence of pulmonary aspergillosis is and the more serious the symptoms are. In cases with hyperactive immune response, allergic bronchopulmonary aspergillosis occurs in patients with asthma and cystic fibrosis. In cases with competent immune response, only planting or temporary residence of aspergillus occurs. Therefore, asymptomatic or slightly symptomatic pulmonary aspergillosis commonly occurs in hosts with competent immunity or slightly suppressed immunity. And the most common type of pulmonary aspergillosis is simplex pulmonary aspergilloma, followed by subacute invasive pulmonary aspergillosis (also known as chronic necrotizing pulmonary aspergillosis). Radiology may demonstrate both with air crescent sign, which indicates the diagnosis. However, subacute invasive pulmonary aspergillosis is radiologically characterized by infiltration opacity around cavity as well as thick and irregular cavity wall. Pathologically, subacute invasive pulmonary aspergillosis is demonstrated as invasion of aspergillus hyphae into lung tissue, while pulmonary aspergilloma only grows in cavity or dilated bronchus and does not invade the lung tissue. The symptoms of simplex pulmonary aspergilloma are slight or absent. But if patients show hemoptysis, it indicates vascular invasion. GM test of Serum and bronchoalveolar lavage fluid (BALF) shows a higher positive rate to subacute invasive pulmonary aspergillosis than to simplex pulmonary aspergilloma, which is related to their invasiveness.

In this section, we introduce three cases of pulmonary aspergillosis with slight or no symptoms. The first case is a patient with acute lymphoblastic leukemia who received bone marrow transplantation. Lung nodule was detected in the postoperative physical examination, and the patient only presented slight cough and expectoration. Thereafter, although anti-aspergillus medication was administered, the condition gradually aggravated with manifestations of fever and breathlessness along with decrease of granulocytes in peripheral blood. The lung nodule enlarged and shrank repeatedly, and the thin-wall cavity progressed into thick-wall cavity till filling of content to form air crescent sign. In this case, the relationship between immunity, clinical symptoms, and radiology is well presented. It should be noted that clinical diagnosis can be made based on radiological changes. Patients with hemoptysis are more likely to be subject to vascular invasion. For them, puncture for biopsy may cause major bleeding, and the decision of its performance should be cautious.

The treatment of pulmonary aspergilloma remains controversial. There has been no agreement on active surgery for asymptomatic simplex pulmonary aspergilloma. In the clinical guideline for chronic pulmonary aspergillosis issued by ERS in 2015, it has been emphasized that treatment of simplex pulmonary aspergilloma is intended to prevent life-threatening major hemoptysis. Therefore, the decision of surgical removal should be made after weighing the benefits and losses. However, some scholars believe that simplex pulmonary aspergilloma just temporarily resides in its host but not pathogenic to the host. Therefore, the decision of surgical removal should be based on possible risk of major hemoptysis and the willingness of the patients. If no leakage of fungal substances occurs during the operation, antifungal medication is not necessary. But for patients with complex aspergilloma, pulmonary basic disease, or failed complete removal of the lesion, antifungal medication is recommended before

The corresponding author of section 15.1 is Yulin He, Email: 33heyulin@163.com.
The corresponding author of section 15.2 is Wendi Huang, Email: vickdi@163.com.
The corresponding author of section 15.3 is Wei Gao, Email: gaomol@sina.com.

G.-X. Cheng (✉)
Shenzhen Hospital of Beijing University, Shenzhen, Guangdong, China

L.-W. Wang
Second Clinical Medical College of Jinan University, Shenzhen, Guangdong, China

C. Qiu et al. (eds.), *Pulmonary Aspergillosis*, https://doi.org/10.1007/978-981-13-3435-1_15

and after the operation. The specific administration is not recommended in the clinical guideline. We recommend the therapeutic course of antifungal medication should be based on clinical manifestations, results of culture for fungi, histopathology, and serology. And regular reexamination every 3 months after the operation is recommended.

Asymptomatic subacute invasive pulmonary aspergillosis tends to be misdiagnosed as lung carcinoma or pulmonary tuberculosis. Based on radiology including PET-CT, the differential diagnosis is challenging. In most cases, the diagnosis is defined based on postoperative pathology. We emphasize that subacute invasive pulmonary aspergillosis is essentially an invasive disease. If it occurs in immunocompetent or slightly immunosuppressed individuals, the clinical course is mild. Without antifungal medication, postoperative relapse is more likely. Therefore, in the clinical guideline issued by ERS, antifungal medication for 6 months is recommended to cure subacute invasive pulmonary aspergillosis. But the therapeutic course after surgical removal of the lesion is not explicit. Individualized therapeutic planning should be formulated by clinicians based on clinical findings.

Generally speaking, this section introduces cases of pulmonary aspergillosis with no or slight symptoms. The introduction and analysis of these cases are intended to expand our knowledge about pulmonary aspergillosis. Pulmonary aspergillosis does occur in individuals with no immunosuppression. In people with normal immunity, pulmonary aspergillosis should be enlisted into differential diagnosis for lung nodule or space-occupying lesion to avoid missed diagnosis and misdiagnosis.

Patients' consents have been obtained for images or other clinical information relating to the cases to be published.

15.1 Case 1: Space Occupying Lesion at the Right Upper Lung for 1 Day

Yulin He, Wanling Qi, Xiaofen Li, Chang'e Jin, Xueyan Liu, and Fei Shi

15.1.1 Presenting Symptom

Space-occupying lesion at the right upper lung for 1 day.

15.1.2 Brief Case History

A 46-year-old woman, a farmer, was admitted to our hospital on July 1, 2009, due to space-occupying lesion at the right upper lung for 1 day. When she received health check in the outpatient department of our hospital, chest X-ray demonstrated solitary nodular opacity at the right upper lung. She experienced no fever, emaciation, cough, and chest pain. To define the diagnosis, the patient was admitted to the thoracic surgery department of our hospital. Her spiritual state, appetite, and sleep were quite good. The urinations and bowel movements were normal. And she experienced no obvious body weight change.

15.1.2.1 Past Medical History

She reported bronchiectasis 15 years ago. At present, she occasionally had sputum with blood streak, but no fever, cough, night sweat, and breathlessness. And she denied histories of diabetes, hypertension, and pulmonary tuberculosis.

15.1.2.2 Physical Examination

By physical examination, the body temperature was 36.6 °C, pulse rate 83/min, respiration rate 20/min, and blood pressure 134/94 mmHg. She was typically developed with average nourishment. And she was well conscious. The skin and sclera showed no yellowish stain. The superficial lymph nodes were not palpable and not enlarged. The skull and five sense organs showed no abnormality. The bilateral tonsils were not enlarged. The thyroid was not enlarged, and the jugular vein showed no distention. The thorax was bilaterally symmetric with no deformity. The trachea was at the midline. By percussion, both lungs showed clear sounds. And the respiration sounds of both lungs were clear, with no dry and/or moist rales. The precordial area showed no protrusion. The heartbeat was 83/min, rhythmic, with no pathological murmur. The abdomen was soft, with no tenderness and rebound pain. The liver and spleen were impalpable under the ribs. The liver and kidney areas were not sensitive to percussion. The shifting dullness was negative. The nervous system showed no abnormality.

15.1.2.3 Auxiliary Investigation

Laboratory Test

By routine blood test, WBC 5.4×10^9/L, neutrophile granulocytes 3.35×10^9/L, lymphocytes 1.35×10^9/L, RBC 4.96×10^{12}/L, Hb 122 g/L, and PLT 209×10^9/L. The liver function test showed Alb 74.6 g/L, TB 12.2 μmol/L, DB 2.5 μmol/L, ALT 10 U/L, AST 22 U/L, and γ-GTT9 U/L. The blood coagulation function was normal.

Radiology

Routine chest X-ray in the outpatient department of our hospital on July 1, 2009, demonstrated solitary nodular opacity at the right upper lung.

15.1.2.4 Initial Diagnosis

The initial diagnosis was nodular opacity at the right upper lung, which was suspected to be peripheral lung carcinoma.

15.1.3 Diagnosis and Treatment

After admission, investigations were performed. The acid-fast staining of sputum showed negative. The antibody against tuberculosis mycobacteria was negative. Fibrobronchoscopic brushing showed no abnormal cells.

After admission, plain chest CT scan was performed on July 2, 2009. It demonstrated an irregular nodular opacity at the apical segment of the right upper lung lobe, in a size of about 2.0 cm × 1.5 cm with surrounding long spikes and a CT value of 33.0 Hu (Fig. 15.1). Chest thin-slice contrast-enhanced CT scan on July 3, 2009, demonstrated SPN CT value of about 36.7 Hu at the vascular phase and SPN CT value of 31.0 Hu at the parenchymal phase. Less small round translucent gas opacities were demonstrated around the nodule (Fig. 15.2). The diagnosis was considered to be solitary

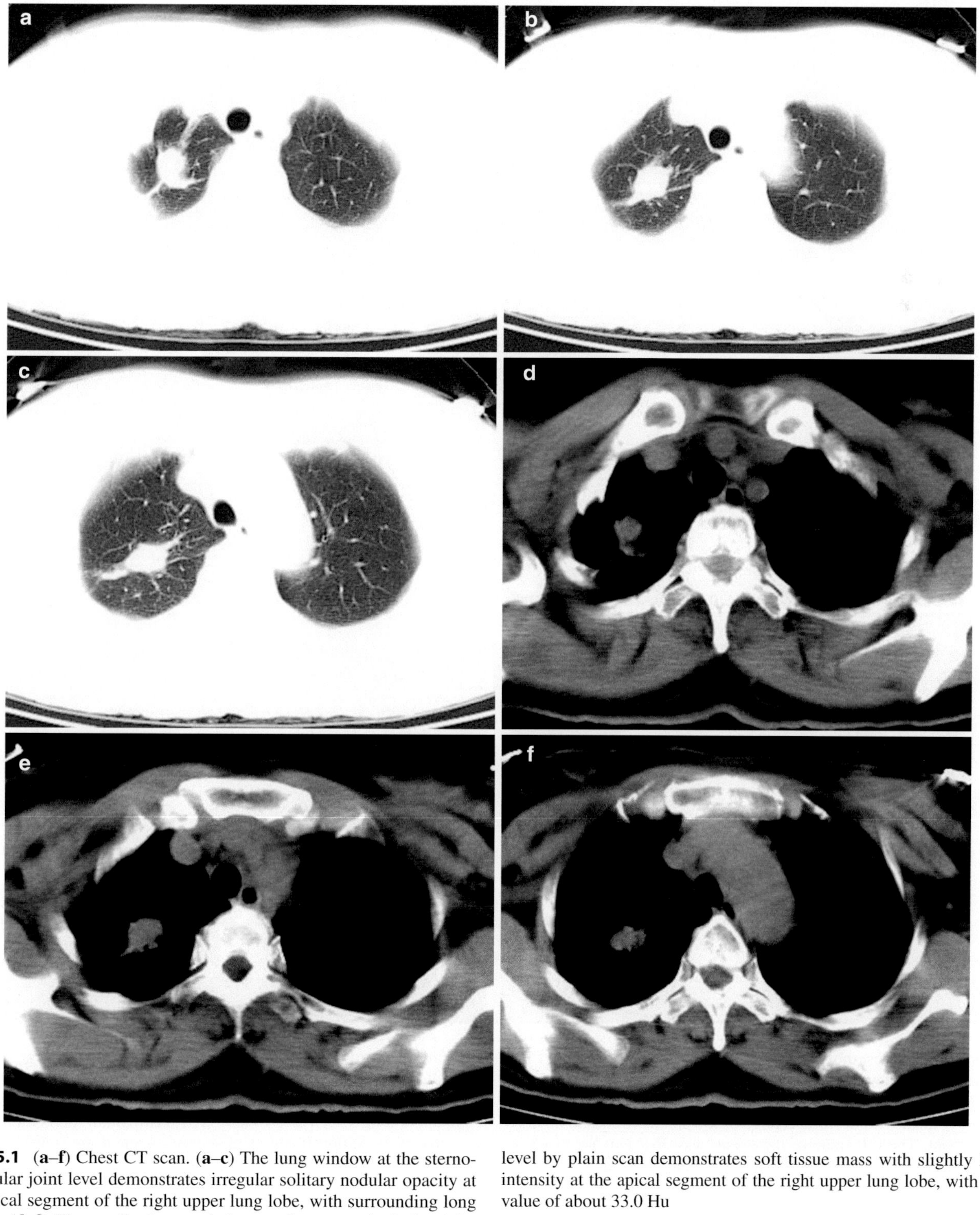

Fig. 15.1 (**a–f**) Chest CT scan. (**a–c**) The lung window at the sternoclavicular joint level demonstrates irregular solitary nodular opacity at the apical segment of the right upper lung lobe, with surrounding long spikes. (**d–f**) The mediastinum window at the sternoclavicular joint level by plain scan demonstrates soft tissue mass with slightly lower intensity at the apical segment of the right upper lung lobe, with a CT value of about 33.0 Hu

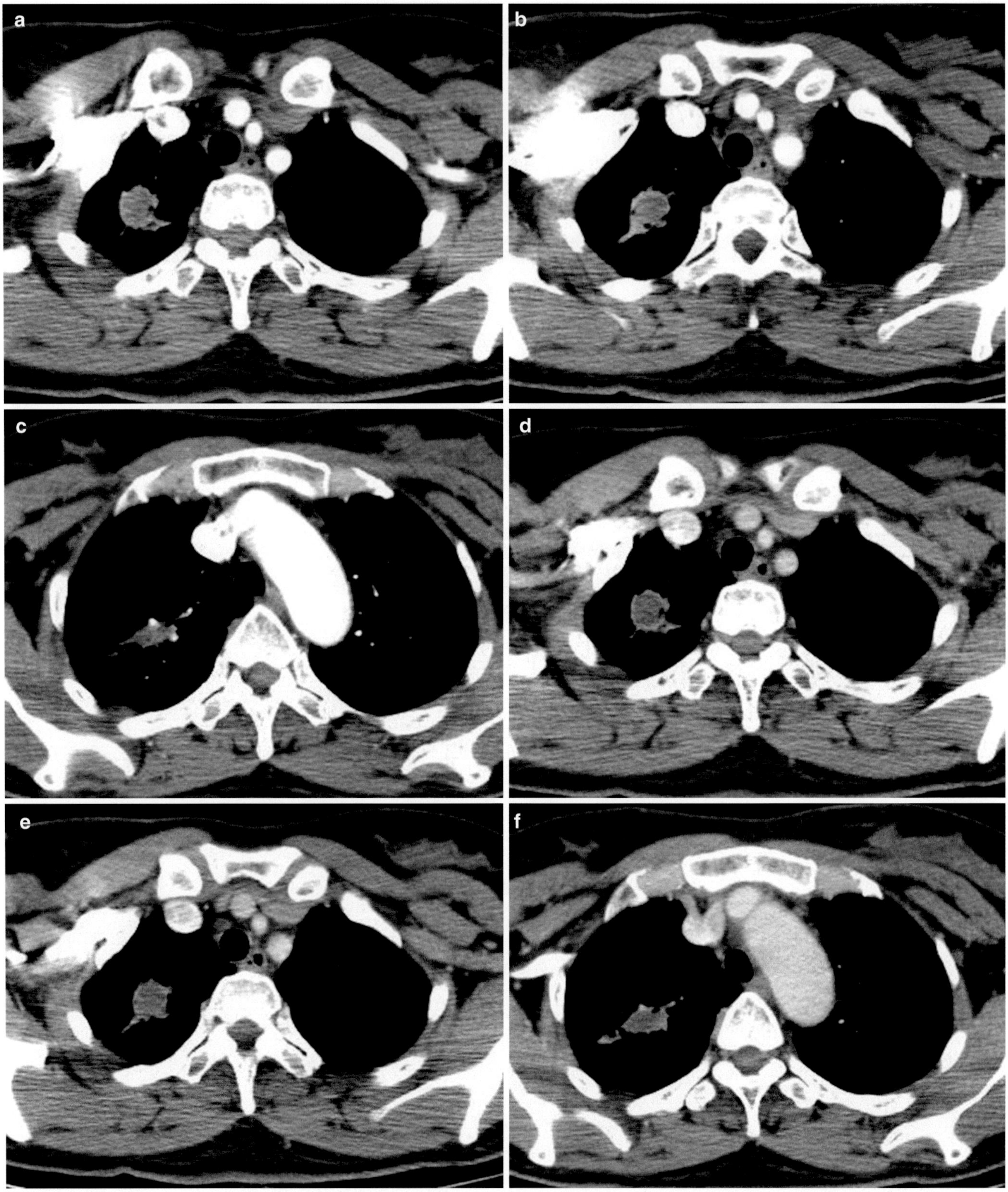

Fig. 15.2 (**a**–**f**) Chest thin-slice contrast-enhanced CT scan. (**a**–**c**) The mediastinum window at the sternoclavicular joint level and arterial phase demonstrates solitary nodular opacity at the apical segment of the right upper lung, with necrotic change of low intensity and no obvious enhancement. The CT value of the lesion was 36.7 Hu. Small round translucent gas opacity is demonstrated at its margin. Around the lesion, there is long cords opacity. (**d**–**f**) The mediastinum window at the sternoclavicular joint level and venous phase demonstrates no obvious enhancement of the solitary nodular opacity at the apical segment of the right upper lung lobe. The CT value is 31.0 Hu. Small round translucent gas opacity is demonstrated at its margin. Around the lesion, there is long cords opacity

nodule at the right upper lung, which was more likely to be peripheral lung carcinoma. But tuberculoma was not excluded.

Due to undefined quality of the nodule, electron bronchoscopy was performed on July 8, 2009 (Fig. 15.3). It demonstrated endobronchial inflammation. Pathological section demonstrated lung tissue, less reddish stained exudates in the alveolar cavity, and less phagocytic histocytes in the interstitium.

Due to radiological indication of peripheral lung carcinoma and not exclusion of tuberculoma, surgical removal of the right upper lung lobe was performed under general anesthesia. The postoperative pathology demonstrated removed lung lobe in a size of 13.0 cm × 8.0 cm × 2.0 cm and a cyst in a size of 4.0 cm × 2.0 cm × 2.0 cm about 2.5 cm away from the bronchial excision margin with grayish-brown bean dregs-like substances inside. Microscopy demonstrated lung tissue, bronchial mucosa coated by pseudostratified ciliated columnar epithelium, squamous epithelial metaplasia in some areas, and subepithelial interstitial fibrosis. There were also focal exudation of many histocytes in the alveolar cavity, widened and fibrotic alveolar septa, and fungal hyphae and spores in focal area. The pathological diagnosis was fungal infection of the right upper lung lobe, specifically aspergillus infection (Fig. 15.4).

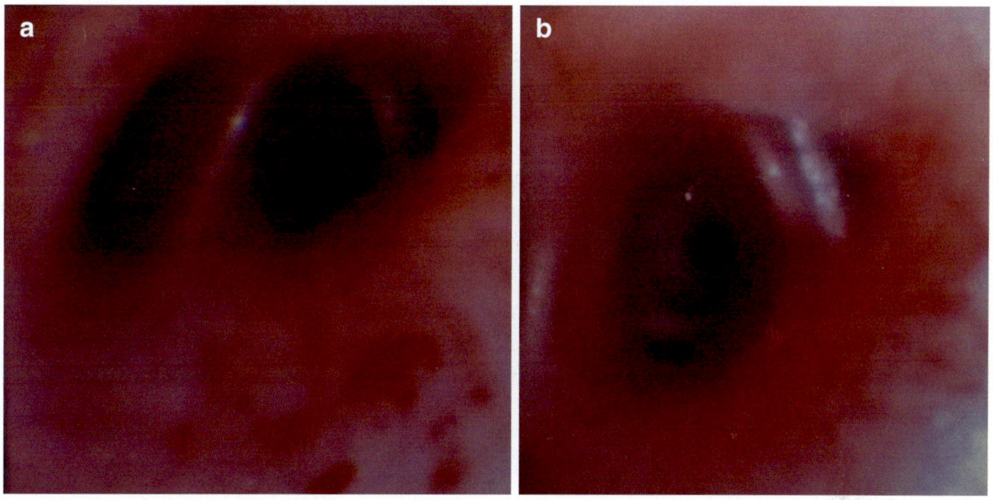

Fig. 15.3 (**a**, **b**) Electron bronchoscopy. (**a**) The segmental openings of the left bronchus are unobstructed, with no neoplasm. The openings of the right upper lung lobe are unobstructed. And specimen for biopsy is harvested, and brushing is performed at the right upper lung lobe. (**b**) The openings of the right middle lung lobe are unobstructed. The mucosa of the right lower lung lobe is congested, with unobstructed openings

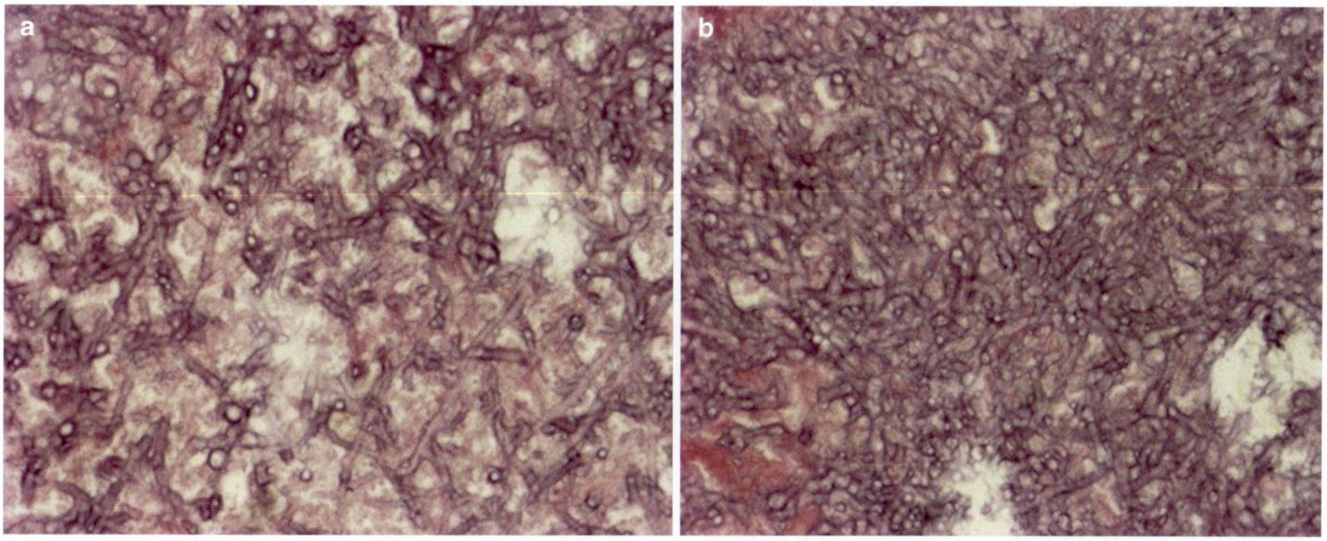

Fig. 15.4 (**a**–**c**) Pathology of lung tissue. (**a**, **b**) Large quantities of aspergillus hyphae and spores are observed. (**c**) There are squamous epithelial metaplasia of bronchial mucosa and widened alveolar septa (H&E staining)

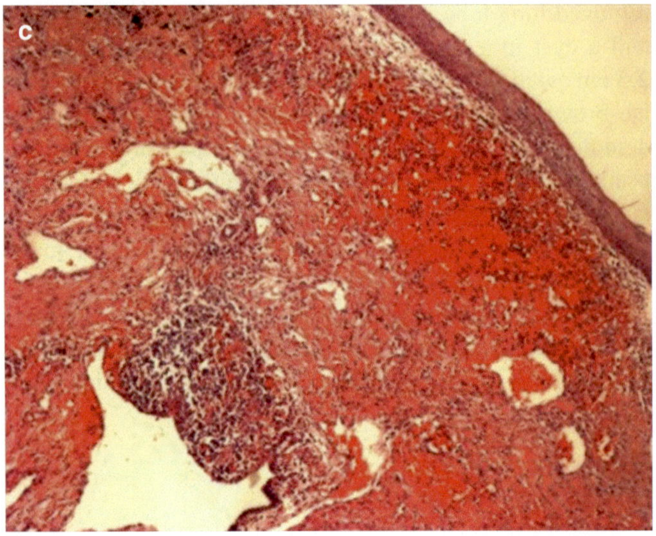

Fig. 15.4 (continued)

After the operation, injection of voriconazole was administered for 1 week, and then the medication was changed to oral intake of itraconazole. After active postoperative antifungal medication for 2 weeks, reexamination of blood test showed no abnormality. The condition was improved and the patient was discharged.

The final diagnosis was chronic pulmonary aspergillosis at the right upper lung (aspergillus nodule). After discharge, the condition of the patient was stable. And the follow-ups showed no relapse of hemoptysis.

15.1.4 Discussion

CPA is a rare pulmonary disease, which refers to chronic aspergillus infection of the lung with an illness course of above 3 months. According to the clinical guidelines issued by ESCMID, ECMM, and ERS in 2015, it can be typed into simplex aspergilloma, chronic cavitary pulmonary aspergillosis, chronic fibrotic pulmonary aspergillosis, aspergillus nodule, and subacute invasive pulmonary aspergillosis. In this case, the patient showed singular solitary nodule with a diameter of less than 3 cm, which was consistent with demonstrations of aspergillus nodule and is a rare type of CPA. Aspergillus nodule is commonly manifested as singular or multiple nodules with a diameter of less than 3 cm. It occurs in immunocompetent patients with past or present medical history of pulmonary disease [1, 2]. It is radiologically characterized by no typical demonstrations of invasive aspergillosis, such as halo sign and air crescent sign [3]. Most of the nodules are round, possibly with central attenuation or cavity. In some cases, the margin of nodule shows spikes. The nodules may be large or small. And occasionally the nodule may be a large mass, commonly with cavity. Aspergillus nodule is commonly subject to necrosis but no invasion to surrounding lung tissue. Radiologically, it resembles to tuberculoma, lung carcinoma, lung metastasis, cryptococcus nodule, coccidioidomycosis, actinomycosis, rheumatoid nodule, and other diseases caused by rare pathogens. It tends to be misdiagnosed before surgical operation. In most cases, the diagnosis is defined via preoperative CT-guided lung puncture for biopsy or postoperative histopathology. If the lesion of aspergillus infection forms nodule with a diameter of above 3 cm with central necrosis, the condition should be more precisely known as mass lesion induced by aspergillus. In this case, CT scan demonstrated solitary nodule at the apex of the lung, with no typical halo sign, and the condition was preoperatively diagnosed as peripheral lung carcinoma and tuberculoma.

The similar manifestations of chronic pulmonary aspergillosis and peripheral lung carcinoma are the main reason for the misdiagnosis. The common manifestations of lung carcinoma include irritating dry cough, recurrent cough and expectoration, sputum with blood streak, chest and back pain, as well as long-term fever. But they are not characteristic manifestations of lung carcinoma [4]. Radiology demonstrates peripheral lung carcinoma as solitary and lobulated nodule or mass with marginal spikes, eccentric cavity due to necrosis, and mediastinal or cervical lymphadenectasis. However, these findings may also be demonstrated in patients with chronic pulmonary aspergillosis or other pulmonary diseases such as tuberculosis [5]. Thus the same radiological demonstrations are shown for different diseases, and the diagnosis, therefore, is challenging. In this case, the condition was preoperatively misdiagnosed as peripheral lung carcinoma of the right upper lung. But by careful reading of the CT images, the lesion can be found with no obvious lobulation, and the surrounding thick long spikes were demonstrated as cords opacity. There was also marginal small round translucent opacity. And contrast-enhanced scan demonstrated no obvious enhancement. These radiological findings did not support the diagnosis of peripheral lung carcinoma but strongly indicated necrotic granuloma. Because the lesion was located at the apex of the lung, the condition was misdiagnosed as tuberculoma.

The diagnosis of aspergillus nodule is commonly defined via removal of the lesion for biopsy, percutaneous lung puncture for biopsy, or other approaches of biopsy. Postoperative antifungal medication is not necessary for immunocompetent patients after complete surgical removal of the lesion. If the singular nodule fails to be completely removed by surgery, the progression of the lesion should be closely monitored. Aspergillus IgG titer, inflammatory indices, and dynamic radiological changes of the lesion should be monitored every 3 months, based on which the necessity of antifungal medication is assessed. For patients with multiple nodules, when one is surgically removed, antifungal medication is recommended for shrinkage of most or all nodules. If the nodule is enlarged, other complications should be considered, such as malignancies. Dynamic radiological changes in the initial 3 months should be closely monitored to ensure no progression of the lesion. For all of the cases, glucocorticoid should be used as less as possible.

15.1.5 Comments

In this case, the patient was a middle-aged woman, with no immunosuppression. Before the surgical operation, radiology demonstrated singular nodule in the lung. Contrast-enhanced scan demonstrated no enhancement. The clinical symptoms were mild. The diagnosis was confirmed to be aspergillus infection by pathology. And the condition should be categorized into CPA, and the typing was aspergillus nodule.

Aspergillus nodule manifests as one or several nodules with a diameter of less than 3 cm and commonly with no cavity, which is a rare type of CPA. Resembling to tuberculoma, lung carcinoma, lung metastasis, cryptococcus nodule, coccidioidomycosis, and other diseases caused by rare pathogens, its diagnosis can only be defined by histopathology. If the lesion of aspergillus infection has a diameter of above 3 cm with central necrosis, the condition should be more precisely known as mass lesion induced by aspergillus. In this case, the patient showed no typical demonstrations of aspergilloma, and the radiological changes resembled to lung carcinoma and tuberculoma. And the diagnosis was preoperatively considered to be peripheral lung carcinoma. The misdiagnosis seemed to be unavoidable. The lesion was peripherally located at the apex of the right lung. Preoperative definitive diagnosis via percutaneous lung puncture for biopsy or bronchoscopy is clinically challenging. In this case, the patient was middle-aged with favorable general conditions, who was a low-risk patient for surgery. Before the surgical operation, a diagnosis of lung malignancy was not excluded. Surgical removal of the lesion as treatment and for diagnosis was a good choice. For patients with competent immunity and singular nodule completely removed, postoperative antifungal medication was not necessary.

In addition, the patient had a past medical history of bronchiectasis. After the aspergillus nodule was surgically removed, the symptoms of hemoptysis were improved. It should be differentiated between bronchiectasis and aspergillus nodule for the reason of hemoptysis.

15.2 Case 2: Space Occupying Lesion Detected in Health Check-Up for 3 Days

Wendi Huang, Wei-Dong Song, Guan-Xun Cheng, Ying-Yun Fu, Xueyan Liu, and Zhijian Yu

15.2.1 Presenting Symptom

Space-occupying lesion detected in health checkup for 3 days.

15.2.2 Brief Case History

A 45-year-old woman from Chongqing of China was admitted to our hospital on August 10, 2014, due to complaints of space-occupying lesion detected in health checkup for 3 days. Three days before her admission, she received health checkup, and chest X-ray demonstrated oval-shaped opacity of high intensity near the mediastinum at the right upper lung. Chest CT scan demonstrated space-occupying lesion at the apex of the right upper lung. She experienced no cough, expectoration, fever, night sweat, chest pain, and chest distress. The spiritual state and appetite were quite good. The urinations and bowel movements were normal. She experienced no obvious changes in physical strength and body weight.

15.2.2.1 Past Medical History

She was in good health and reported no hobbies in smoking.

15.2.2.2 Physical Examination

Physical examination showed temperature 37.1 °C, pulse rate 91/min, respiration rate 18/min, and blood pressure 123/84 mmHg. She was well conscious. The bilateral supraclavicular fossae and the neck showed no palpable enlarged lymph nodes. The respiration sounds of both lungs were clear, with no obvious dry and/or moist rales. The heart and abdomen showed no abnormality. Both lower limbs showed no edema. There was no clubbing finger. The nervous system showed no abnormality.

15.2.2.3 Initial Diagnosis

The initial diagnosis was space-occupying lesion at the right upper lung.

15.2.3 Diagnosis and Treatment

After admission, the investigations were performed. Routine blood test showed WBC 7.01 × 10^9/L, neutrophile granulocytes 59%, hemoglobin 131 g/L, and platelet

304×10^9/L. Routine urine and stool tests showed no abnormalities. The liver and kidney function tests showed no abnormality. The ERS was 6 mm/h. The carcinoembryonic antigen was 2.48 ng/ml (normal range, for non-smoker 0–5.0 ng/ml; for smoker 0–10.0 ng/ml). G test showed 37.36 pg/ml (normal range, <60 pg/ml). The sputum smear for fungi and acid-fast bacilli for consecutive 3 days showed negative. The sputum culture for one time showed no growth of bacteria and fungi.

After admission, levofloxacin and cefminox were administered for infection. Chest contrast-enhanced CT scan on August 12, 2014, is shown in Fig. 15.5.

To define the diagnosis, CT-guided lung puncture was performed on August 13, 2014. The specimen of lung tissue was

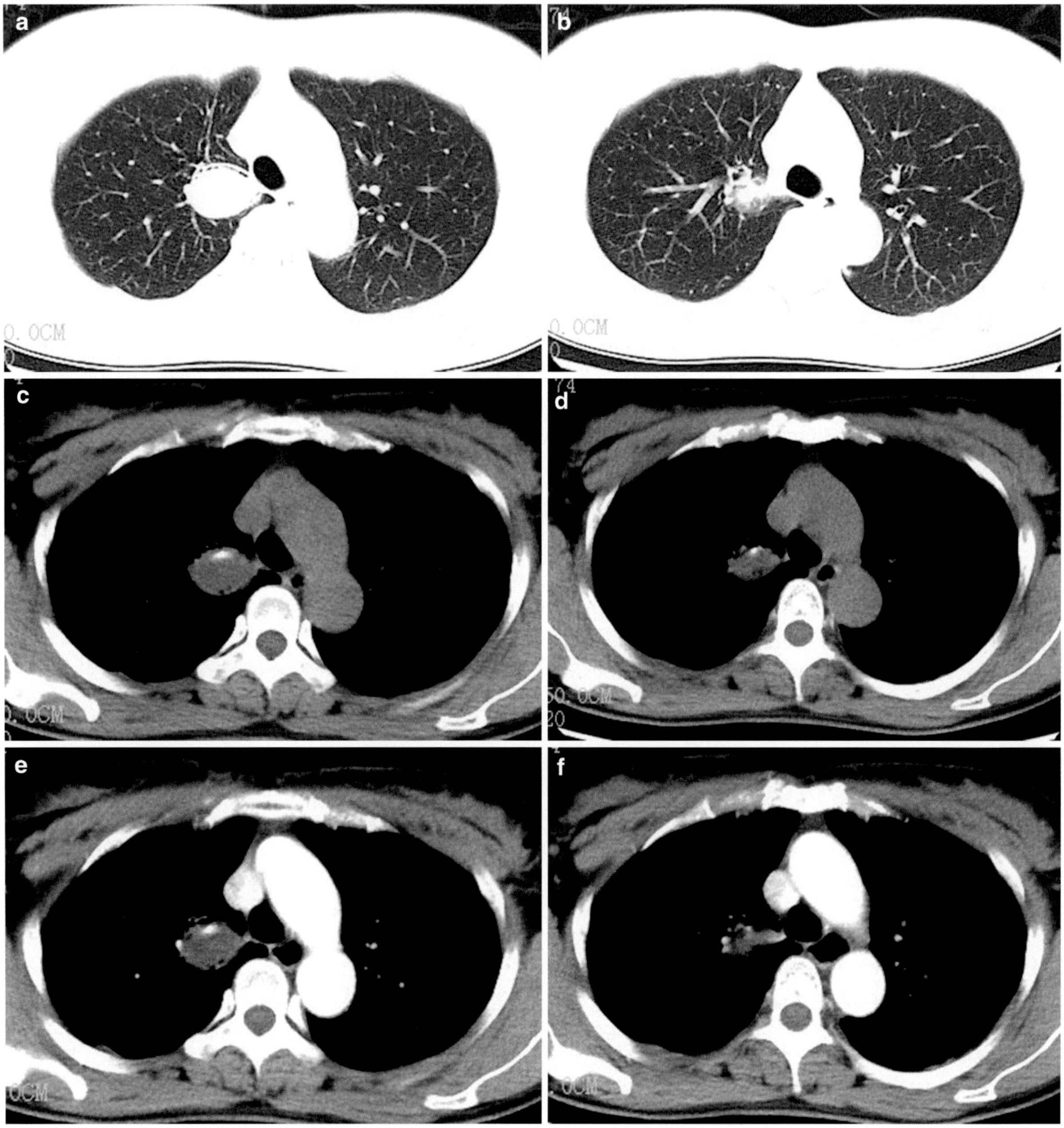

Fig. 15.5 (**a**–**f**) Chest contrast-enhanced CT scan. (**a**, **b**) The lung window at the aorta arch level demonstrates oval round thin-wall opacity with low intensity adjacent to the right upper mediastinal trachea, with spherical dense opacity and superior air crescent sign inside. The oval round thin-wall opacity has smooth and intact margin in size of about 3.4 cm × 2.2 cm. By plain scan, the intensity is homogeneous and the CT value is about 20 Hu. (**c**, **d**) The mediastinum window at the aorta arch level demonstrates spherical dense opacity and superior air crescent sign. There are spots of calcification at the margin. (**e**, **f**) The mediastinum window at the aorta arch level demonstrates oval round thin-wall opacity with low intensity adjacent to the right upper mediastinal trachea. Contrast-enhanced scan demonstrates no obvious enhancement

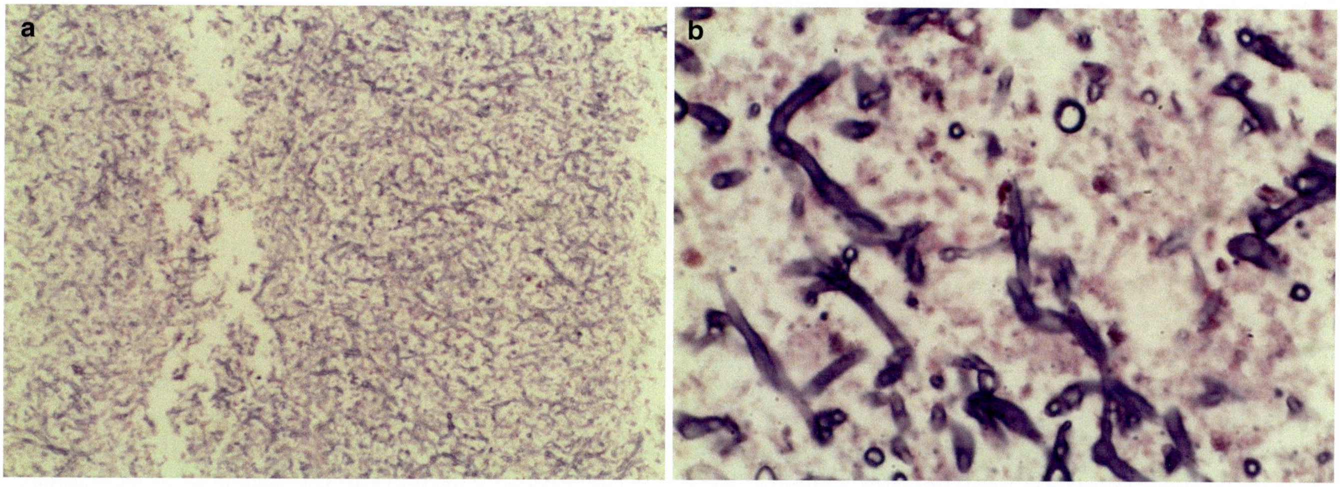

Fig. 15.6 (**a**, **b**) CT-guided lung puncture for histopathology. PAS staining demonstrates many aspergillus hyphae and accompanying infiltration of inflammatory cells in the lung tissue

harvested for pathology, and the pathological diagnosis was pulmonary aspergillosis of the right upper lung (Fig. 15.6).

The final diagnosis was aspergilloma of the right lung. After the diagnosis was defined, surgery was recommended, but the patient refused to receive surgical treatment, and she went to a local hospital in her hometown for treatment.

15.2.4 Discussion

Pulmonary aspergilloma is a type of pulmonary aspergillosis [6], which commonly occurs in primary lesion of basic pulmonary disease, such as cavitary pulmonary tuberculosis, bronchiectasis, congenital pulmonary cyst, and pulmonary abscess. It may also occur in patients with or receiving large doses of antibiotic or hormone as well as systemic compromised immunity. Among the basic pulmonary diseases, pulmonary tuberculosis is the most common. But in recent years, the incidence of pulmonary aspergilloma with no symptoms and no basic pulmonary disease has been increasing [7].

The clinical manifestations of pulmonary aspergilloma are non-specific, and most patients experience chronic cough and hemoptysis. In this case, the patient had no symptoms and no basic pulmonary disease. In health checkup, space-occupying lesion was detected. Therefore, the possibility of pulmonary aspergillosis should also be vigilant in asymptomatic and non-pulmonary basic lesions. Chest CT scan plays an important role in the clinical diagnosis of pulmonary aspergillosis. Typical chest CT scan demonstrations include intrapulmonary cavity [8], spherical high-intensity opacity in cavity, or crescent-shaped low-intensity opacity. In this case, the radiological demonstrations were typically pulmonary aspergilloma. But the condition should be differentiated from pulmonary tuberculosis and cancerous cavity. The cavity formed after liquefaction of tuberculoma or caseous cavity is commonly located at the hilum, with heterogeneous intensity, smooth cavity wall, and surrounding satellite lesions. The cancerous cavity is commonly eccentric, with uneven thickness of the inner wall and peninsula sign. The mass is nodular. Contrast-enhanced CT scan may demonstrate enhancement due to the abundant blood flow and surrounding lymphadenectasis.

If radiological demonstrations are atypical and diagnosis cannot be made, culture for fungi and histopathology should be combined for diagnosis. These are currently the main ways for definitive diagnosis of pulmonary aspergillosis. According to the literature report, the sputum detection shows low positive rate in definitively diagnosed cases of pulmonary aspergillosis, being about 30.0%. But the positive rate of BALF culture is comparatively high [9]. For patients with good physical condition, CT-guided percutaneous lung puncture or thoracotomy can be performed to harvest specimen [10] for H&E staining or special staining such as PAS staining. Microscopy detection of hyphae with branching in sharp angle can define the diagnosis of pulmonary aspergillosis. In this case, the radiological demonstrations highly indicated pulmonary aspergilloma. Because the physical condition of the patient was good, CT-guided percutaneous lung puncture for biopsy was performed, and the following pathology defined the diagnosis.

Because pulmonary aspergilloma is commonly secondary to pulmonary cavitary disease and the cavity wall is thick, the antifungal medication can hardly permeate into the cavity for treatment. Therefore, surgical removal of the lesion is the optimal treatment. Clinically, once the diagnosis of pulmonary aspergilloma is defined, if not contraindicated, surgical operation is recommended to avoid life-threatening hemoptysis [11]. In this case, the patient was good in general condition with a sigle lesion. So surgical treatment was feasible.

15.2.5 Comments

Pulmonary aspergilloma is a clinical type of chronic pulmonary aspergillosis. CT scan of the lungs demonstrates mass in cavity, arch-shaped superior margin that forms air crescent sign with its surrounding tissue. It commonly occurs in the primary lesion of basic pulmonary disease, such as cavitary pulmonary tuberculosis, bronchiectasis, congenital pulmonary cyst, and pulmonary abscess. But in recent years, the incidence of pulmonary aspergilloma with no symptoms and no basic pulmonary disease has been increasing.

In this case, the patient was asymptomatic. But radiology demonstrated typical signs, such as mass in cavity, arch-shaped superior margin that formed air crescent sign with its surrounding tissue. Based on these findings, a clinical diagnosis can be made. But in this case, the condition should also be differentiated from pulmonary tuberculosis and cancerous cavity. Fibrobronchoscopy facilitates the differential diagnosis.

For patients with favorable lung function, surgical removal of the lesion is the optimal choice. Thoracoscopy has reduced chances of complications and shortened hospitalization days. It has been recommended as an alternative treatment for singular aspergilloma and multiple cavities. In this case, the patient was 45 years old and the general conditions were good. She suffered from no basic pulmonary disease, and surgical removal of the lesion should be recommended.

15.3 Case 3: Nodular Opacity Detected in Physical Examination for More than 9 Months

Wei Gao, Guan-Xun Cheng, Yanwei Chen, Xueyan Liu, Chang'e Jin, and Xiongfei Sun

15.3.1 Presenting Symptom

Nodular opacity detected in physical examination for more than 9 months.

15.3.2 Brief Case History

A 13-year-old boy was repeatedly hospitalized due to nodular opacity in the right lower lung detected in physical examination for more than 9 months. Nine months ago after bone marrow transplantation, reexamination demonstrated nodule at the right lower lung. The patient occasionally experienced cough and expectoration. But he experienced no chest distress, breathlessness, chest pain, hemoptysis, low-grade fever, night sweat, and fatigue. Chest CT scan on August 7, 2013, demonstrated nodular opacity at the anterior basilar segment of the right lower lung lobe, which was considered to be fungal infection. Voriconazole, linezolid, and piperacillin sodium/tazobactam sodium were administered then for infection for 5 months. The condition was improved and the patient was discharged. Voriconazole, Bai Yan Jing, and azithromycin were continued, and the symptoms were slightly improved. During the medication, reexamination of chest CT scan demonstrated almost the same lesion at the right lower lung lobe. Chest CT scan on March 21, 2014, demonstrated absorption of the lesion at the right upper lung lobe and almost the same lesion at the anterior basilar segment of the right lower lung lobe compared to the previous CT scan. For further treatment, the patient was admitted again due to complaints of nodule at the right lower lung on March 22, 2014. Since the onset of the symptoms, his spiritual state, appetite, and sleep were average. The urinations and bowel movements were normal. He experienced no obvious weight change.

15.3.2.1 Past Medical History

The patient began chemotherapy on September 26, 2011, due to acute lymphoblastic leukemia (B, MLL+, and IGH+). After the bone marrow showed complete remission, he received hematopoietic stem cell transplantation on March 23, 2012. And the patient was hospitalized on July 6, 2013, due to 15 months after hematopoietic stem cell transplantation for acute lymphoblastic leukemia and liver function abnormality for 2 weeks. The diagnosis was viral myocarditis. Teicoplanin was administered for infection and foscarnet sodium to fight against virus. He denied past medical histories of hepatitis, tuberculosis, and other infectious diseases. And he denied past medical history of hypertension and diabetes.

15.3.2.2 Physical Examination

Physical examination showed a body temperature of 36.9 °C, pulse rate 89/min, respiration rate 20/min, and blood pressure 112/70 mmHg. He was typically developed, with average nourishment. The patient was well conscious, with appearance of chronic disease. He was in active position and well cooperated with the physical examination. The systemic superficial lymph nodes were not palpable and not enlarged. The respiration sounds of both lungs were clear, with no dry and/or moist rales. The heart was not enlarged, with heartbeat of 89/min, rhythmic. The valvular areas showed no pathological murmur. The abdomen was soft, and the shifting dullness was negative. The liver and kidney areas were not sensitive to percussion. And the bowel sounds were normal.

15.3.2.3 Auxiliary Investigation

Laboratory Test

Routine blood test on July 7, 2013, showed WBC 2.63 × 10^9/L, PLT 21 × 10^9/L, N 2.1 × 10^9/L, RBC 3.6 × 10^{12}/L, and Hb 102 g/L. Routine blood test on August 27, 2013, showed WBC 2.03 × 10^9/L, PLT 133 × 10^9/L, N 1.59 × 10^9/L, and RBC 1.06 × 10^{12}/L. Routine blood test on October 19, 2013, showed WBC 1.07 × 10^9/L, PLT 37 × 10^9/L, N 0.53 × 10^9/L, RBC 2.72 × 10^{12}/L, and Hb 85 g/L. Routine blood test on February 23, 2014, showed PLT 308 × 10^9/L, WBC 5.01 × 10^9/L, N 2.12 × 10^9/L, RBC 2.72 × 10^{12}/L, and Hb 88 g/L.

The liver function test on July 7, 2013, showed GPT 106.0 U/L and GOT 70.6 U/L.

The quantification of cytomegalovirus on October 19, 2013, showed lower than 6.82 × 102 copies/ml. The quantification of EB virus on April 2, 2014, showed lower than 500 copies/ml and cytomegalovirus lower than 500 copies/ml. The adenovirus was negative. The herpes simplex virus was negative. And the human parvovirus was negative.

The G test for fungi on August 27, 2013, showed lower than 10 pg/ml; on December 5, 2013, 0.61 pg/ml; and on April 2, 2014, 24.11 pg/ml.

The CRP on October 19, 2013, showed 387.3 mg/L and procalcitonin 7.02 ng/ml. The CRP on November 11, 2013, was 16.2 mg/L and on December 3, 2013, 6.3 mg/L and procalcitonin 0.277 ng/ml. The CRP on December 5, 2013, was 29.3 mg/L and on February 23, 2014, 10.1 mg/L and procalcitonin 0.238 ng/ml. The CRP on April 17, 2014, was 26.3 mg/L and procalcitonin 0.106 ng/ml.

The sputum culture on September 16, 2013, showed growth of *Burkholderia cepacia*.

Radiology

Chest CT scan on July 18, 2013, and March 21, 2014, are shown in Figs. 15.7, 15.8, 15.9, 15.10, 15.11, 15.12, 15.13, and 15.14.

Other Investigations

The lung function test and electrocardiography on April 2, 2014, showed no abnormality.

15.3.2.4 Initial Diagnosis

The initial diagnosis was nodule at the right lower lung, which was suspected to be fungal infection and after bone marrow transplantation for acute lymphoblastic leukemia.

15.3.3 Diagnosis and Treatment

From July 6, 2013 to April 17, 2014, the patient was hospitalized repeatedly for 15 times. Chest CT scan on August 28 demonstrated enlarged nodular lesion at the right lung, and emergence of cavity, which was considered to be fungal infection and aspergillus infection, was highly suspected. Voriconazole was then administered for fungal

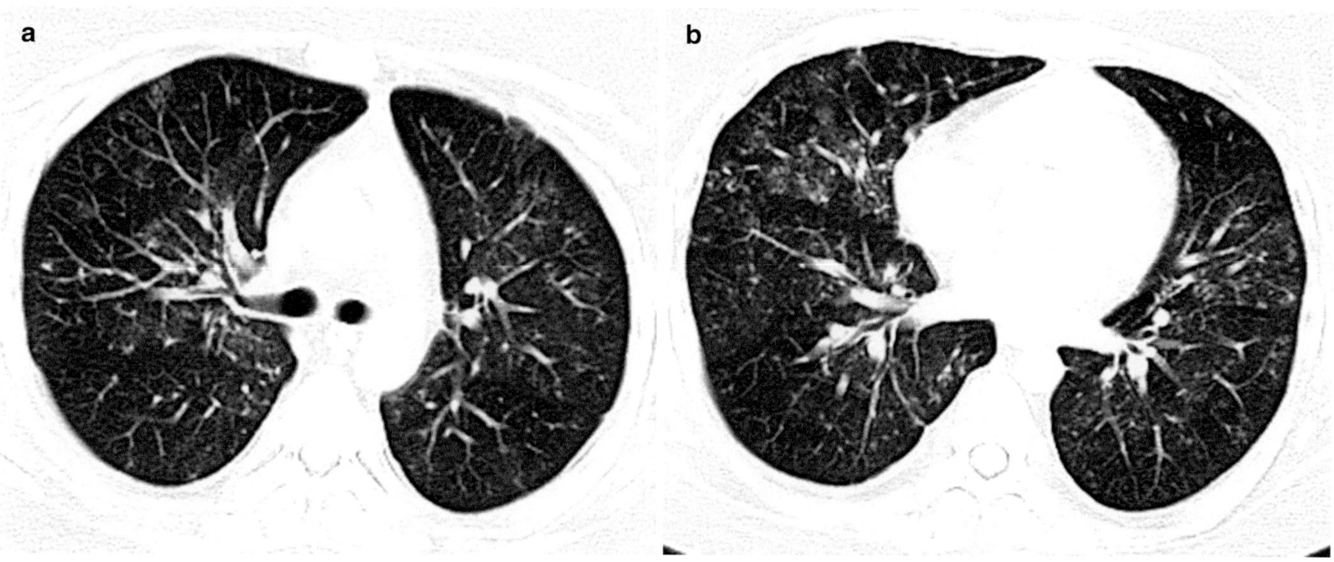

Fig. 15.7 (**a**, **b**) Chest CT scan. (**a**, **b**) The lung window demonstrates diffuse poorly defined patchy, spots and strips opacity of high intensity in both lungs

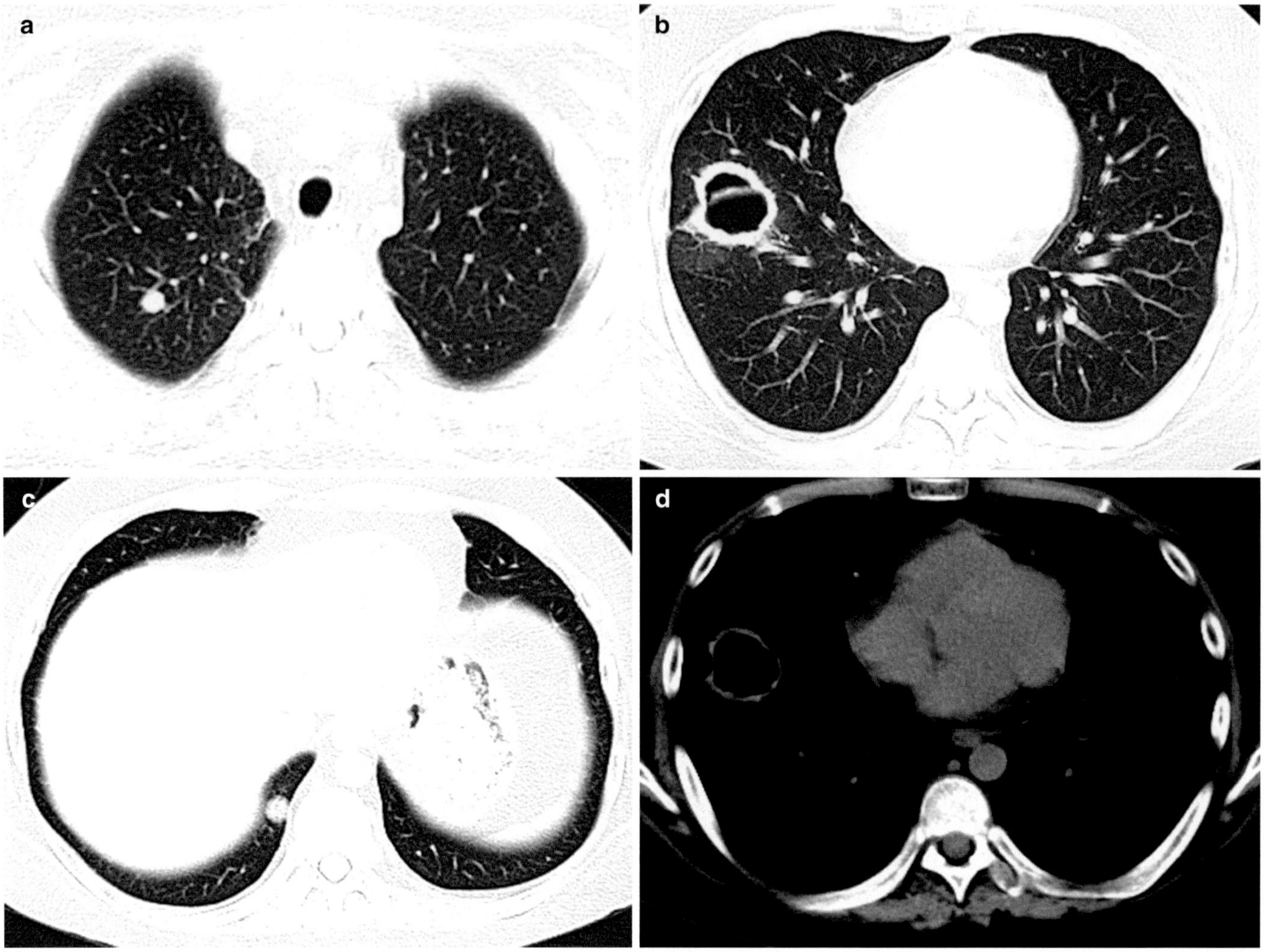

Fig. 15.8 (**a–d**) Chest CT scan. (**a–c**) The lung window demonstrates two new nodular lesions at the apical segment of the right upper lung lobe and posterior basilar segment of the right lower lung lobe, with smooth margins and in diameters of about 0.6 and 1.2 cm. There is central cavity in the lesion at the lateral segment of the right middle lung lobe. (**d**) The mediastinum window demonstrates thin-wall cavity opacity with high intensity at the lateral segment of the right middle lung lobe, with a small flake of opacity with slightly high intensity inside

infection. And its combined use with linezolid and piperacillin sodium/tazobactam sodium was administered for infection. Chest CT scan on September 9 demonstrated enlarged cavity, and the patient experienced aggravation of cough and expectoration. The medication of amphotericin B was added, and the symptoms were improved. The sputum culture on September 16 showed growth of *Burkholderia cepacia*, and then intravenous infusion of piperacillin sodium/tazobactam sodium was administered for treatment. Chest CT scan on September 18 demonstrated thin-wall cavities at the right middle lung lobe and right lower lung lobe, which showed shrinkage compared to the previous scan. But there was content in the cavity. On September 19, amphotericin B was discontinued due to drug-induced renal insufficiency. On September 22, the indices of infection showed improvement, and the patient was discharged. But the patient was admitted again on October 11, 2013, due to cough. Reexamination of blood showed increased quantification of CMV DNA. And reexamination of chest CT scan demonstrated thin-wall cavity with insignificant shrinkage. Voriconazole was administered again, and human immune globulin was given via intravenous infusion. On October 19, the patient began to show fever, with decreased blood oxygen saturation. Chest CT scan on October 20 demonstrated new consolidation opacity at the right upper lung lobe. And the combined use of voriconazole, ganciclovir, teicoplanin, and meropenem was given for infection, and the condition was improved. The patient was then discharged. On December 5, 2013, the patient was hospitalized again, and oral intake of

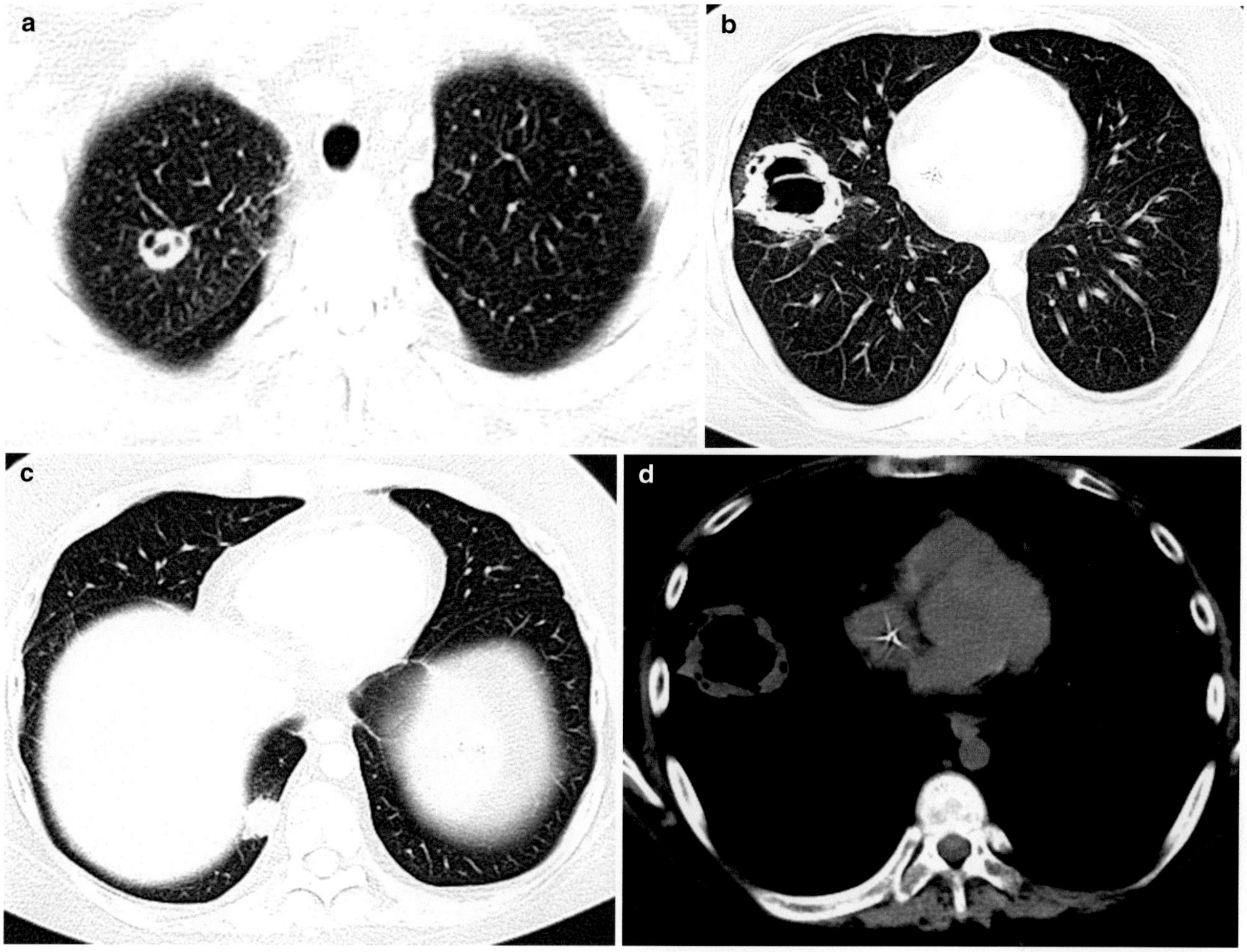

Fig. 15.9 (**a**–**d**) Chest CT scan. (**a**) The lung window demonstrates multiple small cavities in the nodular lesion at the apical segment of the right upper lung lobe. (**b**) The cavity at the right middle lung lobe is demonstrated with thicker wall, and its size shows no change. (**c**) The nodular opacity at the right lower lung lobe is demonstrated to be enlarged. (**d**) The mediastinum window demonstrates thicker wall of the cavity at the lateral segment of the right middle lung lobe, with multiple small translucent areas in the wall

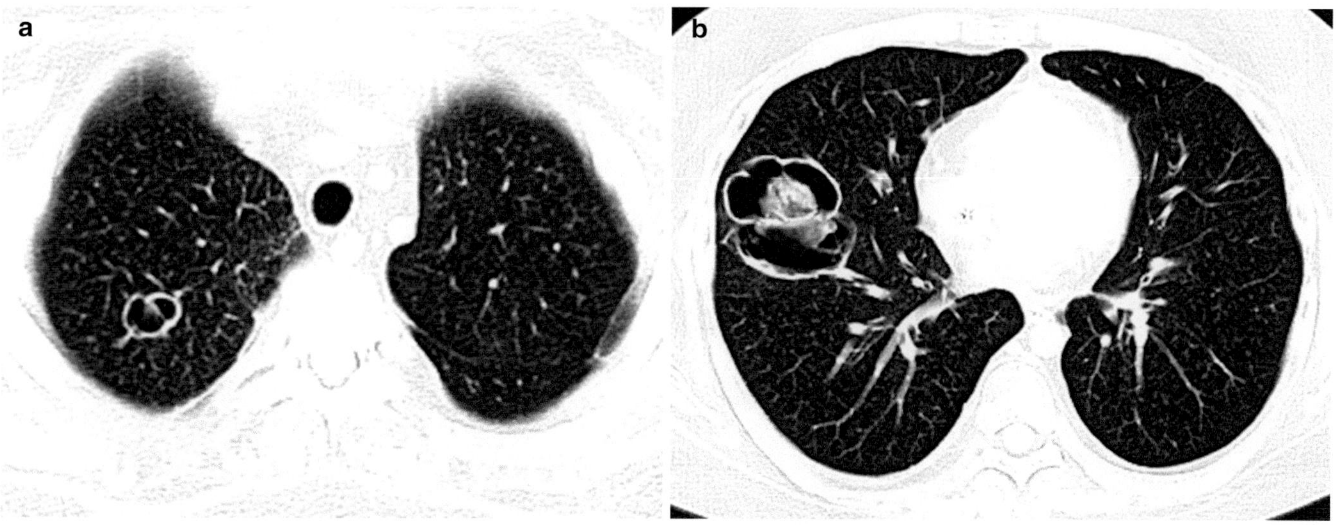

Fig. 15.10 (**a**–**c**) Chest CT scan. (**a**) The apical segment of the right upper lung lobe is demonstrated with thin-wall cavity-like lesions in size of about 4.9 cm × 4.1 cm and 1.5 cm × 1.2 cm, which shows absorption compared to previous CT scan. (**b**) The cavity lesion at the right middle lung lobe shows absorption, with thinner wall but enlarged nodule inside. (**c**) The nodular opacity at the posterior basilar segment of the right lower lung lobe shows obvious absorption, with formation of thin-wall cavity

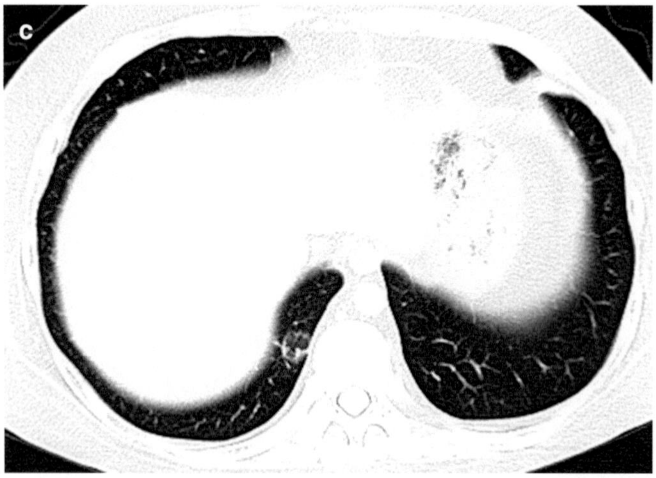

Fig. 15.10 (continued)

voriconazole was prescribed. Chest CT scan on January 2, 2014, demonstrated shrinkage of the thin-wall cavity at the right lung. On February 5 and February 23, the patient was hospitalized, respectively, due to fever and breathlessness. And antifungal treatment was administered. Reexamination of chest CT demonstrated incomplete absorption of the lesions in the lung. Thoracoscopic wedge removal of the right middle lung lobe and the lesion at the right lower lung lobe was performed on April 8 under general anesthesia. Intraoperative frozen pathology demonstrated inflammatory lesions at the right middle and lower lung lobes with necrosis. And the postoperative pathology demonstrated local necrosis of the right middle and lower lung lobes, with a large quantity of fungal hyphae inside. By special staining of F140620-1# and 2#: AAS staining negative,

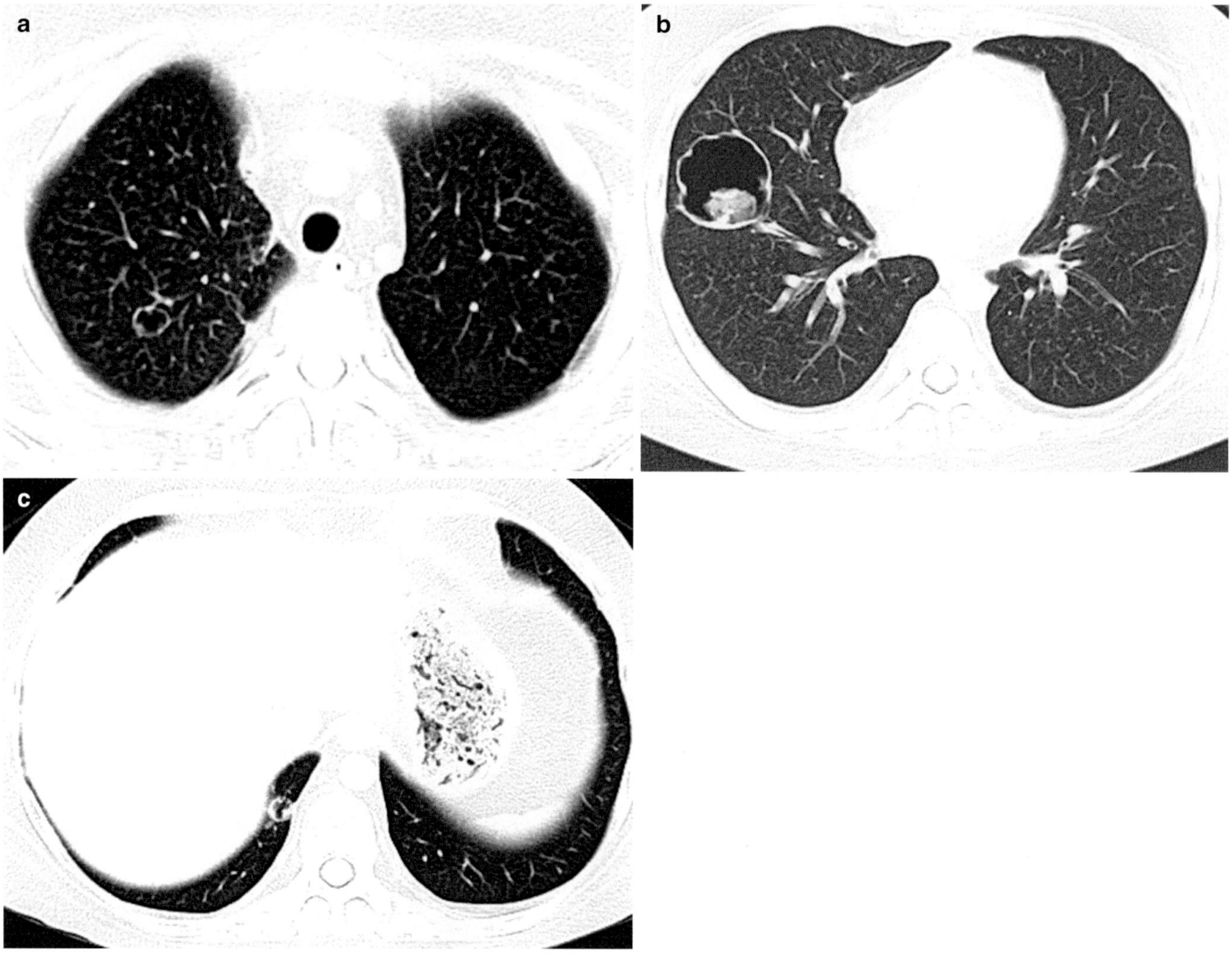

Fig. 15.11 Chest CT scan. (**a**) The cavity at the apical segment of the right upper lung lobe is demonstrated with thinner wall, and the cavity opacity is shown with shrinkage. (**b**) The thin-wall cavity at the lateral segment of the right middle lung lobe is demonstrated with slight shrinkage compared to previous CT scan in size of about 4.3 cm × 4.0 cm. And the nodular opacity inside is demonstrated with slight shrinkage. (**c**) The cavity opacity at the medial basilar segment of the right lower lung lobe is demonstrated with no obvious change

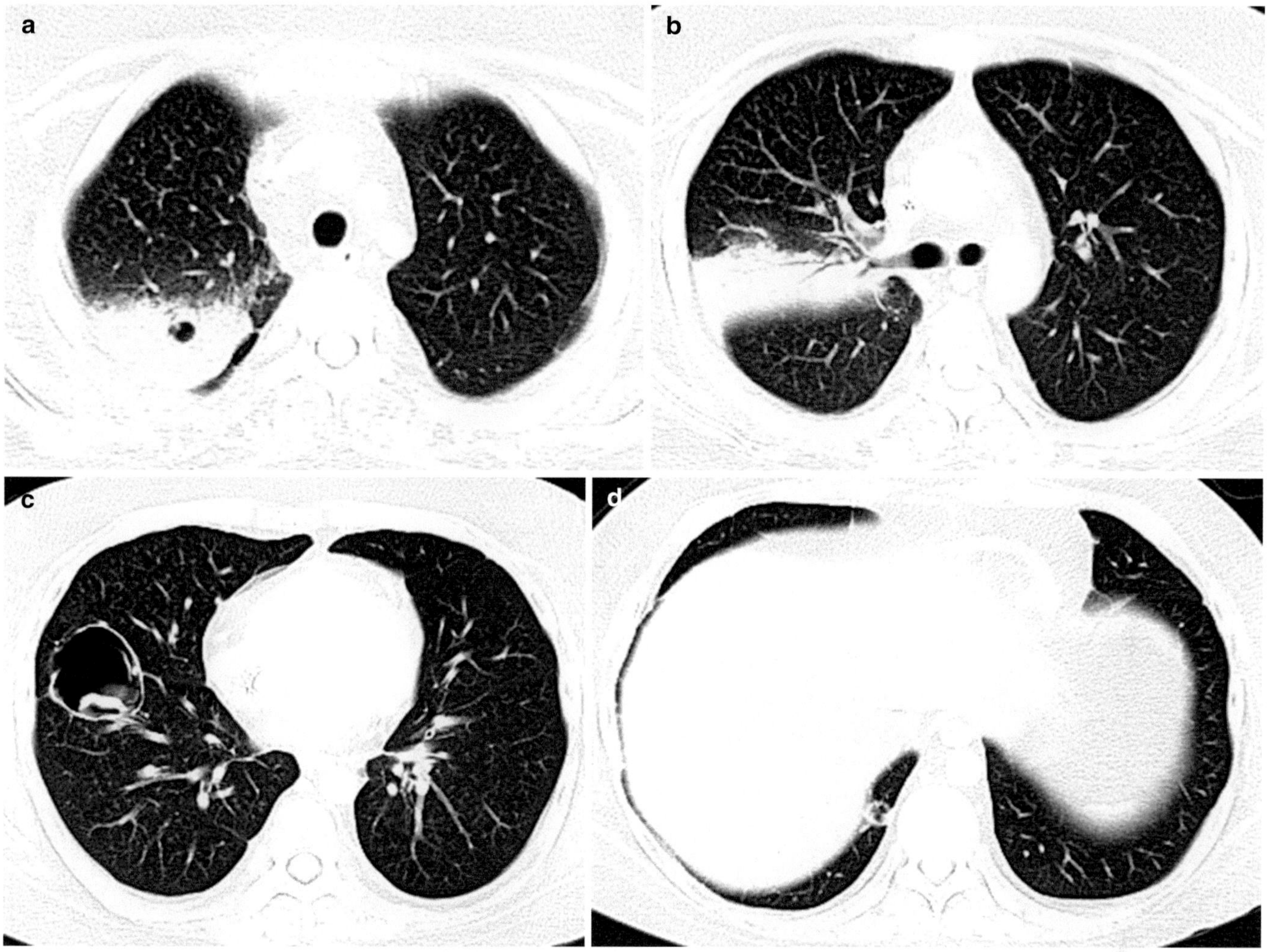

Fig. 15.12 (**a**–**d**) Chest CT scan. (**a**, **b**) The apical segment and posterior segment of the right upper lung lobe are demonstrated with new flakes of consolidation opacity, with cavity and air bronchogram inside. (**c**) The thin-wall cavity at the right middle lung lobe is demonstrated with no obvious change. And the nodular opacity in the cavity shows shrinkage. (**d**) The nodular opacity at the right lower lung is demonstrated the same as the previous scan

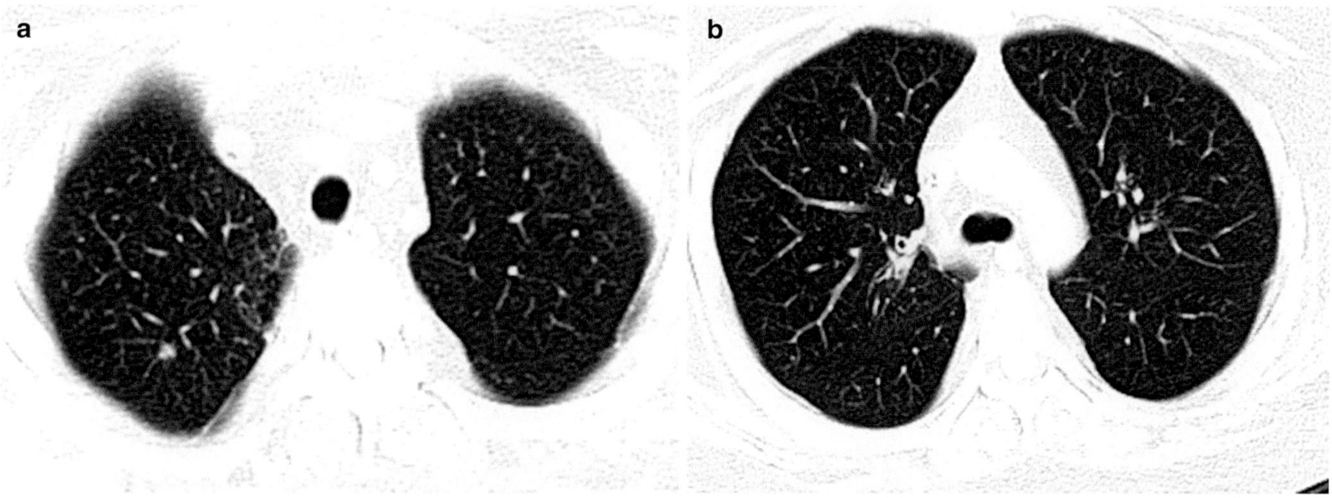

Fig. 15.13 (**a**–**d**) Chest CT scan. (**a**, **b**) The right upper lung lobe is demonstrated with small nodular opacity. And the large flake of consolidation opacity shown in the previous scan is demonstrated with absorption. (**c**) The right middle lung lobe is demonstrated with shrinkage of cavity opacity. And nodular opacity with increased intensity is still demonstrated. (**d**) The right lower lung lobe is demonstrated with thin-wall cavity, which is almost the same as the previous scan

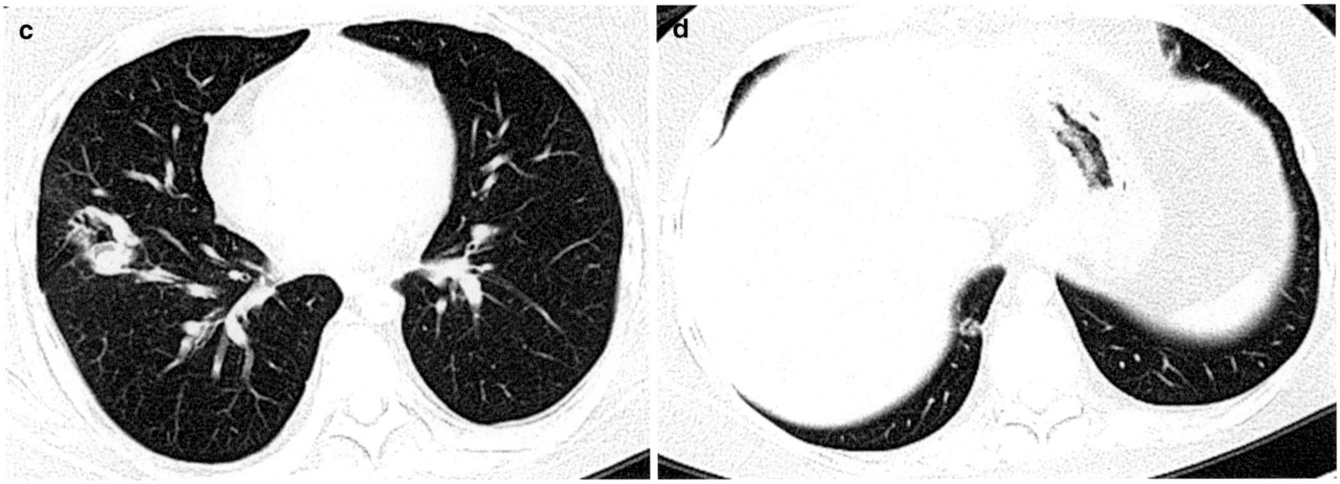

Fig. 15.13 (continued)

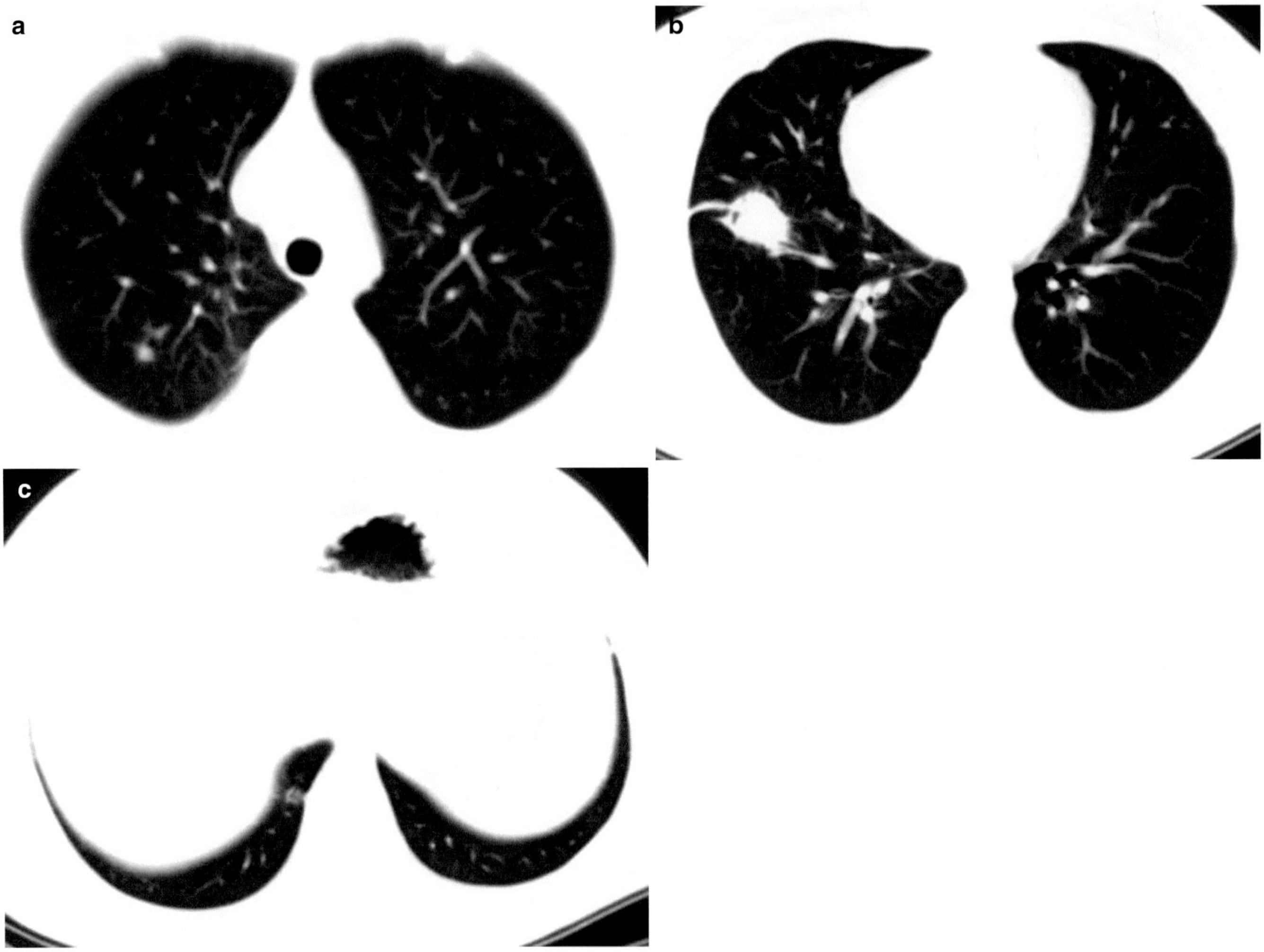

Fig. 15.14 (**a**–**c**) Chest CT scan. (**a**) The apical segment and posterior segment of the right upper lung lobe are demonstrated with spots and flakes of opacity with high intensity, which are absorbed compared to the previous scan. (**b**) The right middle lung lobe is demonstrated with poorly defined nodular opacity with high intensity in size of about 2.8 cm × 2.1 cm. The cavity opacity is shown with shrinkage compared to the previous scan. (**c**) The posterior basilar segment of the right lower lung lobe is demonstrated with cavity-like nodular opacity in a diameter of about 0.4 and 0.9 cm, which is almost the same as the previous scan

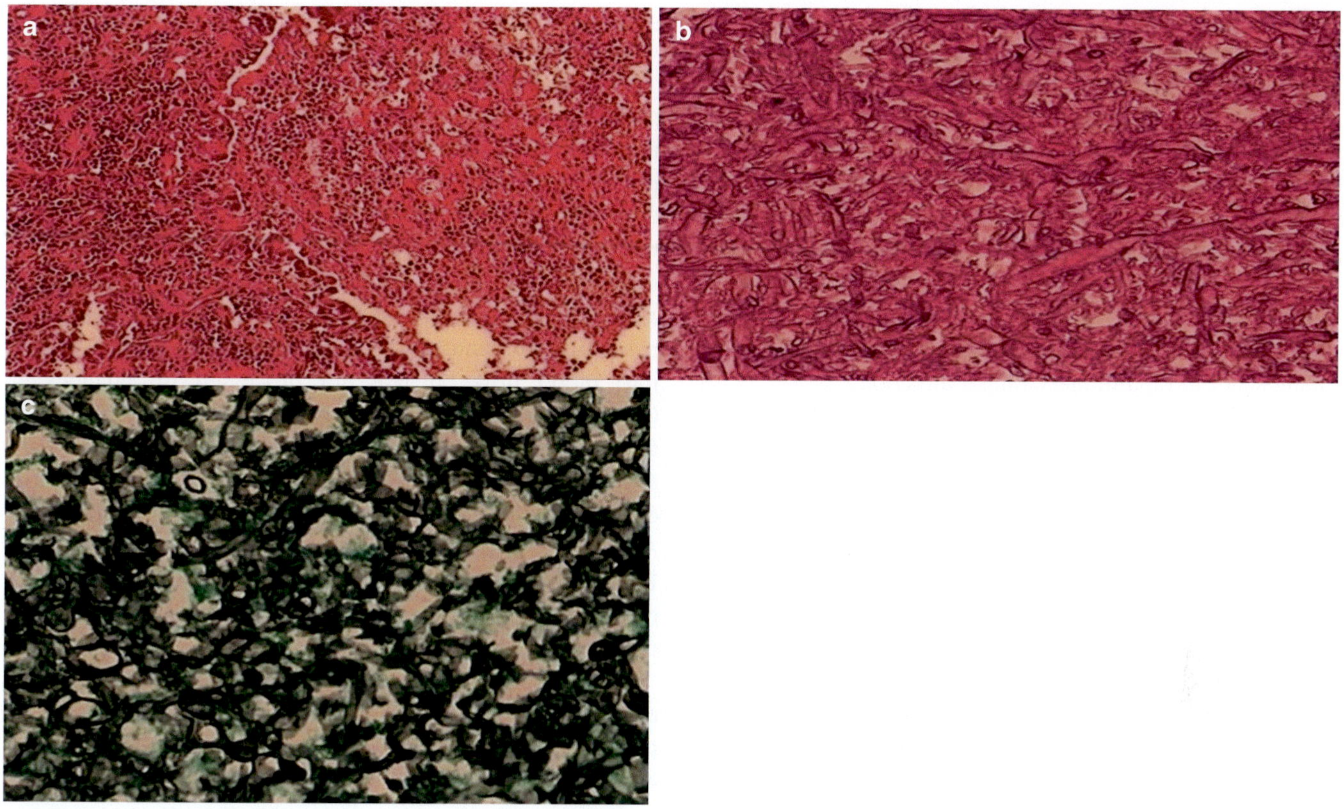

Fig. 15.15 (**a–c**) Pathology of lung tissue. (**a**, **b**) H&E staining. (**c**) PAS staining. (**d**) PASM staining demonstrates aspergillus hyphae and spores as well as infiltration of many inflammatory cells

PSA staining positive, GMS staining positive, and GRAM staining negative. The postoperative pathological diagnosis was fungal pneumonia, which was morphologically consistent to aspergillus infection (Fig. 15.15).

After the operation, the condition of the patient was improved, and the patient was discharged. The diagnosis on discharge was subacute invasive pulmonary aspergillosis, after wedge removal of lesions at the right middle and lower lung lobes, after bone marrow transplantation for acute lymphoblastic leukemia (B, MLL+, and IGH+). After the operation, the patient received long-term follow-ups. And the disease showed no relapse.

15.3.4 Discussion

In this case, the pediatric patient received bone marrow transplantation for acute lymphoblastic leukemia. After transplantation, he received immunosuppression therapy, and neutropenia occurred during the treatment. Therefore, he belonged to immunocompromised population and at high risk of opportunistic fungal infections. This was also the important basis for administration of antifungal medication after detection of intrapulmonary nodular lesions.

In this case, the illness course lasted for up to more than 9 months. According to the 2015 new edition of clinical guideline of pulmonary aspergillosis, the illness course is consistent to that of chronic pulmonary aspergillosis (CPA) [1]. The most common type of CPA is chronic cavitary pulmonary aspergillosis (CCPA). By chest CT scan, it shows diverse demonstrations at different stages, including singular or multiple pulmonary aspergilloma, new and/or progressive cavity lesion with different thickness of wall, accompanying destruction and/or fibrosis of lung parenchyma around the cavity, obvious pleural thickening, and possibly aspergillus pyothorax. In this case, the early lesion was newly emerged nodule. After antifungal medication was given, the lesions progressed, with emergence of cavity and aspergilloma inside, which were consistent to the characteristics of CCPA. However, chest CT scan on October 20, 2013, demonstrated new consolidation and exudation. The patient experienced fever, tachypnea, and decreased blood oxygen saturation, which were consistent to the clinical manifestations of subacute invasive aspergillosis (SAIA). SAIA and CCPA resemble in clinical manifestations and radiology. But SAIA progresses more rapidly. Therefore, for patients with immunosuppression, the anti-aspergillus medication should persist till the lesions are completely absorbed [12].

Serum galactomannan test (GM test) has been well recognized in clinical practice as the diagnostic test of aspergillus infection [13]. The clinical value of BALF GM test has also attracted attention, especially in assessment of antifungal treatment [14]. However, because GM test cannot be performed in the hospital that the patient was admitted, the relevant data was not available, and we thus cannot explore the relationship between GM test results and the condition of the patient. In addition, his parents did not sign the informed consent for fibrobronchoscopy. And the BALF specimen was not obtained. These presented challenges for the definitive diagnosis of intrapulmonary fungal infection.

Biopsy and histopathology of lung tissue have important diagnostic value, which facilitates the differential diagnosis between SAIA and CCPA and more favorable observation of the histological responses after aspergillus infection. In the cases of CCPA, there are hyphae with septa in the excised cavity, which may fill or occlude the cavity. There are also accompanying chronic inflammatory responses, occasionally granuloma, and surrounding fibrosis or infiltration of inflammatory cells. In contrast, SAIA is histologically manifested as invasion of hyphae into lung parenchyma with accompanying acute inflammatory responses or necrosis. In this case, the patient received long-term antifungal medication. Although the cavity showed shrinkage, mass-like lesion remained. Due to suppressed immunity and relapse of the lesions, the condition may progress into invasive pulmonary aspergillosis to cause major hemoptysis. Active thoracoscopic removal of the affected lung lobe is appropriate. Postoperative long-term follow-ups demonstrated stable condition of the patient, indicating surgical operation should be performed when palliative therapy shows unfavorable therapeutic efficacy and there is risk of hemoptysis [15].

15.3.5 Comments

After allogenic bone marrow transplantation for leukemia, aspergillus infection can be staged into super early stage, early stage, and advanced stage. In the super early stage, the count of neutrophile granulocytes is extremely low, and the immunity of the patient remains low, which is the first peak stage of aspergillus infection. In the advanced stage of aspergillus infection, due to graft-versus-host reaction (GVHR), secondary infection of other microorganisms, and use of large doses of hormone and antibiotic, the patient experiences compromised immunity. Thus, the second peak stage of infection emerges. In this case, the period from onset of symptoms to laboratory test is considered to be early aspergillus infection. During the early aspergillus infection, antifungal medication, anti-cocci medication, and macrolides were repeatedly administered. But the lesions gradually enlarged with emergence of cavity. Voriconazole and amphotericin B were administered for up to 8 months, with unfavorable therapeutic efficacy.

During the illness course, G test showed negative. But pathology finally confirmed the diagnosis of aspergillus infection based on findings of hyphae in a large quantity. For patients with compromised immunity, inflammatory indices do not necessarily increase along with fungal infection. In this case, the patient received immunosuppressant after bone marrow transplantation. Repeated routine blood test showed extremely low count of WBC and granulocytic deficiency. In patients with granulocytic deficiency, fungi gain their access into blood flow but are not processed by phagocytes. (1–3)-β-D-Glucan is not or rarely released, which induced false negative in the clinical practice. Therefore, if the condition permits, blood or BALF GM test should be performed, especially BALF GM test, which has a high positive rate. According to research study, the sensitivity and specificity of BALF GM test to aspergillus antigen are 85.7% and 76.3%, respectively. However, the sensitivity of serum GM test is only 23%.

In this case, in addition to fungal infection, infection of other microorganisms should also be screened, including tuberculosis mycobacteria, virus, *Staphylococcus aureus*, and anaerobic bacteria.

In this case, the difficulty is that the lesions were not improved after 8-month standard anti-aspergillus medication. This is also the reason for the decision of surgical removal of the lesions. After the operation, long-term follow-ups showed no relapse, indicating successful treatment.

References

1. Denning DW, Cadranel J, Beigelman-Aubry C, et al. Chronic pulmonary aspergillosis: rationale and clinical guidelines for diagnosis and management. Eur Respir J. 2016;47(1):45–68.
2. Guo X, Song N, Liu Y, et al. Interpretations of the 2015 clinical guideline for chronic pulmonary aspergillosis. Clin Focus. 2016;31(3):325–31.
3. Dabó H, Marinho A, Gomes I. Pulmonary aspergillus nodule—still challenging? Arch Bronconeumol. 2015;51(11):603–4.
4. Luo J, Peng M, Xiao Y. Clinical analysis of invasive pulmonary fungal infection. J Chin Acad Med Sci. 2010;32(02):141–6.
5. Cen Y, Li Y, Huang Y. Pulmonary cryptococcosis: clinical pathology of 25 cases. J Clin Exp Pathol. 2010;26(02):237–8.
6. Soubani AO, Chandraseker PH. The clinical spectrum of pulmonary aspergillosis. Chest. 2002;121:988–1999.
7. Akbari JG, Varma PK, Neema PK, et al. Clinical profile and surgical outcome for pulmonary aspergilloma: a single center experience. Ann Thomc Surg. 2005;80:1067–72.
8. Sharma S, Dubey SK, Kumar N, et al. Monod and air crescent sign in aspergilloma. BMJ Case Rep. 2013; https://doi.org/10.1136/bcr-2013-200936.
9. Trof RJ, Beishuizen A, Debets-Ossenkopp YJ, et al. Management of invasive pulmonary aspergillosis in non-neutropenic critically ill patients. Intensive Care Med. 2007;33(10):1694–703.

10. Bochennek K, Abolmaali N, Wittekindt B, et al. Diagnostic approaches for immunocompromised paediatric patients with pulmonary infiltrates. Clin Microbiol Infect. 2006;12(3):199–201.
11. Moodley L, Pillay J, Dheda K. Aspergilloma and the surgeon. J Thorac Dis. 2014;6:202–9.
12. Walsh TJ, Anaissie EJ, Denning DW, et al. Treatment of aspergillosis: clinical practice guidelines of the Infectious Diseases Society of America. Clin Infect Dis. 2008;46(3):327–60.
13. Leeflang MM, Debets-Ossenkopp YJ, Wang J, et al. Galactomannan detection for invasive aspergillosis in immunocompromised patients. Cochrane Database Syst Rev. 2015;(12):CD007394.
14. Park SY, Lee SO, Choi SH, et al. Serum and bronchoalveolar lavage fluid galactomannan assays in patients with pulmonary aspergilloma. Clin Infect Dis. 2011;52(7):e149–52.
15. Ba PS, Ndiaye A, Diatta S, et al. Results of surgical treatment for pulmonary aspergilloma. Med Sante Trop. 2015;25(1):92–6.

MIX
Papier aus verantwortungsvollen Quellen
Paper from responsible sources
FSC® C105338

If you have any concerns about our products,
you can contact us on
ProductSafety@springernature.com

In case Publisher is established outside the EU,
the EU authorized representative is:
Springer Nature Customer Service Center GmbH
Europaplatz 3, 69115 Heidelberg, Germany

Printed by Libri Plureos GmbH
in Hamburg, Germany